MEDICAL ASSISTING

A Commitment to Service

Administrative Competencies

Margaret Towsend Warren
RN, Ph.D

Charlotte C. Eason
RN, BSN

Pamala F. Burch
BSN

Jeanne Pfeiffer-Ewens
RN, BSN, CMA

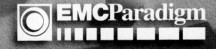

Production Credits

Developmental Editors	Christine Hurney; Jim Patterson, RN, BSN
Editorial Assistant	Susan Capecchi
Production Assistant/Art Coordinator	Courtney Kost
Interior Designer	David Farr, Imagesmythe
Cover Designer	Leslie Anderson; Michelle Lewis
Design Consultant	Joan D'Onofrio
Custom Photography	Encore Color Group
Desktop Production Specialist	Michelle Lewis
Copyeditor	Martin Gerber
Indexer	Terry Casey
Illustrations	Electronic Illustrators Group, www.eig.net
Photo Credits	Follow Index

Special recognition must be given to the editorial team that managed the design, development, and production of this text: Christine Hurney and Jim Patterson. Christine Hurney's dedication, skill, and perseverance ensured that this program meets the highest quality standards for educational textbooks. Jim Patterson's convictions about the need for quality healthcare training ensured a current, accurate, and accessible text. Their shared vision made this program a reality.

Publishing Management Team

George Provol, Publisher; Janice Johnson, Director of Product Development; Lori Landwer, Marketing Manager; Shelley Clubb, Electronic Design and Production Manager.

Library of Congress Cataloging-in-Publication Data

Medical assisting : a commitment to service—administrative competencies /
Margaret Towsend Warren . . . [et al.].
       p. cm.
    Includes bibliographical references and index.
    ISBN 0-7638-1302-8 (text)   ISBN 0-7638-1325-7 (text + CD-ROM)
    1. Medical assistants—Vocational guidance. I. Warren, Margaret Towsend.

R728.8 .A276 2002
610.69'53—dc21

00-050369
CIP

Text + CD-ROM ISBN 0-7638-1325-7
Order Number 12521

© 2002 by Paradigm Publishing Inc.
    Published by EMCParadigm
    875 Montreal Way
    St. Paul, MN 55102
    (800) 535-6865
    E-mail: educate@emcp.com
    Website: www.emcp.com

Printed in the United States of America.

10 9 8 7 6 5 4 3 2 1

Contents in Brief

108653

Contents

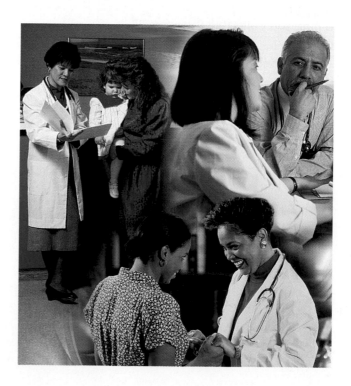

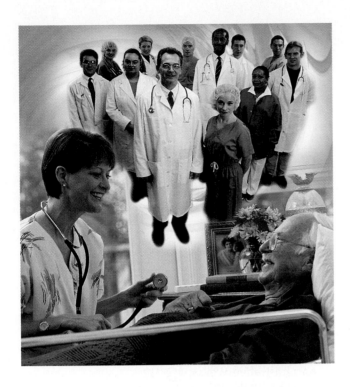

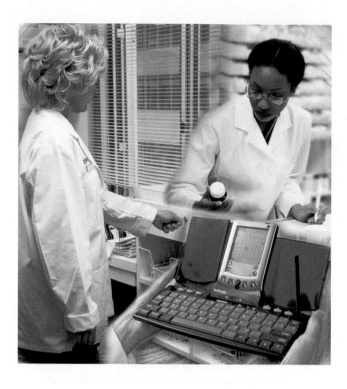

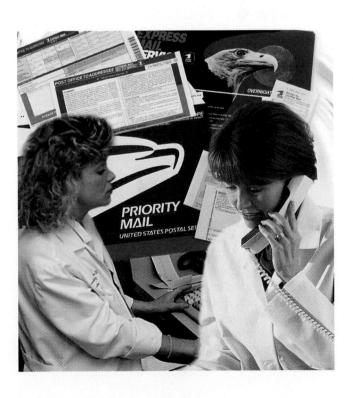

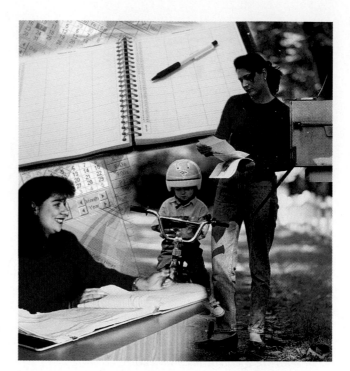

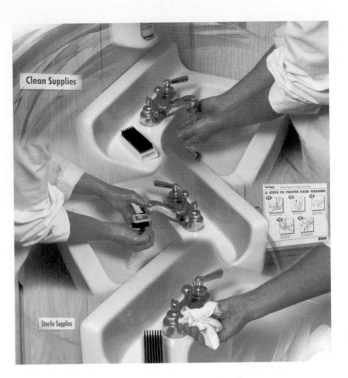

Procedure List

"A healer is no passive observer. She or he sees people whose bodies are disintegrating, whose lives have lost their safety. This kind of courage stands on another, deeper kind: The courage to make oneself responsible for an outcome."

John Poppy

*M*edical Assisting: A Commitment to Service is an extraordinary text that examines both the science and the art of health, healing, and medicine in its remarkable diversity. The text bridges the gap between the science and art of medical assisting, teaching students how to be effective and respectful patient managers by giving them the skills and practice needed to address patient concerns, provide patient education, and communicate well with members of the healthcare team. Never before has it been more imperative to teach medical assisting students how to listen and learn—from their team members, from patients, from family members, and from each other. Integral to this goal is this realization: students need to learn more about themselves. Students need to acquire the intrapersonal intelligence to recognize what they know and what they do not know. They must seek the attitudes of the successful life-long learner.

Our goal is to provide the instructor with a wide array of highly effective curriculum resources for the medical assisting program and to prepare the student for a rewarding career in the field of medical assisting. To accomplish this goal, we detail medical procedures that ensure safe and reliable service, provide teaching sections that build a strong knowledge base, and supply cross-curricular connections that help students develop the communication and problem-solving skills necessary for job success.

Procedures for Safe and Reliable Service

The text and resource guides teach the key competencies in the administrative environment for safe, reliable service. Procedures are included, written in a clear, step-by-step style that fosters respect for the physical, emotional, and cognitive needs of the patient. The hazard notifications, which align with OSHA regulations, are clearly identified by distinctive icons. In addition, rationales are included for all key steps so students learn why the steps are critical to the success of the procedure. Since laws governing the roles of the medical assistant vary by state, the procedures have also been provided in electronic form, allowing instructors to adapt the text to reflect regional and state differences.

Concepts and Skills for the Multiskilled Medical Worker

Medical Assisting: A Commitment to Service is designed around strong, visually oriented teaching sections, building the background knowledge crucial to the medical assistant's success. Ample use of tables, sidebars, and visual elements serve to amplify and extend the text readings. Other learning aids are integrated throughout, helping the student summarize essential concepts: an important tool for long-term memory. Through real-world examples and thought-provoking questions, this program forms caring communicators, effective decision-makers, and problem-solvers who are certain to succeed on the job.

Cross Curricular Connections

In addition to its strong emphasis on procedures and concept knowledge, this program helps the student build effective communication and teamwork skills. In so doing, it builds an appreciation for cultural diversity and individual differences. With the goal of building an appreciation for the views of others, students are asked to consider questions for which there are no right answers and to examine issues from the perspective of others. They are asked to solve problems in teams and to learn to give and receive constructive feedback.

How This Text Is Organized

This text is organized into two main parts.

- Medical Assisting: A Vision of Care
- Administrative Procedures: Systems and Solutions

Each part starts with a list of key competencies, which are highlighted within the part's chapters. These align with the 1999 entry-level competencies identified by

CAAHEP. It is important to keep in mind that mastery of all of these competencies is important for success as a medical assistant and is the basis for certification testing for both the CMA and RMA credentials.

Part I, "Medical Assisting: A Vision of Care," provides an overview of the medical assisting profession. Key legal and ethical issues are introduced early and are examined throughout the text. Also, the importance of effective communication is explained, providing a foundation for successful team-building skills. This section ends with a chapter that looks toward emerging trends in healthcare and includes a discussion of the rise of alternative therapies and holistic methods of healing.

Part II, "Administrative Procedures: Systems and Solutions," introduces the key aspects of working in the front office areas of the medical office. By managing administrative procedures, communications, appointments, medical records, and financial records, the medical assistant keeps the business side of the medical office running smoothly. The importance of customer service is highlighted throughout this section. Customer service includes service to the patients as well as to the other members of the healthcare team. Chapter 13 focuses on managerial responsibilities. Although every medical assistant may not aspire to be a supervisor, all employees in the healthcare setting should be aware of the roles and responsibilities of the front office manager. Chapter 14 presents issues that concern the maintenance of the clinical environment, including handwashing and disinfecting surfaces.

The book concludes with three invaluable reference appendixes, including a "Medical Language Handbook," an "Anatomy Handbook," and a list of the Standard and Universal Precautions. A self-check section provides answers to the end-of-chapter exercises to encourage independent study. In addition, a complete glossary, listing all of the terms, pronunciation guides, and definitions from the key chapter terms is provided as a reference. Because this text will be used as an on-the-job reference tool, the index has been designed to provide quick access to the information in the text.

How Chapters Are Organized

Each chapter begins with a list of "Learning Outcomes" and "Performance Objectives" that help guide the study of the material. The introduction provides a context for the learning that takes place within the chapter and provides a broad overview of the chapter's topics. The "Patient Concerns" feature provides an overview of the selected conditions, illnesses, and complaints that bring patients to the medical office and how these problems are best treated or resolved.

It focuses on developmental differences—conditions associated with stages of life.

Within each chapter, the text discusses the responsibilities of the medical assistant and provides step-by-step procedures. Many procedures include photos to help illustrate complicated steps. Within the procedure steps, levels of notification are indicated to help the medical assistants "think on their feet." Levels of notification teach the medical assistant to anticipate and avoid potential mistakes. The notification levels align with OSHA regulations and include:

- **NOTICE!** may affect the accuracy of the assessment.
- **ATTENTION!** may cause equipment damage if not properly observed.
- **CAUTION!** may cause injury if not observed.
- **WARNING!** may cause serious injury if not observed.

These icons alert students to situations requiring special attention to safety.

Throughout this text the authors have used first-person pronouns for physicians, nurses, patients, and other members of the healthcare team and have made an effort to refer to the male and female genders equally. In most cases, the reader should consider these genders to be interchangeable.

Illustrations, photos, and easy-to-read tables provide additional information as well as visual variety within the page layout. Side bars extend the chapter by providing concrete examples, scenarios, or important points to remember. In addition, "Technology Tips" provide website resources.

End-of-chapter material includes "Challenging Situations," which discusses difficult or unusual situations related to the procedures presented within the chapter. Such situations might include challenges related to age, disability, or cultural background. The "Clinical Summary" highlights the important information learned in the chapter and reinforces the "Learning Outcomes" and "Performance Objectives" that were presented at the beginning of the chapter. "The Language of Medicine" is an alphabetical list of the chapter's key terms, which are set in bold within the text copy where they are first introduced and defined. The vocabulary list includes definitions and pronunciation guides for medical terms. End-of-chapter vocabulary terms and definitions are compiled in the comprehensive end-of-book glossary.

A section called "Signs/Symptoms of Progress" ends each chapter, supplying three different types of exercises. Exercise 1 asks students to recall key concepts from the chapter and to pose questions about those concepts. Then, students are asked to connect that information to other pertinent concepts, contexts, or applications. Exercise 2 provides case studies that emphasize skills related to communicating with patients and patient/family teaching. These situations require not merely the relaying of information, but focus on decision-making and problem-solving. Exercise 3 provides an opportunity for students to form groups to discuss challenging issues presented in the chapter. This exercise addresses problems that have more than one right answer or approach and can be adapted for writing assignments or journaling. Answers for Exercises 1 and 2 are found in the "Self-Check" appendix.

Resources for the Student

Each text comes with a CD-ROM called *The Language of Medicine* that provides definitions and pronunciations for over 1,000 important terms. Together with the end-of-chapter terms lists and end-of-book glossary, this CD-ROM will be a valuable tool to help the student master the language of the healthcare industry.

The accompanying *Student's Resource Guide* provides an opportunity to apply the knowledge learned in the text and provides additional resources to encourage success as a medical assistant. The "Understanding Concepts and Skills" section provides over 140 additional exercises and offers a wide range of exercise types designed to assess the learner's comprehension, problem-solving, and decision-making ability. Some exercises focus on using medical terms and language in context. Other exercises work to develop applied literacy skills such as reading medical documents and forms, documenting and communicating medical decisions, and interpreting numerical data and charts. The "Building Procedural Competence" section provides tips on how to effectively learn procedures and includes worksheets designed for practicing and evaluating all of the procedures in the text. In addition, there is a section providing medical terminology practice. In the "Career Development Handbook," students are given valuable guidelines for preparing a resume, researching the job market, rehearsing for a job interview, and selecting references.

At the EMC/Paradigm website, www.emcp.com, students can visit the *Medical Assisting: A Commitment to Service* page to link to all of the websites mentioned within the text. These useful sites supply up-to-date information and encourage appropriate use of the Internet as a reference tool.

Students may consider supplementing their study with *What Language Does Your Patient Hurt In? A Practical Guide to Culturally Competent Patient Care* by Susan Salimbene. This text helps students develop an understanding of the needs, expectations, and behaviors of a multicultural patient population. By helping the medical assistant integrate the caregiver's treatment with the patient's culturally based expectations, the text provides a foundation for the development of cross-cultural sensitivity, preparing the medical assistant to better encourage patient compliance. The text is also a valuable reference for providing culturally appropriate, high-quality care. Each chapter of this text focuses on a different ethnic group and provides applications for discussion and reflection.

Resources for the Instructor

The *Instructor's Resource Guide* provides innovative suggestions on how to teach *Medical Assisting: A Commitment to Service*. In this comprehensive resource, the authors pay respectful attention to the differences in teaching style, program outcomes, and learner needs encountered in educational institutions today. This compendium of teaching resources includes:

- analysis of course requisites and conditions for learning procedures
- allied health program standards and benchmarks for success
- detailed outline of the student book's chapter contents to support lesson planning
- answer keys and model answers for exercises provided in the student workbook
- tips on teaching and evaluating procedures along with testing sheets
- midterm test and final test examples

The *Instructor's Resource Guide* comes with a CD-ROM that includes files for all of the procedures included in the student textbook. Instructors are free to edit or elaborate the procedure steps to better meet the needs of their specific courses and regional requirements. The CD-ROM also includes medical art and other key illustrations from the student text to support class presentations.

A full-featured computerized testing program on CD-ROM offers instructors a wide variety of options for generating both print and online tests. The testbank offers more than 500 questions that range in difficulty and discrimination levels. Instructors can create custom tests using questions from the testbank provided or can add questions of their own design. All objective question types and constructed response types of items are supported by this program.

WebCT Classroom Connection is a program that allows instructors to create a personalized website for their courses, easily and quickly. It comes preloaded with valuable teacher and student materials including class syllabus information, information about assignments and class changes, full-color art and illustrations, a complete bank of test items, pre-determined unit tests and quizzes, Internet links, E-mail, and an array of discussion forum tools. Instructors can easily adapt or edit the preloaded information to better align the material to their individual courses.

Acknowledgements

The authors would like to thank the editorial team at EMC/Paradigm as well as the following list of reviewers and contributors for their expert advice and opinions on how to make this an effective textbook program.

Julene Bredeson, CMA
Ridgewater College
Willmar, MN

Alice Ettinger, RN, MSN, CPNP, CPON
Division of Pediatric Hematology-Oncology
Saint Peter's University Hospital
Brunswick, NJ

Pat Gallagher Moeck, MBA, CMA
El Centro College
Dallas, TX

Laura Hollinhan
Century College
White Bear Lake, MN

Isabelle Janzen, RHIT, RHIA, BS
Rockland Community College
Suffrin, NY

Virginia Johnson, CMA
Lakeland Medical-Dental Academy
Minneapolis, MN

Karen A. Kittle, CMA, CPT, CHUC
Oakland Community College
Waterford, MI

Bill Larsen, MBA, CMA
Century College
White Bear Lake, MN

Sandy Lehrke
Anoka-Ramsey Community College
Anoka, MN

Kenneth C. Nowak, MD
Stanford University Medical Center
Palo Alto, CA

Vicki Prater, CMA
Concorde Career Institute
San Bernardino, CA

Vicki Scott, MA, MLT, CMA
Medical Institute of Minnesota
Bloomington, MN

Marcia Stevens, RN, Ph.D
St. Cloud State University
St. Cloud, MN

Stephanie Suddendorf, CMA
Globe College of Business
Oakdale, MN

Sylvia Taylor, BS, CMA
Cleveland State Community College
Cleveland, TN

Estelle Lurie Yahes, RN.C, MA
Rockland Community College
Suffern, NY

Susan K. Zolvinski, LPN, RMA
Commonwealth Business College
Michigan City, IN

The Authors and editorial staff encourage your feedback on the text and its supplements. Please reach us by clicking the "Contact Us" button at www.emcp.com.

MEDICAL ASSISTING

Medical Assistant—Entry-Level Competencies

Administrative Competencies

Perform Clerical Functions
- Schedule and manage appointments
- Schedule inpatient and outpatient admissions and procedures
- Perform medical transcription
- Organize a patient's medical record
- File medical records

Perform Bookkeeping Procedures
- Prepare a bank deposit
- Reconcile a bank statement
- Post entries on a daysheet
- Perform accounts receivable procedures
- Perform accounts payable procedures
- Perform billing and collection procedures
- Prepare a check
- Establish and maintain a petty cash fund

Prepare Special Accounting Entries
- Post adjustments
- Process credit balance
- Process refunds
- Post NSF checks
- Post collection agency payments

Process Insurance Claims
- **Apply managed care policies and procedures**
- Apply third party guidelines
- Obtain managed care referrals and pre-certifications
- Perform procedural coding
- Perform diagnostic coding
- Complete insurance claim forms
- Use a physician's fee schedule

Clinical Competencies

Fundamental Principles
- Perform handwashing
- Wrap items for autoclaving
- Perform sterilization techniques
- Dispose of biohazardous materials
- Practice Standard Precautions

Specimen Collection
- Perform venipuncture
- Perform capillary puncture
- Obtain throat specimen for microbiological testing
- Perform wound collection procedure for microbiological testing
- Instruct patients in the collection of a clean-catch mid-stream urine specimen
- Instruct patients in the collection of fecal specimens

Diagnostic Testing
- Use methods of quality control
- Perform urinalysis
- Perform hematology testing
- Perform chemistry testing
- Perform immunology testing
- Perform microbiology testing
- Screen and follow-up test results
- Perform electrocardiograms
- Perform respiratory testing

Patient Care
- Perform telephone and in-person screening
- Obtain vital signs
- Obtain and record patient history
- Prepare and maintain examination and treatment areas
- Prepare patient for and assist with routine and specialty examinations
- Prepare patient for and assist with procedures, treatments, and minor office surgery
- Apply pharmacology principles to prepare and administer oral and parenteral medications
- Maintain medication and immunization records
- Obtain CPR certification and first aid training

Transdisciplinary Competencies

Communicate
- Respond to and initiate written communications
- Recognize and respond to verbal communications
- Recognize and respond to nonverbal communications
- Demonstrate telephone techniques

Legal Concepts
- **Identify and respond to issues of confidentiality**
- **Perform within legal and ethical boundaries**
- **Establish and maintain the medical record**
- **Document appropriately**
- Perform risk management procedures

Patient Instruction
- **Explain general office policies**
- **Instruct individuals according to their needs**
- Instruct and demonstrate the use and care of patient equipment
- Provide instruction for health maintenance and disease prevention
- **Identify community resources**

Operational Functions
- Perform an inventory of supplies and equipment
- Perform routine maintenance of administrative and clinical equipment
- Utilize computer software to maintain office systems

Source: From the 1999 Standards and Guidelines, developed by CAAHEP in conjunction with the Curriculum Review Board of the American Association of Medical Assistants' Endowment. Reprinted by permission.

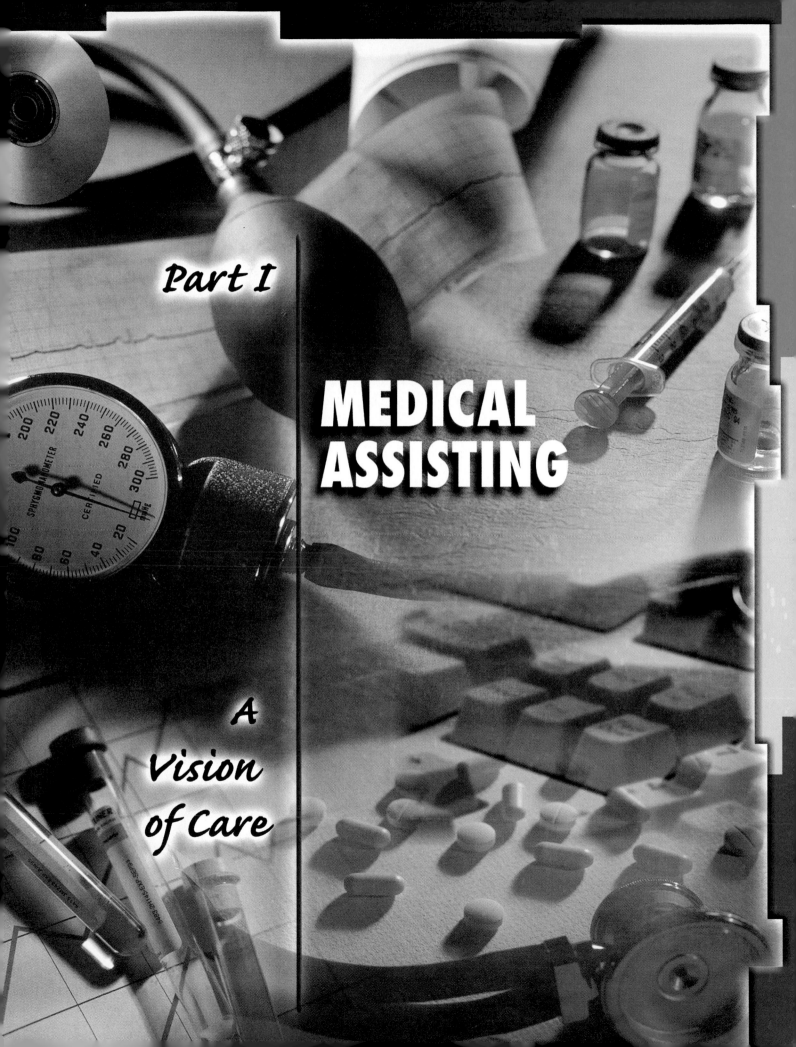

Part I

MEDICAL ASSISTING

A
Vision
of Care

Learning Outcomes

- Define the roles of the medical assistant in the medical office from the perspective of providing quality care and service.
- Describe the major responsibilities of the medical assistant as documented by the American Association of Medical Assistants (AAMA) Role Delineation Study and the American Medical Technologists (AMT) Task Certification Study.
- Analyze the professional and personal attributes required of individuals who choose a career in medical assisting.
- Identify the available avenues of training and education for medical assisting, and understand why it is important to choose an accredited program.

Performance Objectives

- Project a professional manner and image.
- Demonstrate initiative and responsibility in completing administrative and clinical tasks.
- Use the Internet to obtain healthcare information, and assess whether the information is authoritative, accurate, and reliable.

Welcome to the exciting, dynamic career of medical assisting! This chapter gives you an overview of the medical assistant's role in promoting healing, focusing on customer service, educating patients, managing patient care, and assuring that the care is safe and reliable. It explores the professional and personal attributes the medical assistant must possess, such as empathy for others and the ability to work as a member of a team. It gives a brief history of the development of the medical assisting field, and discusses current avenues for training and education. This chapter will help you understand why you should consider obtaining professional credentialing as a medical assistant, and how membership in a professional organization can help you support and strengthen your new skills. The Internet, if used appropriately, can be an excellent resource for the medical assistant. It is a powerful learning and research

chapter 1

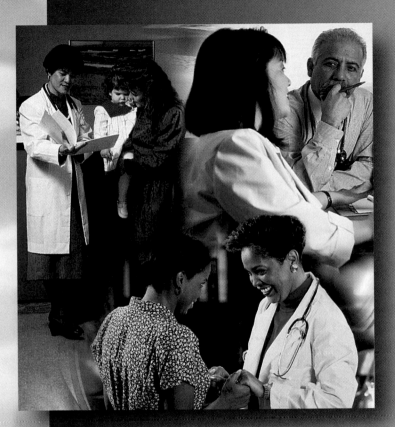

Choosing a Career as a Medical Assistant

tool, but healthcare websites must be carefully scrutinized for accuracy and reliability. The medical assistant can play an important role in helping patients learn how to use healthcare websites effectively.

The Medical Assistant's Role in the Dynamic Medical Office

Imagine a workplace full of people. The space is brightly lit, and colorful posters with statements such as "Eat Right for Health" and "Quit Smoking For Life" hang on several walls. Other walls contain serene paintings of women with children or nature scenes. Several children play with toys and clown stickers at a small table in a corner. Elsewhere in the room, interesting educational brochures are neatly arranged in an attractive display unit.

This place is busy all day long. Some of those who come and go are elderly, some young, and some middle aged. They are of many races, nationalities, and backgrounds, and some speak languages other than English. Some are financially well off, while others must struggle to meet their monthly bills. Some show signs of injury or pain, while others look perfectly healthy and sit quietly reading magazines. If you look closely, you will notice that one of the children playing with toys stops every so often to cough; a teen-aged boy sitting with his mother has a bandage over one eye, perhaps as a result of a sports injury; and an elderly woman has propped up a swollen leg on a nearby chair to elevate it.

As you walk through the halls of the workplace, you see a staff member guide a man using a walker into an examination room. Another staff member gently lifts a tiny baby from her mother's arms and places it on a basket scale, while yet another worker encourages a young boy to try an otoscope on his mother so he can see that it won't hurt him. Several more staff members are on the phone giving advice to callers, answering questions, and setting up appointments. Still others are drawing up injections, handing prescriptions to patients, and explaining to them the possible side effects of their medications. Back at a corner desk in the reception area, a staff member speaks quietly and empathetically to a customer in a wheelchair as he helps the customer schedule an x-ray at a downtown hospital and calls the para-transit provider to arrange transportation for him.

What is this fascinating, dynamic workplace? It is a typical medical office, an exciting, ever-changing, challenging, and sometimes-overwhelming place. Despite their different jobs, the staff members in this office are all committed to the same goal of promoting and sustaining their customers' health through appropriate

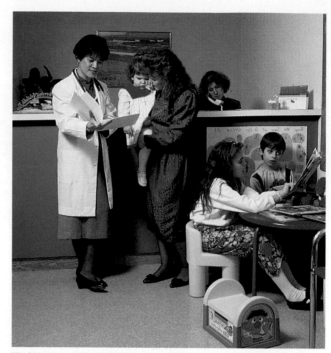

Working in a medical office can be ever-challenging and exciting. The medical assistant will be responsible for both clinical and administrative tasks.

therapies and preventive education. In this office, the medical assistant is an integral part of the healthcare team. She or he possesses multiple skills and talents and, as the scene above shows, often performs a wide variety of clinical and administrative tasks. Indeed, the medical assistant's role in patient care and the smooth running of the healthcare facility is critical since the assistant is often the first provider to serve the patient and the patient's family.

The medical assistant's gentle and confident manner can put the patient at ease and make the visit more pleasant. In addition, the assistant acts as a link between the patient-customer and the physician, a role that calls for both medical skills and communication or "people" skills. The medical assistant has a wide-ranging role, one that is essential to these aspects of medicine: promoting healing, providing exceptional customer service, educating patients, managing patient care, and assuring that the care is safe and reliable.

Promoting Healing of the Whole Person

Of course, the highest goal of any medical professional, including the medical assistant, is to alleviate suffering and promote healing. Physicians learn the Hippocratic Oath, written by the ancient Greek philosopher known as the "Father of Medicine" around 400 B.C. In its essence, this oath states "First, Do No Harm." The meaning of this phrase applies to all healthcare workers.

I swear by . . . whatsoever I hold most sacred, that I will be loyal to the profession of Medicine and just and generous to its members; that I will lead my life and practice my art in uprightness and honor; that into whatsoever house I shall enter, it shall be for the good of the sick to the utmost of my power, holding myself far aloof from wrong, from corruption, from the tempting of others to vice; that I will exercise my art solely for the cure of my patients and will give no drug, perform no operation for a criminal purpose, even if solicited, far less suggest it; that whatsoever I shall see or hear of the lives of men and women which is not fitting to be spoken, I will keep inviolably secret. Now if I keep this oath and break it not, may I enjoy honor, in my life and art, for all time."

Figure 1.1
The Hippocratic Oath

Source: Reprinted with permission from Christopher Tedeschi, © 1999.

It emphasizes the fact that it is better to provide no medical help at all than to provide medical care that will further hurt the patient. Figure 1.1 is a contemporary version of this oath.

Today, we understand that the healing process has both physical and psychological elements. The human body is remarkable in its ability to heal itself after injury or sickness in many circumstances. However, at times, people must seek help from trained healthcare professionals to regain their health. Medical staff members are obligated to strive to assess the patient's physical needs accurately and to prescribe treatments and procedures that target physical illnesses.

But healing only the patient's physical illness is often not enough. Every individual is unique and complex and must be treated as a whole person: body, mind, emotions, and spirit. Healing is greatly promoted, not just by "fixing" the patient's obvious illness, but also by listening to the patient's story, empathizing with the

> **Customer Service**
>
> *"To cure sometimes, to relieve often, and to comfort always."*
> —Anon.
> This fifteenth century approach to medicine is still appropriate for the medical assistant today.

patient's concerns, and establishing a relationship of openness, trust, and respect. In fact, many patients arrive at the medical office with no sign of organic disease or injury. Their need for healing may come from psychological sources such as depression, emotional abuse at home, unresolved conflicts, or other forms of personal trauma.

While the physician has the responsibility of assessing the patient's symptoms and making the final diagnosis, the medical assistant must realize that healing occurs not only because of scientifically based medical treatments but also as a result of the compassionate care given during those treatments. An ability to appreciate the emotional as well as the physical components of the healing process and to see her role as contributing to both components is essential to the medical assistant's work.

Providing Exceptional Customer Service

Have you heard the saying, often used in retail business, that "the customer always comes first"? **Customer service** is important in any business that deals with consumers, but the business that makes a priority of providing *exceptional* service to customers is the business that thrives. In today's society, the healthcare system is intent on striving for excellent customer service. The medical assistant, in particular, plays a key role in ensuring that patients' needs are satisfied. By putting the patients first and meeting their needs, the assistant also finds that his own job becomes more fulfilling.

Patient-customer satisfaction is important for several reasons. In today's healthcare environment, patients have an increasing array of choices, and they rightly demand the best care available. Better educated than any previous generation and taking increased responsibility for their own health, consumers today "shop around" for the best service and prices. If they do not like the service they receive at one clinic or from one physician, they will go to another. Furthermore, the United States's population is aging as the huge number of post-World War II baby boomers are now becoming senior citizens. This older population needs more and better healthcare services. The federal government has recognized the rights of patients as consumers of healthcare by issuing the 1997 Consumer Bill of Rights and Responsibilities. Study Table 1.1 to understand the guidelines of the Consumer Bill of Rights. Consider how they obligate all healthcare workers to strive for the highest quality customer service.

Table 1.1 Consumer Bill of Rights and Responsibilities

Consumer Rights	Consumer Responsibilities
I. Information Disclosure Consumers have the right to receive accurate, easily understood information, and some require assistance in making informed healthcare decisions about their health plans, professionals, and facilities. **II. Choice of Providers and Plans** Consumers have the right to a choice of healthcare providers that is sufficient to ensure access to appropriate high-quality healthcare. **III. Access to Emergency Care** Consumers have the right to access emergency healthcare services when and where the need arises. **IV. Participation in Treatment Decisions** Consumers have the right and responsibility to fully participate in all decisions related to their healthcare. Consumers who are unable to fully participate in treatment decisions have the right to be represented by parents, guardians, family members, or other conservators. **V. Respect and Nondiscrimination** Consumers have the right to considerate, respectful care from all members of the healthcare system at all times and under all circumstances. An environment of mutual respect is essential to maintain a quality healthcare system. Consumers must not be discriminated against in the delivery of healthcare services. Consumers who are eligible for coverage under the terms and conditions of a health plan or program or as required by law must not be discriminated against in marketing and enrollment practices based on race, ethnicity, national origin, religion, sex, age, mental or physical disability, sexual orientation, genetic information, or source of payment. **VI. Confidentiality of Health Information** Consumers have the right to communicate with healthcare providers in confidence and to have the confidentiality of their individually identifiable healthcare information protected. Consumers also have the right to review and copy their own medical records and request amendments to their records. **VII. Complaints and Appeals** All consumers have the right to a fair and efficient process for resolving differences with their health plans, healthcare providers, and the institutions that serve them, including a rigorous system of internal review and an independent system of external review.	■ In a healthcare system that protects consumers' rights, it is reasonable to expect and encourage consumers to assume reasonable responsibilities. ■ Take responsibility for maximizing healthy habits, such as exercising, not smoking, and eating a healthy diet. ■ Become involved in specific healthcare decisions. ■ Work collaboratively with healthcare providers in developing and carrying out agreed-upon treatment plans. ■ Disclose relevant information and clearly communicate wants and needs. ■ Use the health plan's internal complaint and appeal processes to address concerns that may arise. ■ Avoid knowingly spreading disease. ■ Recognize the reality of risks and limits of the science of medical care and the human fallibility of the healthcare professional. ■ Be aware of a healthcare provider's obligation to be reasonably efficient and equitable in providing care to other patients and the community. ■ Become knowledgeable about his or her health plan coverage and health plan options (when available) including all covered benefits, limitations and exclusions, rules regarding use of network providers, coverage and referral rules, appropriate processes to secure additional information, and the process to appeal coverage decisions. ■ Show respect for other patients and health workers. ■ Make a good-faith effort to meet financial obligations. ■ Abide by administrative and operational procedures of health plans, healthcare providers, and government health benefit programs. ■ Report wrongdoing and fraud to appropriate resources or legal authorities.

Source: Summary of the Consumer Bill of Rights and Responsibilities: Report to the President of the United States, prepared by the Advisory Commission on Consumer Protection and Quality in the Health Care Industry, November 1997, U.S. Government Printing Office.

In a clinical setting, there are other customers besides the patients who must be served. These can be classified as internal and external customers. **Internal customers** are all the colleagues that a staff member in the medical office works alongside every day. These include physicians, nurses, office managers, accountants, lab technicians, and medical assistants. **External customers** are those individuals and organizations outside the medical office that supply it with necessary information and products or specialized services. These include managed care organizations, insurance providers, equipment supply agencies, and others with whom the medical office has leases or contracts.

The medical assistant plays a vital role in achieving excellent customer service for patients as well as for other internal and external customers. To do this, she

Technology Tip

The Patient Bill of Rights as written by the American Hospital Association can be seen at its website, www.aha.org/resource/pbillofrights.html. The rights for patients who receive care in the hospital environment are similar to the rights of all patients.

first needs to strive to perform her clinical and administrative duties to her highest possible ability. But she also needs to develop effective communication skills with all the people with whom she interacts. She should be able to listen empathetically and attentively to others, interpret both verbal and nonverbal communication, and respond to others' needs knowledgeably and efficiently. Chapter 4 discusses these communication skills in more detail. Finally, to achieve excellent customer service, the medical assistant must be thoroughly professional in all she does. She must project a professional image in her attitude and appearance so as to gain the respect of others. Also she must do her part to contribute to an open, friendly, polite, and helpful office climate.

Educating Patients

In addition to the critical roles of promoting healing and providing excellent customer care, another important role of the medical assistant is that of educator or "health coach." Numerous times every day, the medical assistant encourages patients to take better care of themselves and to respect their health by such measures as quitting smoking, drinking less alcohol, eating a balanced diet, maintaining optimal weight, getting more exercise, and managing stress. Although physicians and other healthcare workers also help educate patients, the medical assistant in particular is in a prime position to advocate for the health of the whole patient.

Besides promoting general wellness, the medical assistant also dispenses information to patients on medications, procedures, and laboratory results. In some facilities, he is even responsible for evaluating, selecting, and ordering the office's supply of health-related educational materials such as brochures, handouts, and visual aids.

Managing Patient Care

Another role that the medical assistant plays in the medical office is that of helping manage and organize patient care so that it is carried out in the most effec-

tive and efficient manner possible. In a busy medical practice, this is no easy task. In fact, if you have ever been a server at a busy restaurant, the skills you learned there will be a good foundation on which to begin your medical assisting career. As a server, you had to keep any number of tables, individuals, and precise orders in mind at the same time. You had to anticipate your customers' needs and time your work carefully to provide them with each part of the meal on time. You had to serve them with a friendly, positive, helpful attitude, even when they might be disagreeable or express complaints, or when you felt they were demanding too much of you. At the end of each of your customers' meals, you tallied up the bill accurately and presented it to them. To be an effective server, you had to be highly orderly, organized, and efficient in all these separate but related tasks.

The medical assistant must not only be skilled at many tasks and execute them in a focused, efficient, and organized way, she also must be able to perform many tasks at the same time. Depending on the medical office, you may easily serve three dozen or more patients a day. You will greet them, interview them about their medical history, educate them on healthcare matters, assist the physician in the examination room, check blood pressure and vital signs, give injections, and review prescriptions. You will escort the patient back to the front desk and, in some cases, help the patient with insurance or billing issues. This diversity of the medical assistant's tasks ensures that her job is never dull! Rather, the medical assistant's job is challenging, demanding, and exciting. A quick mind, the ability to organize and prioritize many different tasks, and an energetic step will be invaluable to you in this work.

Assuring Safe and Reliable Patient Care

Finally, the medical assistant participates as a team member with other healthcare providers in assuring safe and reliable patient care. In some ways, the healthcare team operates like the U.S. government in which the three branches—executive, legislative, and judicial—check and balance each other to ensure that laws are fair and everyone is represented. Medical offices, too, have a system of checks and balances in treating patients. More than one health practitioner or administrator assesses that medications are accurately dispensed, any allergies are carefully noted, documentation of services is complete and accurate, and patients comply with follow-up procedures or visits to a specialist. As part of this system of checks and balances, the medical assistant may be responsible for updating patients' charts, keeping vaccination records, and recording any lapses in patient compliance.

In addition, the medical assistant is often charged with maintaining the order of charts and other records. He files charts in the central filing system or in the lab if results from tests are pending. He knows how to store the information so that it remains confidential but quickly accessible to other members of the healthcare team when needed.

The Multiskilled Medical Assistant

Medical assistants are multiskilled healthcare practitioners—able to perform a wide variety of distinct tasks knowledgeably—who work primarily in physicians' offices and outpatient clinics. Their tasks involve a broad spectrum of health-related jobs and include both clinical and administrative duties. As a result of such multiskilled training, medical assistants can be employed in many different healthcare delivery settings. While their fundamental role is to assist the physician in providing healthcare, they also facilitate and support other roles such as promoting healing, assuring excellent customer service, educating patients, managing patient care, and assuring that the care is safe and reliable, as we have seen. Study the following three situations to get an idea of the many roles of the multiskilled medical assistant. As you read each situation, note how many tasks the medical assistant performs.

Thirty-five-year-old Carol Smith has been employed as a medical assistant in a general practitioner's office for thirteen years. In this office, she performs primarily administrative and intake duties. She works with one physician, two nurses, and another medical assistant.

When Janice Flood, age twenty-six, phoned the medical office, Carol took the call, listened to Janice's concern that she was experiencing abdominal pain, determined the severity of her discomfort, wrote down Janice's address and phone number, and scheduled an appointment for Janice for that afternoon. When Janice arrived at the office for her appointment, Carol greeted her, obtained a copy of her insurance card, and helped her fill out the patient registration form. She then led Janice to the examination room. After the physician completed Janice's physical examination, Carol reinforced the physician's instructions with Janice, answered Janice's questions about the side effects of her prescribed medication, and gave Janice an educational brochure to take home that discussed her health questions. Carol then scheduled a follow-up visit for Janice and a laboratory test and x-ray to be performed at another facility. Back at the front desk, Carol collected payment for the physician's services and gave Janice a receipt. Once Janice left the office, Carol completed the insurance documents to obtain appropriate reimbursement for Janice from the insurance company. She then filed Janice Flood's chart in the central filing system.

Twenty-eight-year-old medical assistant Jack Montez works in a clinic in a large urban medical center. In this center, Jack's primary responsibilities are of a clinical nature. He works with eighteen physicians, seven nurses, and three medical assistants.

When fifty-six-year-old Steve Wilson arrived at the clinic for his initial visit, Jack greeted him and asked him to complete the registration form. Next, he led Steve to an examination room and obtained a complete medical history. He also took Steve's height, weight, temperature, pulse, blood pressure, and respiration measurements and carefully recorded them on Steve's chart. Following the physician's request, Jack obtained urine and blood specimens, labeled them carefully, and deposited them in the laboratory out-box. When the physician came in to examine Steve, Jack assisted during the physical examination. After the examination, Jack helped reinforce the physician's instructions by explaining the results of Steve's exam and by emphasizing measures Steve should take to prevent future health problems. Jack listened carefully to Steve's questions and answered them, making sure that Steve understood

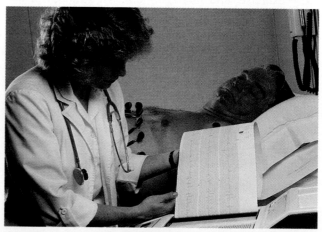

The medical assistant will work closely with the patients during diagnostic testing and will help educate patients as to how to prevent health problems.

fully. He then gave Steve an educational handout, per the physician's instructions, and escorted him back to the reception area. The employee at the front desk collected the appropriate fee and gave Steve a receipt. When results of the urine and blood tests came back, Jack phoned Steve and helped him understand what the results indicated.

Susan Chen is a forty-year-old medical assistant who has worked in a multifunction obstetrical and gynecological clinic for six years. The clinic is large and busy. It employs three physicians, two nurse practitioners, two part-time nurses, and five medical assistants. Three of the medical assistants perform clinical duties in the back office, and two perform administrative duties in the front office. Susan is the clinic's office manager. In this role, she supervises all the staff members. She coordinates their schedules so that the office runs smoothly, and she ensures that there is adequate patient coverage at all times. Susan also screens job applicants, participates on the team that interviews and hires employees, and orients and trains new personnel. She designs and conducts continuing education activities for the staff. In addition, her responsibilities include developing and maintaining personnel, policy, and procedure manuals and managing personnel benefits. In consultation with the physicians and nurse practitioners, Susan develops and maintains patient fee schedules. Finally, she also interacts with insurance companies and other businesses to obtain contracts and renewals and makes sure office records are kept up to date.

In reading about these three situations, how many different tasks of the medical assistants did you note? These situations give you an idea of how the medical assistant operates as a multiskilled healthcare professional. In fact, the medical assisting profession was created to provide a versatile healthcare practitioner who is competent in a wide variety of skills, both clinical and administrative. With the growing complexity of the healthcare delivery system, the medical assistant of the future will no doubt find himself needing even more diverse skills and knowledge to meet the needs of patients. In any healthcare setting, the medical assistant is an indispensable, multiskilled member of the healthcare team, helping ensure that healthcare is delivered in an efficient and effective manner.

The Role Delineation and Job Task Analysis Studies

As we have seen, the role of the medical assistant is a multiskilled one. Two national professional organizations, the **American Association of Medical Assistants (AAMA)** and the **American Medical**

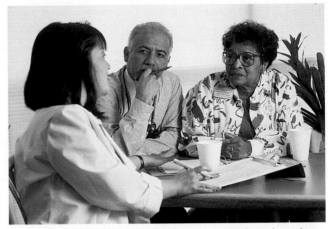

The medical assistant will be responsible for administrative tasks such as holding staff meetings in which office policies and patient care is defined.

Technologists (AMT), have described the skills required to work in the field of medical assisting. In 1979, the AAMA conducted a study on the medical assistant's responsibilities entitled "Developing a Curriculum," or DACUM for short. It updated the study's findings in 1984 and 1990. These studies surveyed practicing certified medical assistants from diverse geographic locations, educational backgrounds, work settings, and practice environments. Their findings formed the basis of the AAMA's recommendations for appropriate educational programs for medical assistants.

In 1996, the AAMA conducted yet another study to once again update its findings. This study, the **Role Delineation Study**, resulted in a model that defined the competencies every medical assistant should have. The competencies were divided into three areas: administrative, clinical, and general (or transdisciplinary). **Administrative competencies** are those practice areas that are generally performed in the "front" office in a healthcare clinic. They include such clerical functions as scheduling patient visits, handling insurance claims, and accounting and bookkeeping procedures. **Clinical competencies** are those generally performed in the "back" office. They include the skills of interviewing patients for medical histories, assisting physicians with examinations, obtaining and processing diagnostic tests, giving injections, and checking patients' charts for accuracy. **General** or **transdisciplinary competencies** are those overlapping skills that are practiced in both the administrative and the clinical areas. They include the skills of professionalism, communication, understanding legal concepts, educating customers, and helping maintain an efficient work environment. Although educational programs for medical assistants include both administrative skills and clinical skills as part of their curriculum, a medical assistant

Table 1.2 Medical Assistant Role Delineation Chart

Administrative			Clinical		
Administrative Procedures	**Practice Finances**	**Fundamental Principles**	**Diagnostic Orders**		**Patient Care**
■ Perform basic clerical functions. ■ Schedule, coordinate, and monitor appointments. ■ Schedule inpatient/outpatient admissions and procedures. ■ Understand and apply third-party guidelines. ■ Obtain reimbursement through accurate claims submission. ■ Monitor third-party reimbursement. ■ Perform medical transcription. ■ Understand and adhere to managed care policies and procedures. ■ *Negotiate managed care contracts. (advanced)*	■ Perform procedural and diagnostic coding. ■ Apply bookkeeping principles. ■ Document and maintain accounting and banking records. ■ Manage accounts receivable. ■ Manage accounts payable. ■ Process payroll. ■ *Develop and maintain fee schedules. (advanced)* ■ *Manage renewals of business and professional insurance policies. (advanced)* ■ *Manage personnel benefits and maintain records. (advanced)*	■ Apply principles of aseptic technique and infection control. ■ Comply with quality assurance practices. ■ Perform and follow up on patient screening tests.	■ Collect and process specimens. ■ Perform diagnostic tests.		■ Adhere to established triage procedures. ■ Obtain patient history and vital signs. ■ Prepare and maintain examination and treatment areas. ■ Prepare patient for examinations, procedures, and treatments. ■ Assist with examinations, procedures, and treatments. ■ Prepare and administer medications and immunizations. ■ Maintain medication and immunization records. ■ Recognize and respond to emergencies. ■ Coordinate patient care information with other healthcare providers.
General (Transdisciplinary)					
Professionalism	**Communication Skills**	**Legal Concepts**	**Instruction**		**Operational Functions**
■ Project a professional manner and image. ■ Adhere to ethical principles. ■ Demonstrate initiative and responsibility. ■ Work as a team member. ■ Manage time effectively. ■ Prioritize and perform multiple tasks. ■ Adapt to change. ■ Promote the CMA credential. ■ Enhance skills through continuing education.	■ Treat all patients with compassion and empathy. ■ Recognize and respect cultural diversity. ■ Adapt communication to individual patient's ability to understand. ■ Use professional telephone technique. ■ Use effective and correct oral and written communication. ■ Recognize and respond to oral and nonverbal communication. ■ Use medical terminology appropriately. ■ Receive, organize, prioritize, and transmit information. ■ Serve as liaison. ■ Promote the medical practice through positive public relations.	■ Maintain confidentiality. ■ Practice within the scope of education, training, and personal capabilities. ■ Prepare and maintain medical records. ■ Document accurately. ■ Use appropriate guidelines when releasing information. ■ Follow employer's established policies dealing with the healthcare contract. ■ Follow federal, state, and local legal guidelines. ■ Maintain awareness of federal and state healthcare legislation and regulations. ■ Maintain and dispose of regulated substances in compliance with government guidelines. ■ Comply with established risk management and safety procedures. ■ Recognize professional credentialing criteria. ■ Participate in the development and maintenance of personnel, policy, and procedure manuals. ■ *Develop and maintain personnel, policy, and procedure manuals. (advanced)*	■ Instruct individuals according to their needs. ■ Explain office policies and procedures. ■ Teach methods of health promotion and disease prevention. ■ Locate community resources and disseminate information. ■ *Orient and train personnel. (advanced)* ■ *Develop educational materials. (advanced)* ■ *Conduct continuing education activities. (advanced)*		■ Maintain supply inventory. ■ Evaluate and recommend equipment and supplies. ■ Apply computer techniques to support office operations. ■ *Supervise personnel. (advanced)* ■ *Interview and recommend job applicants. (advanced)* ■ *Negotiate leases and prices for equipment and supply contracts. (advanced)*

Source: Reprinted by permission of the American Association of Medical Assistants.

may choose to work in an administrative capacity, in a clinical capacity, or as a generalist in both areas.

The AAMA's Role Delineation Study also identified a number of advanced skills for practicing medical assistants who wish to increase their knowledge in the constantly evolving healthcare delivery system. Table 1.2 lists the general and specific skills the Role Delineation Study identified as those the medical assistant needs.

The American Medical Technologists agency in consort with the Accrediting Bureau of Health Education Schools (ABHES), conducted a task analysis of the competencies that medical assistants use on the job. Table 1.3 lists the competencies it identified.

Table 1.3 Medical Assistant Competency Checklist

Professionalism	Communication	Administrative Duties	Office Management
■ Project a positive attitude. ■ Maintain confidentiality at all times. ■ Be a "team player." ■ Be aware of ethical boundaries. ■ Exhibit initiative. ■ Adapt to change. ■ Show a responsible attitude. ■ Be courteous and diplomatic. ■ Conduct work within the scope of your education, training, and ability.	■ Be attentive, listen, and learn. ■ Be impartial and show empathy when dealing with patients. ■ Adapt what you say to the recipient's level of comprehension. ■ Serve as liaison between physician and others. ■ Use proper telephone techniques. ■ Interview effectively. ■ Use appropriate medical terminology. ■ Receive, organize, prioritize, and transmit information expediently. ■ Recognize and respond to oral and non-verbal communication. ■ Use correct grammar, spelling, and formatting techniques in written works.	■ Use basic office skills. ■ Prepare and maintain medical records. ■ Schedule and monitor appointments. ■ Apply computer concepts for office procedures. ■ Perform medical transcription. ■ Locate resources and information for patients and employers. ■ Manage physician's professional schedule and travel.	■ Maintain physical plant. ■ Operate and maintain facilities and equipment safely. ■ Inventory equipment and supplies. ■ Evaluate and recommend equipment and supplies for practice. ■ Maintain liability coverage. ■ Exercise efficient time management.

Financial Management	Clinical Duties	Instruction	Legal Concepts
■ Use manual and computerized bookkeeping systems. ■ Implement current procedural terminology and ICD-9 coding. ■ Analyze and use current third-party guidelines for reimbursement. ■ Manage accounts payable and receivable. ■ Maintain records for accounting and banking purposes. ■ Process employee payroll.	■ Interview and take patient history. ■ Prepare patients for procedures. ■ Apply principles of aseptic techniques and infection control. ■ Take vital signs. ■ Recognize emergencies. ■ Perform first aid and CPR. ■ Prepare and maintain examination and treatment areas. ■ Assist physician with examinations and treatments. ■ Use quality control. ■ Collect and process specimens. ■ Perform selected tests that assist with diagnosis and treatment. ■ Perform and follow up patient tests. ■ Prepare and administer medications as directed by physician. ■ Maintain medical records.	■ Orient patients to office policies and procedures. ■ Instruct patients with special needs. ■ Teach patients methods of health promotion and disease prevention. ■ Orient and train personnel.	■ Determine needs for documentation and reporting. ■ Document accurately. ■ Use appropriate guidelines when releasing records or information. ■ Follow established policy in initiating or terminating medical treatment. ■ Dispose of controlled substances in compliance with government regulations. ■ Maintain licenses and accreditation. ■ Monitor legislation related to current healthcare issues and practices.

Source: Accrediting Bureau of Health Education Schools, *Accreditation Manual, 8th Edition,* June 1999.

The competencies identified in these two tables are mutually reinforcing. Both provide a sound basis on which to plan educational programs for medical assistants.

Professional Attributes of the Medical Assistant

One of the general, or transdisciplinary, competencies that the Role Delineation Study (Table 1.2) and the Medical Assistant Competency Checklist (Table 1.3) specify for medical assistants is that of **professionalism**. At all times, a professional attitude must underscore the medical assistant's work. As defined by the Role Delineation Study, the broad area of professionalism involves nine specific competencies, each of which is described below.

PROJECT A PROFESSIONAL MANNER AND IMAGE A profession is a line of work that requires specialized knowledge and, usually, academic preparation. The medical assistant demonstrates his expertise at and care for his work by his actions, words, and attitudes. He performs his duties to the best of his ability, takes pride in what he does, and emphasizes exceptional customer service. By projecting a professional manner and image, he inspires the respect of others and their confidence in every task he performs.

ADHERE TO ETHICAL PRINCIPLES AND MAINTAIN CONFIDENTIALITY The AAMA has also produced a Code of Ethics that sets forth guidelines for the moral

conduct of medical assistants. It calls for the assistant to be scrupulously honest, act responsibly, and adhere to the medical profession's ethical policies on such matters as maintaining patient confidentiality and respecting patients' dignity. It is crucial that the medical assistant earn the complete trust of the many people who depend on her to act uprightly: patients, their families, other members of the healthcare team, and external customers. Table 1.4 lists the elements of the AAMA's Code of Ethics. A code of ethics for physicians has been provided by the American Medical Association (AMA). The Principles of Medical Ethics delineate the contract of care between physicians and their patients. The medical assistant should also be familiar with this legal contract because he is charged with helping the physician fulfill the requirements of this ethical code. See Table 1.5 for the AMA's Principles of Medical Ethics.

DEMONSTRATE INITIATIVE AND POSITIVE, RESPONSIBLE ATTITUDES An effective medical assistant keeps alert for opportunities to take the initiative in proposing new procedures or other measures that will

Table 1.4 American Association of Medical Assistants' Code of Ethics

The Code of Ethics of AAMA shall set forth principles of ethical and moral conduct as they relate to the medical profession and the particular practice of medical assisting.

Members of AAMA dedicated to the conscientious pursuit of their profession, and thus desiring to merit the high regard of the entire medical profession and the respect of the general public which they serve, do pledge themselves to strive always to

- render service with full respect for the dignity of humanity
- respect confidential information obtained through employment unless legally authorized or required by responsible performance of duty to divulge such information
- uphold the honor and high principles of the profession and accept its disciplines
- seek to continually improve the knowledge and skills of medical assistants for the benefit of patients and professional colleagues
- participate in additional service activities aimed toward improving the health and well-being of the community

Source: Reprinted by permission of the American Association of Medical Assistants, Inc.

Table 1.5 AMA Principles of Medical Ethics

Preamble: The medical profession has long subscribed to a body of ethical statements developed primarily for the benefit of the patient. As a member of this profession, a physician must recognize responsibility not only to patients, but also to society, to other health professionals, and to self. The following Principles adopted by the American Medical Association are not laws, but standards of conduct which define the essentials of honorable behavior for the physician.

I. A physician shall be dedicated to providing competent medical service with compassion and respect for human dignity.

II. A physician shall deal honestly with patients and colleagues, and strive to expose those physicians deficient in character or competence, or who engage in fraud or deception.

III. A physician shall respect the law and also recognize a responsibility to seek changes in those requirements which are contrary to the best interests of the patient.

IV. A physician shall respect the rights of patients, of colleagues, and of other health professionals, and shall safeguard patient confidences within the constraints of the law.

V. A physician shall continue to study, apply and advance knowledge, make relevant information available to patients, colleagues and public, obtain consultation, and use the talents of other health professionals when indicated.

VI. A physician shall, in the provision of appropriate patient care except in emergencies, be free to choose whom to serve, with whom to associate, and the environment in which to provide medical services.

VII. A physician shall recognize a responsibility to participate in activities contributing to an improved community.

Source: From the Code of Medical Ethics, © 1997. Reproduced with permission from the American Medical Association.

improve customer service and the smooth operation of the medical office. She also follows through with the new measures she proposes if they are accepted by others, and monitors and evaluates their results. For example, if the medical assistant learns about new technologies or approaches to patient care in a continuing education class that she thinks might improve the clinic, she should schedule time to talk these over with her supervisor. In this way, the medical assistant makes a valuable contribution to the day-to-day operations of the healthcare facility.

WORK AS A TEAM MEMBER Teamwork is a form of interdependence among healthcare practitioners with each professional bringing different but complementary skills that the team uses together to best serve the patient-customer. A team approach to patient care ensures comprehensive service without expensive duplication of effort. It also addresses the needs of the whole patient. For example, the physician, the nurse, the laboratory technician, the medical assistant, and the front desk manager all work together to provide a single patient with a satisfactory visit to the clinic. Teamwork is also necessary for the smooth operation of the entire medical office. As an important member of the healthcare team, the medical assistant works closely with others to perform the duties that are assigned to him, and he strives to understand how his duties interconnect with those of others on the team. He knows that the role he plays is indispensable in the process of efficient and effective healthcare delivery.

MANAGE TIME EFFECTIVELY Because of the rising cost of healthcare, all healthcare practitioners must manage their time in a way that provides optimal care at the lowest cost. The medical assistant, too, must be aware of this obligation. She must schedule patient appointments with an eye to allowing adequate time for assessment and treatment but also with an eye to ensuring that the time allocated does not exceed the need. When she performs general screening of the patient, she must act in an efficient but relaxed manner, aware that giving too much time to one patient means others may get less time, and that the whole office schedule may be thrown off. She must provide the physician with a succinct summary of the patient's history and symptoms to help the doctor have a focused patient session. Appropriate time management comes with experience, and it is critical to excellent customer service.

PRIORITIZE AND PERFORM MULTIPLE TASKS As a multiskilled worker, the medical assistant must know how to perform his many duties well. These duties may include such clinical functions as drawing blood and administering ECGs, administrative duties such as processing insurance forms and keeping accounts, or a combination of both. To carry out all these tasks, the medical assistant must recognize when and in what order they should be done. He must set priorities and carry out his duties in an orderly and organized manner. By doing so, he will perform his tasks as a member of the healthcare team in the most helpful and effective manner.

ADAPT TO CHANGE A practitioner's ability to learn new ideas, modify her thinking, and adapt to new situations is an increasingly important skill in the evolving and complex healthcare delivery system. The constant development of new technologies and the frequent changes imposed by the managed care environment require constant learning and updating of skills by all healthcare workers. Like their fellow professionals, medical assistants need to be educating themselves continually on such developments. They can do so by reading, taking classes, and merely keeping their eyes and ears open to learn all they can from others in their day-to-day practice. They need to be open to change and able to adapt their thinking to absorb and use new ideas.

PROMOTE PROFESSIONAL CREDENTIALING Medical assistants can promote their profession by obtaining professional certification from a recognized credentialing agency. Both the AAMA and the AMT award national certification to the medical assistant. After the assistant successfully completes a course of training and passes a written examination, certification is awarded. The two credentials, the Certified Medical Assistant (or CMA, for short) and the Registered Medical Assistant (or RMA), will be discussed in more detail later in this chapter. Certification provides professional recognition to the medical assistant and assures healthcare providers that she is proficient in the entry-level skills needed on the job. Promoting the medical assistant credentials is also one of the professional roles of the medical assistant.

CONDUCT WORK WITHIN THE SCOPE OF YOUR EDU-CATION AND ENHANCE SKILLS THROUGH CONTINU-ING EDUCATION As a medical assistant, your education is not complete once you have finished your academic program. In whatever healthcare setting you work, you will have the opportunity and responsibility to continue your learning through independent study

Technology Tip

Visit these websites:
AAMA, www.aama-ntl.org;
AMT, www.amt1.com.

and by taking continuing education seminars or classes. These courses will help you constantly update your skills and learn new ones. Other avenues for continuing education also exist. Many medical assistants read professional journals, both specific to the field of medical assisting and of more general medical interest. Reading professional journals is an excellent way to keep abreast of developments in the field. In addition, a number of professional organizations of interest to medical assistants exist. Their regular meetings provide a forum for networking with others, sharing information and advice, and spotlighting current trends. Many of these organizations also publish their own professional journals. The AAMA publishes the bimonthly *PMA (Professional Medical Assistant)*, a leading journal in the field, and AMT publishes the *Journal of Continuing Education*, another excellent resource. Information and resources can also be found through research on the Internet.

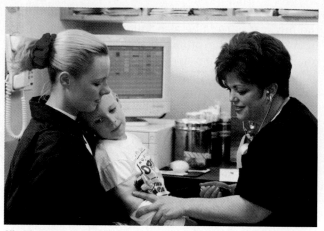

All patients who visit the medical office will benefit from the empathetic care of the medical assistant who understands the needs of the patient and can respond appropriately.

Working Smart

All professionals should engage in a variety of continuing education activities. For the medical assistant, these may include reading professional journals, researching information on the Internet, taking seminars or classes to update medical skills, learning more about the cultures and backgrounds of your customers, or even studying the language of non-English-speaking people you serve.

Personal Attributes of the Medical Assistant

In addition to the professional attributes defined by the Role Delineation Study and the Job Task Analysis Study, the medical assistant needs to have the personal attributes of empathy, diplomacy, reliability, courtesy, a positive attitude, and a professional appearance. These help contribute to the assistant's commitment to excellence in caring for her patients, and also help her serve as an effective liaison between the physician and others and to interact successfully with all staff members in the medical office. These six personal attributes are described below.

EMPATHY Empathy can be defined as conscious identification with another person's concerns or situation. This quality allows the medical assistant to imaginatively see things from the patient's viewpoint and, therefore, understand and appreciate what the patient is experiencing. Empathy helps the medical assistant

evaluate the situation fully and guide the patient through the experience by providing the exact care or information the patient needs.

DIPLOMACY Diplomacy is the art and practice of communicating with others in such a way that little or no ill will results from the conversation. Another word for diplomacy is "tact." The medical assistant is often the first healthcare practitioner a patient encounters. His ability to communicate with the patient effectively during this initial encounter makes a lasting impression on the patient and the patient's family. Patients arrive at the medical office sick, tense, worried, or in pain. The medical assistant needs to communicate with them in a way that calms their fears and eases their minds while still conveying information in a clear, straightforward manner. In the same way, as the medical assistant interacts every day with the other members of the healthcare team, a diplomatic or tactful spirit helps everyone work together to create an optimal professional environment.

RELIABILITY Reliability means that the medical assistant is completely trustworthy. As a team member, he is expected to perform specific functions in an accurate and professional manner. Other members of the healthcare team depend on him. His job is an important link between the physician, the patient, and all the others whom he serves. An unreliable medical assistant hampers the smooth operation of the medical office and may even cause harm to patients. When trust among staff members or between patient and healthcare worker is betrayed, it is exceedingly hard to regain. Therefore, it is important for the medical assistant to set a pattern of reliability by conscientiously delivering his best work at all times.

COURTESY **Courtesy** is polite, gentle conduct that demonstrates respect for and consideration of others. It is a quality that all healthcare practitioners must develop. The medical assistant must know how to treat every person he encounters as a unique, worthwhile human being. Moreover, he must treat everyone with equal courtesy and respect, regardless of the person's race, nationality, religion, or socioeconomic status. Everyone wants to be treated with dignity, and when you demonstrate respect toward others, you receive respect in return. Like the art of diplomacy, treating a patient with courtesy goes a long way in setting the tone for the patient's future interactions with you.

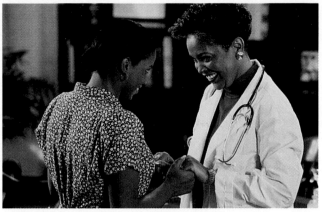

Projecting a positive attitude and a professional appearance will go a long way to make your patients feel comfortable with the healthcare you provide.

POSITIVE ATTITUDE A positive attitude is essential to the medical assisting field. It can be conveyed in many ways. We've all met people who look and act "down in the dumps." They may exhibit stooped shoulders, a shuffling gait, no eye contact, and a cynical or even bitter outlook. Such an attitude has no place in the medical office and will only serve to influence others negatively. We all have stresses in our lives that cause us to be emotionally up one day and down another, but professionals do not let such emotions affect the quality of their work. Rather, they strive to project a positive, caring attitude at all times. The effective medical assistant holds her head high, moves through her rounds energetically, smiles often, looks directly and kindly at those with whom she communicates, and speaks to them in a gentle yet firm tone. It is clear to everyone that she loves her work and is dedicated to the people she serves.

PROFESSIONAL APPEARANCE A professional appearance may seem to be a minor or unnecessary detail, but a person's appearance is a powerful indicator of

Working Smart

The professional medical assistant should make every effort to keep the patient as psychologically comfortable as possible. Most older patients do not understand "body piercing" and may be shocked by it. The medical assistant should not display these adornments while in the medical office environment. Additionally, tattoos should be kept covered while on duty. Earrings should not dangle below the earlobe; tasteful studs are preferred if earrings are worn.

Customer Service

Providing exceptional customer service is a major role of the healthcare professional. Such qualities as courtesy, a positive attitude, and a well-groomed appearance help the medical assistant create a positive first impression of the healthcare available in that medical office or clinic. Always keep in mind that the office is a business and depends upon customers to keep it profitable.

attitude that is directly conveyed to others. Like it or not, others judge us by our appearance. Encountering someone in a professional setting who is clean, neatly and appropriately dressed, and has nicely groomed hair is likely to give us confidence in that person's ability to serve us. His or her appearance communicates a positive attitude. The same holds true with patients who arrive at the clinic and meet the medical assistant for the first time. First impressions are important! The medical assistant should always be clean and neat. In some settings, she will wear a uniform or lab coat over her street clothing; this uniform should be spotlessly clean. Her hair should be groomed, make-up tastefully applied, and any jewelry kept to a minimum. These rules apply to male medical assistants as well. A well-groomed medical assistant promotes confidence in all the people with whom she or he interacts.

The Development of the Medical Assisting Profession

Now that we have discussed the professional and personal qualities the medical assistant needs, let us take a brief look at some landmark events in the history of medicine to understand how the medical assisting profession evolved. Over time, certain historic events have had an impact on the evolution of the practice of medicine. Learning about them helps us understand our current medical environment. Table 1.6 depicts some of the major events in the evolution of medicine.

Did you know, for example, that the first public health laws were established by the Hebrew leader Moses around 1200 B.C.? In fact, the Hebrew scriptures contain laws that guided the ancient Jewish people in many health practices, some of which helped prevent contamination from certain animal diseases. Did you know that the Greek philosopher and physician Hippocrates is considered the "Father of Medicine" because he is credited with establishing its practice as a science and not, as was previously thought, a form of magic? As you read over Table 1.6, note the number of important milestones in the practice of medicine

Table 1.6 Historic Events in the Evolution of Western Medicine

Date	Event	Date	Event
1200 B.C.	Moses established first public health laws by incorporating them into the Hebrew religion.	1895	Wilhelm Conrad Roentgen discovered x-rays.
c.450–370 B.C.	Hippocrates, Greek philosopher known as "the Father of Medicine," wrote the Hippocratic Oath, which serves as the ethical guide for physicians today. He also established the scientific practice of medicine.	1896	Italian physician Scipione Rive-Rocci invented the sphygmomanometer.
		1900	Paul Ehrlich began chemotherapy by using Salvarsan to treat syphilis.
		1901	Willem Einthoven introduced electrocardiography.
129–216	Galen, a Greek physician practicing in Rome, wrote anatomy textbooks and believed in preventive medicine.	1911	Great Britain introduced National Health Insurance.
1270–1280	Glass workers in Venice introduced eyeglasses.	1921	Frederick Banting, Charles Best, James Collip, and John MacLeod discovered insulin.
16th century	Paracelsus introduced the alchemical model, a precursor of chemical pharmacology.	1928	Alexander Fleming discovered penicillin.
1632–1723	Anton van Leeuwenhoek refined the microscope and identified bacteria, protozoa, spermatozoa, and red blood cells.	1933	The causative virus of influenza was first isolated.
1751	Leopold Auenbrugger of Vienna introduced percussion of the chest.	1939–1945	World War II—various medical advances including plastic surgery and treatment of wounds, anesthesia, and widespread availability of blood transfusion.
1790s	Philippe Pinel in France and, later, William Tuke in England founded the era of treating mental illness with kindness and care rather than incarceration and cruelty.	1944–1945	Introduction of wide range of effective medications to treat infections, hypertension, malignant diseases, etc.
1796	Edward Jenner discovered smallpox vaccine.	1948	Establishment of World Health Organization as a special agency of the United Nations.
c.1800	Samuel Hahnemann introduced homeopathy.	1953	James Watson and Francis Crick described the structure of DNA.
1819	Rene-Theophile-Hyacinthe Laennec introduced the use of the stethoscope for auscultation.	1964	Declaration of Helsinki—a landmark in medical ethics, it was the basis for the principle and practice of informed consent in healthcare.
1821–1912	Clara Barton, a nurse in the Civil War, organized the American Red Cross.	1967	Cicely Saunders initiated the hospice movement in London.
1830	John Eliotson used hypnotism in surgery.	1967	Christiaan Barnard performed the first successful heart transplant, in South Africa.
1836	England began recording births, deaths, and marriages.	1980	Endoscopic surgery was introduced.
1844	Horace Wells, a Connecticut dentist, used nitrous oxide as an anesthetic during surgery.	1980s–1990s	The rapid growth of medical genetics and molecular medicine began.
1847	Elizabeth Blackwell entered medical school in Geneva, N.Y., to become the first female physician.	1981–1984	AIDS was recognized as a new disease.
1850	Hermann von Helmholtz invented the ophthalmoscope.	1991	The Office of Alternative Medicine was established in the National Institutes of Health
1854–1960	Florence Nightingale opened the first nursing school in London.	Late 1990s	Biotechnology, including biosensors, computers, and robotics, expanded diagnostic, pharmacologic, and surgical possibilities.
1860	Louis Pasteur began work which, along with that of Robert Koch, laid the foundation for germ theory.	2000	Genome Milestone—full decoding of DNA.
1865	Joseph Lister introduced antisepsis in surgery, followed by asepsis.		

during the nineteenth century, such as the invention of the stethoscope and discovery of x-rays. As you see, the nineteenth century also saw the opening of the medical field to women. The twentieth century witnessed some of the most important advances ever in medical technology, including the identification of DNA structure, increasing skill in transplant surgery, and advances in biotechnology. As we begin the twenty-first century, exciting times are surely ahead for the development of medicine.

In years past, physicians generally treated patients in their own medical offices where they would independently gather needed information, document findings, provide treatments, and charge the patient a fee for their services. However, in the late twentieth century, this system became archaic because of technological advances in healthcare. New technologies made available more-extensive and specialized diagnostic procedures that could not be performed in the general practitioner's office. Physicians, therefore, now needed to refer patients to other healthcare specialists who could perform these sophisticated procedures. As a result, physicians today are increasingly specialized in their training and practice. A physician might opt to become a cardiologist, an oncologist, a urologist, or a pediatric specialist. Table 1.7 lists these and other areas of

Table 1.7 Medical Specialties

Specialty	Description	Specialty	Description
Allergy	concerned with hypersensitivity reactions to intrinsically harmless substances, most of which are environmental	*Obstetrics/Gynecology*	usually grouped together but can be practiced separately; obstetrics deals with pregnancy, labor, and puerperium while gynecology deals with diseases of the female genital tract
Anesthesiology	concerned with pain management, the administration of anesthetics, and monitoring of patients during surgery	*Oncology*	deals with diagnosing and treating cancer
		Ophthalmology	deals with the eye and its diseases
Cardiology	study of heart and blood vessels and their functions	*Orthopedics*	deals with the preservation and restoration of the skeletal system, its articulations, and associated structures
Dermatology	concerned with diagnosis and treatment of skin diseases		
Emergency Medicine	manages the emergency care of patients in both the prehospital setting and the emergency room	*Otolaryngology* (*Otorhinolaryngology*)	concerned with diseases of the ear, nose, and throat
Endocrinology	concerned with diseases and malfunction of glands of internal secretion	*Pathology*	studies the essential nature of disease, especially the changes in body tissues and organs; this specialist does not see patients
Family Medicine	concerned with maintaining the health of all individuals across the life cycle, birth to death; sometimes called primary care doctor or general practitioner	*Pediatrics*	deals with children, their growth and development, and the diseases that affect them
		Physical Medicine	concerned with diseases and disorders that affect physical mobility
Gastroenterology	study of stomach and intestines and the diseases affecting them	*Pulmonology*	concerned with diseases and disorders of the chest, lungs, heart, and blood vessels
Geriatrics	concerned with diseases, disorders, and problems associated with aging		
Immunology	study of all aspects of immunity, including allergy and hypersensitivity	*Psychiatry*	deals with the study, treatment, and prevention of mental illness
Internal Medicine	concerned with diseases and disorders of internal organs; usually for patients in young adulthood or older	*Radiology*	deals with the use of x-rays, radioactive substances, and other forms of radiant energy in diagnosing and treating disease; also interprets radiographic imaging
Nephrology	deals with diseases and disorders of the kidneys	*Surgery*	performs operative and manual procedures to treat diseases, injuries, and deformities
Neurology	concerned with diseases and disorders of the central nervous system		
Nuclear Medicine	diagnoses and treats diseases with use of radionuclides	*Urology*	concerned with the female urinary system and male genitourinary system and the diseases affecting them

specialization that physicians might decide to pursue in the United States today. New areas of specialization are continuing to develop.

During this time that technological advances were mandating increased physician specialization, the insurance industry grew far more complex than in previous years. Increasingly, the physician found that processing insurance claims for reimbursement was a cumbersome and time-consuming duty, taking her away from the primary duty of caring for her patients. To deal with these increased responsibilities, the physician employed a receptionist who, in addition to processing claims, handled other clerical duties such as scheduling appointments and referrals. The physician also hired a nurse who would help interview patients and assess their condition. However, it soon became apparent that one multiskilled individual who could provide both administrative and clinical skills would increase the efficiency of the medical office. Therefore, the position of the medical assistant was created.

The Need for Self-Directed, Continual Learning

In this chapter, we have discussed a number of roles and responsibilities that medical assistants face. To meet the challenges of fulfilling your duties as a medical assistant, nothing will serve you better than a determination to be a lifelong learner. Although no one knows exactly what direction healthcare will take in the future, it is clear that change will be constant and rapid. A medical assistant who is continually learning and adapting will be a prized employee. He must strive to be in tune with not only the state of healthcare in general but also with the changing culture and interests of the population he serves. As a medical assistant, you can expect to be stimulated and challenged by your daily work. You will be called upon to be knowledgeable and confident in a wide variety of functions and skills, from clinical procedures to office administration to human relationships. To perform at your best and keep up with the changing environment, you must develop a plan of self-directed learning. These days, employers are eager to hire professionals who are self-starters: people who do not need constant supervision but can think, act, and learn independently.

Lifelong learning skills are related to success and satisfaction in everything you do. To become a lifelong learner, you first have to know yourself and acknowledge any weakness or lack of understanding you may have in a certain area. Then, form a concrete plan to study or gain the experience necessary to correct this weakness. For example, if you have never used the Internet to see what healthcare sites are posted, you might plan to visit and evaluate ten such sites this month. Or if you are working as a medical assistant and do not understand how your duties interact with those of the medical office's lab technician, you might arrange an interview with the technician to discuss how you can work together more efficiently. Above all, lifelong learning techniques must be real, concrete measures taken to better yourself and make yourself more effective in your job performance. In fostering the habit of lifelong learning, you will not only become a valued member of the healthcare team but also will greatly enhance your enthusiasm for and satisfaction in your work as a medical assistant.

Education and Credentials of Medical Assistants and Other Healthcare Professionals

Today, the job prospects for trained medical assistants are excellent. Medical assistants are increasingly in high demand. In fact, the U.S. Department of Labor's Bureau of Labor Statistics has predicted a 74% increase in the employment of medical assistants from 1996 to 2006—requiring nearly 166,000 people to fill these positions. One of the reasons for this increased need is that the U.S. population is aging. People are living longer than ever before because of advances in medical technology, including earlier and more sophisticated diagnosis and treatment of diseases. Who will fill these new positions? The Bureau of Labor Statistics predicts that medical assistants with formal training and experience will be the best qualified candidates and will find employment in a wide variety of medical offices, specialized clinics, and other healthcare facilities.

The first medical assistants were trained "on-the-job" by their physician employers, and this form of training still remains one of the entries into the profession. However, the effectiveness of on-the-job training depends heavily on the abilities of the physician or other mentor to teach and guide. On-the-job training thus lacks standardization and, in most instances, does not give the medical assistant a comprehensive knowledge of the profession. For the most part, it limits her knowledge to the operation of only one particular medical office, and to the practice of only those tasks that her supervisor deems necessary. Such training, while valuable in itself, restricts the possible settings in which the medical assistant might work.

Formal education is a better choice for a medical assistant's career. Such education is available through proprietary schools, community colleges, technical schools, and hospitals. No matter what the setting, you should seek a medical assisting program that is fully accredited. An accredited educational program means that that program has been evaluated by one or more national boards and has met rigorous standards of quality and specific curriculum guidelines. Accredited programs thus ensure a thorough, comprehensive, and standardized education in the field. Depending on the program, graduates of an accredited medical assisting program may earn a diploma, a certificate, or an associate's degree. The specific award depends on such factors as the length of the program and the content of its curriculum.

In 1997, about 350 medical assisting programs were accredited by the **Commission on Accreditation of Allied Health Education Programs (CAAHEP)**, and over 150 programs were accredited by the **Accrediting Bureau of Health Education Schools (ABHES)**. Just seven years earlier there were only 197 accredited programs. In 1990, the total number of medical assistants was approximately 50,000; by 1996, that number had jumped to over 225,000. These statistics give you some idea of the rapid growth of the medical assisting field.

Accreditation of Educational Programs

As we have noted, program **accreditation** identifies for prospective medical assisting students those educational institutions that meet certain standards of the two nationally recognized accrediting agencies mentioned above. Graduates of a school accredited by one or both of these agencies are assured of:

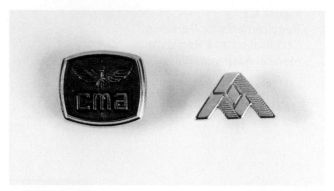

Certified Medical assistants wear these pins to promote the CMA credential.

- having completed a program that meets rigorous national requirements
- having received the knowledge and experience needed to perform their work successfully
- being recognized and respected by their professional peers for their educational preparation
- being eligible for professional credentialing, such as AAMA certification (CAAHEP-accredited program) or AMT certification (ABHES-accredited program)

Both the **Certified Medical Assistant (CMA)** credential, awarded by CAAHEP, and the **Registered Medical Assistant (RMA)** credential, awarded by ABHES, are voluntary in that neither the federal government nor any state requires a medical assistant to have one, and they are national in that the certification tests are given throughout the country. The two credentials are awarded after successful completion of a written examination. Figure 1.2 illustrates the steps required for pursuing certification as a Registered Medical Assistant.

Both certifying boards, CAAHEP and ABHES, require strict adherence to their regulations for the accreditation they provide. Programs that receive accreditation from these agencies must meet or exceed the guidelines, and must continue to meet or exceed them year after year. The major aim of these accrediting agencies is to ensure that the education provided to the medical assistant is thorough, up-to-date, and compatible with the needs of the employment market.

Credentials for Healthcare Practitioners

Professional credentials indicate the level of expertise and experience of the healthcare practitioner and assure healthcare providers that the practitioner is

Figure 1.2
Requirements for Pursuing
Certification as a Registered
Medical Assistant (RMA)

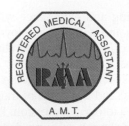

Pass the AMT certification examination

Be a graduate of:
a medical assisant program accredited by an organization approved by the U.S. Department of Education

or

a medical assisant program in an institution accredited by a regional accrediting commission or by a national accrediting organization approved by the U.S. Department of Education

or

a formal medical services training program of the U.S. armed forces

or

Been employed in the profession of medical assisting for a minimum of five years, no more than two years of which may have been as an instructor in a postsecondary medical assistant program

Be a graduate of an accredited high school or equivalent

Be of good moral character

competent in her field. It is important for the medical assistant to understand these credentials because they help to protect patients' rights. Here are two of the credentials healthcare workers may achieve: licensing and certification.

LICENSURE Licensure is a mandatory credential for many healthcare practitioners. It grants individuals who successfully meet certain educational and training requirements the authority to practice in a particular area of the healthcare industry. A license is a legal document that lets the person holding it offer her specific skills and knowledge to the public. Physicians, nurses, and other professional and technical persons must hold individual licenses or other permits from the state or local government in

order to practice. Medical offices are required to keep updated copies of these licenses and permits on hand.

CERTIFICATION Certification, unlike licensure, is usually a voluntary credential that most commonly is national in scope. In most instances, it is sponsored by a nongovernmental agency. Healthcare workers are usually not required to be certified to practice in the profession, although some practitioners, such as paramedics, must be certified. Even if it is not mandatory, however, holding this credential indicates that the practitioner has acquired exemplary expertise and skill in the field. As defined, medical assistant certification offers status and definition to the practitioner; provides a means of establishing a

Professional Organizations and Continuing Education

As a medical assistant, you need to be constantly developing your skills and putting new practices and knowledge into use. All healthcare workers must be involved in continuing education. One recommended way of obtaining ongoing education is by joining a **professional organization**. Professional organizations provide a means by which a healthcare professional can interact with other professionals in the field, read about and discuss issues in the practice, and learn new ideas. Membership in professional organizations is voluntary; however, participating in such an organization can be an invaluable resource and means of support for your career.

The AAMA and AMT are examples of professional organizations that the medical assistant may join. The AAMA's purpose, as stated in its 1997 bylaws, is "to promote the professional identity and stature of its members, and the medical profession, through education and credentialing." The association has developed a creed that defines the medical assistant's commitment to the profession and the individuals served. (See Figure 1.3.) Membership in these organizations is open to both professionals and students. Some of the advantages of becoming a member of the AAMA or AMT organizations include access to up-to-date information about the medical assisting field, reduced rates for the medical assisting examination, discounts on continuing education self-study programs, and networking with other medical assistants at state and national meetings.

national standard of care with regard to the legal duty of the medical assistant to the patient; offers the employer guidelines for hiring qualified staff, as well as a pool of applicants; provides an environment for continuing education of medical assistants; and is cost-effective.

Renewing Credentials

Achieving a license or certification is only a first step. Most credentials must be renewed within a designated period of time. The AAMA offers a five-year recertification program, while AMT has an annual revalidation program. The AAMA requires sixty hours of continuing education credit over a five-year period. AMT requires fifteen hours of continuing education credit each year. The processes are the same; only the time frames are different. Both AMT and the AAMA provide continuing education seminars, workshops, and self-study courses on both national and regional chapter bases.

I believe
in the principles and purposes of the
profession of medical assisting.

I endeavor
to be more effective.

I aspire
to render greater service.

I protect
the confidence entrusted to me.

I am dedicated
to the care and well-being of all people.

I am loyal
to my employer.

I am true
to the ethics of my profession.

I am strengthened
by compassion, courage, and faith.

Figure 1.3
The AAMA Creed

Source: Reprinted by permission of the American
Association of Medical Assistants, Inc.

The Internet as a Healthcare Resource

There is no question that another emerging trend of the twenty-first century will be an explosion in the use of information technologies, especially the Internet. Currently, the Internet contains an overwhelming number of websites from which anyone can glean information about any number of healthcare issues. Consumers thus have many sources online that offer information about health issues, possible diagnoses of medical conditions, and treatment options. Like other online shopping sites, e-pharmacies have recently appeared on the Internet; drugs sometimes seem less expensive on some of these sites than in actual pharmacies, and many consumers appreciate the convenience of ordering online. In addition, chat lines and discussion forums for various medical conditions let patients share their concerns, frustrations, and advice on such issues as weight loss, arthritis, diabetes, and reconstructive surgery with others from around the globe. But healthcare providers and consumers must be aware that the Internet is unregulated: anyone—specialist or non-specialist—may join a discussion or post a website and disseminate information.

Since so many people now have access to the Internet, it will be increasingly important for all healthcare workers, including the medical assistant, to help patients identify those Internet sites that are authoritative and provide accurate and complete information. The following discussion about Internet use will help the medical assistant learn how to use this important resource effectively.

The Internet is a vast collection of computer networks that can provide healthcare professionals and other users with a great wealth of information from libraries, government agencies, universities, non-profit and educational organizations, user groups, and individuals around the world. Originally, the Internet was used almost exclusively by scientists and engineers. Exponential growth in its use, however, came after the invention of the **World Wide Web (www),** often referred to simply as the web. The inventor of the web, Tim Berners-Lee, imagined a worldwide communication system based on hypertext documents. A **hypertext** document is one that contains one or more links, which are represented on the screen by buttons, highlighted text, or icons that send the user to a related, or linked, document. By the system of links, documents on computers all over the world have been connected to one another and can be accessed by a browser, such as Netscape, on a person's computer.

The web is by far the most widely used part of the Internet. Consequently, people often use the terms "net" and "web" interchangeably. There is, however, a difference. Strictly speaking, the Internet is a system of computers, storage devices, and connections, along with the software that lets people use these connections. The web, by contrast, is the total collection of information available on that part of the Internet that contains linked documents. In addition to handling web documents, the Internet also provides the physical basis for a number of other computer communications services, letting people send e-mail, access archives of files, and participate in discussion groups.

Quality Medical Internet Sites

Some Internet sites can provide reliable medical and health information for the medical assistant as well as for patients. The level of information ranges from basic to advanced, and so may be suitable for helping a patient learn more about a subject or learning more about a subject yourself. The cautions regarding healthy skepticism are appropriate, no matter which Internet site you are accessing, but the sites in Table 1.8 are generally regarded as reliable.

Finding Information on the Web

To find information on the World Wide Web, one can simply open a browser and type the complete web

Table 1.8 Reliable Web Sites for Medical Information

URL	Sponsor	Information available	Comments
www.cdc.gov	Centers for Disease Control	health statistics, publications on prevention and incidence	public domain (you can copy it or use it for any reason); offers Spanish-language content
www.fda.gov	U.S. Food and Drug Administration	information about foods, drugs, and cosmetics; includes information about newly approved drugs	public domain
www.medicinenet.com	MedicineNet, Inc.	medical dictionary and detailed information on medications	copyrighted material
www.ncbi.nlm.nih.gov/PubMed	National Center for Biotechnology Information, National Library of Medicine	access to MEDLINE, the National Library of Medicine's database of peer-reviewed research	only the abstract is available
www.merck.com	Merck & Co.	diagnosis and therapy for all but the most obscure disorders	written for health professionals so the vocabulary is quite specialized and specific

address, or URL (universal resource locator), for the site one wishes to visit into a location box. Most URLs are formed by three parts separated by a colon (:), slashes (/), and dots (.) Here is one such URL: http://www.healthcare.com. The *www.* stands for the World Wide Web. The next part of the URL is called the domain name and identifies the person, organization, server, or topic. Following the dot is the domain suffix, *.com*, which identifies the type of organization. Table 1.9 lists common domain suffixes and their meanings. More may be added.

Table 1.9 Key to Internet Domain Suffixes

.com	commercial entity
.edu	educational institution
.firm	business entity
.gov	government agency or department
.info	organizations that provide members with information
.mil	military organization
.net	network resource (administrative site for service providers)
.store	online sales
.nom	personal name
.web	World Wide Web organizations
.rec	recreation/entertainment

Like the yellow pages of a telephone book, a Net Directory is a list of web addresses. Several such directories are available for purchase at bookstores and computer stores, and some are available online. However, a user who does not know the specific address of the company or organization he is trying to visit can use one of several online search engines, such as Yahoo or Alta Vista, to find this information based on key words. Some of the most common search engines and their addresses are listed in Table 1.10.

Internet search techniques use a selection and sort process that is based on Boolean logic. Boolean logic refers to the logical relationship among search terms. To conduct a focused search on the Internet, you use specific Boolean operators, or key words, such as *and, or, not,* and *near.* Depending on what operator you

Table 1.10 Common Search Engines

Name	URL
AltaVista	www.altavista.digital.com
Excite	www.excite.com
Infoseek	www.infoseek.com
Google	www.google.com
Lycos	www.lycos.com
MetaCrawler	www.metacrawler.com
Yahoo!	www.yahoo.com

Table 1.11 Some Boolean Operators Used in Search Strings

Operator	Sample String	Effect
AND or +	computers AND viruses	finds sites dealing with computer viruses but not with computers in general or viruses in general
"..."	"computer viruses"	finds sites containing the entire phrase in quotation marks
NOT or -	"computer virus" NOT hoax	limits search to sites that exclude the keyword after NOT (computer viruses that are not hoaxes)
OR	"WDEF virus" OR "Michaelangelo virus"	finds reference to either the WDEF or the Michaelangelo virus

use, you can expand or limit your search. For example, an Internet search using the key word "virus" would locate websites dealing with computer, human, and animal viruses. A user interested in computer viruses would limit the search by using one of the Boolean operators. Table 1.11 presents a summary of some of the most important Boolean operators and how they work to modify an Internet search.

Evaluating Websites

To conduct research efficiently on the Internet, all users need to understand how to evaluate websites. As noted above, the unregulated nature of the Internet, the huge array of healthcare websites, and the need for consumers to obtain accurate health information make it imperative that you, as a medical assistant, know how to help patients evaluate websites for accurate and safe information. As you scrutinize a particular website, ask yourself the following questions:

- What clues does the website's domain name provide about who is sponsoring the site? Sites that end with *.edu* (educational institutions) and *.gov* (government institutions) are generally reliable. Sites that end with *.com*, however, are commercial sites that, like any commercial institution, are often for-profit enterprises or run by special interest groups that may slant or "spin" information to their advantage.
- Who is the author or developer of the site? Examine any names provided on the site. Investigate the

author's credentials, if given. Do they make him a reliable source? Does the author give you a way to contact her?

- What is the quality of the information? As you examine the site, ask yourself if the information appears accurate, up-to-date, comprehensive, and reliable. Check for a date indicating when the site was last maintained or updated, since many sites on the net are already out of date. Check to see if a bibliography is provided.
- Is the information given without bias? An author with a personal stake in what others think about a subject may withhold or distort information. Read closely and critically to discover whether the author presents the information objectively or is trying to influence how you think. Using loaded, or non-objective, language and ignoring obvious counter-arguments are signs of author bias.
- Examine and follow any hyperlinks embedded in the text. More often than not, a site that itself provides little clue to the bias or slant of its information will have hyperlinks that give strong clues to that bias. What other sources or products does the author promote?

Discussion Forums and Chat Lines

One of the most popular features of the Internet is the many discussion forums and chat lines available. By accessing such clearinghouse addresses as www.dejanews.com, a user can find a wealth of personal interest groups for any topic she is interested in, from Vietnamese cooking to genealogy to the Civil War to fan clubs for soap opera actors. Some discussion forums or chat lines require membership and a fee to join, but many are free. Anyone with a computer and Internet access, therefore, may jump into the conversation, offering personal experience, seeking information, and giving advice. Numerous healthcare chat lines are available, and more are continually being added. On such lines, people from around the world can discuss healthcare matters of concern to them, from controlling stress to identifying the symptoms of a heart attack to comparing alternative therapies for cancer treatment. While excellent information on healthcare is available on many authoritative websites, you as a professional should be extremely cautious of the material presented in these discussion forums and chat lines. Remember that, as with any group of people who gather to discuss an issue, some of what they say may be unproven or untrue. While chat lines can be fun and interesting for personal use, as a general rule, do not recommend them to your patients.

Clinical Summary

- Medical assistants are multiskilled healthcare practitioners who work in a variety of settings including medical offices and clinics.
- Medical assistants fill many roles, including promoting healing of the whole person, providing excellent customer service, educating patients, managing patient care, and assuring that the care is safe and reliable.
- Customer service is of prime importance in today's healthcare environment. It includes treating all internal and external customers with respect and attention to their needs.
- The AAMA's Role Delineation Study defines the competencies that medical assistants must have to practice. They include administrative, clinical, and general or transdisciplinary competencies.
- Professional attributes of a medical assistant are defined by the Role Delineation Study. They are: project a professional manner and image; adhere to ethical principles; demonstrate initiative and responsibility; work as a team member; manage time effectively; prioritize and perform multiple tasks; adapt to change; promote the CMA credential; and enhance skills through continuing education.
- Personal attributes of a medical assistant include empathy, diplomacy, reliability, courtesy, a positive attitude, and a professional appearance.
- A variety of historic events have influenced today's medical practice and led to the creation of the medical assisting field.
- National accreditation of medical assistant programs can be achieved through the Commission on Accreditation of Allied Health Education Programs (CAAHEP) or the Accrediting Bureau of Health Education Schools (ABHES).
- Professional medical assistants may achieve credentialing as a Certified Medical Assistant (CMA) through the American Association of Medical Assistants (AAMA) or as a Registered Medical Assistant (RMA) from the American Medical Technologists Association (AMT).
- One way medical assistants can obtain continuing education is by joining a professional organization such as the AAMA or AMT.
- The Internet will be an increasingly popular medium for healthcare information. The professional medical assistant will be using websites to learn on the job and must know how to evaluate healthcare information on the web for authority, accuracy, and reliability.

The Language of Medicine

accreditation A process by which an outside agency evaluates an educational program and certifies that it meets a set of standard requirements.

administrative competencies Skills that the medical assistant usually uses in the "front office." These may include clerical functions, handling insurance claims, accounting, bookkeeping, greeting patients, answering the telephone, and general office management tasks.

Accrediting Bureau of Health Education Schools (ABHES) An agency that accredits educational programs in either a hospital, private vocational institution, or public post-secondary organization.

American Association of Medical Assistants (AAMA) A national professional organization that represents certified medical assistants and their profession.

American Medical Technologists (AMT) A national professional organization that represents certified medical assistants and their profession.

certification Usually a voluntary credential, most commonly national in scope and sponsored by a non-governmental agency, that indicates that the healthcare practitioner has acquired exemplary knowledge and skills in the field

Certified Medical Assistant (CMA) Title used by medical assistants with a national credential awarded by the Certifying Board of the American Association of Medical Assistants. These graduates have completed a program accredited by the Commission on Accreditation of Allied Health Education Programs and have passed a written examination.

clinical competencies Skills that the medical assistant usually uses in the "back office," which may include assisting the physician with physical examinations, obtaining and processing diagnostic tests, and interviewing patients for medical histories.

Commission on Accreditation of Allied Health Education Programs (CAAHEP) An agency that grants accreditation to programs in medical assisting upon recommendation of its Curriculum Review Board.

courtesy Conduct that provides respect for and consideration of the dignity and needs of others.

customer service Efficient, helpful, and high-quality service provided to the consumer.

diplomacy Tact; communicating in such a way that there is little or no ill will.

empathy An attitude of conscious identification with another person's concerns or situation.

external customers Those individuals and organizations outside the medical office that supply necessary information and products or specialized services to the office.

general or transdisciplinary competencies Skills that are used in both the administrative and clinical areas of the medical office, including professionalism, communication ability, knowledge of legal concepts, instructing, and operational functions.

hypertext A computer document that provides one or more links—icons or highlighted text—that opens related documents.

internal customers Patients and colleagues of the medical assistant in the medical office.

Journal of Continuing Education A professional journal published by American Medical Technologists.

licensure A mandatory credential for some healthcare workers, established by government processes, usually at the state level, which grants individuals who successfully meet the statutory requirements authority to practice in a particular field of endeavor.

professionalism Being skilled at a job that requires advanced educational training; an on-the-job attitude that includes adhering to ethical principles, working as a team member, and adapting to change.

professional organization An organization that exists to support and provide continuing education for a certain profession.

PMA (Professional Medical Assistant) A professional journal published by the American Association of Medical Assistants.

Registered Medical Assistant (RMA) Title used by medical assistants with a national credential awarded by the Cer-

tifying Board of American Medical Technologists. These graduates have completed a program accredited by the Accrediting Bureau of Health Education Schools.

reliability Trustworthiness; capability of being dependable or responsible in action or performance.

role delineation study A 1996 study by the American Association of Medical Assistants that defined the competencies medical assistants must have to practice.

teamwork The ability to work interdependently with others toward a goal.

World Wide Web (web) The collection of Internet information connected by hypertext links.

Signs/Symptoms of Progress

Recall, Question, Connect

Recall
Think of the professional attributes you possess. List those that will help you as a medical assistant.

Question
List the professional attributes you need to develop further to work successfully in the field of medical assisting.

Connect
Describe specific actions you will take to acquire the needed professional attributes to become a skilled medical assistant.

Educating the Patient

After seeing the physician for a routine physical examination, Lisa Babcock stops at the reception desk to pay her bill. You are sitting at the computer as Lisa says, "Aren't these computers great! I've found so much information about my health by just 'chatting' with other people online. I learn more in the chat rooms than I do from my doctor."
1 How would you educate the patient on responsible Internet use?
2 What websites would you recommend for this patient?

Exploring Perspectives in Teams

Perspective involves the discipline of examining how ideas look from different points of view and recognizing that

there are often multiple "answers" to complex questions. In small groups or on your own, reflect on possible alternative views or answers and summarize your findings.

1 The medical assistant is expected to be a multiskilled worker who must "multitask," or do many tasks at once. Think about the terms multiskilled and multitasking. What key skills must the medical assistant possess? Give examples of instances when multitasking is essential to the job. Then discuss whether you can be multiskilled but not able to multitask. Do you know people who can multitask but are not multiskilled?

2 Discuss the concept of customer service. As a medical assistant, who are your internal customers when you work in the administrative office? Who are your external customers? Who are your internal customers when you work in clinical areas? Who are your external customers? Is your patient a customer? Why or why not?

3 The medical assistant has five important roles: promoting health, providing excellent customer service, educating patients, managing patient care, and assuring safe and reliable care. Which role attracted you to the field of medical assisting? In which role will you demonstrate the greatest strengths? In which role do you have weaknesses you will need to work to overcome? Use the competencies listed in Table 1.2 and Table 1.3 to help you identify your strengths and weaknesses.

4 As a long-time medical assistant, you have been assigned to mentor a new medical assistant on her first week on the job. What will you stress as the essential attitudes and qualities a medical assistant needs to do her job? What will you indicate as the most challenging and difficult part of the job?

Learning Outcomes

- Understand the major ways in which the United States's population is shifting and the implications of that shift for healthcare workers.

- Define managed care and discuss its implications for the roles and responsibilities of the medical assistant.

- Describe the role of the medical assistant as a member of the interdisciplinary healthcare team.

- Describe each major type of healthcare delivery setting (ambulatory care, acute care, subacute care, long-term care, public health services) and the role of the medical assistant in each.

- Describe the key types of health insurance and how medical staff members must adhere to managed care policies and procedures.

Performance Objectives

- Coordinate patient care information with other healthcare providers.

- Demonstrate positive and collaborative behavior on departmental and interdisciplinary healthcare teams.

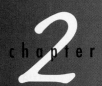

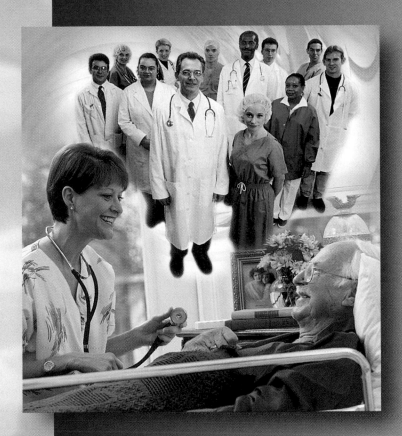

The United States's population is *growing older and more ethnically diverse, a shift in demographics that will require substantial changes in the healthcare delivery system. In response to these changing demographics, as well as to the specific needs of the population, the delivery of healthcare services has evolved over time into a managed care system. This system was created to provide healthcare services in the most cost-effective manner. One of the necessities in this managed care environment is the use of a team approach to healthcare. In this chapter, you will learn the differences between departmental and interdisciplinary teams and the medical assistant's important role as a member of the interdisciplinary team. The chapter also discusses the variety of settings in which healthcare may be provided, including ambulatory care, acute care, subacute care, long-term care, and public health settings. As a medical assistant, you will most likely seek employment in an ambulatory,*

Working in Today's Healthcare Environment

or outpatient, care setting. However, you need to know about all the settings to refer patients to appropriate services and to understand the continuum of care available in the current healthcare system.

This chapter also gives you an overview of the major types of insurance plans available in the United States. The world of managed care and of insurance coverage is changing rapidly, and will no doubt change further throughout this new century. Because she is often charged with processing insurance forms and advising patients on insurance matters, the medical assistant needs a basic understanding of the complex world of insurance benefits to perform these administrative duties skillfully.

The current state of healthcare, under managed care, is extremely complex. An individual has many healthcare insurance options and needs guidance in making the right decision. Some patients are skeptical of the managed care system altogether and may feel more like a "number" than a unique person in dealing with the complex bureaucracy or "red tape" of the system's regulations. Many patients experience difficulty navigating through the many choices available in today's healthcare setting. For example, does a person's elderly parent, just released from the hospital, need subacute or long-term care? If long-term care is needed, should it be given at home, perhaps with the help of a home care agency, or in one of several types of nursing homes or minimal care facilities? Will the person's insurance cover the costs of such long-term care? These are just some of the concerns your patient may have about today's healthcare environment.

The Changing Face of the Patient Population

Our society is rapidly changing, and those changes will probably become even more dramatic throughout this new century. The U.S. population is becoming older and more ethnically diverse. The number of single-parent households has increased dramatically over the last several decades, putting considerable economic pressure on families and altering not only our society's workplaces and daycare structures but also the entire culture. Customers of today's healthcare system are better educated and able to obtain healthcare information from a wide variety of sources. Still, many individuals cannot afford the healthcare insurance needed to obtain adequate care in the present system. In the 2000 presidential election, healthcare matters ranked among the top three concerns for the American people in public opinion polls. The country faces many

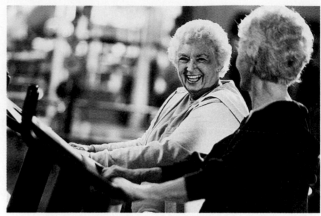

The growing population of the elderly is creating both new challenges and new opportunities for the healthcare professional.

challenges in the twenty-first century if we are to ensure access to healthcare for all Americans.

Today, the elderly are the fastest-growing segment of the U.S. population. Statistics show that the entire population will probably grow 22 percent from 2000 to 2005 but that those age sixty-five and older will increase 78.5 percent. Our country will need to find a way to pay for long-term care, preserve Social Security, improve nursing homes and housing opportunities for the elderly, and provide more help at home for the weak and chronically ill. The current culture, designed for the young with things like bucket seats in cars and small-print newspapers, will be forced to adjust for the new wave of senior citizens. Lights will have to be brighter, signs bigger, and public address systems louder. But within such upheaval, there is also exciting new opportunity.

The members of this growing elderly population are not only better educated than their parents' generation but also increasingly have the power to transform old age into a healthful, active, vibrant stage of life. Medical advances will free many of the elderly from the crippling aches and pains that are experienced today. Among the medical possibilities are cloned organs to replace failing ones, antioxidant cocktails to refresh the body and brain, and technology to detect and eradicate disease. The United States has long been a youth-oriented culture, but as this demographic pattern shifts and medical advances keep pace, old age will become a time of adventure and exploration.

The U.S. Administration on Aging has affirmed that the nation's growing number of elderly residents will vastly increase the number of people requiring healthcare, both formal and informal. This means that the need for skilled healthcare workers will continue to rise, and practitioners and professionals from a variety of disciplines must work together in interdisciplinary teams to provide this population with effective and comprehensive care.

Besides aging, the American population is also becoming more culturally diverse. The U.S. Census Bureau projects that by 2005, non-Caucasian residents will account for 47 percent of the nation's population. Altered immigration laws as well as the desire to improve life circumstances have caused a rapid influx of people from many cultures into the United States. This has led to radical changes in the nation's demographic and ethnic composition throughout the last century, changes that no doubt will continue in this century. The Hispanic/Latino-American community, for example, is growing six times faster than the general population and will surpass the African American population by 2013. The Asian/Pacific Islander-American community also is growing rapidly, with an estimated 30 percent jump in size since 1990. The Native American population now stands at more than two million and is also increasing.

A common metaphor for American society was a "melting pot" where diverse ethnic and cultural groups blended together into a common whole and lost their individual differences. Today we celebrate our ethnic, racial, and cultural differences in this country and do not seek to "melt" them away in a mix. Increasingly, people take pride in their heritage and identify themselves with a certain ethnic background, culture, or race.

In response to these societal changes, health professionals will increasingly need to focus on providing culturally competent healthcare and preventive services that consider an individual's values, belief systems, and response to health and illness issues. Healthcare providers need to understand the ways in which social and cultural backgrounds shape health behaviors and practices in a diverse population. Providers must ensure that patient care is based on sensitivity to the uniqueness of the individual patient and encompasses strategies that facilitate decision-making in health behaviors. Healthcare workers must demonstrate an openness that allows them to learn from others, view situations from another person's perspective, and adapt their strategies to their patients' cultural traditions and values.

Like all healthcare workers of the twenty-first century, the medical assistant will need to become familiar with the various backgrounds and expectations of the patient population she serves. This is especially true in large, urban areas in which the medical office serves a diverse group of people. Differences in spoken language, culture, educational background, behavior preferences, expectations, and assumptions about healthcare can affect the patient's response and cooperation. The medical assistant faces the challenges of learning to understand the cultures of those she serves,

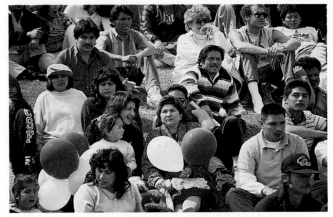

The Hispanic community, part of the changing American demographic, is growing six times faster than the general population.

communicating clearly and effectively with patients from all cultures, and devising methods to break down any barriers that prevent patients from obtaining the highest quality medical care.

A Team Approach to Healthcare in the Managed Care Environment

Healthcare professionals of the twenty-first century face a new world shaped largely by the influence of managed care. The **managed care** system is still in flux, but in general it can be defined as a system of healthcare that seeks to streamline medical services so that patients receive the best care at the lowest financial cost. In the managed care system, all healthcare providers, including the medical assistant, are expected to deliver high-quality services that simultaneously minimize costs. Managed care providers are expected to not only heal their patients but also prevent illness when possible and provide a continuum of care across the patient's life cycle, through the various stages of health, aging, and illness.

Managed care plans began to develop as early as the 1940s. The Health Insurance Plan (HIP) of Greater New York, established on the East Coast, and Kaiser-Permanente, on the West Coast, were the first health insurance plans to consider managed care. The growth of managed care plans, however, was relatively modest until the 1970s, when healthcare costs began to soar. With various adaptations, these plans spread throughout the country. Today, our healthcare continues to evolve toward a managed care delivery system. In 1999, nearly 70 percent of the insured population was enrolled in some form of managed care.

To practice effectively in a managed care environment, healthcare professionals must develop new skills, competencies, and attitudes about the delivery of healthcare. They must be good communicators and adapt to change. They must also work effectively with others in teams.

In 1998, Mark D. Smith, president and CEO of the California Healthcare Foundation, identified the six competencies he felt were most important for healthcare providers to develop to work in the managed care environment over the next ten years:

- excellent communication skills
- appropriate use of research findings in providing patient care
- a team approach to patient care
- a knowledgeable incorporation of information technology in healthcare
- knowledge of how the larger healthcare system works
- appropriate use of cost-effective resources in healthcare

Smith also noted the need for healthcare practitioners to treat patients as valued customers by listening and attending to their needs. To best serve patient-customers, teamwork among healthcare professionals is essential. The specialized contributions of all members of the team in the managed care environment will lead to the most effective patient care.

The purpose of any team is to bring together the talents of skilled individuals to solve a common problem or create a better product. When people work together as a team, they can produce more, use resources more effectively, and solve problems more quickly. Because effective teamwork relies on the expertise and input of each member of the team, it can allow individuals to realize their highest potential and accomplish goals that one person working alone may not be able to reach. For example, teamwork is essential in research that is working toward cures for diseases such as cancer. While the director, the scientists, and the technicians in the lab all perform separate, specialized functions, they are single-minded in working together to solve the same problem. One person could not possibly hope to do each separate job. By pooling their talents and energies, however, such a team may very well achieve success in their endeavor. The same holds true in the healthcare system. Today, a cooperative approach to healthcare provides the most efficient and effective management of patients' healthcare needs.

The Departmental and Interdisciplinary Healthcare Teams

Who are the members of the healthcare team? They are all the healthcare professionals and other members of the office staff who work to meet the patient's needs. The team may include physicians, nurses, medical assistants, front desk personnel, lab technicians, and drug and supply companies. These individuals bring

Customer Service

If your patient expresses a concern:
- Listen to the patient attentively.
- Apologize for errors or misunderstandings, if appropriate, even if you did not cause the problem.
- Do whatever you can to resolve the problem by alerting other appropriate team members.

Remember: Satisfied customers tell others. They are the best ambassadors for the healthcare we provide. Work with the team to solve your patients' concerns.

Working Smart

A major purpose behind managed care is to avoid duplication of services (and thus duplication of expense). Teamwork is one way this can be accomplished. In good teamwork, staff members and specialists come together to coordinate their services and collaborate with others. The goal for any healthcare team, in general, is to serve the patients' needs. The medical assistant is an important link in the team.

together their unique skills to heal the patient. Each performs a separate function, but each is committed to the same goal.

It is also important to keep in mind that the patient himself, and often his family members and friends, too, are essential members of the healthcare team. With multiple healthcare options and better access to health information, patients are playing a greater role as informed decision-makers in their treatment. As discussed in Chapter 1, "Choosing a Career as a Medical Assistant," superior customer service is crucial in today's healthcare environment. If patients do not receive it, they will—rightly—take their business elsewhere. A team approach to the patient's healthcare that involves the patient fully is a major aspect of providing customer satisfaction.

One way to think about teams in the healthcare setting is to consider the two types that are typically formed: a departmental and an **interdisciplinary healthcare team**. A departmental team consists of workers from the same department, group, or set of related specialties who combine their talents to solve a certain problem or deliver specialized patient care.

For example, a departmental team might be a laboratory team consisting of a phlebotomist, pathologist, and medical technologist. Or it might be a mental health team made up of a psychologist, social worker, and substance abuse counselor. Table 2.1 lists some other possible departmental teams and the healthcare professionals who might be members.

Table 2.1 Possible Departmental Healthcare Teams

	Members	Functions
Cardiopulmonary Team	ECG Technician	operates electrocardiographic equipment to record the electrical activity of the heart
	Cardiovascular Technologist	provides supportive services to the cardiologist in the use of sophisticated diagnostic procedures and treatment of diseases of the heart and blood vessels
	Respiratory Therapist (Registered Respiratory Therapist, RRT)	administers respiratory care treatments to patients under the direction of the physician
Direct-Care Team	Registered Nurse (RN)	delivers different types of healthcare services to patients in a variety of settings including hospitals, clinics, agencies, physician's offices, private homes, and other places where people need medical attention
	Licensed Practical Nurse (LPN) or Vocational Nurse (LVN)	works under the supervision of physicians and registered nurses in various healthcare settings to deliver care to the ill and injured
	Nurse Practitioner (NP)	an RN with advanced education and experience who performs in an expanded role and can diagnose, treat, and prescribe under the supervision of a physician
	Pharmacist	advises health professionals and the public about proper selection and use of medicines and dispenses drugs and medicines prescribed by physicians, podiatrists, dentists, and nurse practitioners
	Unlicensed Assistive Personnel (UAP)	auxiliary employee in an entry-level position who assists the professional staff in the care of the sick
	Certified Medical Assistant (CMA) or Registered Medical Assistant (RMA)	coordinates patient care in all areas under the direction of a physician
Emergency-Care Team	Emergency Medical Technician (EMT)	usually the first medical responder at the scene of an accident; responsible for basic life support
	Paramedic	provides advanced life support measures including recognition, assessment, and management of accident victims under the direction of a physician
Information Processing Team	Registered Health Information Technician (RHIT)	serves as technical assistant to the health information manager by handling, organizing, and evaluating the medical record for completeness and accuracy
	Registered Health Information Administrator (RHIA)	directs and controls activities of health information department in various healthcare settings by developing systems for documenting, storing, and retrieving medical information
	Medical Transcriptionist	transcribes, edits, and types physicians' dictated notes of patients' medical procedures and treatments

(continues)

Table 2.1 Possible Departmental Healthcare Teams (continued)

	Members	Functions
Laboratory Team	Medical Technologist (MT)	performs a variety of complex chemical, microscopic, and bacteriologic laboratory procedures to help identify and control disease
	Medical Laboratory Technician (MLT)	assists the medical technologist, and sometimes performs many of the same procedures under supervision
	Pathologist	physician who specializes in the study of disease
	Phlebotomist	an individual with special training in the practice of accessing veins to remove blood
Mental Health Team	Patient Representative	works with patients on a one-to-one basis, acting as a mediator between patients and healthcare agency administration
	Psychologist	provides testing and counseling services to patients with mental and emotional disorders
	Social Worker	assists patients in dealing with the social, emotional, and environmental problems associated with an illness or disability
	Substance Abuse Counselor	helps people who are physiologically or psychologically dependent on alcohol or other drugs to deal with the disease of chemical dependency
Nutritional Team	Registered Dietitian (RD)	responsible for nutrition care and food service; applies principles of nutrition and management to the administration of institutional food service
	Dietetic Technician	assists the dietitian in either food service management or nutritional care services
	Nutritionist	educator on human nutrition; attempts to solve food problems, control disease, and maintain and promote health
Radiologic Team	Diagnostic Medical Sonographer	works under the direction of a physician to provide quality imaging in ultrasound diagnosis
	Nuclear Medicine Technologist	assists with the administration and detection of radioactive materials in diagnosis and therapy
	Radiation Therapy Technologist	uses radiation-producing equipment, mainly to treat cancer patients
	Radiologic Technician or Radiographer	assists the radiologist in using x-ray equipment in the diagnostic imaging of such medical problems as broken bones, ulcers, and tumors
Rehabilitation Team	Art Therapist	works with patients, generally on a one-to-one basis, in the treatment and rehabilitation of mental and emotional disorders
	Dance Therapist	incorporates dance and movement in the rehabilitation and treatment of physical, behavioral, and mental disorders
	Music Therapist	organizes and conducts medically prescribed musical programs to assist in the rehabilitation of patients suffering from mental or physical illness or disability
	Occupational Therapist (OT)	attempts to restore a patient's health, independence, and self-reliance by evaluating needs and teaching how to compensate for disabilities through planned activities and therapy
	Occupational Therapy Assistant (OTA)	works under the supervision of a professional occupational therapist helping to plan and implement the rehabilitation program

(continues)

Table 2.1 Possible Departmental Healthcare Teams (continued)

	Members	Functions
Rehabilitation Team (continued)	Orthotist and Prosthetist	designs, fabricates, fits, and repairs supportive appliances (orthoses) and artificial limbs (prostheses)
	Physical Therapist (PT)	evaluates the extent of the patient's disability in such areas as neuromuscular, musculoskeletal, sensorimotor, cardiovascular, and respiratory functions and plans, implements, and evaluates appropriate treatment plans
	Physical Therapy Assistant (PTA)	works under the supervision of a professional physical therapist in the rehabilitation of disabled persons
	Recreational Therapist	plans, organizes, directs, and counsels medically approved recreation programs
	Recreation Assistant	assists the recreational therapist in carrying out recreation rehabilitation programs in hospitals and other healthcare settings

Unlike the departmental team, an interdisciplinary team is composed of workers from a widely varying set of disciplines or areas of expertise in the healthcare professions. They bring together a diverse range of skills and expertise to provide coordinated and high-quality services to patients. Patients and their families are also members of the extended interdisciplinary team. An interdisciplinary team, then, can consist of the patient, her family members, the physician, a nurse, a medical assistant, and specialists to whom the patient is referred, such as a nutritionist or a respiratory therapist. Since no one area possesses all the skills and knowledge needed to provide comprehensive care in the multifaceted healthcare system, it is only through the coordinated efforts of all professionals that cost-effective care of the patient can be realized. In the current managed care environment, interdisciplinary teams are becoming more and more essential to the delivery of healthcare services.

Collaboration and Coordination of the Healthcare Team

To function as a member of either type of team, you will quickly learn that collaboration and coordination are key elements in the team's success. Since teamwork involves interaction with others in order for skills or viewpoints to be shared, team members must respect, support, and encourage the contributions of every other member. In this way, the collaboration will bring about positive results. Members of a successful working team know each other, trust each other, are open to each other's ideas, and know when and how to compromise. Each member is committed to the goals of the team and contributes fully to achieving those goals. Depending on the situation, team members

collaborate on performing work, sharing information and resources, developing procedures, monitoring and evaluating outcomes, and making recommendations for improvements.

Team members must also work to coordinate their separate actions or functions. They must know how their individual work fits into the larger picture in achieving the team's goals and how and when to perform their work so that others may do their own jobs thoroughly and competently. Both collaboration and coordination serve to optimize the level at which the team operates, even as it allows individual members to thrive in their unique capacities.

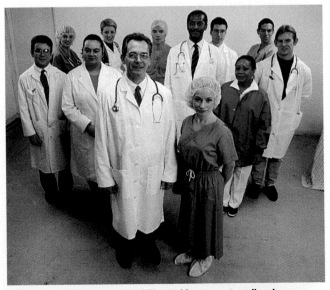

Teams of members with varied skills combine to meet cardiopulmonary, mental health, emergency care, and a wide range of other patient needs.

The Medical Assistant's Link in the Healthcare Team

While working under the direction of the physician in a clinic or medical office, the medical assistant is in a unique position to coordinate interdisciplinary teams. He works closely with the patient and has access to the patient's medical record and the physician's diagnosis. He helps assess the patient's needs and works to involve the patient and the patient's family in the prescribed treatment plan.

The fact that the medical assistant, as a multiskilled worker, exercises both clinical and administrative skills places him in the advantageous position of seeing the patient's health problems from a unique perspective that is not always available to other members of the healthcare team who provide more-specialized services. For example, the medical assistant interviews the patient about her health history and obtains ECG and laboratory screening results; he also prepares the patient's bill, processes the insurance claim, and files her records. He interacts with the patient from the beginning of her presentation of her concern through to the end of her treatment.

Because the medical assistant has a broad understanding of every aspect of the patient's needs, his responsibility is to coordinate the members of the interdisciplinary team and collaborate with them to provide the most efficient approach for the patient's treatment. He is familiar with the services available to the patient through insurance coverage and community resources, and he arranges referrals when needed. Through his efforts at coordination and collaboration, the interdisciplinary team works together harmoniously and productively to bring about patient healing. In fact, in a real sense, the medical assistant is the "glue" that holds the team together!

Working Smart

Teamwork can help accomplish goals that individuals alone cannot achieve. Think of an instance in your life when you worked with someone else or more than one person to accomplish a goal. In what ways did you collaborate and coordinate your efforts? What other qualities are necessary for effective teamwork? As a medical assistant, you will be working closely in teams to provide excellent customer service.

Now, let us see how a successful interdisciplinary healthcare team operates. Read over the following situation, and consider how each member of the team must collaborate with others and coordinate his or her efforts to be a successful team member. Also, note carefully the vital role the medical assistant plays in the smooth operation of the healthcare team. List or highlight each role or function that the medical assistant performs.

Fifty-one-year-old accountant Richard Thompson decides to make an appointment with a general practitioner for a complete physical examination. When he calls the doctor's office, medical assistant Rona Cortez answers the phone; obtains basic information from Richard including his address, phone number, and insurance coverage; and schedules a morning appointment. She tells him he should not eat or drink anything after midnight or in the morning before his appointment so that routine blood samples can be obtained and food digestion will not alter the results of any lab tests taken.

When Richard arrives for his appointment, Rona greets him, asks him to complete the patient registration form, and requests his medical insurance card to photocopy. After Richard returns the completed registration form, Rona tells medical assistant Camille Alfonso, who works in the office's clinical area, that Richard has arrived.

Camille greets Richard and escorts him into the examination room. She explains what procedures are part of the physical examination and answers his questions. Then she interviews him to obtain a complete medical history. She notes Richard's weight in his medical record, as well as the fact that he gets very little exercise. Camille then measures his vital signs including blood pressure, temperature, pulse, and respiratory rate.

She then gives Richard an examination gown and shows him the bathroom where he can change. Camille also instructs him on how to provide a urine sample and where to place it so that the laboratory technician will take it promptly to the clinical lab for analysis. After Richard completes these steps, Camille obtains a venous blood sample for laboratory analysis and performs an ECG; she then escorts him to the x-ray area where a technician will take a chest x-ray.

When Dr. Harry Ferres arrives, Camille briefs him on the measurements she has taken and the results she obtained. She then assists Dr. Ferres during the physical exam. The doctor notes that Richard's blood pressure was elevated when Camille measured it but tells him he wants to wait for the results of the other tests before prescribing a treatment plan. He asks Richard to stop by the registration desk as he leaves the office and make a follow-up appointment to discuss the results of the tests.

When Richard returns for the follow-up visit, Dr. Ferres takes his blood pressure again and discusses

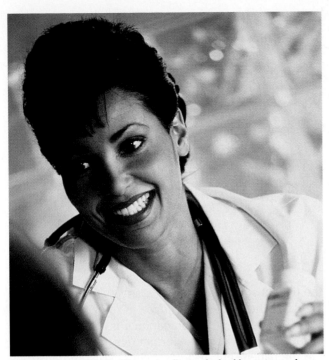

Medical assistant Camille Alfonso coordinates the healthcare team whose combined efforts help Richard and Helen Thompson achieve a happier and healthier life.

the results of his tests with him. He explains that he is concerned that Richard's blood pressure has been elevated on both visits, and that his ECG indicates some changes from one done five years ago. Dr. Ferres tells Richard that his blood cholesterol and glucose levels are also elevated. He gives Richard prescriptions for his elevated blood pressure and cholesterol and tells him he wants additional testing for the elevated blood glucose level and a stress test to further evaluate Richard's heart activity. Back at the reception desk, Rona helps Richard schedule the additional tests at a local hospital. Rona contacts the cardiopulmonary department to schedule the stress test and also contacts the laboratory department to schedule the additional blood test. Camille sets up an appointment for Richard with a nutritionist whom the office employs as a consultant.

Accompanied by his wife, Helen, Richard returns to the office to meet with the nutritionist. Camille is present at the meeting. The nutritionist recommends that Richard adopt a low-calorie, low-cholesterol, low-sodium diabetic diet. As the nutritionist explains the diet, Camille notices that Helen appears uneasy. Camille asks a few questions to determine her concerns and discovers that Helen is afraid her husband might suffer a heart attack. Camille helps reinforce the fact that the diet the nutritionist is recommending will reduce that possibility. Since Dr. Ferres has also prescribed a cardiac rehabilitation program for Richard, Camille tells Helen she can help her husband by work-

ing through the program with him. Since Helen continues to be anxious about her husband's condition, Camille makes an appointment for her to meet with the social worker who is a member of the cardiac rehabilitation team.

At the next office visit several months later, both Richard and Helen Thompson meet with Dr. Ferres. Camille joins them in the consultation room. During the meeting, the Thompsons discuss the outcome of their joint efforts to meet the prescribed treatment plan. Richard expresses delight that he has lost fifteen pounds since his initial visit and has considerably more energy. His diet, while somewhat difficult to maintain at first, is now easy to follow. Helen and Richard shop together for food and are careful to eat only what the prescribed diet allows. They have adopted a walking plan that gives them both sustained daily exercise.

Through the combined efforts of all the members of Richard's healthcare team, and the close coordination of medical assistant Camille Alfonso, his health has improved significantly in an optimal period of time. Richard's blood pressure is now within the normal range, and his cholesterol level, while slightly elevated, is lower than before. He has lost weight, improved his diet, is getting regular exercise, and has a new outlook on life. Even Helen, a member of his healthcare team, feels happier and healthier from the effort!

Working Smart

An alert medical assistant can be aware of potential health concerns in other family members who accompany the patient to the medical office. For example, in the situation describing the visit of Richard and Helen Thompson, Camille noted that Helen's concerns about her husband were significant enough to require the intervention of a social worker who was part of her husband's cardiac rehabilitation team. In helping Helen, Camille also helped her primary patient, Richard.

Healthcare Delivery Settings

Healthcare delivery services occur in a number of distinct settings under the direction of a variety of healthcare professionals. Although as a medical assistant you will most likely be employed in an outpatient care setting, you should become familiar with other healthcare settings so you can give patients referrals to them as is necessary and appropriate. These settings include ambulatory care, acute care, subacute care, long-term care, and public health settings. It is very important for the medical assistant to gain a broad overview of the entire continuum of healthcare services available to the public to meet the needs of individual patients.

Ambulatory Care

Ambulatory care includes a wide range of services that are provided to non-institutionalized patients. Office-based physicians constitute the majority of ambulatory care providers. Services the patient can receive in an ambulatory care setting include routine treatments such as checkups, immunizations, tests, x-rays, and therapies. Traditionally, ambulatory care services have been viewed as the primary contact most people have with the healthcare system. Table 2.2 describes the various ways in which the office-based physician may elect to practice.

Ambulatory care services play a key role in healthcare delivery. They include primary care, outpatient surgery, emergency centers, specialized testing facilities, and other types of services. Many services that were previously performed on an inpatient basis, including minor surgical procedures, patient maintenance care, and some technical procedures, are now performed in the ambulatory care setting.

PRIMARY CARE One way to differentiate ambulatory care services is by the different levels of care given. Medical care that is oriented toward the daily, routine needs of patients, such as the initial diagnosis and continued treatment of common illnesses, is called **primary care**. The primary care practitioner serves as

Working Smart

As a multiskilled worker, the medical assistant has a wide variety of choices as to the healthcare setting in which she chooses to work. She might, for example, seek employment in a freestanding outpatient surgery center, an emergency center, or a center of particular interest to her such as a reproductive health clinic or mental health clinic.

the patient's advisor, advocate, and evaluator for referrals and other treatment. In fact, in some managed care plans, the primary care practitioner is termed the "gatekeeper" because of his important role in not only assessing the patient but also controlling costs and ensuring that services are used appropriately. Secondary and tertiary level care involving more complex treatment and more sophisticated equipment are usually provided by specialists and other highly trained support personnel. Secondary care often includes routine hospitalization and specialized outpatient care, whereas tertiary care involves the most complex services.

These different designations of levels of care have resulted from the evolution of technology and our increased ability to intervene in illness. Although secondary and tertiary care were initially provided on an inpatient basis, today they may be given in an ambulatory care setting. In fact, at times, no clear lines exist

Table 2.2 Medical Practices

Type	Description	Advantages	Disadvantages
Solo Practice	one physician practicing in the office	physician has to satisfy only the patient, who gets individualized care and attention; confidentiality maintained	fees for service set by physician or insurance; physician not accountable to partners for comprehensiveness or quality of care
Group Practice	a number of physicians with either the same specialty or multiple specialties, including nurse practitioners or physician assistants	consultation, intellectual stimulation, coverage on nights and days off, sharing of expenses and resources	individual physician may be liable for practice of all partners; close relationship with individual patients might be lost
Corporate Practice	large number of physicians and other healthcare practitioners	income and tax advantages; variety of specialists to treat patients	loss of autonomy and independent decision-making for physician; patients may feel care and attention are not individualized

between these levels of care, particularly between secondary and tertiary care.

OUTPATIENT SURGERY Recent years have witnessed a dramatic rise in the amount of surgery performed on an ambulatory basis. Advances in anesthesiology as well as other sophisticated technologies make it possible to perform increasingly complex operations on an outpatient basis. The number of hospital patients who go home the same day as their surgery is growing, as is the performance of outpatient surgery in freestanding surgical centers. Most of these are independently owned, many by surgeons who are competing with the very hospitals in which they perform more-complicated procedures. The medical assistant is well prepared to practice her administrative skills in these freestanding surgical centers and is also trained to provide direct patient care before and after the surgical procedure.

EMERGENCY CENTERS Freestanding emergency or urgent-care centers that provide episodic emergency care services twenty-four hours a day are also on the rise in the United States. If emergency care is needed, patients do not have to wait for an appointment with their regular physician or visit the hospital emergency room but instead can go to the urgent-care center to be helped immediately. Such centers, in fact, compete with local hospitals in providing emergency care. Many patients find them more conveniently located and providing quicker care than the hospital emergency room. Freestanding emergency centers are yet another setting in which the medical assistant may choose to work, often performing both administrative and clinical duties.

SPECIALIZED TESTING FACILITIES Routine laboratory analyses to facilitate diagnosis and treatment may be carried out in the physician's office, but specialized testing is often done in either the hospital outpatient laboratory or in a freestanding clinical lab run by a pathologist or registered medical technologist. In a specialized testing facility, the medical assistant may be assigned to collect routine blood and urine specimens and complete the necessary forms, or may perform basic diagnostic procedures. The sophisticated analysis of specimens will be performed by the medical technologist who has been trained in analyzing these specimens.

OTHER AMBULATORY CARE SERVICES Many other types of ambulatory care services exist. They include

family planning clinics, voluntary health agencies, renal dialysis centers, mental health centers, community or neighborhood health centers, and ambulance services, each of which is briefly described below. The medical assistant should be aware of these services and their availability in her community to provide patients with appropriate referrals. She may also choose to seek employment in one of these centers.

Family planning centers provide gynecologic examinations, breast and cervical cancer screening, contraceptive information and supplies, and other services related to reproductive health. Funding for these centers usually comes from the federal or state government, private donations, fund-raising, and a sliding scale of client fees.

Voluntary health agencies are typically oriented toward a specific disease such as AIDS or cancer, and are financed largely by charitable contributions. Examples of these agencies include the American Heart Association, the American Cancer Society, and the National Society for the Prevention of Blindness. Through these agencies, patients can sometimes receive direct services such as diagnostic tests, clinic consultations, financial assistance, and education.

In 1972, Congress extended Medicare coverage to all persons, regardless of age, who had chronic kidney disease and required periodic dialysis treatment. As a result, renal dialysis centers were established to treat these patients. The centers may be freestanding and owned by physicians or for-profit organizations, or may be located in a hospital. Individuals who are employed in these settings require special training to operate the dialysis equipment and monitor patients during treatment.

Mental health centers care for outpatients who are mentally ill. Community hospitals, state and county psychiatric hospitals, and private psychiatric hospitals fall under this category. Mental health patients may also seek services privately by contacting mental health professionals such as psychiatrists (who are physicians), psychologists, psychiatric nurses, or social workers.

Community or neighborhood health centers provide comprehensive ambulatory care for a defined group of people with no other access to healthcare. Their purpose is to make healthcare available to everyone, especially those who cannot access traditional healthcare services. They are subsidized by government agencies. These centers provide a wide range of support

Technology Tip

Helpful information is available through the websites of the American Heart Association, www.americanheart.org, and the American Cancer Society, www.cancer.org.

services, including non-medical services such as social events. Part of the philosophy behind these centers is the belief that consumers should be involved in their management. However, over time, government priorities have shifted to other areas and funding has decreased. Today, the demand for services far exceeds availability. The future of these community centers is uncertain and depends on the federal government.

Ambulance services are provided by a variety of organizations including police and fire departments, hospitals, volunteer groups, and private ambulance companies. Ambulance crews are specially trained to deal with all types of emergencies.

Acute Care

Unlike ambulatory care services, **acute care** services are usually provided in a hospital. Acute care is the treatment a patient receives for an abrupt episode of illness, for complications from an accident or other trauma, or during recovery from surgery.

The modern hospital remains a key resource for and the organized hub of the American healthcare system. Its role is central to the delivery of healthcare, the training of health personnel, and the conducting and dissemination of health-related research. Many times, the hospital is the first place the customer thinks of in relation to healthcare. In fact, today's hospital is even expanding its services to meet consumers' needs for convenience, adding restaurants, banking services, and dry cleaning services!

Over the last few decades, with the rapid advances in technology and the increasing costs, hospitals have found a need to merge into larger systems to render services efficiently with limited duplication. Many

smaller and rural hospitals have closed or become part of larger multihospital systems. This has led to the need for many healthcare providers to become multiskilled practitioners, competent in a variety of skills beyond their original profession. Such multiskilled professionals fill in whenever circumstances require, exercising additional skills when their basic role is not needed. For example, a respiratory therapist might be expected to draw venous blood samples for testing or take routine ECGs. Or a dietitian may be asked to take blood pressure readings while instructing patients about their low salt diets. Providing these additional skills helps

> ### Working Smart
> Medical assistants put their many skills to use in acute, subacute, and long-term-care settings. Each healthcare setting has its own duties and responsibilities, some of them clinic-related and others administrative. A medical assistant should become familiar with each of these healthcare venues before choosing where to work.

maintain comprehensive care for the patient. Moreover, being a multiskilled worker helps ensure job security for the healthcare professional.

Hospitals are regulated by both public and private organizations. Federal controls are mandated by regulations of **Medicare** and **Medicaid**, the government programs to help the elderly and the poor, respectively, with their healthcare costs. (See Chapter 12, "Processing Insurance Claims," for more information about these programs.) The **Joint Commission on Accreditation of Healthcare Organizations (JCAHO)**, a voluntary accrediting agency, establishes quality standards and surveys hospitals and other healthcare organizations to ensure that the standards are met. Each state licenses its hospitals to maintain minimum standards of operation. Furthermore, state agencies ensure that the healthcare provided in these facilities meets minimal requirements for quality through certification. Certification by state healthcare agencies is required to participate in Medicare and Medicaid programs.

Medical assistants may seek employment in the acute care setting of a hospital. For example, they may be employed in the outpatient clinic, the admitting department, the billing department, the emergency room, the ECG department, or the laboratory department, to name just a few possibilities. As a multiskilled healthcare provider, the medical assistant is trained to perform a wide range of functions in the acute care setting, and her flexibility is viewed as an asset there.

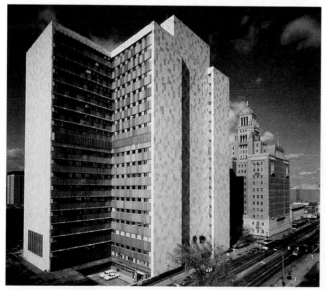

The modern hospital is able to meet patients' increasingly complex needs—but it has become increasingly complex itself in the process.

Subacute Care

Subacute care is the level of healthcare between the type provided in an acute care hospital setting and the several forms of long-term healthcare discussed below. With the advent of managed care, insurance companies began examining the length of hospital stays and re-evaluating the financial reimbursement for services in a hospital setting. Since some patients cannot return directly home after leaving an acute care center, managed care plans sought a cost-effective way to provide the care they needed. The result was subacute care, the level of healthcare that provides services for patients who, by managed care program criteria, are well enough to leave an acute care setting but too ill to be included in the long-term-care environment.

In its 1995 Survey Protocol for Subacute Programs, JCAHO defined subacute care as goal-oriented, comprehensive, inpatient care designed for the person with an acute illness, injury, or exacerbation of a disease process. This care may be provided immediately after or instead of acute hospitalization and may include treatment for one or more specific, active, or complex medical conditions. Subacute care facilities may also administer one or more technically advanced treatments. Generally, subacute care does not depend on high technology or highly specialized procedures.

Subacute care is coordinated by an interdisciplinary healthcare team. Members are knowledgeable about and trained in assessing and managing specific conditions and in performing many necessary procedures. Subacute care often requires frequent, daily to weekly, assessment and review of the patient's clinical course and treatment plan, for a limited period of time. The timeframe may be several days to several months, depending on both stabilization of the patient's condition and the prescribed course of treatment.

Two examples of subacute care services are those that meet the needs of ventilator-dependent patients and those designed for spinal cord injury patients. Some members of the interdisciplinary team assigned to such patients may include physical, occupational, and respiratory therapists. The physical therapist is concerned with the patient's mobility and must provide for either active movement of the patient or passive movement provided by the physical therapy staff. The occupational therapist is responsible for making sure the patient can perform the routine activities of daily living, such as eating, washing, and dressing. The patient may also need assistive devices for these routine activities. The respiratory therapist ensures that the patient can expand her lungs to the fullest extent possible to prevent respiratory complications such as pneumonia. It is through the interaction of these and other members of the interdisciplinary subacute care team that the patient will return to the most satisfying and productive life possible.

Long-Term Care

Long-term care includes a range of healthcare and social services that some patients need to compensate for functional disabilities. Although this type of care serves individuals of any age with conditions such as birth defects, spinal cord injuries, mental impairment, or other chronic debilitating illnesses, most people who receive long-term care are elderly and experiencing difficulty functioning independently. The goal of long-term care is to help each patient function at the highest level possible. This is accomplished through the coordination of appropriate health, social, and support services. Individuals needing long-term care can receive it in a number of settings including their own homes, adult day care, and assisted living long-term care facilities.

In recent years, long-term care has grown dramatically because of the aging of the U.S. population. However, components of the long-term care delivery system still need to be integrated to create a well-organized, efficient, consumer-oriented continuum of healthcare.

HOME CARE An ideal situation for a patient needing long-term care is receiving it in her own home. For this to happen, one or more individuals must accept responsibility for the patient's day-to-day care. Optimally, a home care giver is someone who is close to the patient, perhaps a spouse, a family member, or a friend. Home care givers often require occasional assistance with patient care. This can be provided by **home healthcare agencies** that can be contracted with to provide both medical and social services such as changing dressings, monitoring medications, and assisting with bathing and cooking.

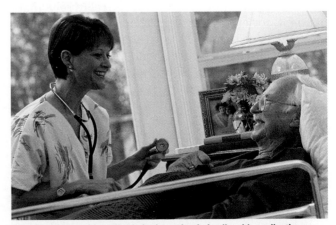

Home healthcare aides often help the patient's family with medications, dressings, and other domestic and social needs.

NURSING HOME CARE Nursing homes are another option for long-term care. They provide two levels of assistance: skilled nursing care and intermediate nursing care. A **skilled nursing facility** provides a level of care closely resembling that of a hospital, with around-the-clock nursing service available. An **intermediate care facility** provides less extensive healthcare and services and may have, but is not required to have, twenty-four-hour nursing care. While both types of nursing homes are privately owned, they must be certified as meeting federal standards. Their size may vary dramatically from three beds to more than 1,000.

ADULT DAY CARE Long-term care is also available to people who, because they are physically or mentally impaired, require supervision that family members cannot provide. Adult day care centers let such individuals remain in their community while being supervised by healthcare professionals. They provide a range of activities for patients to promote their well-being. One advantage of adult day care is that it lets members of the patient's family keep their jobs by having others care for the patient during the day. Many adult day care services are privately paid-for facilities.

HOSPICE CARE Yet another venue for long-term care is a **hospice**. Hospice care is designed for patients whom conventional treatments are no longer helping and who are dying. It emphasizes the management of pain and allows the dying person to spend his last days in a peaceful, supportive, open atmosphere. The vast majority of hospice users are cancer patients and their families. Many hospices offer only home services, but some are increasingly adding bed care facilities.

ASSISTED LIVING FACILITIES Very recently, **assisted living facilities** have been developed for long-term care. They provide a continuum of levels of care, from primary independent care to nursing home care. An older individual who is relatively independent, for example, might choose to live in one of these facilities to have his meals provided and housekeeping chores taken care of and to participate in the social atmosphere of group living. As he ages and needs more assistance, supervision, or medical care, the facility has the resources to accommodate his changing needs.

As a multiskilled healthcare practitioner, the medical assistant employed in a long-term-care environment assists with routine health screenings and assigns referrals when appropriate. She is well qualified to work in any of the long-term-care settings, providing support and encouragement for the patient with a chronic illness or disability as well as for his or her family.

Public Health Services

Public health services are a critically important part of our healthcare system. The efforts of public health professionals emphasize the prevention of disease, disability, and premature death through the organized efforts of federal, state, and local agencies. Although the emphasis has shifted somewhat over the years, the fundamental concern of public health officials is to improve the health of the general population.

In the early twentieth century, public health efforts were directed at preventing or mitigating the effects of infectious diseases such as smallpox, yellow fever, venereal disease, and tuberculosis. Now, the efforts of public health professionals are directed at improved access to healthcare and providing quality healthcare for everyone.

By necessity, public health agencies have always had a larger or broader mission than the private physician or the HMO system. Public health facilities are expected to coordinate and ensure services that will improve the quality of health for community members at large, while private physicians are responsible for the health of individual patients or members of their specific HMO organizations.

On the federal level, there are a variety of public health agencies. The National Institutes of Health is the federal agency that focuses on medical research. The Alcohol, Drug Abuse, and Mental Health Administration works toward the prevention of alcoholism, drug addiction, and mental illness and is concerned with improving treatment and rehabilitation methods. The Food and Drug Administration ensures the safety of foods, biologic devices, and drugs. The Centers for Disease Control seeks to prevent and control infectious and chronic disease; prevent disease, disability, and death associated with environmental and workplace hazards; and reduce health risks through educational programs. The Health Resources and Services Administration works to improve and assure access to basic and preventive health services for the uninsured and underinsured and to address disparities in health indicators among races and population groups. Table 2.3 lists the public health agencies within the U.S. Department of Health and Human Services. The services and programs of these and other public health agencies encompass areas of environmental health, health education, maternal and child health, nursing services, vital statistics record-keeping, dental health, and communicable disease control. Funds for these services and programs are generated from tax revenues and are distributed through the federal, state, and local governments.

The thrust of these public activities takes place at the local level since each state, and in some cases each

Chapter 2
Working in Today's Healthcare Environment

Table 2.3 Federal Public Health Agencies within the Department of Health and Human Services

Administration on Aging
Administration for Children and Families
Agency for Health Care Policy and Research
Agency for Toxic Substances and Disease Registry
Centers for Disease Control and Prevention
Food and Drug Administration
Health Care Financing Administration
Health Resources and Services Administration
Indian Health Service
National Institutes of Health
Office of Public Health and Science
Office of the Surgeon General
Substance Abuse and Mental Health Services Administration

region of the state, encounters a unique set of health concerns. Boards of health are found at the city, county, and state levels, and it is their responsibility to plan, provide, and evaluate medical services. These services are generally available to the entire community and may involve sliding fees based on income.

Public health agencies have three specific responsibilities: assessing the overall health status of the community and the availability of community health resources; developing health policy and recommending programs to address the health gaps they identify; and assuring that the services provided are high quality and effective in meeting community needs. This includes assuring that those who need the services have access to them. Figure 2.1 illustrates the core public health functions at the federal, state, and community levels.

Assessing the health of the community, though complicated, is done by systematically collecting data on key statistical indicators such as the infant mortality rate, incidence of diseases such as AIDS, proportion of children immunized, and number of teen-agers and adults who smoke, as shown in Table 2.4. Factors similar to the ones listed in the table are also tracked at the federal level by the Department of Health and Human Services and are reflected in the goals of the Healthy People 2010 initiative. Health indicators for each community are then compared with benchmarks or goals derived by earlier statistical comparisons. Once the population is statistically identified, federal officials study the health and medical resources available, develop a health policy, and recommend and implement programs to align community members with the necessary services. When services have been provided and received, the officials evaluate their effectiveness and determine if the program goals were met.

More and more, private physicians and public health professionals realize that they share the same health goals. In the past, health and medical care was paid for by those individuals who were able to pay and those physicians and hospitals who could afford to charge little or nothing to those unable to pay. Because of the greater costs required by technological advances and the increased regulation by insurance companies, this payment process has changed significantly. Public health programs such as Medicare and Medicaid, together with other community-based programs for people with low incomes, have lessened, but have not solved, the problems concerning access to quality healthcare for everyone. Medicare does not pay for all expenses incurred by the elderly, nor does Medicaid pay all expenses incurred by the poor. Many people still never see a primary physician except in an emergency.

There are two major problems to be solved: improving access to medical care for every individual and controlling costs. Private physicians are realizing that they have to take more responsibility for the health of the community at large, and public health professionals are realizing that they also have to take more responsibility for the health of individuals by identifying health needs as they occur and assuring access to quality services. Both managed care and the government health system realize that their shared goals of improved access and better quality care can only be met through more joint and coordinated planning.

As a medical assistant, you should be aware that the public health agencies are an excellent resource for health education materials. Contact your local health agencies to obtain free materials on a variety of contemporary health topics. You are in the position of monitoring the needs of the population you serve. If specific healthcare or educational needs surface for an

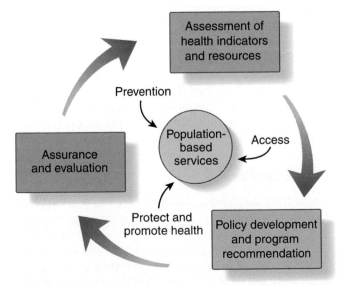

Figure 2.1
Core Public Health Functions

Table 2.4 Proposed Indicators for a Community Health Profile

Socio-Demographic Characteristics

- distribution of the population by age and race/ethnicity
- number and proportion of persons in groups such as migrants, homeless, or the non-English speaking, for whom access to community services and resources may be a concern
- number and proportion of persons aged twenty-five and older with less than a high school education
- ratio of the number of students graduating from high school to the number who entered the ninth grade three years previously
- median household income
- proportion of children younger than fifteen living in families at or below the poverty level
- unemployment rate
- number and proportion of single-parent families
- number and proportion of persons without health insurance

Health Status

- infant mortality rate by race/ethnicity
- numbers of deaths or age-adjusted death rates for motor vehicle accidents, work-related injuries, suicides, homicides, lung cancer, breast cancer, cardiovascular diseases, and all causes, by age, race, and gender as appropriate
- births to adolescents (younger than eighteen) as a proportion of total live births
- number and rate of confirmed abuse and neglect cases among children

Health Risk Factors

- proportion of two-year-old children who have received all age-appropriate vaccines, as recommended by the Advisory Committee on Immunization Practices
- proportion of adults aged sixty-five and older who have ever been immunized for pneumococcal pneumonia; proportion who have been immunized in the past twelve months for influenza
- proportion of the population who smoke, by age, race, and gender as appropriate
- proportion of the population aged eighteen and older who are obese
- number and type of U.S. Environmental Protection Agency air quality standards not met
- proportion of rivers, lakes, and estuaries that support beneficial uses (e.g., fishing and swimming approved)

Health Care Resource Consumption

- per capita healthcare spending for Medicare beneficiaries (the Medicare-adjusted average per capita cost)

Functional Status

- proportion of adults reporting that their general health is good to excellent
- during the past thirty days, average number of days for which adults report that their physical or mental health was not good

Quality of Life

- proportion of adults satisfied with the healthcare system in their community
- proportion of persons satisfied with the quality of life in their community

Source: Michael A. Stoto, editor. "Sharing Responsibility for the Public's Health: A New Perspective from the Institute of Medicine." Journal of Public Health Management Practice, 1997, 3(5), 22-34. (page 31).

individual or a group, you need to contact the local health department and inform officials there of those needs. If, for example, you find that there are children who have not been adequately immunized for childhood illnesses or elderly persons with health needs that are not being met, you should report these cases to the appropriate health department official. Through these efforts, you contribute to instituting healthcare programs that promote and protect the health of those in your community.

Health Insurance Plans in the United States

Healthcare focuses upon the prevention, treatment, and management of illness across the life cycle and on a continuum of care that ranges from those in excellent health to patients with serious or chronic illness. In what direction is the healthcare delivery system of the twenty-first century headed? Although we can learn from the past evolution of healthcare, it is clear that the growing complexity of today's healthcare environment will not mirror the past. Healthcare costs are skyrocketing. Who is paying for it? In many instances, employers subsidize part of their workers' healthcare insurance, while employees also contribute to it. For both the employer and employee, insurance costs are increasing steadily.

Because of the rise in insurance costs, many Americans cannot afford adequate healthcare insurance. An astonishing forty-four million people are uninsured in the United States today—one person in every six. These people include working parents and wage earners whose employers do not offer health benefits. The United States's healthcare system is in need of overall reform, and the twenty-first century will no doubt bring many changes.

The world of insurance is very complex; however, medical assistants should be familiar with the major types of healthcare insurance now available. Insurance is explained in depth in Chapter 12, but an overview of insurance options is discussed here.

Managed Care Plans

As we have discussed, managed care is a term applied to plans that seek to contain healthcare costs by monitoring services and emphasizing preventive care, with the goal of keeping people healthy, functional, and independent. This means not only providing needed healthcare services but also intervening early in the disease process, avoiding the complications of illness, and managing catastrophic episodes in a cost-effective manner. Some physicians, though, believe that managed care is, by definition, the equivalent of diminished care.

Traditionally, healthcare was based on the fee-for-service plan. Simply put, the consumer was able to choose virtually any provider, and submit the bill to the insurance provider. The patient was responsible for a deductible each year and the first twenty percent of the medical bill. The insurance coverage was for the remaining 80 percent. However, preventative care was not normally covered.

In 1973, the federal government took the initiative to control healthcare costs with the passage of the Health Maintenance Organization Assistance Act. This act provided financial incentives for the development of what became **Health Maintenance Organizations (HMOs)**. These are organizations that contract with businesses or other groups to provide healthcare for employees or enrollees. Members must use the plan's physicians, and they usually need a primary care physician's referral or plan approval before tests, surgery, visits to specialists, or hospitalization. Members must pay a **copayment** that today may vary from $10 to $30 for each visit.

Customer Service

When helping your patients identify their healthcare options, remember that the government also provides insurance for the elderly through Medicare and for the low-income population through Medicaid. These forms of medical coverage are discussed in Chapter 12.

Throughout the 1980s and 1990s, HMO enrollment continued to increase as employers found it the least expensive way of covering their employees' insurance costs. Like all managed care plans, HMOs are administered mostly by business and insurance companies who, of course, want to make a profit. Some people believe that the rising cost of healthcare, which they attribute in part to the performance of many unnecessary procedures, must be controlled, or "managed," and that therefore, HMOs are the best way to keep costs low. However, others maintain that HMOs put pressure on doctors to avoid expensive procedures or drugs and to cut corners to minimize costs, rather than being guided by the patient's needs. Each patient's care is unique, some physicians say, and HMOs do not encourage individualized diagnoses

and treatments. One woman's gallbladder operation, for example, might keep her hospitalized for a week and a half, while the same operation on a similar woman might require only a few days' stay in the hospital. Under the HMO system, it would be strongly recommended that both women be hospitalized for the shorter amount of time. Because of this standardization of care, some healthcare providers express concern that managed care has taken the doctor out of the decision-making process.

Preferred Provider Organizations (PPOs) are loose forms of managed care that began to surface in the 1980s. A PPO arranges with a limited number of healthcare providers to serve a defined group of individuals. Enrollees who use a network healthcare practitioner receive discounted service and must make a copayment. However, the patient is free to seek care from any other provider—at greater out-of-pocket expense.

A much more restrictive arrangement is the **Exclusive Provider Organization (EPO)**. This type of plan provides coverage only when services are provided by contracted providers. These plans provide a cost-savings alternative for employers. However, the restricted choice of providers has the effect of attracting healthier (and therefore less-expensive) enrollees. Potential enrollees who have complicated or chronic health problems are reluctant to "start over" with new healthcare providers.

In the managed care system, the medical assistant works collaboratively with all other members of the healthcare team to educate consumers about maintaining wellness and to provide accessible care to those needing medical assistance. Under managed care, health professionals, including the medical assistant, play a major role in delivering care that improves the quality of life, lowers costs, and enhances patient satisfaction throughout the continuum of care.

Government-Sponsored Plans

When working as a medical assistant, you will find that many of your customers are covered by some type of insurance offered through the federal or state government. As mentioned previously, the federal government administers Medicare, a national insurance plan that covers the elderly and disabled, including those who suffer from kidney failure. Eligible persons can enroll at the local office of the Social Security Administration. Another government program is the Civilian Health and Medical Program of the Uniformed Services (CHAMPUS), which covers the dependents of military personnel and military retirees. If you work in a health care facility near a military base, you may see patients with this kind of insurance, since its purpose is to provide them with access to civilian healthcare facilities. If a person injured on the job seeks medical treatment, you may find that he is covered by Workers' Compensation insurance. This is provided to employees and may be administered by either the state or federal government. The Medicaid program, which provides insurance for the needy, is administered through the joint efforts of local, state, and federal governments. Persons who qualify for this program must apply through their local welfare office.

Individual and Group Insurance Plans

Many private insurance companies offer insurance to individuals or groups of people. A patient may be covered by a group policy plan where he works or may buy health insurance on an individual basis. Some organizations may offer a group plan to their members. Blue Cross/Blue Shield and Aetna are examples of insurance companies that operate in many areas and provide group coverage through employers and organizations.

Helping Patients Choose a Health Plan

Because she serves both patients' clinical and administrative needs, the medical assistant may be in a position to advise them about insurance needs. She should, therefore, be aware of the various insurance options available and be prepared to discuss them with her patients. Patients who do not understand how their insurance works—for example, the deductible and copayment—and what services their plan covers may challenge the medical office staff about payments or services. It is important to establish good communication with patients on insurance matters. Questions you should stress to patients choosing a health plan include:

- How important is it for the patient to have the flexibility to choose her physician, where she wishes to be treated, and her own specialist?
- What is the patient's current level of health? What is her health history? If pre-existing conditions are present, does the insurance plan cover them?
- What is the patient's age?
- What are the overall costs of the various insurance plans? What are the monthly costs? What is the deductible, and what is the copayment? What can the patient afford to pay for coverage?
- Does the plan cover the patient when she is out of the state or country? Is this coverage important to the patient?

Think about how to help advise patients on their insurance needs and consider the choices and costs of healthcare insurance plans. In general, as the number of choices in a healthcare insurance plan increases, the cost also increases. Patients will need to balance the level of choice and cost that is most appropriate for their needs, and you may be in a position to help them analyze this balance. Some experts recommend that a medical office develop a type of "cheat sheet," or one-page chart of health plans, procedures covered, and phone numbers for contacts which can be kept handy at the front desk. It will also be useful to have a separate file for each health plan that contains the plan's reference manual and other information for easy access. Most important, whenever a question about healthcare coverage arises with a patient, make sure that the service given and the conversation is documented. Write down what service was performed, to whom it was done, the date of the service, and the name of the person who disputed the coverage or had the question. Insurance companies require careful documentation when they review cases and pay claims upon appeal. The medical assistant is often called upon to perform all these tasks involving the complexities of healthcare insurance in her day-to-day work.

> ### Customer Service
> The medical assistant is in an optimal position to assist patients in making the most of their health benefits. He can help educate patients so that they make informed decisions and can also help them negotiate their way through the variety of services and requirements of the managed care system.

Clinical Summary

- Healthcare practitioners of the twenty-first century are challenged to meet many changes, including an ever-changing healthcare delivery environment, a more culturally and ethnically diverse and older population, technological advances in diagnostic and treatment modalities, and better-informed customers.
- Healthcare delivery is evolving toward a managed care system in which healthcare plans seek to monitor the use of physicians and healthcare services in order to minimize costs.
- To work in today's managed care environment, the medical assistant needs to perform effectively as a member of the healthcare team.

- The interdisciplinary team functions by bringing several variously skilled healthcare professionals together to treat the patient. The patient and her family are also members of this team.
- Within the interdisciplinary team, the medical assistant provides an important link between the patient, his family, and the various other team members.
- Ambulatory care services are those provided for non-institutionalized patients in primary care facilities, outpatient surgical centers, freestanding emergency centers, specialized testing centers, and other facilities.
- Public health efforts emphasize the prevention of disease, disability, and premature death through organized efforts of federal, state and local governments.
- Acute care is administered in a hospital setting. The hospital also serves as a training site for health personnel and a site for conducting and disseminating research.
- Subacute care has recently developed as a specialty providing patients with needed professional healthcare after discharge from a hospital.
- Long-term care consists of health and social services that are provided for individuals with a functional disability or chronic illness. Long-term care may be administered in a variety of settings, including the patient's home, nursing homes, and hospices.
- There are a variety of healthcare insurance plans. The medical assistant should have a basic understanding of these plans to help patients choose the most appropriate one for their healthcare needs.

The Language of Medicine

acute care Healthcare in which a patient is treated for an abrupt episode of illness, for the complications of an accident or other trauma, or during recovery from surgery, usually given in a hospital.

ambulatory care (**am**-byoo-la-tor-ee kayr) A wide range of services provided to non-institutionalized patients which generally include primary care treatments such as check-ups, immunizations, tests, x-rays, and therapies. Ambulatory care settings include physician's offices, outpatient surgery centers, and freestanding emergency centers.

assisted living facilities Long-term-care facilities, used primarily by the elderly, which provide living assistance and a range of available healthcare services on a continuum of care. A resident who requires more services as time passes can arrange to increase the level of care given.

copayment Fixed fee paid by the patient at the time medical service is rendered with the remaining cost paid by insurance.

Exclusive Provider Organization (EPO) A healthcare plan that provides coverage only when services are provided by contracted or preferred providers.

Health Maintenance Organizations (HMOs) Managed care in which the patient must use the plan's physicians and generally needs a primary care physician's referral or plan approval before visits to specialists, tests, surgery, or hospitalization.

home healthcare agencies Long-term-care agencies that provide a combination of medical and social services in the patient's home, including changing dressings, monitoring medications, and assisting with bathing and cooking.

hospice Long-term care that emphasizes the management of pain and other symptoms when conventional treatment is no longer of value and the patient is dying.

interdisciplinary healthcare team A group of workers from different disciplines who bring together diverse skills and expertise to provide coordinated, high-quality services for the patient.

intermediate care facility A nursing home that provides care for patients who need minimal professional nursing care.

Joint Commission on Accreditation of Healthcare Organizations (JCAHO) A voluntary accrediting agency that establishes quality standards and surveys hospitals and other healthcare organizations to ensure that the standards are met.

long-term care A range of health and social services that compensate for the functional disabilities of people or care for the chronically ill.

managed care Healthcare plans that provide services and stress early intervention in the disease process, avoidance of complications of illness, and managing catastrophic episodes in a cost-effective manner.

Medicaid Governmental medical insurance for individuals with reduced incomes.

Medicare Federal medical insurance for the elderly and some disabled recipients.

Preferred Provider Organizations (PPO) A loose form of managed care that arranges with providers to serve a defined group of patients who pay reduced fees (plus a copayment) and also can see other providers if they pay more.

primary care Medical care that is oriented toward the daily, routine needs of the patient.

skilled nursing facility A nursing home that provides twenty-four-hour professional nursing services.

subacute care Healthcare that falls between the level of care provided in an acute care hospital setting and the various forms of long term healthcare.

Signs/Symptoms of Progress

Recall, Question, Connect

Recall

Think of an elderly patient who is having trouble managing in his home. List two or three potential environments or sites that might provide care for that patient.

Question

List at least six questions a person should consider when deciding between the types of long-term care you have listed above.

Connect

Why should you, as a medical assistant, be familiar with long-term-care options? State how you can educate yourself about these options, and describe how you might act as a "link" in helping patients choose among options.

Educating the Patient

Cynthia Radice is a twenty-three-year-old recent college graduate who has just begun working at a large graphic design firm. As a new employee, she has been given information discussing her medical coverage options. She may select either a PPO or an HMO.

1 Ms. Radice asks you what the major differences between the two plans are. How do you respond?
2 Her medical record indicates to you that Ms. Radice has been generally healthy, and has been seen in the medical office only occasionally with minor complaints. The physician in the office does not participate in the HMO or PPO plans from which she may choose.

She asks you which plan would be best for her. What would you say? What questions would you ask her?

Exploring Perspectives in Teams

Perspective involves the discipline of examining how ideas look from different points of view and recognizing that there are often multiple "answers" to complex questions. In small groups or on your own, reflect on possible alternative views and summarize your findings.

1 If you were critically ill, what type of healthcare team would you prefer managing your care, an interdisciplinary team or a team of specialists from the same department? Debate the advantages and the disadvantages.
2 Review the healthcare settings discussed in this chapter. What type of health setting attracted you to the field of medical assisting? Why? With what type of healthcare specialists do you want to work? Are there particular types of patients you would prefer to serve or health problems you would prefer to help resolve?
3 What are the key issues involved in choosing a health plan? Consider how a person's perspective on these issues changes if she or he is young and single, married with three children, or seventy years old with heart problems.
4 Research the latest developments in managed care plans. What are the advantages of managed care plans for both the physicians and the patients? What are the disadvantages? What types of illnesses and conditions are effectively served by managed care plans, and which ones are less effectively served?

chapter 3

Learning Outcomes

■ Explain the importance of knowing the fundamentals of law in the medical office.

■ Identify the legal basis for the principle of confidentiality.

■ Apply a working knowledge of the ethical issues involved in AIDS, abuse, and advance directives such as the living will, durable power of attorney for healthcare, and healthcare proxy.

■ Define the terms negligence, statute of limitations, *respondeat superior, res ipsa loquitur,* Good Samaritan law, consent, and torts.

■ Explain the types of consent used in medical practice situations.

■ List the ethical and legal considerations for physicians regarding controlled drugs, DEA regulations, AIDS, and child, domestic, and elder abuse.

■ State the importance of accurate documentation for defending malpractice claims.

Performance Objectives

■ Use appropriate guidelines when documenting information.

■ Use appropriate guidelines for releasing information.

■ Maintain awareness of federal and state healthcare regulations.

■ Adhere to ethical principles.

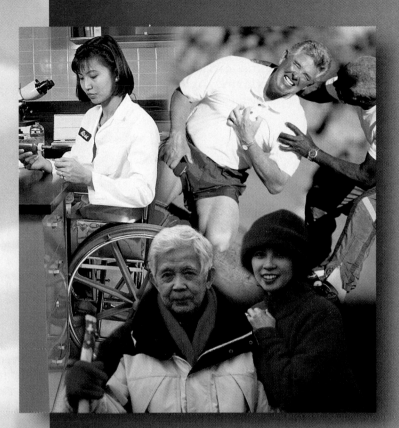

Understanding Legal and Ethical Issues

The medical assistant must *have a working knowledge and understanding of legal, moral, and ethical issues involved in the practice of medicine. You must perform your duties in accordance with the law and take precautions to prevent possible lawsuits and other legal and ethical difficulties. You act within the law in order to protect yourself, your employer, and your patients.*

Laws and ethical standards have been enacted to protect the patient and to guide physicians and other healthcare workers. These laws and guidelines safeguard patients' rights and protect the healthcare professional. In addition, the laws also protect the public.

Certain health matters, for example, deaths, births, vulnerable adult abuse, and some communicable diseases, must be reported to the state.

The American legal system is complex and multifaceted and is sometimes difficult to understand. However, a familiarity with the basic laws that apply to the medical professional enables the medical assistant to perform duties assigned by the physician employer safely, effectively, and responsibly within the legal and medical context.

Ethics, Morals, and the Law

Ethics are the principles that govern right behavior. Ethical principles may be upheld by the law, but not always. For example, if a cashier gives you back too much change when you pay for an item, you are not required by law to return that money. However, the moral or ethical response would be to correct the cashier's mistake by returning the money. You do this because it is *the right thing to do*, not because the law requires you to do it. The extra change situation is an ethical dilemma, not a legal event. When working in the healthcare setting, it is best to always try to follow the highest medical and ethical standards.

Morals are personal codes of conduct. These will vary from person to person. Morals are based upon personal beliefs, religion, and cultural values. Ethics are an extension of morals.

Many laws are intended to support the ethical principle of justice. For example, the **Americans with Disabilities Act (ADA)**, passed by Congress in 1990, protects persons with physical or mental disabilities in employment, public services, public accommodations, and telecommunications. This law provides clear, inclusive national directives to end discrimination against individuals with disabilities so that they can enter into the economic and social mainstream of daily life. **Disability** is defined as a physical or mental impairment that considerably limits one or more of the major life activities of the individual. The ADA protects individuals with disabilities, patients with a record of such an impairment, or people who are thought to have such an impairment. It applies to people with the AIDS virus, cancer, or mental retardation. The act also guarantees the disabled access to the workplace and places of business such as a medical office. The law protects the rights of patients by stating that healthcare facilities must be fully accessible to persons with disabilities.

Legal Issue
Laws establish minimal standards of behavior, while ethics provide standards we should work toward attaining.

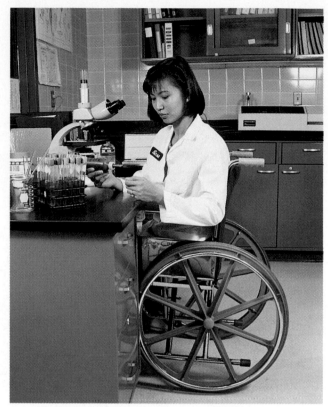

The Americans with Disabilities Act helps people with disabilities to participate in the country's economic and social mainstream.

Medical Ethics and Bioethics

Ethics are concerned with standards of behavior and the understanding of right and wrong beyond what is legally required. They are based on moral values that have been formed through the influences and beliefs of family, culture, and society over thousands of years. **Medical ethics** are those standards of behavior that apply in the medical setting. Strict adherence to medical ethics assures that optimum healthcare is provided to all patients. Chapter 1, "Choosing a Career as a Medical Assistant," discussed the ethical standard of showing respect for a patient's dignity and privacy that the medical assistant follows by having a patient disrobe in a private room and using proper draping so that the patient is minimally exposed during an examination.

Bioethics is the study of moral and ethical questions evolving from the multitude of new biological and research findings that affect the practice of medicine. As medical technology has prolonged life, most patients and their families have become more aware and better informed about healthcare and are more involved in making choices and decisions concerning medical treatment and end-of-life issues.

Patient Self-Determination Act

Decisions about terminating life by stopping or refusing treatment can be difficult for patients and their families. To assist with these concerns, Congress passed the **Patient Self-Determination Act** in 1990. This law requires that patients receive written information about their right to make medical decisions and execute advance directives. An **advance directive** may be in the form of a living will, durable power of attorney for healthcare, or healthcare proxy. These directives should be executed in consultation with healthcare providers, family members, and others who are important to the patient. An advance directive helps ensure that the patient's preferences are known if the patient becomes incapable of participating in decisions affecting treatment or end-of-life care.

The medical assistant and other members of the healthcare team can help patients be informed about the various types of advance directives by:

- complying with state laws regarding advance directives
- having advance directive forms available for patient use
- educating patients about advance directives

LIVING WILL The **living will** is a document that a competent person writes stating what he wants done if a terminal illness or catastrophic injury leaves him comatose or incompetent. Living wills provide instructions for treatment, such as a request to discontinue it if a terminal illness is diagnosed. The will may specifically state that no unusual measures or life support systems should be used to prolong life. The living will also

Working Smart
A patient's advance directive should be filed as part of her permanent medical record.

may address a patient's desire to donate any organs that can be used. This is a legal document and must be signed in the presence of two witnesses. A patient may save the family and medical professionals enormous difficulty and anguish by putting her wishes in writing before an emotional situation arises. Figure 3.1 is an example of a living will that can be modified to express the wishes of an individual patient. The wording of a valid living will varies from state to state.

DURABLE POWER OF ATTORNEY FOR HEALTHCARE AND HEALTHCARE PROXY A **durable power of attorney for healthcare** is a legal document that allows another person, usually a spouse or other relative, to act on behalf of the individual. The person signing a power of attorney must be competent at the time for it to be legally binding. The main reason for signing a power of attorney is to ensure that someone is empowered to act for a person who becomes physically or mentally impaired. A signed durable power of attorney remains in effect until revoked or the person dies.

The healthcare proxy is a specific type of power of attorney that applies to *medical* decisions. With a **healthcare proxy**, patients designate an individual to make medical decisions for them when they cannot make those decisions because of an inability to reason or communicate.

ORGAN DONATION There has been much publicity in recent years about the gift of the body or body parts after death. In 1968, the **Uniform Anatomical Gift Act** was approved by the National Conference of Commissioners on Uniform State Laws. All 50 states have adopted this act. It declares that any mentally competent adult may donate any part or all of her or his body after death for research, transplantation, or storage in a tissue bank. The act says that the survivors of the deceased person, in the legal order of consent, may donate any part of the decedent's remains if the decedent did not oppose a donation before dying. Donation documents for bodies or organs free physicians from the risk of civil or criminal proceedings. However, if a physician or hospital official knows that the deceased opposed donation, or if the survivors object, the donation must be refused. The anatomical gift act further states that hospitals, surgeons, physicians, accredited medical or dental schools, colleges and universities, and tissue banks or storage facilities may accept anatomical gifts for research, advancement of medical or dental science, therapy, or transplantation. The donor's attending

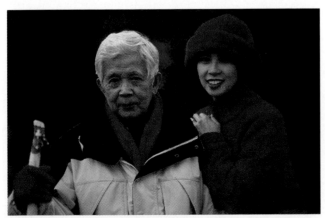

Talking openly with family members and executing a living will are ways the elderly can ensure that their wishes will be followed concerning medical treatment and end-of-life care.

Living Will

If I am not able to make an informed decision regarding my healthcare, I direct my healthcare providers to follow my instructions as set forth below. (Initial those statements you wish to be included in the document and cross through those statements which do not apply.)

A. If my death from a terminal condition is imminent and even if life-sustaining procedures are used there is no reasonable expectation of my recovery:

_____ I direct that my life not be extended by life-sustaining procedures, including the administration of nutrition and hydration artificially.

_____ I direct that my life not be extended by life-sustaining procedures, except that, if I am unable to take food by mouth, I wish to receive nutrition and hydration artificially.

_____ I direct that, even in a terminal condition, I be given all available medical treatment in accordance with accepted healthcare standards.

B. If I am in a persistent vegetative state, that is, if I am not conscious and am not aware of my environment nor able to interact with others, and there is no reasonable expectation of my recovery within a medically appropriate period:

_____ I direct that my life not be extended by life-sustaining procedures, including the administration of nutrition and hydration artificially.

_____ I direct that my life not be extended by life-sustaining procedures, except that if I am unable to take food by mouth, I wish to receive nutrition and hydration artificially.

_____ I direct that I be given all available medical treatment in accordance with accepted healthcare standards.

C. If I am pregnant, my decision concerning life-sustaining procedures shall be modified as follows:

_____

By signing below, I indicate that I am emotionally and mentally competent to make this Living Will and that I understand its purpose and effect.

_____ (Signature of Declarant)   _____ (Date)

The declarant signed or acknowledged signing this Living Will in my presence, and based upon my personal observation, the declarant appears to be a competent individual.

_____ (Signature of Witness 1)   _____ (Date)
_____ (Signature of Witness 2)   _____ (Date)

Figure 3.1
An Example of a Living Will Approved for Use in Maryland

Source: Department of Legislative Reference, General Assembly of Maryland.

physician is not allowed to be a member of the transplant team.

The gift may be made through a will or an affidavit that is filed with the state motor vehicle department. Some states supply space on drivers' licenses for anatomical gift designations, along with an "organ donor" sticker in a bright color to alert emergency personnel to the donor's wishes.

Uniform donor cards can be obtained from the American Medical Association, the Coalition on Donation, the American Kidney Fund, or local health-related agencies. Regardless of who supplies the card, an anatomical gift donation is valid if the authorization is properly witnessed. Figure 3.2 is an example of a donor card.

Even if a patient signs a donor card, many states require that a close family member give permission

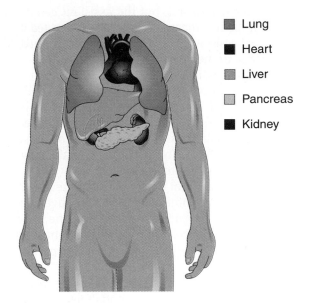

Lung
Heart
Liver
Pancreas
Kidney

Figure 3.3
Organs Needed for Transplantation

before organs can be removed. For this reason, it is important for a patient to discuss his desire to be an organ donor with family members. Figure 3.3 lists the organs that are typically needed for transplantation.

In 1984, Congress passed the National Organ Transplant Act (NOTA) establishing a nationwide system for organ sharing. The act set up the Organ Procurement Transplantation Network (OPTN) to develop a system for allocating donated organs. In 1986, the United Network for Organ Sharing (UNOS) was awarded a contract to register all organ donations.

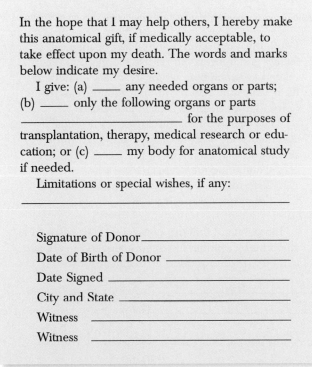

In the hope that I may help others, I hereby make this anatomical gift, if medically acceptable, to take effect upon my death. The words and marks below indicate my desire.

I give: (a) _____ any needed organs or parts;
(b) _____ only the following organs or parts
_____ for the purposes of transplantation, therapy, medical research or education; or (c) _____ my body for anatomical study if needed.

Limitations or special wishes, if any:
_____

Signature of Donor _____
Date of Birth of Donor _____
Date Signed _____
City and State _____
Witness _____
Witness _____

Figure 3.2
Donor Card
Source: Reprinted by permission of the American Kidney Fund.

The Medical Assistant's Legal Responsibilities

The medical assistant is the link between the patient and the doctor in arranging office visits and scheduling laboratory procedures, radiology tests, outpatient clinic appointments, and inpatient hospital admissions. Skillful, kind, and confident performance of these duties is critical to the development of good relations between the physician and the patient. In addition, your understanding of the legal issues involved in all these aspects of medical practice can help avoid misunderstandings and unpleasant situations.

As a medical professional, you will be expected to conduct your interpersonal relationships in a responsible manner that does not lead to harm. The medical assistant must practice safe procedures and must know the difference between what can and cannot be done from both legal and moral standpoints. For example, the medical assistant must *not* practice medicine. It is against the law for a medical assistant to diagnose a patient either over the telephone or during an office visit. You may *never* dispense drugs. An order for medication may be given to a patient only if it is signed by the physician, nurse practitioner, or physician's assistant, depending on state law. Laboratory testing or scheduling of x-rays may *never* be ordered by the medical assistant, but the assistant can schedule them if the healthcare provider has requested them. The medical assistant always works under the direction and authority of the physician.

The medical assistant may sometimes answer questions regarding how drugs are to be taken and side effects to look for, but this information must be based on a thorough understanding of drugs dispensed for most common ailments. While you cannot prescribe procedures or treatments, you may explain how different procedures and treatments work.

The medical assistant must take accurate telephone messages, set up appointments that are convenient for the patient, and determine the length of the appointment based on a description of the patient's symptoms. Diagnosing or prescribing is never a part of the assistant's role.

The medical assistant must practice safe procedures for the operation of all medical modalities, such as the electrocardiograph, physical therapy instruments, and glucometers. This requires that general maintenance procedures be followed regularly for the continued safe operation of all office equipment.

The medical assistant needs to be current with the constantly changing trends in healthcare and in the responsibilities of his position. Reading the bimonthly magazine published by the American Association of Medical Assistants and other professional magazines, attending seminars and local, state, and national meetings, and participating in continuing education courses will help you stay up to date with emerging medical trends and issues. The medical assistant must know and follow standards of care and procedures according to current local and state laws.

Etiquette

The medical assistant acts as the physician's representative. When speaking with patients and other persons, the assistant must be tactful, courteous, and patient. She must observe the rules of etiquette that define good behavior. While you may think of etiquette as simply how to hold your fork at dinner, etiquette in the medical office covers a broad range of activities. When you display good manners or proper etiquette, you set a positive tone for the office. When you treat people who are sick, hurting, and upset with compassion, respect, and politeness, you convey to them the fact that you care. This is part of the public image that makes people feel comfortable in your office. Conversely, rude or impolite behavior by medical staff members will drive patients away. In the extreme, bad behavior could cause a patient to bring a legal action against the practice rather than trying to discuss a dispute first.

Confidentiality

Physicians and all medical personnel are obligated to keep information about their patients confidential. In other words, the medical information must be kept private and not disclosed to any unauthorized individuals. The understanding that no member of the medical staff will disclose private information about the patient provides a foundation for trust in the therapeutic relationship. Respect for confidentiality is firmly established in codes of ethics and in law. The physician should disclose only that information necessary to help the patient or to prevent harm and should reveal it only to those who need to know for those reasons.

Patients who do not trust that their disclosures will be kept confidential may withhold personal information that would aid the physician's efforts to treat them effectively. Even though a patient's medical record is the property of the physician or facility that compiles it, the patient has the right to control the use of the information in the record.

Because a patient's records are absolutely confidential, the patient's authorization is needed for disclosure of this information to a third party, even the patient's insurance company. Unauthorized release or use of medical information is prohibited. A sample of an authorization to release patient records to a third party is shown in Figure 3.4. The release form must

I authorize and request <physician or medical facility and address> to release the medical records related to <condition and/or treatment identified> from <day/month/year> to <day/month/year> to <physician or medical facility and address>.

The purpose of this disclosure is for (initial statements you wish to include and cross through statements that do not apply):
____ Continuing medical care
____ Referral
____ Other, please specify _____

I understand that this consent may be revoked at any time by sending a written notice to the above-named provider of this information.

_____ (Signature of Declarant)
_____ (Date)

_____ (Signature of Witness)
_____ (Date)

Figure 3.4
Consent to Release Medical Information Form

specify which information is to be released, to whom, and for what purpose. The patient or the patient's legal guardian must sign the form. Once a release is obtained, it should be kept in the patient's medical record. Some medical facilities may not recognize a signed release that is older than one year. An example of a release form used for sharing billing information with insurance companies is included in Chapter 12, "Processing Insurance Claims."

The physician and the medical assistant may never release confidential information without the consent of the patient except when it is legally required. For example, it is mandatory to report certain incidents to law enforcement agencies, such as gunshot or knife wounds and certain communicable diseases. In the case of mentally impaired individuals, law enforcement or protective services agencies must be notified if there is a possibility of life-threatening injury to themselves or others.

With the use of the computer in the medical office, there is always the possibility that a computerized database could become accessible to people not employed in the office. The medical assistant must protect the confidentiality of all medical records in the computer. Table 3.1 provides guides for ensuring that information in the computer is kept confidential.

Public Duties

The medical assistant generally acts as a spokesperson for the physician and must never discuss a patient's medical condition, disease, or illness with the media, either press or television, without permission of the attending physician and the written consent of the patient.

MEDIA Sometimes, the physician, or the medical assistant with the approval of her employer, may release information that is in the public domain. This includes births, deaths, accidents, and police cases that are part of the public record and of concern to civil authorities.

Table 3.1 Guidelines to Ensure Computer Confidentiality

- Restrict the access of outside sources to your computerized database.
- Never divulge your password unless the office manager requests it.
- Prohibit users from walking away from the terminal while online.
- Ensure that adequate security precautions are in place to safeguard data and the system.
- Make backup files and store them securely elsewhere in case of fire, burglary, or other events that could threaten the records.

The physician and other staff members may cooperate with the media to ensure that medical news of this sort is available more promptly and more accurately than would be possible without their assistance. Some examples are multiple births such as septuplets, injuries received in either auto or industrial accidents, or the death of a public official.

Physicians and their employees are legally and ethically required to protect the personal privacy and other legal rights of the patient. Confidentiality must always be maintained, but the physician may assist the media in circumstances where confidentiality will not be breached.

REPORTING OF VITAL STATISTICS An important function of the medical office is the recording of births and deaths. These data are reported on certificates that are legal documents and as such require truthfulness, accuracy, and promptness. The specific type of certificate required varies among states. All live births must be reported to the state registrar, but neither a birth certificate nor a death certificate is required for the stillbirth of a fetus that has not passed the 20th week of gestation.

A death certificate states the date, time, place, and cause of death, and whether the physician signing was present at the time. As a courtesy to the family, it is imperative that the death certificate be completed and signed by the physician as quickly as possible so that funeral and financial arrangements can begin. Many states require that the death certificate be filed within 24–72 hours of death.

Statutory Law

Law is defined as a rule established by authority, society, or custom. Legislative bodies enact **statutory laws**, which are broken when a crime is committed. Some laws apply to events that occur only within a certain period of time (statute of limitations). Thus, it is imperative for the physician and the medical assistant to understand how the law affects the practice of medicine and the legal limits on the filing of suits.

Civil Law

Civil law is defined as the body of law dealing with the rights of individuals in their relationship with each other rather than with government. Under civil law, a person can sue another person or business. Restitution for a civil wrong is generally monetary. Court judgments in civil cases usually involve payment of damages. Most lawsuits brought against medical practices are civil in nature. Civil law falls into two classifications: contracts and torts.

CONTRACTS A **contract** is an agreement between two or more parties; it may be written, oral, or implied. It is a voluntary agreement in which specific promises are made in exchange for something of value. A contract establishes a legal relationship between the parties. When a contract—which is like a promise—is broken, a legal action may be started. The contract between a physician and a patient is usually based on an offer, an act of acceptance, and payment of consideration. The offer is made when a physician opens a medical office. The patient accepts the offer by requesting an appointment with the physician, making an appointment, arriving for the appointment, and allowing the physician to conduct an examination. The patient completes the contract by paying for the services the physician provides. The physician's consideration is providing services, and the patient's consideration is paying the physician's fees.

A major cause of legal actions against medical personnel stems from the perception by a patient of non-performance of a contract. For example, when a physician agrees to treat a patient, there is an implicit contract to care for that patient. A physician who, for any reason, refuses to treat the patient may be sued for breach of contract. A patient who feels that a physician has not provided adequate care may claim **abandonment**. However, if a patient refuses the treatment the physician recommends, the physician may terminate the patient/physician relationship. To legally terminate a patient so that a claim of abandonment cannot be filed, the physician must give the patient a **letter of withdrawal** stating why she is withdrawing from the patient's care. The letter should give a termination date that allows the patient sufficient time to find another physician. A sample letter of withdrawal is shown in Figure 3.5. In this example, the patient refused the physician's recommended care and did not come to subsequent appointments.

Although the physician is responsible for issuing the letter of withdrawal, the medical assistant will have to ensure that documentation of the patient treatment, appointment cancellations, and other relevant data is complete and up-to-date. The notice of withdrawal should be sent by certified mail, return receipt requested, so that the physician can prove it was sent and received. A copy of the letter along with the returned mailing receipt must be kept with the patient's record. In addition, it is also a good idea to mail a copy of the letter by regular mail delivery. If the postal carrier attempts the delivery when no one is available to sign for it, some patients will not or cannot make a special trip to the post office to sign for a certified letter.

At your last appointment on February 4, 20XX, we discussed further treatment and possible surgery for your medical condition.

You have not kept subsequent appointments for any follow-up of this condition. Therefore, I find it necessary to withdraw as your physician effective July 7, 20XX. It is very important that you have continued medical care and treatment, and I urge you to select another physician to treat you after July 7. We will supply your new physician with all information necessary to continue your care upon receipt of your written request.

If you desire or require medical care before July 7, I will be available to you.

Figure 3.5
Sample Letter of Withdrawal

TORTS A **tort** is defined as a wrongful act committed willfully or negligently by one person against another person or against property that results in damage or injury but does not involve a breach of contract. A tort is not necessarily a crime. A tort can include physical injury caused by substandard care on the part of the physician or medical assistant or deprivation of a patient's personal liberty and freedom.

Intentional torts are deliberate wrongs in violation of a person's legal rights. Generally, actions that are considered deliberate (willful) torts do not involve medical treatment but develop from the physical and private nature of the physician/patient relationship. Allegations of deliberate wrongdoings normally have little to do with the quality of medical care. When they occur, they often could have been avoided if the physician or the medical assistant had respected the patient's rights.

Common torts that may occur in the medical office are assault, battery, defamation of character, invasion of privacy, fraud, and false imprisonment. These actions are illegal and inappropriate and must not be tolerated in the medical office.

Assault is the intentional threat to do something to the patient that the patient does not want done. An example would be a threat to give an adult patient medication against his wishes. Medical personnel should always obtain the patient's consent before performing any procedures.

Battery is any bodily contact with another person without permission. Battery is unlawful. When it occurs, the patient's right has been violated. It does not matter if the procedure constituting the battery will improve the patient's health. For example, taking a blood sample from an unwilling patient could be considered battery even though it was intended to help the patient. Other procedures that could be considered battery if performed against the patient's will are incision and drainage, proctoscopic or vaginal examinations, and inoculation. Again, it is imperative that the patient's consent be obtained before a procedure is performed.

Defamation of character is the speaking or writing of false and malicious words that injure a person's reputation. Damages are usually in the form of money. A patient may bring a claim of defamation in the following examples:

- A medical assistant, aware that a socially prominent patient was having an extramarital affair because of information the patient revealed during an examination, tells the receptionist and other personnel in the office.
- A medical assistant, knowing that a patient who owned a restaurant was tested for HIV, writes a letter to a friend saying she would not eat there because she knows that the owner has been tested for HIV and probably has AIDS.

Defamation of character can occur in two forms: **libel**, which is written, and **slander**, which is spoken. Strict care should be taken to avoid gossip. As a medical assistant, you must keep all information about patients confidential, even non-medical information. Failure to be discreet in this regard could lead to serious legal consequences.

Invasion of privacy is the inappropriate forcing of oneself into a person's private affairs and interfering with a person's right to be left alone. Invasion of privacy includes such acts as publicly disclosing private facts about a person, giving false publicity, or using the name of another person without permission. The medical assistant needs to be especially watchful concerning the proper use of medical records to avoid revealing any personal or medical information about patients. Medical records and treatment data cannot be released without the patient's written permission. An invasion of privacy claim could be made in these situations:

- The medical office releases the results of HIV testing without the patient's written consent.
- A medical assistant shows photographs of a patient with domestic abuse injuries without the patient's permission.

- A medical assistant discusses medical test results with a friend of a patient's without the patient's consent.

Fraud consists of deliberate and deceitful practices intended to misrepresent or hide the true nature of a situation and to thereby deprive a person of her rights. In most legal applications, "fraud" and "deceit" are interchangeable terms. A physician may be charged with fraud if he tells a patient that a procedure involves no serious risks but knows otherwise. The physician/patient relationship legally binds the physician to disclose completely and voluntarily to patients all the facts related to their health conditions.

> *Legal Issue*
> *Medical office employees act as the physician's agent in performing duties ordered by and supervised by the employing physician. The medical assistant must be careful not to make promises that cannot be kept.*

> *Legal Issue*
> *Charges against physicians for defamation of character are closely associated with charges of invasion of privacy or disclosure of confidential information.*

False imprisonment is the unlawful violation of the personal liberty of an individual. This tort involves the unlawful detention or restraint of another person. Most charges of false imprisonment develop when patients are involuntarily committed to hospital psychiatric wards. All states have statutes governing and preventing involuntary commitment. In most states, there is a 72-hour limit after which a patient being held involuntarily must be released unless a judge permits further confinement. False imprisonment could occur in a medical office if:

- The physician or other medical personnel threaten a patient who continually refuses to pay a due bill or keep the person in the office for a given time while trying to coerce payment.
- A patient is forcibly forbidden to leave the office for a non-medical reason.

Intentional torts can be prevented through attention to legal practices and ethical behavior. Integrity must be of paramount importance, and the standard of care provided by all medical personnel must be excellent. The medical assistant must protect the privacy and reputation of all patients by always showing respect for their bodies and personal possessions, such as their clothes or jewelry.

UNINTENTIONAL TORTS The duty to provide reasonable care is one of the many obligations that physicians owe to their patients. To do this, the physician and medical assistant must have the proper medical education and training, good communication skills, and access to safe and appropriate equipment. In addition, they are obligated to keep up-to-date with advances in medicine.

The failure of medical practitioners to perform their professional duties competently is called **negligence.** Failing to act with reasonable care constitutes an unintentional tort, the tort of negligence. A tort action lawsuit asserts that the physician failed to meet the standards of reasonable care.

Under the doctrine of **respondeat superior,** or "let the master answer," physicians are legally responsible for negligent acts of the medical assistants they employ as well as for their own acts. A case of negligence could result from the following situation.

During a telephone call, a patient tells a medical assistant that the medication the physician prescribed is not working. The assistant passes the information on to the physician, who tells her to call the patient and ask him to return to the office for reevaluation. The medical assistant forgets to call and goes home. Later that evening, the patient's condition worsens, and he requires hospitalization.

The patient may sue the physician because the physician is legally responsible for the medical assistant's negligence in forgetting to call. Even though it was the assistant who acted negligently, it is the physician who is charged with the negligence. However, the patient may sue the medical assistant as well.

The doctrine of **res ipsa loquitur** states that, "The thing speaks for itself." This applies to an act that was clearly under the control of the physician and was one in which the patient did not contribute to the injury. It means that negligence is obvious, and the result would not have happened if reasonable care had been used. Some examples of *res ipsa loquitur* are:

- causing infection by using unsterilized instruments
- unintentionally leaving a foreign body, such as a sponge, inside a wound and then suturing the incision
- removing the wrong body part

The physician is held legally accountable if the action or omission fits the **four Ds of negligence,** the requirements necessary to meet the legal definition of negligence. These are described in Table 3.2.

Legal Issue
Allegations of negligence by healthcare professionals often result in malpractice lawsuits.

Table 3.2 The Four Ds of Negligence

- **Duty** refers to the establishment of a patient/physician relationship. The patient makes an appointment to see the physician and sees the doctor, then makes another appointment for a future visit.
- **Dereliction** refers to the claim that the physician did not comply with the standards of the medical profession.
- **Direct cause** refers to the allegation that the physician's dereliction, or breach of duty, was the immediate and direct cause of an injury that resulted.
- **Damages** refers to the fact that the patient suffered injuries as a result of the doctor's actions.

CRIMINAL LAW **Criminal laws** deal with the punishment of individuals who violate the law by committing crimes. They affect the relationship between the individual and the government. Criminal acts are offenses against the safety and welfare of society. A criminal act may be either a misdemeanor or a felony, and may range from littering (misdemeanor) to burglary (felony) to murder (felony). The punishment for criminal acts is a fine, prison sentence, or both. Perpetrators of criminal acts are prosecuted by the state. An example of a violation of criminal law by a physician would be practicing medicine without a license or illegally dispensing drugs.

CONTROLLED SUBSTANCES Federal and state governments regulate the sale and use of certain drugs. The federal agency charged with this responsibility is the **Drug Enforcement Administration (DEA).** Some general regulations apply to all physicians who purchase, dispense, administer, prescribe, or in any other way handle controlled drugs, any drug whose manufacture, distribution, and use the DEA has chosen to regulate. As part of the federal regulation of controlled drugs, a physician must register with the DEA and receive a DEA number. When pharmacies call the medical office seeking authorization to fill or refill a prescription for a controlled substance, the medical assistant should have this number handy. Registration with the DEA must be renewed every three years.

The physician must keep records relating to the administration or dispensing of a controlled drug on file for at least two years. The record must include the patient's full name and address, why the drug was prescribed, the date the prescription was written, the name of the drug, the dosage and amount given, and whether the medication was administered in the office or dispensed through a pharmacy. The medical assistant is responsible for checking the patient's record to see that this information is accurate and up-to-date. The DEA may inspect a physician's records at any time concerning all drugs dispensed. In addition, the medical assistant should make sure that all drugs are kept in a locked safe or cabinet. If a theft should occur, the nearest DEA office or the local police department must be notified immediately.

Drugs are subject to varying categories of restriction, which are called schedules. Table 3.3 provides examples of the drug classification schedules, with Schedule I drugs having the highest potential for abuse and addiction and Schedule V drugs having the least probability. Schedule I drugs are not permitted to be prescribed in the U.S., though they may be used for research with DEA approval. Schedule II drugs have a relatively high probability of abuse or addiction, and thus receive a great deal of scrutiny. Schedule III drugs have low-to-moderate potential for addiction. Schedule IV drugs have less probability of addiction than Schedule III drugs, and Schedule V drugs have the least probability of addiction. Schedule V drugs may be dispensed without a prescription if permitted by state regulations. The guidelines in Table 3.4 will help the medical assistant comply with the regulations governing the handling of controlled substances.

NOTIFICATION OF COMMUNICABLE DISEASES, INJURIES, AND ABUSE Communicable diseases are reportable when public health is at stake and the disease is a potentially pathological condition that is transmittable. Because they are mandated by state rather than federal law, the reporting requirements for communicable diseases vary from state to state. The list of reportable diseases is long and varied. Communicable

Table 3.4 Guidelines for Controlled Substances

- Keep DEA license up-to-date and renew at least two months before expiration.
- Keep accurate records of prescriptions for and administration of scheduled drugs, including documentation of phone orders for refills.
- Maintain accurate inventory records of scheduled drugs in the medical office.
- Keep the necessary stock of scheduled drugs in inventory.
- Assure the security of scheduled drugs that are kept in the medical office.
- Keep prescription blanks in areas that are not accessible to patients.

diseases most likely to be categorized as reportable are meningitis, tuberculosis, AIDS, infectious and serum hepatitis, tetanus, measles, and chickenpox. Table 3.5 lists infectious diseases designated as notifiable at the national level.

Table 3.3 Schedules of Controlled Substances

Schedule	Addiction	Abuse Potential Examples
I	high	heroin, lysergic acid diethylamide (LSD), mescaline
II	moderate	amphetamines, barbiturates, codeine, cocaine, opium, morphine
III	low-moderate	certain opiates, some depressants
IV	low	chloral hydrate, meprobamate, phenobarbital, librium
V	lowest	small amounts of codeine in cough preparations and pain relievers

Table 3.5 Infectious Diseases Notifiable at the National Level

Acquired immunodeficiency syndrome (AIDS)	HIV infection, pediatric
Anthrax	Legionellosis
Botulism	Lyme disease
Brucellosis	Malaria
Chancroid	Measles
Chlamydia trachomatis genital infections	Meningococcal disease
Cholera	Mumps
Coccidioidomycosis (regional)	Pertussis
Cryptosporidiosis	Plague
Cyclosporiasis	Poliomyelitis, paralytic
Diphtheria	Psittacosis
Ehrlichiosis, human granulocytic	Rabies, animal
Ehrlichiosis, human monocytic	Rabies, human
Encephalitis, California serogroup	Rocky Mountain spotted fever
Encephalitis, eastern equine	Rubella
Encephalitis, St. Louis	Rubella, congenital syndrome
Encephalitis, western equine	Salmonellosis
Escherichia coli O157:H7	Shigellosis
Gonorrhea	Streptococcal disease, invasive, group A
Haemophilus influenzae invasive disease	*Streptococcus pneumoniae* drug-resistant invasive disease
Hansen's disease (leprosy)	Streptococcal toxic-shock syndrome
Hantavirus pulmonary syndrome	Syphilis
Hemolytic uremic syndrome, post-diarrheal	Syphilis, congenital
Hepatitis A	Tetanus
Hepatitis B	Toxic-shock syndrome
Hepatitis C	Trichinosis
	Tuberculosis
	Typhoid fever
	Varicella deaths
	Yellow fever

Source: CDC MMWR Weekly, June 4, 1999.

Physicians are obligated to follow the reporting guidelines in their state. The information required includes the disease or suspected disease, date of onset, name of the physician reporting the disease, and name, address, age, and occupation of the patient. This information is valuable in determining the incidence of the disease and helps the local health department determine the source of infection and mode of transmission.

Certain sexually transmitted diseases (STDs) must be reported whenever they are diagnosed. State requirements vary, but the generally reportable STDs include chlamydia, gonorrhea, syphilis, and genital warts.

Technology Tip

The Association of State and Territorial Health Officials (ASTHO) is a non-profit public health organization that provides Internet links to state and territory public health resources. At these links, you can learn about state laws concerning the reporting of communicable diseases. The association's site is at www.astho.org/state.html.

Though state requirements vary, government authorities must be informed about **reportable injuries** because they concern the public welfare. These include injuries caused by lethal weapons such as guns and knives. Usually, patients with this type of wound will be treated in emergency facilities, though they may be seen in a medical office for follow-up.

Rape victims or battered persons will sometimes seek treatment in your medical office. When this occurs, a number of questions arise. If an adult rape victim comes to your office for medical care, must the assault be reported? Statutes vary from state to state. The physician needs to consider the patient's vulnerability to future assaults and should respect the patient's right not to report the rape, *if permissible by law*. A physician who treats the patient must follow law enforcement agencies' guidelines regarding reporting such incidents and obtaining, securing, and handling medical legal evidence.

The medical assistant, as well as the entire office staff, should be familiar with the community's resources for battered persons and be able to refer patients to them when appropriate. In addition, the medical assistant can help make a difference to these victims by being supportive and treating them with respect and dignity.

Abuse—defined as hurting, insulting, misusing, or deceiving a person—can be emotional, physical, or verbal. When abused patients are seen in the physician's office, the symptoms of various types of abuse are often evident. Emotionally and verbally abused persons generally have a very poor self-image and try to please everyone. Often, the patient is accompanied by another adult (husband, wife, or significant other) who will interrupt and answer the questions that are asked. The patient sometimes has a very withdrawn attitude or personality and will agree by nodding or mumbling an answer.

Physical abuse is easy to see, as there generally are bruises, cuts, and scars suggesting that mistreatment has occurred. Emotional and verbal abuse are harder to detect. Children suffer most from all three, as in this example:

> The patient was a three-year-old boy. In the presence of the physician and medical attendant, he was referred to as "dumb, clumsy, and a trouble-maker" (verbal and emotional abuse). He also appeared to suffer from malnutrition and be underweight and frightened. His appearance was dull and apathetic. Scars (showing physical abuse) were visible on his back and legs.

Elderly patients may be abused by either their adult children or their caregivers. Signs of this include injuries attributed to frequent falls, malnutrition, dirty clothing, body odors, poor oral hygiene, and a general disheveled appearance.

Domestic abuse patients generally are seen in a hospital emergency room, but sometimes there are follow-up visits to a physician's office. These cases, if initially seen in the medical office, present somewhat of a dilemma. Other patients who are waiting will either try to ignore the injured patient or become very inquisitive. The medical assistant should try to escort the patient to an examining room as quickly as possible. Each situation requires that the assistant attempt to remain as objective as possible.

Medical assistants, as well as other healthcare providers, are identified as "mandated reporters" under state statutes. This may sometimes cause personal conflict for a physician or other members of the healthcare team who have been caring for an entire family. It is important for the medical assistant to maintain interpersonal relationships with both the patient and other family members despite the possibility of having to testify against a family member.

In private life, anyone—family member, neighbor, or concerned adult—may file an abuse complaint with a protective agency. In the physician's office, within the scope of employment, the medical assistant may file a complaint only when delegated to do so by the physician.

Statute of Limitations Law

The **statute of limitations** in the law sets a time limit within which a lawsuit must be filed. It applies to injuries, accidents, and patient suits in medical and surgical cases resulting from malpractice or negligence. Statutory time limits also apply to other legal actions such as bad debt collections and wrongful death claims, as well as requirements for retention of medical records. While the length of time varies among states, it is usually a year or two from the time the alleged malpractice or negligence takes place, or from the time a patient discovers the malpractice or negligence. Patients may not sue a physician for negligence or malpractice if this length of time has elapsed.

It is very important to know the period of time set by the statute of limitations in a particular state because the statutory period does not necessarily begin at the time of treatment. A state's law will indicate how to calculate the statutory period. Even if the negligently caused injury occurred some time earlier, the clock may only begin to run when it is discovered. The most common occurrences for starting the statutory period are:

- the day the allegedly negligent act was committed
- when the injury resulting from the act was discovered by the patient
- the day the physician/patient relationship ended
- the day of the last medical treatment in a series

> **Legal Issue**
> Remember that careless talk in a medical office could result in a serious lawsuit.

> **Technology Tip**
> For a listing of the medical malpractice laws for each state, visit the McCullough, Campbell & Lane law firm's website at www.mcandl.com/states.html.

In some states, the statutory periods are modified for minors, the legally insane, and incarcerated persons, or in cases where foreign objects are left in the body during surgery. Because statutes of limitations vary, medical office personnel must become familiar with the specific laws in their state of employment. Knowing the statute of limitations in each state in part determines how long patients' medical records must be kept.

Professional Liability

The medical assistant is an agent of the physician—in other words, employed and insured under the physician's policy. However, the assistant is responsible for his own actions, and should also carry his own liability insurance. A patient may sue an individual medical assistant as well as the employing physician.

It is crucial that the medical assistant keep all information confidential. This means that she does not talk about patients and their conditions in the office where other patients may be able to hear. Discussion of anything that has happened in the workplace should be kept at a minimum. The medical assistant must always remember that most lawsuits are caused by careless behavior. Something as simple as an overheard conversation can cause a lawsuit.

The medical assistant must never make statements concerning a physician or other employee that could be construed as admission of fault for an undesirable outcome. The assistant's duty concerning a lawsuit is to say nothing to anyone except as required by the physician's attorney or by the court. The only exception occurs if a medical assistant has seen the physician act illegally. In this situation, the assistant has an ethical and moral responsibility to be truthful. Additionally, remaining silent to protect the physician in this case could result in a liability action against the medical assistant.

The physician may be subpoenaed to testify about the patient's medical record in court. The patient's history, diagnosis, treatment, and prognosis may be discussed with the patient's lawyer if the patient or the patient's legal representative has given written consent. Insurance companies may have access to medical information when investigating an insurance claim. However, the medical assistant may never share this knowledge without prior consent from the physician.

Patient Files

Progress notes, x-rays, laboratory reports, referrals, and all correspondence relevant to the patient's condition must be kept up-to-date in the patient's chart. Although medical records are the property of the physician, patients have the right to examine them and copy the information they contain.

RECORDS AND DOCUMENTATION You must make sure that actions are properly documented in the record. Entries in the medical chart must be objective, concise, clear, and legible. Particular attention to referrals is needed to ensure that the patient understands whether the referring physician's staff will make the appointment and notify the patient or if the patient must make the call. Written notes on details of the referral process should be placed in the patient's chart. These should include the date the patient was seen by the physician and given the referral, who made the referral appointment, the date of any follow-up phone call regarding the appointment time, date, and place, and whether the patient kept the appointment.

Documentation of the referring physician's consultation and recommendations concerning the care of the patient are kept in the patient's file. The medical assistant should document all missed appointments and follow up with a phone call to ask the patient why an appointment was not kept. Figure 3.6 provides an example of documentation in a patient's record concerning an appointment. Table 3.6 provides guidelines for documentation in a patient's chart.

SEPARATION OF FILES Most patient files will concern medical matters. Certain types of information should be kept in separate files. For example, a patient complaint should be filed in a separate folder, and a file relating to an accident in the medical office should be kept separate.

Accidents that happen on the job are covered by worker's compensation laws. To process a claim, an injured employee will need medical records of the

Table 3.6 Guidelines for Chart Documentation

- Enter specific information on the patient's chart with a black ink pen.
- Enter only objective data, not personal opinions or observations.
- Put all patient statements in quotation marks (" ") for clarity in case of possible litigation.
- Enter information about the referral including date, time, physician referred to, facility, address, and phone number.
- Place all referral sheets and results of consultations in the patient's file.
- Recheck all your entries for legibility and accuracy.

injury. When an insurance company or employer seeks information, only the treatment, after-care, and referrals relating to the injury may be released. For this reason, documentation related to accidents that happen to patients in the workplace should be kept separate from the patient's standard medical record. Worker's compensation will be discussed in more detail in Chapter 12, "Processing Insurance Claims."

Separation of files becomes important in the event of a legal action. In most lawsuits, a demand is made that the physician produce certain patient documents. This is called a **subpoena duces tecum**. In most cases, only those files specific to the legal issues of the case need to be produced.

Patient Consent

Patients are entitled to make decisions about their medical care, and have the right to be given all available information relating to such decisions. **Consent** is the patient's permission to be examined, for diagnostic tests to be performed, or for a medical condition to be treated by the physician. Obtaining consent is not a distinct event but rather a process that should occur throughout the physician/patient relationship. Although the term "consent" suggests acceptance of treatment, the idea of consent applies equally to the refusal of treatment. A patient has the right to refuse treatment and to be given all available information relevant to that refusal.

TYPES OF CONSENT Consent may be written, oral, or implied. **Implied consent** occurs when the patient indicates a willingness to undergo a certain procedure or treatment by appearing in the physician's office at the appointment time scheduled for the treatment or procedure. Consent for venipuncture is implied, for example, when the patient rolls up a sleeve and presents an arm for the withdrawal of blood.

Certain medical and surgical procedures always require the patient's signed consent. The physician is responsible for determining whether a written consent is necessary. The physician is responsible for explaining

12/12/XX Referred patient to Lakeside Hospital ENT clinic. Referral sent via fax (334-9857). Appointment, 12/20/XX 9:15 AM with Dr. J. Black, Ophthalmologist. Appt. verified with Jane Clark, RN. Patient given written instruction as to appt. time and place. Mary Jones, CMA

12/21/XX 8:30 AM phone call to Lakeside Hospital ENT clinic. Jane Clark, RN, states that patient did not keep appointment. Mary Jones, CMA

12/21/XX 8:50 AM Telephone call to patient. States "It was too early in the morning to go to the doctor and I was tired and must have overslept." Mary Jones, CMA

12/21/XX 9:20 AM new appointment made for 1/05/X5 1:30 PM with Dr. J. Black, confirmed with Jane Clark, RN. Mary Jones, CMA

12/21/XX 9:30 AM, patient notified of new appointment time by phone call and states, "I will be there at 1:30." Mary Jones, CMA

Figure 3.6
Sample Documentation

to the patient exactly what the procedure is, how it will be performed, what risks are involved, the expected results, alternative procedures or treatments, and the expected result if no treatment is given. Permission given with an understanding of the nature, risks, and alternatives of a procedure is called **informed consent**. The physician's obligation to obtain patient consent to treatment is founded in the ethical principles of patient self-protection and respect for the person. An example of a patient consent form for a surgical procedure is shown in Figure 3.7. Physicians may require signed consent for less invasive procedures and treatments as well, depending on the litigious nature of the patient community. Signed consent forms are always witnessed and signed by someone in addition to the doctor or patient, usually the medical assistant. If the physician

Customer Service

Research has shown that the process of obtaining consent can improve patient satisfaction and compliance and ultimately the health outcome for the patient.

does not request a signed consent for a procedure, the physician and medical assistant should document in the patient's chart whether oral or implied consent occurred.

WHO CAN GIVE CONSENT? A person who is a **legal incompetent** cannot provide consent for a medical procedure. Such a person, for the purposes of legal and binding consent, has been defined as a minor or an individual who is cognitively delayed or under the influence of a drug that alters his mental status.

The age of majority, at which a person ceases to be a minor is either 18 or 21, as defined by state law. Legally, a minor is incapable of giving effective consent for any type of medical treatment; therefore, permission of a parent or guardian is required. However, an **emancipated minor** is not considered a legal incompetent and does not need consent from a parent or guardian, even though the individual is under the age of majority. This person is defined as a minor who is self-supporting, married, in the armed services, or no longer living under parental control.

If a legal guardian provides oral consent on behalf of a patient, the guardian's relationship must be documented on the signed consent form or in the patient's chart.

EXCEPTIONS TO CONSENT REQUIREMENTS Common law recognizes emergency treatment of incapable persons as an exception to the requirement for consent. Such treatment might take place in a professional environment such as a medical office. It also could take place outside the medical office and be administered by either an off-duty medical professional or a layperson.

Emergencies occurring in the medical office could include, for example, a patient's collapse and hemorrhage from a severe laceration. Because it is imperative that the bleeding be controlled, the doctor may suture the wound without consent being required. Or a patient who stops breathing may be intubated by the physician without oral or written consent.

Healthcare professionals are protected by common law when they respond to an emergency situation.

I hereby authorize Dr. _____ to perform the following surgical procedure _____.
If any unforeseen conditions arise during this surgical procedure that, in the physician's judgment, call for procedure(s) not currently contemplated in addition to or different from this procedure, I give Dr. _____ authorization to do whatever is deemed advisable.

   The nature and purpose of this surgical procedure, as well as possible alternative methods and treatment, risks, and possible consequences involved, including the possibility of complications, have been explained to me and are clearly understood.

   I certify that I have read this form or have had it read to me and I fully understand the above consent for the surgical procedure.

_____ (Signature of Patient)   _____ (Date)
_____ (Signature of Witness)   _____ (Date)
_____ (Signature of Witness)   _____ (Date)

Figure 3.7
Sample Consent to Surgical Procedure Form

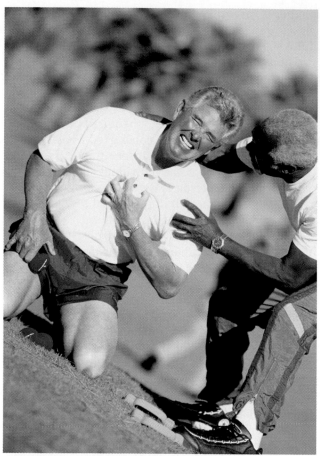

A trained person who volunteers medical assistance in an emergency is protected by Good Samaritan laws against being sued in most circumstances.

the limits of her skills and training. All healthcare professionals should know what and who the Good Samaritan law in their state covers.

Clinical Summary

- The medical assistant must follow ethical standards adopted by the medical profession.
- Legal requirements for and restrictions on the practice of medicine are determined by the laws of each state.
- The physician is responsible for the actions and omissions of the medical assistant, but the medical assistant also can be sued.
- A basic understanding of the legal principles governing the performance of professional duties is essential to avoid legal action.
- Medicine and law are joined in a common concern for the rights and health of the patient.
- The medical assistant must stay knowledgeable about medical-legal issues for self-protection and to protect other healthcare professionals from legal action.
- Malpractice suits can be prevented by performing clinical tasks safely, effectively, and responsibly.
- Clear, concise, correct documentation is essential if medical records are subpoenaed by a court.
- The physician is obligated to obtain a patient's consent to treatment. Consent can be written, oral, or implied. The medical assistant should document the patient's consent in the medical record.
- Lawsuits can and will be avoided if attention and energy are directed toward positive healthcare.

The basis for this exception is the belief that a reasonable person would consent to the treatment and that a delay in treatment would lead to death or serious harm. A physician should not administer emergency treatment without consent if there is reason to believe the patient would refuse the treatment if she could.

Emergency care by a volunteer, either an off-duty trained medical person who happens to be present or even a minimally trained passerby is protected by the **Good Samaritan law**. Versions of this law exist in all 50 states. Good Samaritan statutes provide immunity to volunteers at the scene of an accident if they do not intentionally or recklessly injure the patient further. Although the specifics of the law vary among states, the basic premise is to encourage all healthcare professionals to render emergency first aid to accident victims without fear of liability.

Depending on the state law, physicians or healthcare professionals may not have a legal obligation to stop and give first aid in a life-threatening situation. However, a health professional who chooses to help in an emergency situation is required to act only within

The Language of Medicine

abandonment A physician's halting of treatment without proper notification to the patient.

advance directive A living will, durable power of attorney for healthcare, or healthcare proxy specifying what treatment the patient wants or doesn't want if the patient cannot voice those decisions, and/or designating a person to make those decisions at that time.

Americans with Disabilities Act A federal law prohibiting discrimination against the disabled in the workplace and mandating full accessibility for them in all public places.

assault A threat to inflict harm.

battery Bodily contact with another person without permission.

bioethics The study of moral and ethical questions evolving from new research and medical advances.

civil law The body of law dealing with the rights of individuals in their relationships with each other rather than with government.

communicable diseases Diseases that may be transmitted from one person to another.

consent Permission from a patient, expressed either in oral or written form or implied, for medical examination, testing, or treatment.

contract A voluntary agreement between two or more parties in which specific promises are made in exchange for something of value.

criminal law The legal area dealing with offenses committed against the safety and welfare of society.

defamation of character Damaging a person's reputation by making false and malicious statements.

disability Physical or mental impairment that considerably limits one or more of the major life activities of the individual.

Drug Enforcement Administration (DEA) The federal agency that regulates the sale and use of controlled drugs.

durable power of attorney for healthcare A legal document that allows another person to make healthcare decisions on behalf of a person who is physically or mentally impaired.

emancipated minor A person younger than the age of majority who is married, in the armed services, self-supporting, or no longer living under parental control. Such a person does not need the consent of a parent or guardian to obtain medical treatment.

ethics Principles governing the right thing to do.

false imprisonment The unlawful restraint of another person's freedom of movement.

four Ds of negligence The elements necessary to meet the legal definition of negligence: duty, dereliction, direct cause, and damages.

Good Samaritan law A statute protecting a volunteer who administers emergency medical treatment from liability in most circumstances.

health care proxy A document transferring the authority to make medical decisions for a patient who cannot reason or communicate.

implied consent Willingness to undergo a medical procedure that the patient indicates by appearing for the procedure at the scheduled time and place.

informed consent The patient's permission for a procedure given with a full understanding of its nature, risks, and alternatives.

invasion of privacy Interference in a person's private affairs, encroachment on a person's right to be left alone.

law A rule established by authority, society, or custom.

legal incompetent A person under the legal age or one who is cognitively delayed or under the influence of mind-altering drugs.

letter of withdrawal A letter informing a patient of the physician's intent to withdraw from care of the patient and setting a deadline by which the patient must find alternative medical care.

libel The damaging of a person's reputation through written words or pictures.

living will A document in which a person gives instructions for treatment in the event the person becomes comatose or incompetent.

medical ethics Principles of right or wrong conduct that apply in the medical setting.

morals Personal codes of conduct based on individual beliefs, religion, and cultural values.

negligence Failure to meet the standards of reasonable care.

Patient Self-Determination Act A federal law requiring that patients receive written information about their right to make medical decisions and execute advance directives.

reportable injuries Injuries that concern the public welfare because they were caused by lethal weapons or resulted from abuse.

res ipsa loquitur "The thing speaks for itself." Indicates obvious negligence.

respondeat superior "Let the master answer," a legal doctrine that holds the employer physician responsible for acts performed by employees acting within the scope of their duties.

slander The damaging of a person's reputation through spoken words.

statute of limitations A time limit fixed by state laws within which a lawsuit must be filed.

statutory laws Laws enacted by a legislative body.

subpoena duces tecum A court order to produce documents.

tort A wrongful act committed by one person against another person or against property that results in damage or injury but does not involve a breach of contract.

Uniform Anatomical Gift Act State laws facilitating the donation of bodies or body parts for use in transplant surgery, tissue banks, or medical research or education.

Signs/Symptoms of Progress

Recall, Question, Connect

Recall
Identify three ways that an individual can indicate her wishes regarding medical treatment and end-of-life issues.

Question
Write down three questions you have about advance directives. Research the answers and document how you and others in the office could learn more about advance directives.

Connect
Explain how a thorough understanding of advance directives will help your employer and your patients.

Educating the Patient

Alma Jacobson, a patient for many years, has terminal cancer. Although she knows she is not expected to live more than another three months, she has never spoken about dying. Moreover, you do not have an advance directive in her file.

1 What can you ask Alma to determine if she has any special care requests for her final days? What questions should you avoid asking?

2 What information could you give members of Alma's family to help her prepare for her death?

Exploring Perspectives in Teams

Perspective involves the discipline of examining how ideas look from different points of view and recognizing that there are often multiple "answers" to complex questions. In small groups or on your own, reflect on possible alternative views or answers and summarize your findings.

1 How is the physician liable for your actions as a medical assistant? Do you share liability? Why or why not?

2 Explain the difference between ethics and law, and give five examples. Then discuss three instances in which an ethical situation could result in a legal concern.

3 A badly bruised and distraught woman comes to your office unannounced. She is with a man who is using loud and abusive language. The woman asks to see a doctor. As far as you can determine, she is not a patient of the practice. What do you do? Would your actions change if you recognized her as a patient of the practice?

Learning Outcomes

- Recognize the importance of effective communication in the medical office.

- Name the three primary modes of communication and give examples for each of effective and ineffective interactions.

- Recognize that stress can be a barrier to effective communication.

- Discuss how issues related to patient diversity affect response to treatment and how cultural sensitivity can be fostered in the medical office.

- State several strategies that can improve communication with both internal and external customers.

Performance Objectives

- Demonstrate the effective use of active listening, questioning, and feedback in oral communications.

- Recognize and respect cultural diversity.

- Use effective written communication and precise writing skills.

- Promote the medical practice through positive public relations.

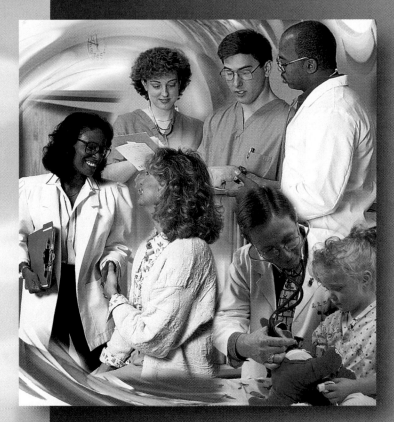

Effective communication *is one of the most important skills the medical assistant must develop to be a successful member of the healthcare team and promote positive public relations. The importance of effective communication within the healthcare community cannot be overemphasized. The ability to communicate with patients and their families, with coworkers, and with the general public is essential to efficient healthcare delivery. Effective communication is especially important in light of the dominance of managed care as the primary deliverer of healthcare in the United States. The logistics involved in navigating the healthcare system are complicated, and patients often feel overwhelmed. Treating patients and their family members as valued and unique customers is essential to the communication process.*

Communicating with Patients, Physicians, and Staff

During your career as a medical assistant, you will work daily with many people. Your body language, your spoken words, and your written words are all important means of communicating the message that patient healthcare is the top priority of the medical system. At all times, the medical assistant must be aware of her role as a member of the medical team. She is part of a wide web of professionals serving the patient-customer, and as such, she must ensure the accuracy, completeness, and professionalism of her communications with all other team members.

Patients often arrive at the medical office worried or in pain. Even if they have come for a routine physical, visiting a doctor is stressful for many people. If they have come with a specific health concern, the stress is heightened. Furthermore, patients often worry that their doctor or other healthcare provider will not understand their concerns. They realize that they often do not understand complicated medical terminology, and too many patients have had the experience of providers not really listening to them or truly caring about their needs. In a complex managed care environment, some patients feel more like a "number" than an individual with unique needs. All these worries are greatly multiplied if a patient does not speak English well or has a cultural background that makes him wary of the way we practice medicine in this country. For the medical assistant, good communication is essential in easing patients' fears and making them receptive to medical treatment.

Understanding Communication

Communication is central to human life and civilization, but communicating well is an art and a skill that must be learned and practiced. In our modern society, the exchange of thoughts, opinions, and information among people has become increasingly complex and multifaceted. Through computer technology, international media, and entertainment networks, we are bombarded daily with an ever-increasing amount of information. In spite of these technological advances, there are still essentially only three modes of communication: oral, written, and nonverbal.

Three Ways to Send a Message

The most common way to communicate with those around us is through **oral communication**, or spoken words. From the moment we wake up in the morning, we communicate by talking to others in the household. As we listen to the news on the radio on our way to work, we are receiving oral messages. In the office, we

communicate orally when we use the telephone and when we have conversations with other members of the staff. Patients use oral communication to reveal health problems and concerns when they are interviewed and to explain the reason for their visit. The ability to converse with patients using simple and direct language that avoids misunderstanding but is not patronizing is vital to the medical assistant in his role as liaison between the patient-customer and the physician-provider. In this role, you are responsible for collecting, assessing, and relaying information that is critical in promoting wellness or diagnosing and treating disease. You are often the first and the last person the patient sees when visiting the physician's office. Patients who have not been to a doctor for a few years or are new to your office will be more comfortable and receptive to your instructions if they are met with friendly professionalism. That first contact will set the tone for the visit. A pleasant and genuine greeting conveys a sense of care and interest. By speaking in a positive and professional manner, the medical assistant can set a nervous or fearful patient at ease.

Nonverbal communication refers to the many messages people send and receive without the use of spoken words. Gestures, body movements, tone of voice, facial expressions, eye contact, and spatial relationships send powerful, nonverbal messages to others. We learn nonverbal communication intuitively. As infants, before we can speak, we learn that this form of communication will get our mother to meet our needs. As we grow up, we often subconsciously adopt the mannerisms and expressions of those around us, and we often remain unaware of what those mannerisms are communicating to others. One of the keys to

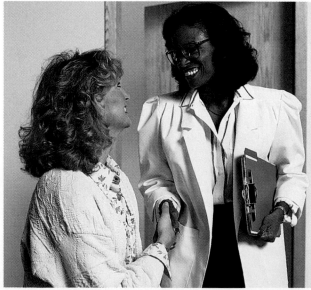

A medical assistant's friendly greeting helps the medical practice meet the patient's healthcare needs.

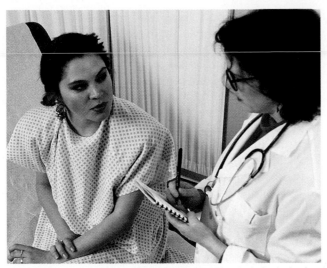

The medical assistant's communication with the patient includes both what is said and many nonverbal messages as well.

effective communication, therefore, is becoming aware of what we are communicating nonverbally. The medical assistant should always speak in a calm, gentle tone of voice. She should listen attentively and maintain eye contact when talking to others. She should be aware that brusque or harsh gestures and a scowling face communicate lack of care and unfriendliness to patients, and those patients' trust. Even the medical assistant's appearance sends a strong message to others. Neat, professional attire and well-groomed hair combine with a positive attitude to communicate a sense of confidence, efficiency, and caring. The medical assistant should also remember that nonverbal signals may vary from culture to culture, as we will explore later in this chapter. These cultural differences may lead to unintentional misunderstandings.

Finally, the third and last basic mode of communication is written communication. Like all healthcare professionals, the medical assistant is responsible for perfecting his writing so that it is clear and accurate. In the medical office, the medical assistant is responsible for a number of different written communications. Certainly, the most important of these include the patient's chart and vital records, lab reports, treatment plans, and all other permanent records of patient care that can be accessed by other members of the healthcare team.

On the patient's chart, the medical assistant must be able to describe the symptoms, treatments, and other important information in order to document them accurately and communicate them to the other members of the team who will interact with the patient. An expression in the medical field goes something like this: "If you haven't written it down, you haven't done it." Of course, this is not literally true, but the spirit of the saying holds true when considering the extreme importance

of leaving accurate information for others to read and for legal documentation purposes. What if a child's immunizations were never recorded in her chart and her parents cannot remember if she has had certain shots? What if prescribed medication for an elderly person was not recorded in his chart and the physician prescribes another medication that interferes with what he is already taking? Such failures to record vital health information clearly may lead to a patient's death and legal charges of negligence by the healthcare team.

Medical language is complex. It is essential that the medical assistant not only record information but do so precisely. For example, 50 milligrams of a medication is one tenth of 500. What if the prescription were for 50 milligrams but the medical assistant erroneously wrote down "500" instead? Because the *ilium* is a completely different part of the body than the *ileum*, what if the two terms were mixed up in the record? (See Figure 4.1.) Omissions, inaccuracies, and even misspellings in writing can be deadly in the medical field.

Working Smart

Misspelled words or incorrect grammar or sentence structure may distort written communication. For example, if the word "ilium" is used when "ileum" should have been written in the patient's record, a completely different part of the body is indicated. This may lead to harmful patient treatment.

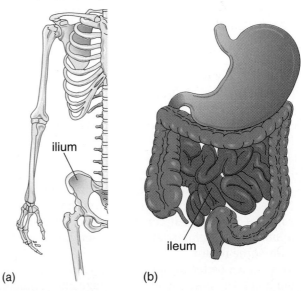

(a) (b)

Figure 4.1
Ilium vs. Ileum

(a) The ilium is the wide, flared bone that forms the upper portion of the pelvis. (b) The ileum is the lower portion of the small intestine.

Other forms of written communication that the medical assistant will encounter in her work include routine memos, letters, computer data, instructional materials, policies and procedures, and e-mail correspondence. Each type of communication has its own conventions, and how those conventions are applied often depends on the culture of the particular medical office. In your first few weeks on the job, you should study how the office staff composes these materials. What tone of voice—very formal or less formal—is used? How are patients and other customers addressed? What layouts are used in these documents? In all her writing, the medical assistant must strive for clarity and accuracy.

Communication Modes in Practice

We have discussed the three basic modes of communication: oral, written, and nonverbal. Let us now take a closer look at how oral and nonverbal communication operate together to forge strong patient-provider relationships. Study the following situation:

> Paula Anderson, a medical assistant at a large urban medical center, is very busy. The waiting room is full, and appointments are running behind. In addition, it is almost the end of her shift, and Paula is tired. Her next patient is a teenage girl named Susan Blake who is here for her first pelvic exam. Moving quickly, Paula brings Susan into an examination room, sits down with the chart in front of her, and grabs the blood pressure cuff to take Susan's blood pressure. Susan is sitting with her arms crossed in front of her and will not look up. When she does not readily extend her arm for the blood pressure cuff, Paula impatiently pulls her arm out and puts on the cuff. She lets the systolic mercury rise to 220 out of irritation, which is not necessary and hurts the girl's arm. Susan bursts into tears.

What has gone wrong in this situation? Because she is focused on her own need to hurry and her own feeling of fatigue, Paula has failed to focus on her patient, Susan, and therefore, has not noticed Susan's nonverbal signals of distress. She has not seen the tears in Susan's eyes or noticed how nervous she is about the pelvic exam. Paula thus misinterprets Susan's actions as resistance, not fear. In turn, her brusque and preoccupied manner gives clear nonverbal signals to Susan that Paula is not concerned with her, does not care about her feelings, and may even be angry with her for some reason.

How much better would this interaction have been if Paula had taken a moment to recognize and respond to the patient's nervousness? Probably much better. If Paula had understood that Susan was anxious, she could have communicated empathy and caring through a kind, gentle touch, a smile, and focused eye contact.

Moreover, she could have used her words—her oral communication—to explain the pelvic exam procedure to Susan in a calm and reassuring tone. Many patients are put at ease by a combination of friendly and caring body language and oral communication that helps them understand what the medical assistant is doing and why. All Paula succeeded in doing in the above situation was increasing Susan's fear and, most likely, blocking the trust that is essential to a successful relationship between the patient and the healthcare practitioner.

In the medical setting, both a patient's personal body space and privacy are routinely invaded. This can be very disconcerting for many people. It is all the more important, then, that all healthcare providers, including the medical assistant, put into practice reassuring and positive nonverbal communication. Eye contact, posture, facial expressions, and even gait can set a professional, compassionate tone. With experience, you will learn how to put the patient at ease with your caring, focused attention, even if you have only five minutes to spend with that patient. Part of this nonverbal caring attitude is taking a few minutes to listen to patients as they tell their story. Do not hesitate to allow for a few moments of silence which also can go a long way in calming patients and letting them understand that you are focused on their needs. Silence implies a willingness to listen and an unhurried attitude. For example, if a patient expresses despair over the loss of a job, a simple "That must be difficult for you" accompanied by silence lets the patient gather herself to continue the interview. Take the time to listen and observe what each patient is communicating. This will help you improve your relationships with your patients and will make your daily work more fulfilling.

The Communication Process

For communication to take place, a process of give and take between a sender and a receiver must occur. The sender has an idea, decides how to present the idea, and sends the message. The message is then received and interpreted by the receiver. The receiver may respond to the sender. Each step in this process can be communicated either orally or nonverbally. Oral messages use words, which are symbols whose meanings can vary according to backgrounds, values, or assumptions of the people communicating. Nonverbal signals such as gestures, negotiation of space, and tone of voice also vary in meaning according to the backgrounds, values, and assumptions of the communicators. If the sender chooses incorrect words to convey his idea or sends his message with inappropriate nonverbal signals, the receiver may misinterpret the information. For your message to be interpreted accurately,

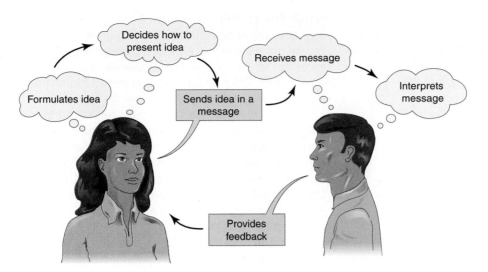

Figure 4.2
The Process of Communication

you must say what you mean clearly, choose precise words, and make your body language correspond to and emphasize your words. The more people involved in the chain of communication—such as when you speak to a group of people—the greater the chance that your message will be distorted or misunderstood. **Feedback**, the oral or nonverbal response of the receiver, is the best indicator of whether the message received was the same as the message sent. Figure 4.2 illustrates this communication process.

As you see, communication is not easy! Any stage in the process may break down and misunderstandings may occur. It is critical, therefore, that the medical assistant learn to speak clearly and concisely to everyone he interacts with in his job. When discussing patient concerns with the physician, he must report only the most pertinent details and must do so concisely. What is most essential? Patients may share with you any number of concerns and facts about their lives. It is important that the medical assistant discern and extract from the conversation only the most essential complaints when briefing the physician on the results of the patient interview.

As an example of the need for clear and precise communication, consider this situation:

A medical assistant is reporting the results of a patient interview to a nurse practitioner. "She's angry and crying," the medical assistant states, "and she said she might have a fever. Her boyfriend left her, so I really think that's her main problem." The nurse practitioner tries to focus the medical assistant's remarks by asking, "What brought her in today?" The medical assistant replies, "Her hand hurt and then her dog bit her child and she had to go to the emergency room with the baby." Once again, the nurse practitioner asks, "But why is she here today?" Finally, the medical assistant states, "She thinks her wrist is broken from an accident at work. A box of gears fell on her arm. She thought she

was all right when it happened, but she couldn't sleep last night from the pain. The wrist and hand are swollen."

Notice how the last remarks represent the concise and necessary information the provider was waiting for. The medical assistant's first words only served to distort the impression of the patient's chief complaint, and, moreover, wasted the nurse practitioner's valuable time.

Stress: A Barrier to Communication

Stress, the physical and psychological tension caused by certain events and situations, can be a huge barrier to effective communication. Both positive and negative events can cause stress, and people react to stress in very different ways. Negative events such as losing a job or getting a divorce tend to cause more stress for most people than positive events such as having a baby or moving into a new home. Also, events we can control or predict usually cause less stress than those we cannot control or predict. Table 4.1 lists events that

Table 4.1 Stressful Events

■ death of a close family member	■ mortgage or major loan
■ divorce	■ change in responsibility at work
■ personal injury or illness	■ beginning or ending of school
■ getting married	■ change in personal habits
■ loss of job	■ trouble with boss
■ retirement	■ change in work hours or conditions
■ decline in the health of a family member	■ change in residence
■ pregnancy	■ change in school
■ sex difficulties	■ vacation
■ financial problems	■ minor violations of law
■ death of a close friend	
■ change in jobs	

are commonly considered stressful, from the most down to the least stressful.

Stress is a fact of daily life, and a certain amount of stress is necessary to motivate most people to function at their best. In most daily situations, we learn to **cope** with or manage stress effectively. However, sometimes the amount of stress in our lives reaches a level at which we are unable to cope, and as a result, begins to affect our mental and physical health in negative ways. Today, stress is recognized as a major contributing factor in hypertension, lowered resistance to disease, hormonal changes, depression, and other disorders. If we can successfully manage stress, we are better able to preserve our physical and emotional well-being. By understanding the causes of stress and learning techniques to reduce it, we can live happier, healthier, and more productive lives.

The work of all healthcare workers, including the medical assistant, is often very stressful. Each day, the medical assistant is called upon to perform a vast array of duties and to answer the needs of patients, providers, external customers, and administrative staff members. She must use her utmost physical, emotional, and mental abilities to do her job well. Furthermore, in most medical settings, the medical assistant works very closely with others on the healthcare team. Personal space is limited, and little time exists for privacy or relaxation during the work day. At times, the fast pace and intensity of the job may seem overwhelming. The medical assistant must learn to cope with the demands of her work while minimizing stress.

Stress in the medical environment is caused by a number of factors. In the healthcare field, you encounter stress as you work with patients who are ill, in pain, or even dying. Few other professions must cope with life and death issues on a daily basis. Furthermore, the first few days or weeks on the job may be extremely stressful for the medical assistant until he has become familiar with the demands of the position and feels confident performing routine duties. Not

being able to perform assigned tasks efficiently and well because of insufficient knowledge or preparation can be quite stressful. Yet when a coworker is ill or on vacation, or when a staff member is not pulling his own weight, others must pick up the added responsibilities as well as attending to their own tasks.

Stress in the workplace may also be related to your personal circumstances. The personal decisions we must make, our relationships with family and friends, and major life changes affect our daily moods. The death or serious illness of a loved one; financial or family problems; or even positive changes such as marriage, pregnancy, or a promotion can affect the level of a medical assistant's stress.

Stress can negatively affect our ability to communicate with others. Our tone of voice, our words, and our body language are all affected by our stress level and emotional state. A medical assistant who is impatient or irritated because of stress may use an angry tone of voice that will confuse the receiver of the message. The receiver may misunderstand the tone and think the medical assistant is upset about something the receiver has done. If the assistant continues to let her stress level affect her communication with others, she will spread a negative atmosphere over the entire medical office. When tempers flare because of an individual's stress, issues in the workplace can easily become distorted and difficult to resolve. In addition, sadness caused by the stress of grief or depression can cause a medical assistant to be lethargic in her work, disinterested in customer service, and unable to communicate in an effective manner.

In all these cases, if the medical assistant does not work to control her stress, she may forget information or needed procedures. Unhealthy levels of stress are related to forgetfulness and inattention to detail which, in the medical profession, cannot be tolerated.

To combat stress, the medical assistant must first be aware of its cause in his life. Then, he needs to manage it by resolving negative sources of conflict or seeking help if necessary. If the source of stress is at work, communicating openly with coworkers about feelings can help alleviate the stress. For example, if confusion about duties or procedures arises, the medical assistant should make it a point to schedule time to talk to his supervisor to clarify those roles and responsibilities. Or if the clinic is not operating as smoothly as it could be and this is causing stress among the staff, the medical assistant, alone or with others, should discuss the matter with the supervisor and form a plan to improve the situation. Since stress often results from a feeling of lack of control, confronting a situation directly and working toward a solution is one of the best ways to eliminate or reduce stress in our lives.

Finally, to work to the best of her ability, the medical assistant must be healthy herself. She should take care of her health needs so that she can best help her patients do the same. She should get enough sleep and exercise; she should practice good nutritional habits; and she should work to minimize personal stress by cultivating healthy relationships with family and friends.

Here are some techniques that can help you manage or prevent stress in the workplace:

- Make sure you are prepared to handle the responsibilities of your job. When confronted with unfamiliar tasks, seek instruction and advice from your supervisor.
- Be organized. You can get more work done if you plan your day. Prioritize your tasks and do the most important things first. Less important things can be done as time permits.
- Set realistic goals and accept your limitations.
- Share ideas for solving problems such as work overload with your supervisor and other staff members.
- Maintain your physical health. Get plenty of rest and eat a balanced diet. Exercise regularly and allow sufficient quiet time in your life for such "centering" activities as yoga, prayer, or meditation.
- Allow time to relax alone and with family and friends.

In summary, while stress in our daily working lives is inevitable, we can take measures to understand its sources and to cope with it and reduce its effect on our lives. In this way, you as the medical assistant will be better able not only to perform your job accurately but also to communicate with others both orally and nonverbally in a warm, caring, and professional manner.

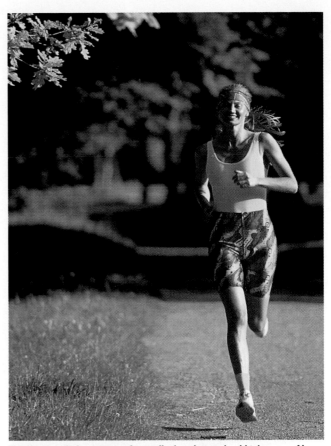

To reduce workplace stress, the medical assistant should take care of her physical needs, including getting sufficient exercise.

Understanding Patient Diversity and Its Effect on Communication

Today, we in the United States value and celebrate our **diversity**. A primary reason our nation is a vital one is the fact that people in this country come from a wide variety of cultural backgrounds. Those different backgrounds and experiences strongly affect the way individuals view the world. What is the impact of this diversity on the medical staff? What special awareness must the medical assistant have to communicate effectively with all of his patients?

One important way individual differences affect the medical staff is that people respond very differently to office visits and to treatments. Some people dread going to the medical office for even routine visits. Moreover, when a person is faced with a health problem, this sense of dread is often compounded by feelings of anxiety, fear, frustration, and confusion. Some people who are ill will not admit it, preferring a state of denial. If a patient is in pain, these feelings are heightened. Some patients feel uncomfortable when revealing intimate information or are embarrassed when answering personal questions. For many people, phys-

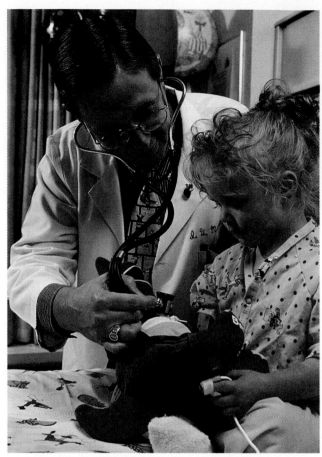

To calm a child's fears, demonstrate by using your medical instrument on a doll or stuffed animal before the procedure.

ical examinations and procedures are a stressful invasion of privacy and personal space. Medical terminology is unfamiliar to most people and this adds to feelings of lack of control. Worries about paying for healthcare and feeling lost in the maze of the healthcare system are sources of frustration and fear for many people.

All of these factors can cause tremendous stress for an individual patient. How a patient responds to this stress depends on his or her background, experiences, and emotional makeup. The medical assistant should be aware of the diverse factors that shape the way a person responds to an office visit, such as the patient's age, gender, language and culture, economic status, and the presence of disabilities. By being aware of these factors, the medical assistant can better learn to communicate effectively with each individual and meet that person's needs.

Age

Age is one of the first factors the medical assistant should consider when communicating with the patient. Children may pose special challenges. Very young children may not comprehend what you are saying but will quickly respond to your tone of voice, your facial expressions, and your gestures. Smiling and talking quietly to a child makes him feel secure and less afraid of the unfamiliar environment. As the child develops language skills, your explanations and directions should be simple but firm, using words the child can understand. Explain clearly what you are going to do. Let the child touch the instrument you are about to use, and perhaps "practice" with it first on a doll or stuffed animal. This will help calm the child's fears and establish the child's trust in you. Teen-agers should be given the opportunity to spend some time with the healthcare provider without their parent or guardian present. This gives them the chance to ask questions or volunteer information they may be reluctant to divulge with someone else present.

Communication with older adults may be difficult if physical and mental changes have taken place as part of the aging process. However, the medical assistant should always assume that the older person is of sound mind and body unless she has information about any special needs from the medical record or the patient's family. Older people do not like to be patronized or "talked down" to. If the patient has difficulty hearing, communication should take place with a family member present. You will need the patient's approval for the family member to be in the examination room. If the family member is included in the conversation, never speak to the family member as if the patient were not present. Instead, include the patient in the conversation by facing her, maintaining some eye contact, and speaking alternately to both her and the family member.

Gender

In perhaps more subtle ways than age, gender also plays a role in a patient's response to a healthcare environment. It can be a dynamic factor in the interaction between caregiver and patient. Men and women are conditioned by society to respond in certain predictable

Customer Service
Some adults dislike being addressed by their first names by people who are younger than they are. To show respect, always ask an adult patient how she prefers to be addressed, and then remember to use that form of address on each visit.

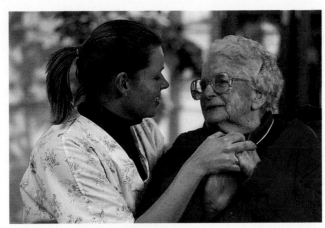

When communicating with others, you can signal your concern and care nonverbally at times with a friendly, non-invasive touch.

ways, although it is always dangerous to generalize too extensively about what those responses are. However, the medical assistant should be aware that differences between the sexes are often apparent in terms of responses to healthcare. In general, men have a tendency to use the system less. They are sometimes more resistant than women to admitting to illness and seeking medical help. In addition, it is sometimes harder for men to talk about their feelings, especially to a stranger with whom they may feel vulnerable. As a group, women tend to be more "tuned in" to their bodies and aware of their healthcare needs. They more readily seek professional care, and are more comfortable than men in describing in detail how they feel and what their concerns are. Both sexes, however, often feel more comfortable confiding intimate details about their health to a member of the same sex. Some women, therefore, prefer female practitioners and men prefer male practitioners. If practical, the patient's wishes should be honored in these matters of gender preference. However, if it is not possible, the issue should be honestly discussed with the patient, and the medical assistant should do his or her best to put the patient at ease.

Furthermore, in spite of increased understanding and acceptance in many communities, discrimination and even violence against those who live alternative sexual lifestyles still continues. However, the medical setting is one place in which openness about sexuality is critical to providing quality healthcare. As with any patient, those who are homosexual, bisexual, or transgender must be allowed to express issues related to their lifestyle and healthcare in order to receive appropriate medical care.

Economic Status

A person's economic status may also affect his response to healthcare. In spite of the United States's continued economic prosperity, it is a sad fact that more Americans than ever are living in poverty. In fact, the disparity between the rich and the poor has grown in the last few decades. The richest fifth of Americans have seen a 43% increase in their income over the last twenty years, while the poorest fifth, a group that includes many single working mothers, have seen their incomes fall by 9%. In other words, our country now has a small number of extremely wealthy people, and a growing number of the very poor.

Even as the number of lower middle class or poor Americans increases, the cost of healthcare is rising dramatically. Upper middle class or wealthy patients may well be able to afford expensive insurance premiums for excellent, comprehensive coverage and may therefore have few concerns about healthcare costs. However, in today's managed care system, many Americans must struggle to pay high insurance premiums, deductibles, and copayments, or, if not insured, high out-of-pocket expenses for office visits or treatments. The cost of visits, medicines, and procedures may greatly concern a patient and reduce his willingness to accept a physician's recommendations. The medical assistant should be aware, if possible, of these patient concerns and be able to refer the patient to sources of government financial aid or community assistance. In this way, the medical assistant acts as an important link and patient advocate in the healthcare system.

Customer Service

Locating appropriate government-sponsored and community services for patients, including those that offer financial assistance for low-income patients, is an important responsibility of the medical assistant. Make it a point to find out what services of this type exist in the community you serve.

Disability

Among the patients practitioners see every day are those with a variety of disabilities. These patients, as with any patient, need to be treated with compassionate care, with courtesy, and with respect, but they also do not want their special needs ignored. Patients with a vision loss for example, depend more on oral messages because they may not be able to see your nonverbal communication. When working with such patients, you should be especially aware of your tone of voice. As with any patient, speak clearly and at a

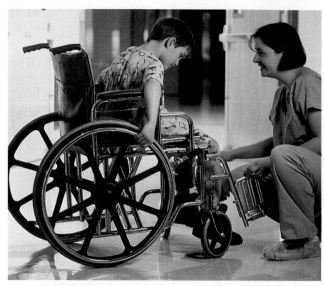

The medical assistant must be aware of a disabled person's special needs but should always ask how much help the patient would like.

normal speed. Sometimes, touching a visually impaired patient, such as offering him your elbow, may be necessary to guide him around an unfamiliar environment or demonstrate an unfamiliar procedure. However, be careful not to startle a patient by touching him unexpectedly. Never assume that a person with a disability needs help. In all cases, first ask the patient honestly and respectfully what assistance, if any, he or she would like from you. Over time you will learn how best to interact with such patients in this way.

Working Smart

Never assume that you know exactly how to assist a disabled patient. Do not, for example, grab a sight-impaired person's arm to guide her or him into the examination room or yell into the ear of a hearing-impaired person. Always ask what assistance the patient would like from you first, or wait until the patient gives an appropriate cue. Always respect the patient's wishes.

Language and Culture

A major source of patient diversity is the many cultural and language backgrounds from which they come. Such differences in **culture**—the ways of living of a group of people passed down through the generations—

and language can present challenges to patient-provider communication. If you have ever visited a country where you did not speak or understand the language, you can easily empathize with the difficulty experienced by patients whose primary language is not English. Even a strong accent can lead to a breakdown in communication.

If your patient does not understand English, an interpreter should be present. However, if the patient has some understanding of English, there are certain strategies you can use to convey your message. Many times, gestures and a few key words may be all that is needed. Speak slowly and pronounce words distinctly. Use formal English and avoid slang or colloquial expressions. Demonstrate what you want the patient to do, and use visual aids such as pictures, diagrams, and signs. Often, a person can read a language better than he can speak it, so keep a notebook and marker handy to write down key words to show the patient. Watch for signs that the patient understands what you are attempting to get across.

A medical practice that serves a large population from a certain language group should consider hiring at least one staff member fluent in that language who may, in difficult cases, act as a translator. However, if a staff interpreter is not available, other options exist. With the patient's permission, a family member or friend who is more fluent in English may remain in the examination room to act as interpreter. Professional interpreters can also be hired on an hourly basis, and, in an emergency, telephone interpretations can be arranged. In addition, patient forms and health education materials in the target language should be kept on hand.

Like language, a person's cultural background or **ethnicity** can considerably affect patient-healthcare worker communication. As a medical assistant, you should be aware that nonverbal signals that are acceptable in American culture may be interpreted very differently by those from other cultural groups. For this reason, nonverbal messages are especially susceptible to distortion. For example, the common American "thumbs up" or "OK" signs are considered to be obscene gestures in some Mediterranean and South American countries. For some cultures, pointing with the index finger is considered very rude. In yet other cultures, lowering one's eyes and refraining from eye contact indicates respect for authority, not, as in American culture, evasion, deceit, or extreme shyness.

Although it would be impossible for the medical assistant to learn all the cultural interpretations of all nonverbal signals, he can certainly make the effort to learn those of the cultural populations he serves. This may even become the basis of a fruitful office educational seminar in which members of the Latino community, Hmong community, Somalian community, or even later. While most clinics will need to reschedule a patient who arrives so late, it is important not to upbraid the patient for lateness. Instead, realizing that the issue may be a cultural one and not a matter of laziness or irresponsibility, explain the misunderstanding in a clear but kindly manner.

Although the need for understanding each unique cultural background is valid, medical assistants who treat all patients in a respectful, professional manner will have very few, if any, problems with misunderstanding caused by cultural differences. Instructions, directions, and other factual messages should be presented as clearly and concisely as possible in any given situation. By incorporating these habits into an everyday routine, the medical assistant ensures that miscommunication will be a rarity.

other groups served are invited to speak to the office staff about practices in their culture. Perhaps the best advice, however, is that the medical assistant who is in doubt about how certain signals may be interpreted should simply avoid making informal nonverbal gestures such as the "thumbs-up" sign or pointing a finger at a person, in exactly the same way he would avoid those actions in any formal situation. The assistant should act in a responsible, professional manner at all times. Informal gestures, remarks, or slang are not considered appropriate in a medical setting.

Cultural differences may also affect how a patient approaches healthcare. Some cultures believe it is a sign of weakness to admit to pain. This makes it difficult to diagnose a patient's health problem. In some cultures, the extended family may insist on accompanying a patient into the examination room or to the hospital. Some cultures are strong believers in homeopathic or folk remedies, or ritualized healing ceremonies; people from these cultures may harbor deep suspicions about Western medicine and thus be resistant to drug therapies or invasive treatments.

Other aspects of cultural background that affect how a patient approaches healthcare include the accustomed level of formality and perception of time. U.S. culture is relatively casual and egalitarian. Medical staff members are trained to speak to patients with efficient, direct language. We tell the patient, for instance: "Please urinate in this cup." Such frank directness may embarrass and offend patients from cultural backgrounds where indirection or more subtle language is the norm. Perception of time also can be a troublesome difference between cultures. Here in the United States, we expect a patient to arrive on time for his appointment or perhaps even a few minutes early. In fact, a patient who is ten minutes late may lose that appointment, especially if there is no good excuse for his tardiness. However, other cultures perceive time in much different ways. For some cultures, a 2 o'clock appointment really "means" arriving at 2:15, 2:30, or

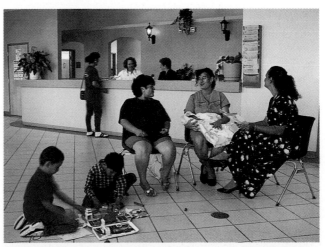

Treating all patients with respectful professionalism will minimize problems resulting from varied cultural backgrounds.

While these brief comments about language and cultural differences make clear that they are key aspects of patient-caretaker communication, it is important for you as a medical assistant never to assume that all people from a certain background will exhibit the same responses. Do not rely on **stereotypes** or generalizations when interacting with someone from another culture, race, or ethnic group, but as much as possible be intent on treating each person as an individual. Be sensitive to sources of miscommunication. If you think you have done or said something that has offended someone, be direct in asking that person if indeed this is the case. Most people are more than willing to forgive or explain misunderstandings if they know the other person is making a sincere effort to understand and remedy mistakes.

Here are some additional suggestions for improving cross-cultural communication:

- Pay attention to what your patients' nonverbal signals—their body language, facial expressions, tone of voice, and eye contact—are communicating.
- Be open-minded toward people who do things differently from you. Try to understand why these differences might be occurring.
- Follow the example of your patient regarding formality, distance when speaking, and touch. Base your response on the other person's comfort level with these factors.
- Be aware that gestures and expressions you commonly use may not have the same meaning for others as they do for you.
- Create an unhurried atmosphere by giving the necessary time to listen carefully to a patient who does not speak English fluently. Arrange for a translator, if necessary.
- Speak clearly and note signs of patient comprehension.
- Use pictures and diagrams when needed to get your message across.
- Learn as much as you can about the language, cultural background, and expectations of the people you serve.

We have only touched on some of the many factors illustrating ways diversity can affect patient-healthcare worker communication and the way a person responds to healthcare. As we have seen, a person's age, gender, economic status, disability, and language and cultural background are some of the factors involved when considering patient differences. Such differences lend richness to the medical assistant's job, especially when he regards each patient he treats as a unique individual. On any given day, his first patient may be a 20-year-old African American Marine with a skin rash, his second a 90-year-old Serbian woman complaining of dizziness, and his third a 3-year-old malnourished child accompanied by her homeless mother. It is absolutely essential that the medical assistant respect, appreciate, and strive to understand the differences affecting communication and response in the people he serves.

One of the great strengths of American culture is its diversity. Today, we rightly celebrate such diversity, and all people, especially professionals who serve the public, must work to understand the backgrounds, habits, and customs of the people with whom they interact. Understanding others—seeing the situation from their point of view—is the basis of **empathy,** an all-important quality that you as a medical assistant must develop. By striving to increase your understanding of cultural and language differences, you can greatly increase the quality of your work and the satisfaction you find in meeting others' needs.

Avoiding Prejudice in the Medical Office

Prejudice refers to unreasonable feelings, opinions, or attitudes directed against others. It usually involves one person's need to feel superior to another. Prejudice often leads to **discrimination**, the treating of a person or group unfairly based on age, gender, race, religion, sexual orientation, handicap, country of origin, cultural background, or other characteristic. Prejudice in the

---

Cultural Differences

Did you know that:

- In Japan, to be diagnosed with cancer is often considered shameful and a death sentence.
- Many Koreans refrain from laughing or smiling because they believe it makes them appear unintelligent.
- In the Middle East, it is common for people to stand much closer together when conversing than in the United States.
- Many Asians would never consider sending their aging or ill parents or grandparents to a long-term-care facility. Instead, the elderly person would be cared for by the family, in the home.

Remember that while all these statements are generally true, any individual you meet may be an exception.

medical office is completely unacceptable. It can interfere with medical care and cause friction among the staff. Our attitudes influence our actions and can be quickly discerned by others.

If we are honest with ourselves, we may discover that certain types of people trigger feelings of dislike, resentment, or scorn in us even though we do not think of ourselves as prejudiced. For example, we may have trouble showing empathy for the patient who weighs 350 pounds and is complaining of fatigue and chronic lower back pain. Secretly, we may say to ourselves: "Well, no wonder! Why doesn't he just lose weight and his problems will go away? He must be too lazy to go on a diet." In fact, such "hidden" prejudice is common to many people. Expression of prejudice is never acceptable. The medical assistant should be sensitive to her own sources of prejudice, try to understand where those prejudicial feelings may have come from, and act to develop new habits that eliminate the prejudice. It is important to approach all patients with compassion and not to allow prejudice to affect your professional responsibilities.

Legal Issue

The Civil Rights Act of 1964 and its 1972 amendments make it illegal to discriminate in the workplace because of race, color, national origin, religion, gender, age, handicap, or family status.

Prejudice usually results from stereotyping or "grouping" people rather than knowing and appreciating them as individuals. We often absorb prejudiced feelings toward certain groups from our family, our friends, or our culture. When you sense negative feelings about a person because of her physical appearance, her disability, her religion, her sexual preference, or her race, pause and ask yourself where you might have acquired those negative ideas about an entire group of people. Did a family member joke about them or make derogatory remarks? Have you heard members of that group "put down" in the media such as by a radio DJ? Ask yourself what you have actually experienced in your interactions with such people. Did you have a negative encounter with a person of a certain race or culture that has now made you feel prejudiced toward all people of that race or culture, or have you, in reality, had little or no experience with such people? Distinguish between fact and opinion, reality and stereotype. Recommit yourself to treating all people as individuals, with dignity, compassion, and respect. Challenge yourself to "walk a mile in the other person's shoes." Try to imaginatively see things from the viewpoint of members of that group and experience life the way they do. In your on-the-job interactions with others, take advantage of opportunities to learn something new about those people whose culture, beliefs, or lifestyle may be unfamiliar to you. Try to find common ground with all people you serve, and then enjoy learning about the differences among you!

Building Strong Communication Skills and Techniques

Although nearly all humans can communicate on some level, the breakdown of communication among people has led to tremendous pain and destruction in our society and our world. At least some of the blame for high divorce rates and for ethnic wars, for instance, can be attributed to poor or hostile communication among individuals or countries. In any profession, an individual with excellent communication skills is a highly valued employee.

Once you are on the job, you will find that daily practice will help you improve your communication skills over time. The medical assistant must work to gain expertise in key techniques of communication such as active listening, questioning, assertiveness, timing, feedback and observation, and precise writing. Although you already use these techniques in your everyday interactions with others, do not take for granted your ability to apply these competencies skillfully in your work with patients and colleagues in the medical office. You should constantly try to improve your skills in each of these areas.

Active Listening

Have you ever known a person who talks constantly but never seems to listen to what others have to say? Or a person who appears to be listening but really isn't? Hearing is not the same as listening. **Active listening**—consciously seeking to understand what another person is expressing—is a necessary skill in

Working Smart

All professional work environments have a clearly defined policy against all forms of discrimination. Make sure you know what that policy states, and abide by its code of behavior. Use respectful language with everyone with whom you interact, and object firmly to any racist or sexist jokes or other remarks. They cannot be tolerated in the workplace.

the medical setting. What the patient tells you is essential to his treatment. In active listening, the other person has your undivided attention. You maintain eye contact with the person and do not interrupt him when he speaks. You ask questions to elicit further information or get clarification if necessary. A variant to active listening, known as **reflective listening**, can also help communication. In reflective listening, the listener also repeats or restates what the patient says back to him to confirm your mutual understanding of what is being communicated. This brief dialogue illustrates an example of reflective listening:

> *Patient:* "This is my first pelvic exam and I'm nervous. My friends told me it will hurt really bad."
> *Medical Assistant:* "Your friends told you about their experiences and now you're nervous about your own exam?"
> *Patient:* "That's right."

Active and reflective listening can lead the medical assistant to a better understanding of the concerns and mental outlook of the patient. In addition, use of these techniques helps the assistant communicate empathy to her patient. As discussed in Chapter 1, "Choosing a Career as a Medical Assistant," empathy is an awareness of and insight into another person's feelings and behavior. It is an important component of active listening. Through listening empathetically, you can put yourself in another person's shoes and understand her viewpoint even though you may not agree with it.

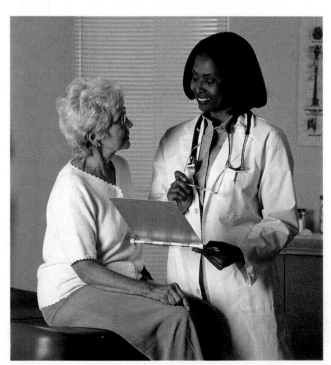

Active listening includes eye contact and giving the speaker your undivided attention.

Showing the patient that you understand her builds trust in the relationship.

Questioning

Another way to practice good communication skills is by paying attention to the way you ask the patient questions. There are two basic types of questions: closed-ended and open-ended. **Closed-ended questions** can be answered with a short, definitive reply. For example, "When did you first notice the nausea?" can be answered with "last night" or "two weeks ago." **Open-ended questions**, on the other hand, encourage the patient to elaborate on her statements and reveal more details. They encourage more substantial patient feedback, which is often a necessity in diagnosing a patient's illness. For example, in response to the question, "Can you tell me how this problem began?" a patient might say, "Last week I ate at a fast food restaurant because I was upset after my boss yelled at me. I don't usually eat food like that, and I haven't felt the same since. I've had stomach cramps and nausea every day since then. I'm sure it began in that restaurant!" When asking open-ended questions, use phrases like "explain to me," "tell me about," or "describe for me" to elicit information from patients in a non-threatening, conversational manner. In this way, the patient will not feel as if he is being cross-examined and will be comfortable enough to tell his story.

When interviewing a patient, also bear in mind that the distance between you and the patient can affect the success of your communication. Positioning yourself at about arms' length from the patient conveys the message that the other person has your complete attention and interest. Your body language should indicate openness and acceptance. Maintain some eye contact with the patient even as you write your notes on the chart. Never rush a patient, and do not stand up to leave before the interview is over. Doing so will only communicate impatience and lack of caring to the patient.

Assertiveness

Displaying confidence without being aggressive or defensive is an important aspect of communication with other members of the healthcare team as well as with patients. **Assertiveness** is the firm, honest expression of information and opinions, and involves standing up for what you believe. It also involves taking necessary action when action is needed. It is the opposite of fear or hesitancy. Defined in this way, assertiveness does not involve an aggressive or overbearing attitude; one can—and should—be gentle, calm, and assertive at the same time in the medical setting. Assertiveness when dealing with patients helps

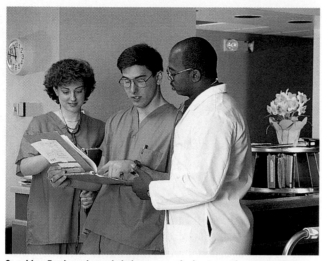

Speaking firmly and openly helps ensure the best care for your patients.

gain their respect and helps focus communication on the necessary issues. It can also be crucial when helping educate patients about their healthcare. Moreover, assertiveness with other members of the healthcare team is also important when you as the medical assistant are concerned about a patient's care. When the patient's health is at stake, you need to bring this concern to the attention of the provider in an assertive manner. In more serious cases, the medical assistant might notice a possible error in the patient's diagnosis or treatment. Whenever a patient's health is in jeopardy, it is the medical assistant's responsibility to convey the situation to the attending physician immediately. By speaking and acting assertively, the assistant contributes her best effort to the healthcare team and ensures her patients the best possible care.

Timing

Timing is yet another important consideration in your communication with others. When you wish to convey a message to another person, true communication cannot take place unless that person is receptive to your message. A person who is not in the mood to receive your message will not listen to or understand it, and your attempt at communication is futile. When dealing with both patients and coworkers, this often means you should pause to consider whether the time is right to speak, or whether delaying your message a bit might improve communication. For example, you would not admonish a coworker for not cleaning up a minor spill in the staff lounge on her first day back from leave to attend her mother's funeral. You would not counsel a patient on weight control when he arrives at the clinic with chest pain and fears that he is having a heart attack. You would not discuss birth control methods with a teen-aged girl who arrives at

your office scared and alone with an unwanted pregnancy. In each of these examples, it is best to wait until the situation is stabilized and the receiver is calmer to convey your message. There are many such examples of the need for timing in communication in the medical office. As a medical assistant, you will soon develop an intuitive and common sense approach to picking the best time for patient teaching, problem-solving with colleagues, and assertiveness.

Feedback and Observation

When sending a message, you can never be sure it has been understood unless you get the right feedback. This may be either oral or nonverbal; that is, the receiver may reply to you in words or in actions. For example, if you tell a patient the doctor has ordered an injection, and he rolls up his sleeve, the patient's nonverbal response tells you your message was understood. To obtain oral feedback, especially after giving instructions or explanations, it sometimes helps to ask the patient to repeat the information to make sure he understands the most critical aspects of what you have said. You might also ask the patient follow-up questions about your teaching. Clarification of your message may be necessary. For example, imagine that you need to tell a patient she must not drink alcohol while taking a particular drug because of the risk of an adverse reaction. Because this information is vital to her health, you might then ask, "What can't you do while taking this drug?" If the patient cannot answer, the information must be repeated and more feedback sought.

As you speak with patients, watch for the nonverbal cues they give you. Learn to be a careful observer. A patient's body language and facial expressions, for instance, may not be compatible with her words. If this seems to be the case, you need to ask open-ended questions to try to accurately understand the patient's response. For example, if you begin the conversation by asking, "How are you feeling today?" the patient might answer, "Okay." However, you notice that her eyes are red and swollen as if she has been crying. You could then say, "You seem upset. Would you like to talk about what's bothering you?" Careful observation of your patient's communication will help you become a more skillful, more compassionate communicator.

Precise Writing

We have now explored several techniques of oral and nonverbal communication: listening, questioning, assertiveness, timing, and feedback and observation. Along with oral and nonverbal communication skills, excellent written communication skills are also important in the medical office. The medical assistant should be concerned about her writing and strive to improve it, because inaccurate or confusing writing in the medical setting not only irritates others but also may well lead to harmful patient care.

Although the medical assistant will often be responsible for many kinds of writing, including memos, e-mails, and educational materials, in her daily work she is mostly responsible for maintaining the patient's chart and other records. It is of paramount importance that what she writes on these records be clear, brief, and accurate. Mechanical matters such as spelling, grammar, and punctuation must be correct, for errors in these aspects of writing can lead to misunderstanding in the same way that inaccurate technical documentation can. Consider the following example from a medical assistant's writing on a patient's chart: "Patient complains of ake in stomach now hurts more last week." The spelling and sentence structure errors in this sentence make it difficult to read and obscure the meaning for other members of the healthcare team. A better-written statement would read: "Patient complains of a stomach ache that hurts more this week than last week."

Here is another example of how even a misplaced comma can obscure a record's meaning and lead to miscommunication. A medical assistant writes on a patient's chart: "Patient complains of joint pain and throbbing, headache." Does the patient have throbbing pain in her joints, or does she have a throbbing headache? Because of the placement of the comma, it is hard to tell. Probably, the sentence should read, "Patient complains of joint pain and throbbing headache." Guessing cannot be tolerated in a medical office where accurate documentation is critical to patient care and is, moreover, a legal issue. The medical assistant should strive at all times for exceptionally clear, accurate, and to-the-point writing, and should seek instruction if she needs additional help in this area of communication. Figure 4.3 is an example of a clear note added to a patient's chart.

Figure 4.3
Example of Precise Writing in a Patient's Chart

beyond the immediate office setting). For effective interaction with each of these different types of customer, the medical assistant needs to build specific skills in effective, sensitive communication. Such communication will establish trust and respect between the patient and the medical assistant and between the medical assistant and her colleagues, both internal and external. Let us now look at each of these types of customers and how the medical assistant can communicate with them effectively.

Communicating with Patients and Their Families

Today's medical practice emphasizes the patient's active participation in his own healthcare. Therefore, to make wise choices, the patient must be fully informed about his condition, treatment options, complications that may occur, and what he may expect if he refuses prescribed treatment. Armed with this knowledge, the patient can determine what his options are and decide on a course of action. You as the medical assistant can do much to alleviate the patient's anxiety and communicate the information he needs in a way he thoroughly understands. Your goal in working with your patient is to meet his needs on an individual basis. These patient communication techniques should help you achieve this goal:

Legal Issue
The patient's medical file is a legal document that must clearly and accurately record the treatment provided.

Communicating Effectively with Customers

Within the healthcare setting, a unique relationship is established between the healthcare providers and patients, and between coworkers on the healthcare team. As we have seen in Chapter 1, the medical assistant should consider each person she interacts with in her daily work as a customer. Her customers are both internal (patients, their families, office coworkers) and external (members of the larger healthcare team

- Be warm and friendly in both your speech and your nonverbal interaction with the patient. These qualities go a long way in inspiring a patient's confidence in you and in the healthcare he receives.
- Strive to make each patient feel important.
- Be absolutely sure the information you give the patient is accurate. If he asks a question you cannot answer, do not guess. Be honest. Tell him you don't know the answer but will find out for him. Then, follow through and do it.
- Show confidence and assertiveness in dealing with the patient. Patients appreciate caregivers who

know what they are doing. Over time, you will gain the confidence and expertise that puts patients at ease.

- Avoid minimizing the patient's source of anxiety, no matter how trivial the concern may appear to you.
- Take the time to explain procedures to the patient. Give her an overview of the procedures, and tell her why they are necessary. This will help relieve the patient's stress.
- Your positive attitude will encourage the patient to accept instructions or procedures he may be uneasy about.
- Ask the patient for feedback to be sure she is listening and understands what you are saying. For example, ask her to repeat back essential instructions, or ask follow-up questions about your teaching.
- Praise positive behavior. Patients look to healthcare professionals for guidance and support in health and wellness issues such as weight loss, smoking cessation, and medication regimen compliance.

By following these guidelines, you will soon become skilled at communicating with your patients. You will be able to quickly set them at ease, and they will be more comfortable with you in revealing information about their health problems. You will thus be in the

Customer Service

The medical assistant may be responsible for developing written information that can reinforce or back up oral instructions or explanations. Handouts, brochures, and other materials help prevent misunderstandings by clarifying instructions and answering questions the patient may have after leaving the medical office. Here are some topics for handouts you may wish to have available for patients in your office:

- instructions on preparing for treatments or lab tests
- possible side effects of medications
- post-surgery instructions
- information on specific medical conditions
- wellness promotion, such as smoking cessation, fitness, nutrition, and birth control

The physician should review all educational material before it is made available to patients.

Ethical Issue

To protect a patient's privacy, do not discuss details of his health with his family or friends without the patient's permission.

best possible position to be an active participant in their healthcare.

Often, a patient visits your office accompanied by a spouse, family member, or friend. You should always acknowledge a companion's presence with a pleasant greeting. The patient has the option of choosing whether the other person will accompany her into the examining room. In every case, the patient's preference is the most important factor. Honor the request, unless the physician directs otherwise. Communicate with a family member or friend in the room in the same manner you use with the patient. Be warm, open, clear, firm, and responsive to questions but be careful not to let the person accompanying the patient turn your attention away from the patient and in a sense "become a patient." The medical visit must focus on the health needs of the patient.

You should be aware that there are certain instances in which the patient should be seen alone by you and the physician in the examining room. For example, a patient with a controlling, or perhaps even abusive, spouse may be too intimidated to disclose necessary information to the provider if that spouse accompanies the patient into the examination room. Be sensitive to such situations and strongly urge, if necessary, that the spouse remain in the waiting room.

Finally, keep in mind that unless a family member or friend has been involved in the physician's examination of the patient, the medical assistant must never discuss details of the patient's illness with that other person. As with all healthcare workers, the medical assistant should be extremely careful in abiding by the rules of patient confidentiality.

Communicating with Internal Customers: Physicians, Nurses, and Other Coworkers

The medical assistant's communication skills must extend to all other internal customers. These include physicians, nurses, other medical assistants, laboratory technicians, and office coworkers. Since all staff members have the same primary goal—optimal patient care—effective communication among them is extremely important in reaching that goal.

As a medical assistant, your relationship with your supervisor is different from your relationship with other coworkers. For one thing, your supervisor is also your evaluator: She is in a position to judge how you do your job, and she will give you a formal, written and/or oral evaluation of your progress at regular intervals. Your raises and any possible promotions will be based on these evaluations. Your supervisor is also often your most important teacher. You can learn a great deal from her about how to become expert at your job. Go to your supervisor first when you are unclear about how to carry out a task, when you do not understand what is expected of you, or with other questions about your work. In addition, schedule time with her periodically to communicate in an open and relaxed manner about any suggestions you have or concerns that arise. Keep her informed of how things are going for you. By establishing regular lines of communication with your supervisor, you will develop a better understanding of your role in the office and how to perform your duties more skillfully.

In most medical offices, the medical assistant's primary responsibility is to act as a link between the physician and the patient. Because the assistant often does the initial intake of the patient, conducts the patient interview, and performs general screening tests, such as taking weight and blood pressure measurements, the patient often feels more comfortable talking to the medical assistant than to the doctor. The physician, however, bears the full responsibility for the treatment of the patient. It is therefore essential that the medical assistant learn how to convey the pertinent information obtained from the patient to the physician in a precise, brief, yet accurate manner. If you have specific concerns about a patient, be sure to mention them to the physician before she sees the patient. As with your supervisor, you may also wish to set a specific time at regular intervals to discuss with the physician any suggestions or concerns you have about patient care or administrative matters. This will allow you to get to know the physician more informally and will help establish good communication between you.

In the medical office, staff members come from a variety of backgrounds. In some instances, conflicts may develop because of differences in habits, values, and personalities among coworkers who must work closely together in a busy setting. Here are some helpful guidelines to avoid this friction and assure positive communication between you and your coworkers:

- Never gossip or make uncomplimentary statements about a coworker.
- Be polite and friendly to all members of the office staff.
- Remember to say *please* and *thank you.*

- Keep your work space neat and organized. Do not violate others' personal space or property.
- Be willing to help a coworker when needed even though the task may not be your responsibility.
- Make sure you bear your share of the workload and carry out all your duties completely and responsibly.
- Use tact and diplomacy when trying to resolve problems.
- Avoid arguments by speaking calmly and respectfully to others at all times. Never let anger or defensiveness into your communication, as this will only trigger anger and defensiveness in the other person.
- Do not let issues that bother you fester. Be assertive about your feelings and opinions, and be open to discussing them.
- Be willing to compromise, if necessary.
- Do not judge others.

Just as it is important to use appropriate names and titles of respect with patients, it is also important to use correct names and titles when speaking to your coworkers or when referring to external customers. Always address others by the name and title they prefer, and make it a point to ask what is preferred if you do not know. In most offices, the physician will be addressed as "Doctor." Moreover, when you speak to patients about certain members of the healthcare team, make sure you use their titles with their names, such as "Doctor Smith," "Nurse Wu," or "Medical Assistant Peter Barnes," so that the patient better understands these individuals' roles in her healthcare.

As we have discussed in Chapter 2, both intradepartmental and interdisciplinary healthcare teams exist within the medical setting. For a team to work together to achieve its goal of excellent patient care, members of the team must be skilled in communicating with others, and the team should meet regularly as a group to exchange information and ideas. Each team member has a significant and unique contribution to make to the group, and, therefore, each member must be encouraged to speak her mind freely and know that her ideas are welcome. As a team member, the medical assistant should voice her suggestions and concerns assertively in the group and should listen respectfully and actively to those of others. She should adopt a positive approach toward change and new ideas and be open to **constructive criticism** of her work, the positive or negative feedback from others that will help her improve. These are some suggestions for communicating well together as a team:

- Respect group norms and culture. Most office teams have norms or rules that govern appropriate behavior for their members, and you must first accept or adapt to those norms before effecting needed change.

■ Understand group roles. When working as a team, it is important to understand not just your own role in the group dynamic but also the role of every other member. For what duties is each person responsible? Is there a "harmonizer" who tries to help others reach a compromise if there is disagreement? Are additional roles needed for smooth and effective interaction?

■ Take turns participating. Everyone should have a chance to say what is on his or her mind. Some people will naturally talk more than others, but a gentle reminder that everyone should contribute will let more voices be heard.

■ Help foster a positive, professional **group climate**. This refers to the degree of warmth or coolness group members feel toward each other. A warm group climate is achieved by encouraging every team member to speak, by listening carefully to others, by supporting others' ideas, by empathizing with others, by treating them as equals, and by remaining open to new ideas and information. Many professional groups develop a type of "ice-breaker" activity to warm the group up. Such activities take only a few minutes and have proven to go a long way in setting a positive and friendly tone for the remainder of the meeting. One such "ice-breaker" is having members take turns in relating one "good thing" that happened to them since the previous meeting. This "check in" time provides an opportunity for each group member to share feelings about work or personal life and promotes group bonding and team spirit.

As a medical assistant, remember that while you have certain duties and responsibilities that are unique to your job, you are also part of a team of medical practitioners who are working together toward a common goal. To be an effective member of the healthcare team, you must learn to communicate skillfully with all other team members.

Communicating with External Customers

The medical assistant encounters numerous occasions that require interaction, either in person, over the telephone, or by e-mail, with professionals outside the immediate office environment. These external customers are also members of the extended healthcare team. They provide you with information and services that are necessary for treating patients. Such outside customers include laboratories, school clinics, drug and medical supply companies, and social and mental

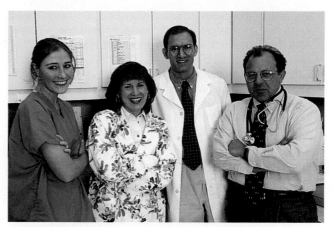

A warm, supportive atmosphere helps turn a group into a team.

health services such as child protection agencies or grief counselors. When communicating with these external professionals, you must first understand their roles in the field and how the resources they provide interact with your medical office. When the laboratory calls with results from a patient's test, for example, the medical assistant should be aware of how critical the information is and what action should be taken. She should also know whose responsibility it is to take the call, document any abnormal results, and call the patient with the information. She should follow through exactly with the physician's or nurse's requests about receiving such outside information. For example, the physician may tell you she is waiting for a call from a child protection agency and that she wants you to interrupt her to take the call even if she is in the exam room. Most physicians, however, do not want to be interrupted for a routine or less essential call such as one from a medical supply company.

When communicating with all external customers, be aware that your attitude and manner reflect on not only yourself but also the office in which you work. At all times, be pleasant, courteous, respectful, and helpful in your interactions with others.

Clinical Summary

■ Precise and accurate communication in the medical office is crucial to effective and safe patient care.

■ Communication can be oral, written, or nonverbal.

■ Stress can be a barrier to communication with patients and coworkers.

■ Nonverbal signals such as gestures and eye contact convey strong messages to others.

■ A patient's response to treatment often depends on diversity factors such as age, gender, economic status, disability, or culture.

■ Cultural and lifestyle diversity among patients and staff plays a significant role in the communication process.

- The lack of a common language may be a substantial obstacle to communication and may require use of an interpreter.
- Prejudice can interfere with medical care and cause friction among staff members.
- Strong communication skills can be built by using techniques of active listening, questioning, assertiveness, timing, feedback and observation, and precise writing.
- Active listening involves giving the other person your undivided attention, looking directly at her or him, clarifying what was said to be sure there is no misunderstanding, and responding to feedback.
- Open-ended questions invite the patient to reveal more information than closed-ended questions.
- Feedback is the best indicator of whether the message received was the same as the message sent.
- Using written material to back up oral information helps answer questions and prevent misunderstandings.
- The medical assistant should work to build strong communication with all internal and external customers.

The Language of Medicine

active listening A form of listening in which a person listens closely to what another says with few interruptions, seeking to understand what is being communicated.

assertiveness Displaying assurance and confidence without being aggressive.

closed-ended questions Questions that elicit a short, definitive answer.

communication The exchange of thoughts, opinions, or information between two or more people.

constructive criticism Criticism aimed at helping a person perform better.

cope To manage or adapt to a situation.

culture Ways of living developed by a group of people and passed down from one generation to another.

discrimination Acting toward others in a prejudiced manner; treating one group or person differently than another.

diversity Variety; the state of being different.

empathy An attitude marked by conscious awareness of and insight into another person's actions and behavior. Understanding and being sensitive to another person's feelings.

ethnicity The cultural or racial background of a people or country.

feedback The oral or nonverbal response of one person to another person's actions or words.

group climate The atmosphere or comfort level in a group of people or a team.

nonverbal communication Messages that are sent and received without using spoken words.

open-ended questions Questions asked in a way that invites the receiver to respond at length.

oral communication Communication using spoken words.

prejudice Unreasonable feelings, opinions, or attitudes directed against others.

reflective listening A type of active listening in which the listener asks the speaker questions that mirror the speaker's own statements.

stereotypes The mistaken concept that all members of a cultural, ethnic, or other group are the same and lack substantial individual differences.

stress Physical and/or psychological tension caused by events or situations.

Signs/Symptoms of Progress

1 Recall, Question, Connect

Recall
Identify at least three factors about a patient that may affect communication in the medical office.

Question
What questions do you have about your role as a medical assistant when these factors affect communication?

Connect
Explain the connection between your successful communication with the patient and effective treatment by the physician.

2 Educating the Patient

Jane Freeman is a 19-year-old who has just been diagnosed with diabetes. The doctor tells you to instruct her in administering her own insulin injections. Jane tells you she is afraid of shots and cannot stick herself with a needle.
1 How might you use oral, nonverbal, and written communication skills to relieve her anxiety and complete the instruction?
2 How can you determine whether she understands what you have taught her?

3 Exploring Perspectives in Teams

Perspective involves the discipline of examining how ideas look from different points of view and recognizing that there are often multiple "answers" to complex questions. In small groups or on your own, reflect on possible alternative views or answers and summarize your findings.
1 How do culture and language affect the way different groups think and act? Propose three examples and then discuss whether you think each of them involves stereotyping and/or prejudicial thinking, or represents genuine cultural differences.
2 Write a paragraph summarizing an incident from your own experience involving oral or nonverbal miscommunication. Discuss the incident and offer at least two alternative explanations for the miscommunication.
3 Consider this scenario: Your coworker shows a strong prejudice against the two American Indians on the staff. You think her behavior is obvious and that your boss should confront her. When you talked to your boss, she said that things will work out over time as the coworkers get to know each other better. Six months have passed, and things have gotten worse. What should you say to your boss? What if the prejudiced person were your boss, not your coworker?

Learning Outcomes

- Identify the emerging disease conditions and challenges that face the medical community today.

- Summarize the emerging technologies and therapies designed to diagnose and treat new diseases.

- State why the field of biomedical ethics is receiving increased attention.

- Discuss several types of alternative therapies included in National Center for Complementary and Alternative Medicine's designation "alternative systems of medical practice," such as acupuncture, ayurveda, and homeopathy.

- Describe several forms of mind-body therapy used in today's healthcare environment.

Performance Objectives

- Adhere to ethical principles.
- Adapt to change.
- Enhance skills through continuing education.

The twenty-first century promises to be an exciting and challenging one for healthcare practitioners. As a medical assistant, you will encounter a variety of emerging trends, and you must learn to expect and adapt to rapid change. This chapter explores some of these trends and describes their impact on the medical community. As we discussed in Chapter 2, "Working in Today's Healthcare Environment," the U.S. population is growing older and more ethnically diverse, and this shift in demographics will require substantial changes in the healthcare delivery system. In addition, although many diseases have been conquered, new medical threats including new viruses and resistant strains of bacteria are on the rise. Yet even as such new threats emerge, powerful new research, diagnostic, and surgical technologies are also being developed. Genetic research, brain research, and cancer research are particular areas to watch for rapid advances over the next several decades.

chapter 5

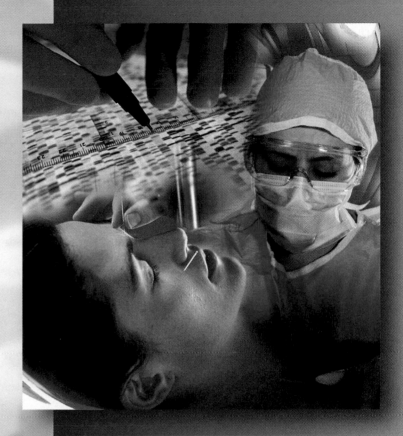

Scanning the Future: Emerging Trends

Another important trend in medicine today is the rise of alternative and holistic therapies. Americans are increasingly interested in these therapies as alternatives or complements to traditional Western medicine, and all healthcare workers need to be aware of their impact on the traditional approach to healthcare delivery.

Clearly, many challenges and opportunities lie ahead for the medical community, and all healthcare workers, including medical assistants, must be prepared to undertake the continuing education needed to keep abreast of these exciting advances.

Explosive Changes in Modern Medicine

Chapter 1, "Choosing a Career as a Medical Assistant," provided a quick tour through some landmarks in the history of medicine. Before we consider the challenges facing the healthcare industry in the future, let us return to aspects of that history to give us some helpful perspective. As we review the history of medicine, we must give credit for major advances to a diverse group of scientists and healers. Hippocrates of ancient Greece is considered the "father" of modern medicine; he was one of the first individuals to teach that diseases are natural processes, not caused by magic or the influence of demonic spirits. As technology improves, we continue to develop new ways to learn about and practice medicine. As new diseases emerge, the world-wide medical community responds with research. Our knowledge of chemistry, biology, human physiology, and the origins and treatment of diseases has developed through many centuries of trial and error, experimentation, and cycles of advances and setbacks taking place in many countries.

Conquered Diseases of the Twentieth Century

In 1546, the Italian researcher Girolamo Fracastoro suggested that sickness was caused by tiny germs—particular kinds for each disease—that multiplied in the patient's body. However, his findings were ignored because he had no proof. A few generations later, with the introduction of the microscope in the early 1600s, people could actually observe tiny parasites and bacteria. However, most early scientists believed those microorganisms were merely symptoms of disease rather than its cause. In the late 1800s, Louis Pasteur proved that the air was full of tiny microbes, too small for the human eye to see. From this discovery, he concluded that germs floating through the air could spread contagious diseases.

The knowledge gained about the transmission of disease increased dramatically throughout the twenti-

eth century. The century witnessed such significant medical advances as the discovery of penicillin to combat bacterial infection, the formulation of insulin to control diabetes, and the development of a vaccine against polio.

Penicillin, the first antibiotic, was discovered by a young doctor named Alexander Fleming. In 1928, Fleming was working with a sample of staphylococcus. He left the cultures growing while on vacation, and on his return, noted a fuzzy circle of mold growing in one of the cultures. The staphylococcus surrounding the mold had died. From this beginning, several other scientists purified the substance that Fleming named penicillin, a substance not unlike the mold that grows on bread that is several days old.

Insulin for diabetes control was discovered by a team of scientists at the University of Toronto in 1921. Unlike infectious diseases, diabetes is not caused by a virus or by bacteria. A person with diabetes cannot metabolize glucose; his pancreas, the organ that produces a hormone to perform this action, does not work properly. The person's body tries but fails to get energy by converting fat into glucose, but eventually, without treatment, the person will lapse into a coma and die. Frederick Banting, Charles Best, James Collip, and John MacLeod discovered that the necessary pancreatic hormone could be reproduced by using the same hormone produced by animals. They called the substance insulin, and its discovery has saved the lives of millions of diabetics around the world.

On April 12, 1955, the American scientist Jonas Salk announced to a news conference of eager observers that a vaccine he had discovered prevented poliomyelitis, an infection of the intestinal tract that can progress to inflict paralysis and even death. Over the next decade, the dreaded childhood disease, polio, was all but eradicated from the Western Hemisphere. However, today the disease is still widespread in such Third World countries as India, where approximately 10,000 children are afflicted each year. The failure of recent efforts to immunize enough children in Bangladesh, Sri Lanka, and Pakistan have resulted in the continual spread of polio in this area.

These are just a few of the significant medical advances of the last century in controlling disease. As with all medical breakthroughs, these remarkable twentieth century medical advances and their continued refinements resulted from the persistent research of many, many scientists who combined their expertise to achieve these important goals.

Emerging Threats: New Viruses and Resistant Diseases

Even while medical advances have greatly reduced or eradicated certain diseases, new ones are emerging.

Over the past decade, many new viruses have been identified. These include Ebola Ivory Coast, Hepatitis G, and Black Lagoon. Some of these newly identified viruses cause devastating fatal diseases. Moreover, the growing urbanization that demographers predict for the twenty-first century will increase the already-dense concentrations of people in the large cities of less-developed countries. The potential is great for the birth of even more new viruses in locations where sanitation facilities and medical care are diminished.

The HIV virus is a particular worry. Although this virus is no longer new, it is now a growing threat to international health. This modern plague will certainly be with us for several generations despite major scientific and social advances in its detection, prevention, and treatment. By January of 2000, the AIDS epidemic had killed fifteen million people and left forty million others living with a viral infection that slowly but relentlessly erodes the immune system. In the United States and Europe, powerful drugs now exist that can extend life and improve its quality for AIDS patients. But for those in the developing world, the situation is much more bleak. By the year 2025, it is predicted that AIDS will be the major killer of young Africans, decreasing life expectancy to as low as forty years.

Another great concern of the medical community is that we are now also facing a number of resistant strains of formerly susceptible bacteria. The reason for this is the overuse of antibiotics. In the past, antibiotics were more commonly preemptively prescribed for upper respiratory infections even though such illnesses are frequently caused by viruses. Viruses do not respond to antibiotic treatment. However, bacteria pass through many generations in a matter of days or weeks, and defenses evolve rapidly. When bacteria are exposed to an antibiotic and survive the treatment, they evolve by mutating, thus becoming resistant to future attacks by that antibiotic. The inappropriate use of antibiotics has led to ever-more antibiotics becoming ineffective. Today, other treatments for symptomatic relief are being used because of fears about the overuse of antibiotics, which promotes the development of resistant strains. For example, when treating acute bronchitis, antibiotics are only prescribed for patients whose cough is persistent.

Emerging Technologies

Even as new diseases appear, new technologies designed to combat disease are also emerging. Today, the diagnosis of disease has become a finely tuned, highly precise pursuit. Current trends in medical research point to a growing reliance on so-called "smart" technology including sophisticated diagnostic, surgical, or health-monitoring tools. One example is the use of sleepwear to monitor infant sleep apnea. This sleepwear has technical circuitry embedded in it that senses when a baby is distressed and sends that message via a monitor to the parents' room.

SURGICAL TECHNOLOGIES The field of surgery has also undergone significant changes during recent decades. It was once standard for a physician to open

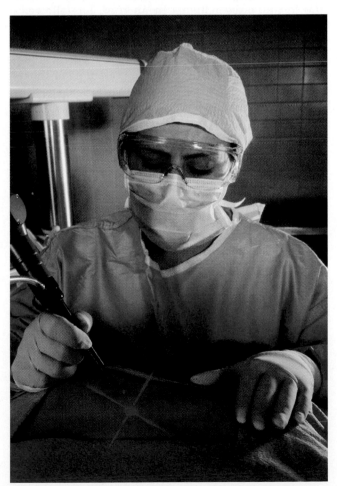

The development of laser techniques has allowed for less-invasive surgeries with shortened recovery times for patients.

the patient's abdomen surgically to see the operating field and perform the operation. Today, the physician is more likely to slide a miniature camera, light, and special tools through a small incision and watch his work on a television screen. Laser technology has turned microsurgery into a routine procedure. In some instances, doctors can perform "virtual" surgery by using remote-controlled robotic arms. A surgeon may also talk directly to the tools she or he is using through a voice recognition system, telling the instrument, for example, to move to the left or to apply more pressure. Engineers will soon perfect tools that let surgeons simulate an operation realistically—down to the resistance of skin against scalpel. These significant advances in surgical technologies have resulted in minimizing the trauma of large incisions, thereby reducing pain and recovery time. In turn, the trend toward doing more surgery with less cutting and much less bleeding has led to the redesign of operating rooms to accommodate the sophisticated technological equipment used.

DIAGNOSTIC TECHNOLOGIES Telemedicine, the use of video and computer technology to let physicians in one location see patients in another, has allowed a patient to access the care of a medical specialist without actually being in his or her presence. In a room with sophisticated TV cameras and medical equipment, a specialist can examine a patient even though the patient is in another city or country. The specialist views the patient and the patient's doctor on a video screen and can hear heartbeats or auscultatory sounds through stethoscopes wired to phone lines. During radiologic examinations, such as MRI or ultrasound, the specialist can also receive diagnostic information over long distances. In fact, the future of the on-call "cyberdoctor" has just begun, and the possibilities for effective use of such remote diagnostic tools are just now being imagined.

Furthermore, with the introduction of microtechnologies such as computer chips, diagnostic tools will only continue to become more precise and more comprehensive. Presently, researchers are working on what is called "nano technology," with "nano" representing a billionth part of a unit. In fact, a patient may someday soon be able to ingest a germ-sized robot that can travel through the body measuring vital signs and providing other data that can be analyzed for signs of disease.

New Research and Treatment Modalities

The more we know about an illness, the greater our potential for preventing and treating it. This is the premise behind all medical research. The following sections discuss several areas of modern medicine in which recent research has greatly enhanced our under-

standing of the workings of the human body and our potential for curing its illnesses. Throughout the twenty-first century, research will continue to shape diagnostic techniques, treatments, pharmacologic options, and the state of the medical practice itself.

GENETIC RESEARCH Our understanding of human physiology, chemistry, and microanatomy has expanded to include the largest portion of the human genetic map, usually called a **genome**. A genome is all of the DNA in an organism, including its genes. Many illnesses are caused by a defect in one **gene**, a single segment of the body's hereditary material. If undamaged copies of a defective gene could be introduced into the patient's body, the activity controlled by that gene could be corrected. Someday, gene-spliced medicines will be perfectly engineered to fit the needs of the individual patient. Unlike many traditional pharmacologic treatments, gene-based medicines do not just relieve symptoms but actually cure the condition. Eventually, researchers may be able to determine what proteins a defective gene is supposed to be making and replace just those proteins instead of replacing the whole gene. New drugs may be designed on computer screens using gene information as a blueprint.

In 1953, Francis Crick and James Watson demonstrated the double-helical structure of DNA. The order of DNA's base pairs forms a code specifying the structure of all proteins in every cell of an organism. This cracking of the genetic code has led to the Human Genome Project (HGP), formally begun in 1990. The goal of the HGP is to identify the 100,000 genes in the human DNA and to determine the sequence of the 3 billion chemical pairs that make up human DNA. The first mapping sequence of human chromosome 22 was completed in December 1999. In addition to sequencing the genes, the HPG is addressing the ethical, legal, and social issues that may arise from the availability of personal genetic information. The significance of this DNA work cannot be underestimated since scientists believe they will find that many more diseases are genetically linked than those they know of now.

With each new milestone reached, the science of genetics must reinvent itself. In the 1970s, genetic science was used to diagnose rare diseases that caused mental retardation and deforming physical handicaps.

Technology Tip
For information about the Human Genome Project, visit www.ornl.gov/hgmis.

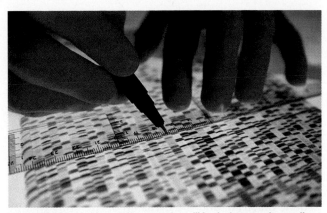

Information provided from DNA sequencing will be the key to understanding the structure, organization, and function of DNA in chromosomes. If used wisely, this knowledge will reap fantastic benefits for humankind.

In the 1980s, genetics led to new reproductive technologies for the prenatal diagnosis of both common and rare birth defects. In the 1990s, genetic tests were used for an ever-widening range of human conditions, including cancer, diabetes, heart disease, auto-immune disorders, premature aging, and Alzheimer's disease. In the twenty-first century, it will be possible to test every person for any number of deleterious effects imposed by his or her genetic code. These findings may then be recorded on a personalized computer chip and used to predict susceptibility to debilitating disorders. Genetic research will thus be able to help physicians in the early diagnosis of conditions affected by genetics, and will enable them to recommend gene therapy, genetically engineered pharmaceuticals, or other advanced techniques for mediating tissue and organ rejuvenation. In addition, it is expected that genetic science will be able to identify a person's predisposition to emotional or behavioral disorders, and allow specialists to treat such conditions early to ensure patients a healthy and satisfying life.

Finally, what might be the role of transplant and replacement surgery in the twenty-first century? Indeed, it is difficult even to imagine the range of regenerative possibilities that may be available for diseased organs or damaged or missing limbs. Increasingly, tissues from the breast, liver, skin, and nervous system can be grown in the lab and transplanted into patients. These astonishing developments may soon be as common to us as cataract or hip replacement surgery is now.

BRAIN RESEARCH As we have noted, the number of elderly individuals in this country is expected to double by the year 2025, and researchers project that the incidence of Alzheimer's disease and other age-related

Technology Tip

Visit these websites for up-to-date information on breast and colon disease: www.breastdisease.net, www.colondisease.net.

conditions will increase proportionally. Therefore, a key area of current research deals with the causes, prevention, and treatment of Alzheimer's disease. This research has found that in patients with the disease, certain plaques have developed that fill the brain's memory centers, resulting in misshapen proteins that cause brain damage. Stopping or reversing this process may result in delaying or preventing symptoms of the disease. In the future, this may be done effectively with gene or drug therapy. Research into a vaccine that targets these proteins and into other drugs that keep them from forming is progressing, and a strong possibility exists that by the time the population has aged substantially, drugs will be widely available to cure these neurologic diseases.

In another exciting development, discussion is proceeding about neural transplants and extending brain stem cell transplants for brain repair. Scientists are researching transplantation of embryonic tissue and big brain cells into humans for the treatment of Parkinson's, Alzheimer's, and Huntington's diseases. Amazingly, it was recently discovered that neural stem cells can grow into any kind of brain cell. The theory is that the cells, when injected into a damaged adult brain, will turn themselves into replacements for cells that are dead or diseased.

CANCER RESEARCH Much of the cancer research in recent decades has focused on how various cancers can be prevented or how certain populations can, at the very least, decrease the risk of developing cancer. Of course, we know that smoking can predispose an individual to a number of cancers. We now also know that excess animal fats may predispose people to colon cancer and that eating lots of vegetables and other fiber-rich foods may protect against the development of cancer. Extensive research has been done to determine if post-menopausal use of synthetic estrogen increases a woman's risk of breast cancer, even as it protects her from heart disease. The search for a cure for cancer continues. However, it is, in fact, unlikely that a single cure for all cancers will ever be found, since each type of cancer is unique. However, significant new developments in cancer treatment have recently evolved, and good reason exists to hope that by 2025, new drugs will be discovered that can suppress or even cure many common cancers.

For a cure to take place, though, a cancer must first be detected. As in all areas of medical science, the mapping of human genes increases the possibility of detecting the "cancer genes" specific to a particular type of cancer in a certain individual. Blood tests have been developed for the early detection of prostate cancer and ovarian cancer, and tests for breast disease, colon disease, and head and neck cancers are being developed. Furthermore, clinical trials are being conducted on a device that removes a sample of breast cells through the nipple to determine the presence of cancer. Soon, in fact, a fecal sample may be all that is needed to search for cells on their way to becoming colon cancers.

DRUGS AND VACCINES Despite medical advances, we still have a long way to go in eliminating infectious diseases. Though diseases such as measles and polio are now almost nonexistent in the United States because of widespread childhood vaccination, they still menace some developing countries. Malaria remains a concern in much of the developing world. The mosquito that carries the parasite that causes this disease has become resistant to the pesticides formerly used to control it, and the disease may, therefore, increase, especially with the worldwide rise in temperature due to global warming. Today, we desperately need a vaccine for malaria.

Cancer treatment, too, will improve with the use of new drug and gene therapies. Vaccines are being developed that use cancer cells to boost the body's immune system so that the body will be able to fight cancer. In the future, perhaps a gene might be "carried" by a virus into cancer cells, causing them to die. Or a drug that inhibits the growth of blood vessels may be able to cut off a tumor's blood supply, thus killing the cells and the tumor. Chemical inhibitors may also be introduced into the patient's bloodstream that will block the production of enzymes the tumors need to spread.

Perhaps the greatest change we will see in the research and development of new pharmacologic modalities is the genetic engineering of medicines and vaccines to fit each person's physical features. Most drugs and medicines have been designed to address the disease or the symptoms, not the health needs of the individual patient. However, we know that medicines, by themselves or when combined, cause adverse and potentially dangerous side effects for many people. The genetically engineered drugs of the future will be designed for the patient as an individual. Atenolol, for instance, a beta blocker used in treating hypertension and prescribed to heart patients, can cause serious kidney problems for some patients. A special version of atenolol designed to reduce the variance in effects on patients is just one example of treating the patient,

Technology Tip
Visit the National Bioethics Advisory Commission website at bioethics.gov/ cgi-bin/bioeth_counter.pl .

not the disease. These same drugs will increasingly replace the scalpel in the operating room.

Ethics and Social Policies

We as health professionals in the twenty-first century are clearly living in exciting times. We are on the verge of astonishing advances in the medical field, but together with these advances come new ethical issues as research and technology break barriers formerly thought to be unsurpassable, or even sacred. For example, the test tube baby, the elaboration and mapping of genetic material, and the invasion of the body by tiny neuron simulators present ethical dilemmas for both the researcher and the philosopher. What limits should be set? Who will suffer if we do or do not proceed? Is there such a thing as going "too far" in increasing medical capabilities? If so, what is "too far"? Is it desirable, for example, for humans to be able to "design" their children by using genetic material from fashion models or astronauts? Is it desirable to increase the human life span to well over 100 years when overpopulation and the possibility of resources unable to meet the needs of this population may pose real threats to the delivery of adequate healthcare? Genetic technology has been identified as a phenomenally vital resource in the detection and treatment of many diseases, but healthcare practitioners today, including the medical assistant, must be prepared to deal with the inevitable collision between scientific advances and society's moral and ethical values.

In fact, **biomedical ethics** was created as a field of academic study and research to ponder this intersection between science and morality. In addition, many hospitals and clinics have established committees on biomedical ethics. Some countries, as well, are forming national bioethics commissions to which national dilemmas in these areas could be referred, and which would suggest possible legislation or codes of professional conduct. The United States has already established a body of this kind.

The Rise of Alternative Therapies and Holistic Methods of Healing

While scientifically based diagnoses and treatments have dominated Western medicine for several hundred years, healthcare consumers in the United States have recently shown increasing interest in an array of alternative approaches to healthcare, including the practice of holistic healthcare. Such alternative therapies represent an emerging trend in today's healthcare environment. So widespread is this interest, in fact, that the U.S. National Institutes of Health (NIH) established the **National Center for Complementary and Alternative Medicine (NCCAM)** in 1991. This office is responsible for investigating holistic healthcare practices and other complementary and alternative therapies. As part of its investigation, NCCAM has categorized these therapies into specific fields of practice:

- alternative systems of medical practice, including traditional Asian medicine, ayurveda (a system of healing from India), homeopathy, naturopathic medicine, and environmental medicine
- mind-body medicine or bio-behavioral interventions such as biofeedback, relaxation, imagery, meditation, hypnosis, prayer, mental healing, art and music therapy, yoga, and t'ai chi ch'uan
- biofield and bioelectromagnetics, two distinct areas that explore how living organisms interact with electromagnetic fields for a variety of applications, including bone repair, wound healing, and immune system stimulation
- manipulative and body-based systems such as osteopathy, massage therapy, chiropractic, physical therapy, and therapeutic touch used as diagnostic and therapeutic tools
- biologically based therapies including drugs and vaccines not yet accepted in mainstream Western medicine
- lifestyle and disease prevention that focuses on practices designed to prevent the development of illnesses and to identify and treat health risk factors including lifestyle therapies such as diet and stress management that are applied in unconventional ways

Holistic healthcare is a term used for a type of comprehensive treatment that covers the patient's physical, emotional, social, economic, and spiritual needs. Many alternative therapies are holistic. Holistic healthcare emphasizes the fundamental wholeness and integrity of the individual and considers the body, mind, and spirit as inseparable and interdependent. In this type of healthcare, all behaviors, including health and illness, are viewed as manifestations of the life process of the whole person. The condition of health itself is considered a dynamic, constantly evolving state and not merely the absence of signs or symptoms of disease. In holistic healthcare, the individual is responsible for her own well-being. She is aware of her needs, and she makes choices about how to promote wellness and healing in

Technology Tip
Visit the NCCAM's website at altmed.od.nih.gov.

Working Smart
Consumer interest in alternative and holistic methods of healing is at an all-time high and will be a growing trend throughout the twenty-first century. Some hospitals, clinics, and universities are responding to this interest by opening special clinics that stress the integration of the mind and body in healthcare. Fairview-Riverside Medical Center in Minneapolis, for example, opened its Mind Body Spirit Clinic in 1999, providing such alternative healthcare services as acupuncture, massage, herbal remedies, and spiritual counseling.

each aspect of her life, choices that allow her to exert control over the direction of her life and health.

Although the concept of holistic healing has only recently emerged in the West, it has been an important aspect of other world cultures, especially certain Eastern cultures, for many thousands of years. Early healers treated their patients holistically, viewing them as both physical and spiritual beings. These early healthcare providers developed forms of healing that are in use today, such as acupuncture, meditation, massage, and herbal remedies. Hippocrates treated patients holistically. His philosophy of medicine, which was based on the close relationship between disease and the physical environment, was widely accepted until the advent of the germ theory of disease in the late nineteenth century. Although the understanding that diseases are caused by specific agents advanced the technologic aspects of healthcare delivery, it also resulted in fragmentation of the delivery system into a multitude of specialty practices. As a consequence, the holistic perspective and practice in treating and preventing illness was diminished.

Today, as consumer interest in holistic healthcare has grown, medical and allied health schools are beginning to take steps to include courses in these areas. These courses focus on various aspects of holistic treatment including acupuncture, massage therapy, therapeutic touch, homeopathy, and herbal medicine. Since the holistic philosophy promotes the well-being of the whole person, matters of faith and spirituality are also included in some of these courses.

Concern exists in both the educational and research environments that some holistic therapies are not based in science, are not proven, and may even harm patients.

However, because of increased consumer interest, healthcare providers must continue to seek additional knowledge about these holistic therapies, and insurance policies are beginning to include provisions for reimbursement of some of these services. The efficacy and safety of these new approaches to healthcare must continue to be researched and evaluated.

Let us now consider some of the therapies among the NCCAM categories. As you read each description, note that many of them are holistic, emphasizing the comprehensive healing of the patient and her role as an active player in maintaining a balance of body, mind, and spirit.

Alternative Medical Systems

As defined by NCCAM, alternative systems of medical practice include traditional Asian medicine, ayurveda, homeopathy, naturopathic medicine, and environmental medicine. Each of these is described below.

TRADITIONAL CHINESE MEDICINE: ACUPUNCTURE AND ACUPRESSURE Traditional Chinese Medicine (TCM), which is rooted in Chinese culture, has been practiced for many thousands of years. Like other alternative therapies, use of TCM is an emerging trend in the United States. The focus of Traditional Chinese Medicine is on prevention. In this practice, the patient takes responsibility for his or her own well-being, and the doctor serves as a role model and resource, providing guidance and offering help in the form of herbs, acupuncture, massage, and other therapies.

At the heart of Chinese medicine is the concept of *qi* (pronounced "kee"), which may be translated as "energy" or "life force." Shen Nung, the "father" of Chinese medicine, theorized that the body has energy forces running throughout it. This energy force known as *qi* exists in all essential life activities, including a person's spiritual, emotional, mental, and physical aspects. An individual's health is influenced by the flow of *qi* in the body in combination with the universal forces of *yin* and *yang*. *Yin* and *yang* represent opposing but complementary forces. All forces and elements in the universe may be categorized as either *yin* or *yang*: for example, cold and hot, female and male, passive and active. *Yin* and *yang* are constantly interacting and changing in relation to each other, and one or the other of these forces will predominate. The body, too, is seen as a complex system of interconnected *yin-and-yang* forces. Good health requires a balance of *yin* and *yang* throughout the body.

Qi travels throughout the body along **meridians**, or special pathways. The meridians, or channels, are the same on both sides of the body. There are fourteen main meridians running vertically up and down

the surface of the body. Of the 14 meridians, there are 12 on each side of the body. There are also two unpaired midline meridians. Connections between the meridians ensure that there is an even circulation of *qi* and a balance between *yin* and *yang*. If the flow of *qi* is insufficient, unbalanced, or interrupted, *yin* and *yang* become unbalanced, and illness may occur. If such an imbalance happens, a therapy is applied. Table 5.1 lists a variety of therapies that may be used in Traditional Chinese Medicine.

Many Americans are familiar with the form of traditional Asian healing called **acupuncture**. Acupuncture originated in the Far East over 5,000 years ago and has gained increasing attention in the West since the

Table 5.1 Therapies Used in Traditional Chinese Medicine

Therapy	Definition
Acupressure	stimulation of acupuncture points by applying direct pressure on *qi* meridian points with hands or fingertips
Acupuncture	insertion of thin needles at specific points on the body that relate to the *qi* meridians
Cupping	applying suction created by warming the air in a glass jar and placing the overturned jar over the part of the body requiring treatment; the vacuum dispels dampness, warms the *qi*, and reduces swelling
Diet	foods are organized into groups based on their energetic qualities such as heating, cooling, and moistening
Herbal remedies	use of over 3,000 herbs as well as animal and mineral substances
Massage	practiced on specific parts of the body associated with meridians to restore the balance of *qi*
Moxibustion	burning of a mound of the plant moxa (*Artemisia vulgaris*) on specific points of the body near *qi* meridians; the heat produced penetrates deep into the body, restoring the balance of *qi*
Qigong	consists of various forms of exercise, breathing techniques, and meditation that are aimed at balancing *qi*

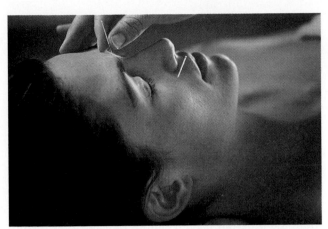

Acupuncture is being recognized in the United States as an effective treatment for a variety of conditions.

early 1970s. Today, it is commonly practiced in many medical settings in the United States. Acupuncture is a method of relieving pain or altering the functioning of a system of the body by inserting fine, wire-thin needles into the skin at specific sites on the body along the series of meridians. The needles may be twirled, energized electrically, or warmed. Although states vary widely regarding the credentialing and permitted scope of practice of acupuncturists, most states have laws for licensing or registering of acupuncture professionals. The NIH has determined that acupuncture is an effective treatment for a variety of conditions, and the federal Food and Drug Administration (FDA) has begun to regulate acupuncture needles in the same fashion as other medical instruments such as scalpels and syringes.

Acupressure is less familiar than acupuncture to most Americans. It uses the same points and meridians as acupuncture, but instead of applying needles, the practitioner uses gentle, firm pressure of the fingers and hands on the body. The belief behind acupressure is that stimulation of the points results in the relief of muscle tension and release by the brain of **endorphins**, neurochemicals that, among their other properties, can relieve pain. Acupressure is used to relieve stresses within the body before they affect the patient's overall health. The patient lies fully clothed on a massage table while the practitioner presses gently on the points on the body. Acupressure may also include gentle stretching and corrective exercises.

AYURVEDA **Ayurveda** is a holistic system of healing that evolved in India some 3,000 to 5,000 years ago. It is similar to Traditional Chinese Medicine in that it stresses the interdependence of the body, mind, and spirit of the individual and the importance of maintaining them in balance. The practice of ayurveda places great emphasis on preventing disease and on the individual's responsibility for achieving health through such things as proper nutrition, exercise, and sleep habits.

Within ayurveda, there are three *doshas*, known as *vata*, *pitta*, and *kapha*. *Doshas* can be described as fundamental biologic energies that regulate all the life processes of an individual. In ayurvedic medicine, all individuals are perceived as consisting of these *doshas*, and each person contains them in a unique proportion. In each individual, one of the three types of *doshas* usually predominates. Each *dosha* is associated with specific body organs, and also with the environmental elements of space, air, fire, water, and earth. The predominant *dosha* determines the individual's body type, personality traits, and the types of illness that will affect that individual. A person who is aware of his *dosha* type and its characteristics can make appropriate lifestyle changes to restore balance and maintain health.

Once the ayurvedic healer has determined the patient's *dosha* imbalance, a treatment plan will be recommended to restore equilibrium. Dietary changes or *panchakarma*, a series of complex steps to rid the body of physical impurities or toxins, may be recommended. These steps may include massage with herbs, steam treatments, therapeutic vomiting, bowel purging, enemas, or nasal inhalation of herbal potions. Meditation, yoga, and breathing exercises are also used in ayurveda to help the mind reach a higher level of functioning.

> ### Technology Tip
> You can visit the American Academy of Medical Acupuncture website at www.medicalacupuncture.org. The site provides general information about medical acupuncture as well as a search tool for finding physicians who practice acupuncture in a specific state and area code.

HOMEOPATHIC MEDICINE **Homeopathy** is a type of holistic medicine that was founded in the late eighteenth century by Samuel Hahnemann, a German doctor who was searching for a medical treatment that did not involve the then-popular medical practice of bloodletting and purging. Hahnemann thought disease was caused by an imbalance in the body's "vital force," a disturbance that affected the individual's pattern of physical, mental, and emotional responses.

Homeopathy is based on the notion that "like cures like." In homeopathy, minute doses of a remedy that would produce disease-like symptoms in healthy persons are administered. This, in fact, is quite similar to the approach used to desensitize patients with allergies. The homeopathic practitioner prepares medicines from raw herbs and other natural substances derived from animal and mineral sources. The substances are crushed and dissolved in water or grain alcohol. Each compound is diluted many times, depending on the patient's presenting symptoms. The FDA regulates homeopathic medicines and recommends those safe enough to be sold over the counter.

Homeopathic first aid kits are available in many health food stores. Some of the basic remedies recommended by homeopaths to treat everyday accidents and ailments include:

- apis (honeybee venom) for insect bites and bee stings
- arenicum (arsenic) for upset stomach, food poisoning, diarrhea, and vomiting
- aconite (monkshood) for swelling or fever
- belladonna (nightshade) for sore throats, colds, headaches, and earaches
- ipccacuanha (ipecac root) for nausea and bleeding

Technology Tip You can reach the Council on Homeopathic Education at www.chedu.org.

There are various levels of training for practitioners of homeopathy from self-taught to formal programs. The Council on Homeopathic Education (CHE) reviews and certifies course material for homeopathic education.

NATUROPATHIC MEDICINE Naturopathy, an alternative therapy that emphasizes health maintenance, disease prevention, patient education, and the patient's responsibility for her own health, is an American approach to healthcare that was developed in the late nineteenth century. In many ways, naturopathic doctors are similar to medical physicians. They study the same sciences, including anatomy, physiology, biology, and epidemiology, and use similar diagnostic evaluations, including laboratory tests.

The difference lies, however, in the philosophy behind naturopathy and its method of treating medical conditions. The overriding philosophical principle of naturopathy is *vitalism*, the belief that the body naturally strives to obtain a maximum level of health. Naturopathic doctors believe that disease is caused by the body's attempt to defend itself against pathogens. They also believe that individuals with strong immune systems can ward off illness whereas those with high levels of stress or poor nutrition will develop illness. However, just because an individual is disease-free does not mean that she is healthy. Naturopathic doctors maintain that a healthy lifestyle promotes wellness,

Technology Tip You can visit the website of the Council for Naturopathic Medical Education at www.cnme.org.

while an unhealthy lifestyle can lead to disability and early death.

Practitioners of naturopathy complete a four-year graduate program from a school that is either regionally accredited or approved by the U.S. Department of Education. Graduates must complete 4,500 hours of academic and clinical training that includes body work, clinical nutrition, herbal medicine, homeopathy, Oriental medicine, psychological medicine, and minor surgery. The Council for Naturopathic Medical Education is the national accrediting agency for education and training programs leading to the Doctor of Naturopathic Medicine (ND or NMD) degree.

ENVIRONMENTAL MEDICINE Environmental medicine is concerned with responses of individuals to environmental factors. This alternative therapy focuses on the chemicals, dust, molds, and certain foods that cause allergic reactions in individuals and that may result in or aggravate more-severe medical conditions. Exposure to these environmental substances may result in chronic or cyclical conditions and may involve one or more body organs.

Food allergies are one major form of environmental illness. In an individual, a specific food apparently triggers an adverse immune system response, which results in a rash or breathing problem. A second form of environmental illness is chemical sensitivity to items in the environment. Some petroleum products, insecticides, and household cleansers, for example, cannot be broken down by the body into harmless elements and, therefore, threaten the health of persons in an environment where these products are used frequently. Environmental medicine specialists believe that toxins from these elements accumulate in the body over time and eventually result in diseases affecting neurologic, gastrointestinal, and mental functions. They may also predispose an individual to certain forms of cancer.

LIGHT THERAPIES In the 1970s, scientists first proposed the theory that the chronic depression that affects people primarily in the long winter months of

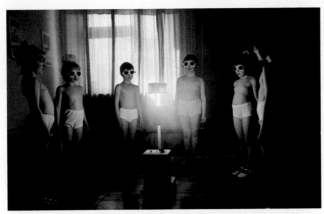

Light therapy is used in northern climates in order to help shift circadian rhythms but it may have additional therapeutic effects.

northern climates was due to insufficient exposure to sunlight. Today, this condition is termed Seasonal Affective Disorder (SAD). **Light therapy** has become an accepted form of treatment for patients with SAD. In treatment sessions, patients spend time daily sitting in artificial light that is similar to outdoor light. Exposure to intense, artificial, bright light suppresses the secretion of the nighttime hormone melatonin, helping to shift circadian rhythms. This form of light therapy helps people remain awake and more alert during the day.

Practitioners of this form of alternative healing believe that light therapy can also be used to treat a variety of other illnesses, including bulimia, psoriasis, and cancer. Different types of light therapy are recommended for different illnesses. Ultraviolet light therapy, colored light therapy, photodynamic therapy, syntonic optometry, and cold laser therapy are some of the forms of artificial light used for therapeutic effects.

Mind–Body Medicine

A second category of alternative therapies designated by NCCAM is that of **mind-body therapies**. As noted above, healthcare practitioners today are increasingly concerned with holism, or healing the whole person. The complex relationship between the mind and the body is especially under scrutiny to help us understand how our thoughts and emotions influence our health. This mind-body relationship will no doubt be an exciting and innovative area of research in the new century.

Mind-body therapies are based on the theory that the mind is a powerful influence on our physical health, and that stress, depression, or even a negative attitude may lead to illness. One example of the close interaction between mind and body can be seen in the individual who is confronted with a real or perceived threat. In such a high-stress confrontation, the nervous system reacts with the "fight-or-flight" response, releasing adrenaline and other hormones to either fight the threat or run from it. In this instance, just the thought or fear of a perceived or actual threat triggers a powerful physical response in the body. Mind-body therapies consider that, in many usually less extreme ways, our minds control our physical health. Some of the mind-body therapies explored below include meditation, hypnosis, yoga, prayer, and mental healing.

MEDITATION **Meditation** is a form of mind-body therapy in which the individual seeks to arrive at a state of deep relaxation with attention focused on one thing at a time. A number of techniques are used to clear the mind of all stressful outside interferences. Most meditation practices can be categorized as either concentrative or mindful meditation. In concentrative meditation, the patient achieves relaxation and the expanding of consciousness by focusing intently on a *mantra,* or a key word, sound, or image. The patient is instructed to notice other thoughts when they enter the mind but to continue to return to the mantra. In mindful meditation, the patient remains peacefully aware of all sensations, such as feelings, images, thoughts, and sounds that pass through her mind without consciously focusing on them. The aim of this form of meditation is the achievement of a calmer, clearer, non-reactive state of mind.

Meditation has been used in the medical profession to treat a variety of conditions, including hypertension and anxiety. It has also been credited with enhancing the immune functions of cancer patients and AIDS patients. In the 1970s, Harvard Professor Herbert Benson researched the physiologic effects of Transcendental Meditation, a form of concentrative meditation in which the patient silently repeats a mantra over and over while sitting in a comfortable position. In his research, he found decreases during meditation in oxygen consumption, metabolism, and heart and respiratory rates, and that alpha waves (which are associated with a feeling of well-being) increased in intensity and frequency. In addition, levels of blood lactate (a substance produced by skeletal muscles during anxiety) decreased. Since then, instruction in meditation has been added to the curriculum of many universities and medical schools.

HYPNOSIS **Hypnosis**, another form of mind-body therapy, is the achieving of a relaxed, heightened state of awareness. It is usually induced by the monotonous repetition of words and gestures while an individual is completely relaxed. While under hypnosis, a patient is very susceptible to suggestion—but nevertheless cannot follow suggestions that are contrary to his wishes.

Hypnosis can be used to treat almost any problem that can be affected by the mind. It has proven effective

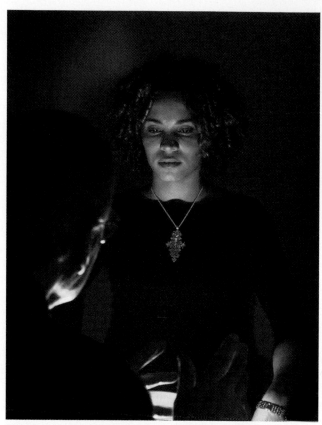

Hypnosis can be an effective therapy for reducing a patient's pain and anxiety.

GUIDED IMAGERY The mind-body therapy of **guided imagery** uses consciously chosen healing images along with deep relaxation to reduce or manage stress, prevent illness, and help patients deal with the effects of disease. Patients are directed to concentrate on a positive image, figure, or idea which may involve any of the five senses. Guided imagery uses mental images to promote physical healing and to change negative attitudes and behaviors. Imagery incorporates specific visualization exercises and can be used as a self-help tool. It can be used to change negative emotions into positive ones and enhance problem-solving. Like hypnosis, it can be used to control chronic pain and enhance the immune system. Guided imagery has also been used successfully in cancer patients to treat the nausea and vomiting associated with chemotherapy and to relieve the pain and stress these patients experience.

MUSIC THERAPY Music therapy is used to address a patient's physical, psychological, cognitive, and social needs. Through the rhythmic sound of music and musical activities, music therapists attempt to help their patients create a general feeling of well-being. The therapy may involve creating, singing, moving to, or listening to music. Music therapy can provide an avenue of communication for those who find it difficult to express themselves in words. Furthermore, it can be effective in facilitating movement and overall physical rehabilitation, motivating patients to cope with treatment, and providing emotional support and an outlet for feelings.

PRAYER AND MENTAL HEALING Throughout the ages, people have used prayer and mental healing to seek assistance from a higher being for a wide range of problems, including illness. Regardless of the practitioner's particular religion, the underlying belief of those who use prayer for healing is the same. This belief is that God, or a powerful higher being, exists, and that people can communicate with God through prayer. Prayer, like meditation, can calm the mind and relieve stress. It can produce positive states of mind that enhance physical health. Several recent interesting studies have demonstrated the efficacy of a patient's prayer or the prayer of family members and friends in promoting healing. These studies concluded that those who prayed or were prayed for healed more quickly than those who did not involve prayer in the healing process.

T'AI CHI CH'UAN The mind-body therapy, t'ai chi ch'uan (or, more commonly, **tai chi**) is a form of exercise that combines physical movement, meditation, and breathing. It is performed to induce relaxation and tranquility of mind, and to improve balance, posture, coordination, endurance, strength, and flexibility. Tai chi

in managing pain, reducing anxiety, and enhancing the immune system. Pregnant women who receive hypnosis before delivery have shorter and less painful labor and deliveries. Hypnosis is also used during dental surgery, either as a complement to or replacement for anesthesia, and it has proven effective in helping certain patients stop smoking or lose weight.

YOGA Yoga, a Sanskrit word meaning "union," is a mind-body therapy that involves the integration of physical, mental, and spiritual energies in promoting health and wellness. It is based on the Hindu principle of mind-body unity. Yoga practitioners believe that it can combat poor health and decreased mental clarity and can restore optimal emotional and physical health. Yoga consists of a series of exercises that involve proper breathing, movement, and posture. While performing specific postures and stretching exercises, an individual pays close attention to her breathing, exhaling at certain times and inhaling at others. These breathing techniques are believed to help maintain the postures as well as promote relaxation by enhancing the body's flow of vital energy known as *prana*, which is similar to the Chinese concept of *qi*.

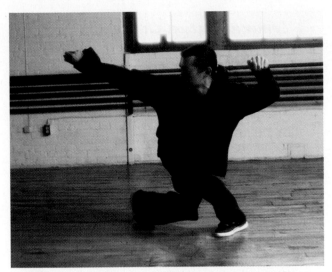

The goal of tai chi is achieve harmony through exercise that combines simple physical movement, meditation, and regulated breathing.

is based on the principle of *yin-yang*, which, as noted earlier, is the basis for the Chinese understanding of health and sickness. Good health requires a balance of *yin* and *yang*, or the opposing forces within the body.

Tai chi movements are carried out in pairs of opposites to balance the negative (*yin*) and positive (*yang*) forces. For example, a movement that begins to the left will typically end with a movement to the right. Tai chi movements are simple, involving the bending and unbending of the knees while raising or lowering the arms. The coordination of movement and breathing patterns is what constitutes tai chi. The ultimate goal of tai chi is to achieve harmony among the body, mind, and spirit.

ART THERAPY Art therapy is a mind-body therapy that uses art media, images, the creative process, and response to artwork to help patients release the creative energy that can lead to physical, emotional, and spiritual healing. Like music, art often appeals to people on a profound level, one not available to everyone through words. Through the use of art therapy, for example, patients can access and express memories, trauma, and psychological conflicts that exist in their subconscious and will not surface until released by creativity.

Biofield and Bioelectromagnetics

Biofield medicine studies the energy fields in and surrounding the body. **Bioelectromagnetics (BEM) is** the study of the interaction of living organisms with **electromagnetic fields**. Bioelectricity refers to the electric current that is generated by living tissues, such as the nerves and muscles. Devices outside the body can record the electrical potentials of human tissues.

Traditional medical practice uses electrocardiographs, electroencephalographs, and similar sensitive devices to diagnose the conditions of various vital organs. The human body is also affected by externally produced electromagnetic fields that can be detected outside the body. The influence of these external fields may alter the body's own bioelectromagnetic activity and cause physical and behavioral changes. This potential influence is the basis for BEM therapies. Electromagnetic and magnetic therapies involve the use of magnetic fields, magnets, and magnetic devices to treat various physical and emotional conditions. These therapies are based on the premise that electrical activity exists in the body at all times, particularly as the heart beats or during bone production.

ELECTROMAGNETIC THERAPY Electromagnetic therapy involves the application of electrical current, either directly through wires or indirectly through a magnetic field, to affect body tissues. Electromagnetic therapy is believed to alter the body's own electromagnetic activity enough to cause physical and behavioral changes. Electroconversion of the heart muscle during a dysrhythmia, implanted cardiac pacemakers, and electroconvulsive therapy for severe depression are additional examples of the use of electrical therapy in medicine today. Bioelectromagnetic therapies are also being used to help heal bone fractures and wounds that fail to heal spontaneously. In addition, alternative practitioners are also using some electromagnetic fields to enhance traditional acupuncture, stimulate the immune system, and combat cancers.

MAGNET THERAPY Magnet therapy, also called magnetic field therapy, is a treatment modality using small magnets that are placed on the skin to increase energy flow in the body. The goal of this therapy is to restore a person's internal bioelectric magnetic balance. Practitioners of magnet therapy range from self-healers to licensed healthcare professionals who report benefits in a wide range of conditions from acute and chronic pain to systemic illness. Most recently, magnet therapy has been used in sports medicine to relieve sprains and strains.

Manipulative and Body-Based Systems

In **manual healing therapies**, a fourth type of NCCAM-designated alternative therapy, the holistic practitioner uses her hands to treat the patient and, in some cases, to diagnose the patient's condition. Most of these therapies involve physical manipulation or pressure of some sort applied to the body. Some, however, do not involve physical touch but rather the moving of energy fields over and around the patient.

Other practitioners use both physical touch and energy-based movement. Manual healing therapies attempt to improve or maintain health by restoring the physiologic integrity of the body. Most of these therapies are aimed at enhancing well-being rather than curing specific diseases.

There are four main categories of manual healing:

- energetic healing, which focuses primarily on the flow of energy through the body (as in acupuncture or therapeutic touch)
- movement repatterning, which aims at altering patterns of body movements (Alexander technique, Feldenkrais method)
- adjustment-based techniques, which are concerned with manipulation of the musculoskeletal system (craniosacral therapy, chiropractic methods)
- pressure-based techniques, which focus on the use of pressure and similar techniques (massage, reflexology)

Rather than relying on a single method, many manual healers use a combination of these techniques on their patients. We have already discussed the manual healing therapies of acupuncture and acupressure. Others include osteopathy, chiropractic therapy, and reflexology.

OSTEOPATHIC MEDICINE **Osteopathy** is a manual healing therapeutic approach that also uses all the common forms of medical therapy and diagnosis, including drugs, surgery, and radiation. However, osteopathy places greater emphasis than traditional medicine on the influence of the relationship between the organs and the musculoskeletal system. Osteopathy originated in the late nineteenth century as a reaction to the practice of traditional Western medicine and its ineffectiveness in treating patients. Osteopathic physicians recognize and correct structural problems by manually manipulating the body. The role of the osteopath is to assist the body in the process of self-healing. He may use a range of manipulation therapies, including gentle mobilization, articulation, muscle energy technique, positional release method, and cranial techniques. All of these are designed to treat the patient's symptoms and restore health. Osteopathy is an alternative therapy that has been approved by the American Medical Association.

CHIROPRACTIC THERAPY Chiropractors are the fourth largest group of health professionals in the United States, after physicians, dentists, and nurses. **Chiropractic therapy** is a form of manual healing based on the belief that most medical problems are caused by misalignment of the vertebrae and can be corrected by

Communication Challenge

Chiropractic therapy is sought by patients with a wide variety of complaints. A patient may visit the chiropractic office with excruciating back pain. As part of the assessment process, the chiropractor may take x-rays and devise a treatment plan that involves manipulation of the spine. Conventional medicine, however, might treat the same patient with rest, cold applications, and muscle relaxants. Differences in these treatment plans may be difficult for the patient to understand. The medical assistant may be challenged to explain the rationale behind each of the treatment approaches.

manipulating the spine. Chiropractors maintain that the two major benefits of chiropractic treatments are the relief of musculoskeletal pain and disability and the re-establishment of internal organ functions.

The founder of chiropractic treatment, Daniel Palmer, believed that the human body seeks to maintain a state of homeostasis, or balance, and has an innate ability to heal itself. He believed that all body functions are regulated through the nervous system and that, since nerves originate in the spine, displaced vertebrae disrupt the nerve transmissions. Palmer called these disruptions *subluxations*, and maintained that they caused almost every illness, but that manipulation of the spine could correct them. Today, chiropractic practice involves the detection and correction of vertebral misalignment, although few chiropractors believe that all diseases can be treated in this manner.

Although traditional Western medical practice repudiated chiropractic therapies for many years, today many patients seek out chiropractors for pain relief and treatment of injuries, as well as some internal ailments. Chiropractors can obtain licensing in all states after a five-year course of study. Moreover, chiropractic services are covered by Medicare and many other insurance providers. Traditional medical physicians also have recognized the benefit of chiropractors' treatments and refer patients to them. Like osteopathy, chiropractic therapy has been approved by the American Medical Association.

REFLEXOLOGY **Reflexology** is a form of manual healing that derives from the principle that certain reflexes in the feet and hands correspond to organs and glands in the body. This therapy dates back 3,000 years to the folk medicine traditions of Egypt, India, and

China. An American otolaryngologist, William Fitzgerald, found in the early 1900s that it reduced pain during surgery if he first applied pressure to specific points on the soles of his patient's feet or the palms of the hands. Eunice Ingham, a physical therapist, expanded on Fitzgerald's work in the 1930s by studying whether applying varying levels of pressure on the feet and hands could also bring about other health benefits.

Reflexology relieves stress and muscle tension and produces relaxation. Reflexologists say the treatment can also be effective in relieving skin disorders, gastrointestinal disorders, hypertension, migraines, anxiety, and asthma. During treatment, the therapist uses thumbs and fingers to apply gentle but firm pressure to the reflex zones, paying more attention to those zones that are tender to the touch. Working on the foot, for example, the therapist proceeds systematically, beginning with gentle pressure on the toes and working across the foot to end at the heel. On the hand, he works from the fingers to the wrists.

THERAPEUTIC MASSAGE **Therapeutic massage** is an ancient form of healing used mainly to improve blood circulation. With improved circulation, toxins are removed from muscle tissue and excreted from the body. Improved circulation also increases the blood supply and the oxygenation of tissues. It may also assist in releasing endorphins in the brain. Today, massage is used to relieve pain and tension and to promote a general state of well-being. It can also help relieve the pain and stiffness of arthritic joints and speed the healing of broken bones.

THERAPEUTIC TOUCH Dolores Krieger, a nursing professor at New York University, and Dora Kunz, a natural healer, developed **therapeutic touch** in the early 1970s. Therapeutic touch is a complementary therapy that is commonly believed to relieve pain and anxiety. It is used to treat many stress-related conditions such as tension headaches, ulcers, hypertension, and emotional problems. Practitioners also find it effective in easing discomfort and speeding the healing process of patients with wounds or infections.

Therapeutic touch treatment begins with the practitioner achieving a calm, relaxed, meditative state that allows her to be sensitive to the patient's problems. This is called "centering." The practitioner then moves her hands over the patient's body approximately 5 to 10 centimeters from the skin. This is done to detect any alterations in the patient's so-called "energy field." These alterations might be feelings of cold or heat, vibration, or blockages. If alterations are found, the practitioner will perform interventions, such as smoothing a tangled field or eliminating congestion, to return the patient's energy field to a state of balance.

Biologically Based Therapies

Biologically based therapies consist of the use of active biological or chemical compounds, and are usually invasive. In the United States, traditional medical practitioners often regard these therapies as questionable. They maintain that no evidence of their effectiveness has been demonstrated, especially as curatives for critical conditions such as cancer and AIDS. Some physicians fear that seriously ill patients will seek these forms of treatment instead of conventional medical treatment, to the detriment of their health. However, other individuals hold that these treatments, because they consist of nontoxic, natural compounds, offer hope for patients with life-threatening diseases that do not respond to traditional medicines.

HERBAL REMEDIES **Herbal remedies** are used primarily to treat minor health problems such as nausea, colds, flu, coughs, headaches, aches and pains, constipation, diarrhea, menstrual cramps, and skin disorders. Some herbalists have also reported success in treating certain chronic conditions such as peptic ulcers, colitis, hypertension, and respiratory problems. Herbs are available in a wide array of forms, depending on their medicinal purpose. They may be bought individually or in mixtures formulated for specific conditions. Herbs may be prepared as tinctures or extracts, capsules or tablets, lozenges, teas, juices, vapor treatments, or bath products. Some herbs are applied topically with a poultice or compress. Others are rubbed into the skin as an

Dangerous Situation

Patients who seek alternative healthcare therapies may be reluctant to tell their traditional physicians or other caregivers about their participation in these forms of treatment, but withholding this information from a physician can harm the patient. For example, herbal remedies, although safe for some patients, may conflict with or counteract the effects of physician-prescribed medicine. Medical assistants should be sure to question patients about the use of alternative healthcare therapies when they obtain their medical histories.

Technology Tip

More information about herbal medicine can be obtained from the American Botanical Council's website at, www.herbalgram.org or the Herb Research Foundation's website at www.herbs.org.

oil, ointment, or salve. Furthermore, herbs and plants may be valuable not only for their active ingredients but also for their minerals, vitamins, volatile oils (used in aromatherapy), glycosides (a sugar derivative), alkaloids, and bioflavonoids. Herbalists may select leaves, flowers, stems, berries, seeds, fruit, bark, roots, or any other plant part for medicinal uses.

In the United States, traditional medical practitioners remain largely unaware of the successful use of herbal remedies, and patients are sometimes reluctant to reveal their use of such remedies. However, herbal medicine has been practiced since the beginning of recorded history, and specific remedies have been handed down from generation to generation. Today, herbal remedies are still largely unregulated. The FDA regulates them only as dietary supplements, not as drugs. This means it can recall an herbal product that is shown to be harmful but that manufacturers are not required to provide information about their products' contents or adverse effects, or to prove their safety or efficacy.

APITHERAPY Apitherapy is a pharmacologic therapy that uses products derived from honeybees to promote health and healing. Bee venom is the most popular form of treatment and is administered either by injection or by live bee stings to treat chronic inflammatory diseases such as arthritis. Apitherapists believe that the inflammation that occurs at the injection site triggers the production of anti-inflammatory substances that help relieve pain and swelling. Other bee products, available as pills or capsules, contain honey, royal jelly, pollen, and propolis (the coating on the inside of beehives and honeycomb cells).

Apitherapists maintain that bee venom can alleviate lower back pain, migraine headaches, symptoms caused by multiple sclerosis, and certain dermatologic conditions such as psoriasis. Bee pollen and raw honey are also sometimes used to increase energy and endurance.

AROMATHERAPY Aromatherapy, the inhalation or application of essential oils distilled from plants to heal the body, mind, and spirit, is a pharmacologic therapy that has been practiced since ancient times. As it is used today, the therapy is founded on the work of French chemist Rene-Maurice Gattefosse, who began studying the healing effects of plant oils in the 1930s after burning his hand in his family's perfume factory. For relief, he plunged his hand into a container of lavender oil and found that his wound healed quickly and without a scar. Aromatherapy is popular in both Europe and the United States.

Aromatherapists treat specific ailments with oils that are inhaled, massaged into the skin, or placed in bath water. Besides creating pleasant sensations and promoting relaxation, aromatherapy may be useful in treating bacterial and viral infections, anxiety, pain, muscle disorders, arthritis, skin disorders, premenstrual syndrome, headaches, and indigestion. But because there is no scientific evidence indicating that aromatherapy prevents or cures disease, it is typically used as a complementary therapy. Table 5.2 lists

Table 5.2 Therapeutic Uses of Essential Oils for Aromatherapy

Essential Oil	Proposed Therapeutic Use
Chamomile	muscle relaxant, anti-inflammatory, antifungal, and antibacterial effects; relieves mental or physical stress
Eucalyptus	antiseptic, deodorant, skin conditioner, insect repellent, antiviral and expectorant effects; soothes irritable bowel, relieves nausea and motion sickness
Fennel	antiseptic, muscle relaxant, soothing agent
Geranium	astringent, skin conditioner, antiviral and antifungal effects; improves circulation, relieves pain
Lavender	anti-inflammatory and antibacterial effects; treats burns, insect bites, and minor injuries; relieves toothache and teething pain; relieves physical and mental stress
Peppermint	antibacterial and antiviral effects, decongestant and expectorant effects; relieves nausea and motion sickness; soothes irritable bowel
Rosemary	antibacterial, antifungal, and antiviral effects; restores energy and alleviates stress
Tea tree	anti-inflammatory, antibacterial, and antiviral effects; treats burns, insect bites, and minor injuries; calming, sedative effects

Patient Teaching
Many patients take the safety of the foods and drugs they buy for granted. However, a patient who is taking, or considering taking, any herbal remedy needs to be aware that these products are not reviewed by the FDA for quality, dosage, safety, or efficacy.

some of the proposed therapeutic uses of selected essential oils.

Lifestyle and Disease Prevention

Lifestyle and disease prevention techniques use integrated and cross-disciplinary approaches to help manage chronic disease. Some of the treatments involve research on electrodermal diagnostics; unconventional therapies for drug addiction, obesity, or stress; and epidemiologic research on healing. This area of alternative medicine is divided into three categories or perspectives of study: clinical preventative, lifestyle therapies, and health promotion.

Clinical Summary

- A number of health threats will continue to dominate medicine in this century, including the AIDS virus, malaria, new emerging viruses, and resistant strains of bacteria.
- Emerging diagnostic and surgical technologies include telemedicine and microsurgery.
- Emerging research and treatments include genetic research, brain research, cancer research, and the development of new drugs and vaccines.
- The field of biomedical ethics was created to deal with the collision between medical science and ethics as new boundaries are crossed by medical advances.
- Alternative therapies and holistic healthcare are emerging trends in the United States. Holistic healthcare emphasizes the fundamental wholeness and integrity of the individual and views the body, mind, and spirit as inseparable and interdependent. The National Institutes of Health established the National Center for Complementary and Alternative Medicine to investigate these alternative therapies.
- Alternative systems of medical practice include traditional Chinese medicine systems such as acupuncture and acupressure, ayurveda, homeopathy, naturopathy, environmental medicine, and light therapy.

- Mind-body therapies are based on the belief that stress leads to illness and stress reduction restores health. Meditation, hypnosis, yoga, guided imagery, music therapy, prayer and mental healing, t'ai chi ch'uan, and art therapy are examples of mind-body therapies.
- Bioelectromagnetic therapies, based on the influence of internal and external electromagnetic fields on living organisms, are used to treat illness such as cancer and to stimulate the immune system.
- Manual healing therapies involve the holistic practitioner's use of hands to treat and, in some instances, diagnose a patient's condition. Forms of manual healing include acupuncture, acupressure, osteopathy, chiropractic therapy, reflexology, therapeutic massage, and therapeutic touch.
- Pharmacologic therapies are those that use active biological or chemical compounds in treating illness or promoting well-being. Forms of pharmacologic therapies include herbal remedies, apitherapy, and aromatherapy. Some medical practitioners in the United States generally regard alternative pharmacologic and biological therapies as questionable remedies with no proven evidence of their effectiveness.

The Language of Medicine

acupressure (**ak**-yoo-presh-er) A method of relieving pain or altering the function of a system of the body by applying gentle, firm pressure with the fingers and hands.

acupuncture (**ak**-yoo-pungk-cher) A method of relieving pain or altering the function of a system of the body by inserting fine, wire-thin needles into the skin at specific sites on the body along a series of lines, or channels, called meridians.

apitherapy (ap-ch-**ther**-ah-pee) The use of products derived from honeybees to promote health and healing.

aromatherapy (ah-rO-mah-**ther**-ah-pee) The inhalation or application of essential oils distilled from various plants to heal the body, mind, and spirit.

art therapy A mind-body therapy that uses art media, images, the creative art process, and patient response to artwork as tools for healing.

ayurveda (ah-yoor-**vay**-dah) An Indian holistic system of healing that stresses the interdependence of the individual's body, mind, and spirit and the importance of balancing these aspects.

bioelectromagnetics (BEM) The study of the interaction of living organisms with electromagnetic fields.

biomedical ethics An area of academic research that studies the intersection between science and morality.

chiropractic therapy (kI-rO-**prak**-tik **ther**-ah-pee) A therapeutic system based on the belief that most medical problems are caused by misalignments of the vertebrae and can be corrected by manipulating the spine.

electromagnetic fields Electrical potentials that may be created either within or outside the body.

endorphins (en-**dor**-finz) Neurochemicals released in the brain that can relieve pain.

environmental medicine A form of alternative medical intervention concerned with the responses of individuals to substances in the environment that include chemicals, dust, molds, and certain foods.

gene (jeen) A single segment of the body's hereditary material.

genome (**jee**-nOm) All of the DNA in an organism, including its genes.

guided imagery A mind-body therapy that uses consciously chosen positive and healing images along with deep relaxation to reduce or manage stresses, prevent illness, and help patients deal with the effects of disease.

herbal remedies The use of various herbs to treat minor health problems.

holistic healthcare Healthcare that emphasizes the fundamental wholeness and integrity of the individual and views the body, mind, and spirit as inseparable and interdependent.

homeopathy (hO-mee-**op**-ah-thee) An alternative medical approach based on the notion that "like cures like"; treatment includes the administering of minute doses of a remedy that would, in healthy persons, produce symptoms similar to those of the disease.

hypnosis Mind-body therapy that produces a relaxed yet heightened state of awareness during which individuals are more open to suggestion.

light therapy Use of exposure to various forms of artificial light to treat illness.

manual healing therapies Alternative therapies in which the practitioner uses his or her hands to treat the patient and, in some cases, diagnose the patient's condition.

meditation A profound form of deep relaxation during which attention is focused on one thing at a time.

meridians (meh-**rid**-ee-anz) Channels that run up and down the surface of the body, as well as deeper inside, along which acupuncture and acupressure is performed.

mind-body therapies A form of non-traditional medicine based on the theory that stress leads to illness and stress reduction helps restore health.

music therapy An alternative therapy that uses creating, singing, moving to, and/or listening to music to address a patient's physical and emotional needs.

National Center for Complementary and Alternative Medicine (NCCAM) 1991 office established by the National Institutes of Health to investigate alternative and holistic methods of healthcare. It was originally called the Office of Alternative Medicine.

naturopathy (nay-chur-**op**-ah-thee) An alternative therapy that emphasizes health maintenance, disease prevention, patient education, and the patient's responsibility for his or her own health; the overriding principle is vitalism, the belief that the body naturally strives for a maximum level of health.

osteopathy (os-tee-**op**-ah-thee) A therapeutic approach to medicine that uses all the usual forms of medical therapy and diagnosis but also places greater emphasis on the influence of the relationship between the organs and the musculoskeletal system.

reflexology (ree-fleks-**ol**-O-gee) A form of manual healing based on the principle that reflexes in the feet and hands correspond to various organs and glands within the body.

tai chi (tI-**chee**) A form of exercise built upon the mind-body connection that combines physical movement, meditation, and breathing.

telemedicine Using video and computer technology to let physicians in one location see patients in another, providing an expanded means for patients to access healthcare.

therapeutic massage The use of various motions and pressures on the body to improve circulation and remove toxins.

therapeutic touch A complementary therapy used to relieve pain and anxiety in which the practitioner moves her hands over the patient's body without touching the skin to detect any alterations in the patient's energy field.

Traditional Chinese Medicine (TCM) An alternative therapy in which the patient is responsible for his own health and the doctor serves as a guide and role model, offering aid in the form of herbs, acupuncture, and massage.

yoga (**yO**-guh) A Hindu mind-body therapy that involves the integration of physical, mental, and spiritual energies to promote health and wellness.

Signs/Symptoms of Progress

1 Recall, Question, Connect

Recall
Review the alternative healing therapies mentioned in this chapter and state which two are acceptable today to almost all traditional medical physicians in the United States.

Question
What questions do you have about why some alternative therapies are accepted and some are not?

Connect
Explain why you, as a medical assistant, need to be knowledgeable about alternative therapies.

2 Educating the Patient

Liya Si, a Chinese-born American professor, comes to the general practitioner's office with complaints of gastrointestinal disturbance. She states that she has been experiencing periods of diarrhea and has lost her appetite. She informs you, the medical assistant, that the problems started two weeks ago and have progressively worsened. You weigh her and take her vital signs. Based upon her medical record, you note that she has lost ten pounds since her last visit six months ago. Her vital signs are within her normal range. As you interview Liya regarding her chief complaints, she states that she has been experiencing an imbalance in her *qi* that most likely is causing her problems.

1 How would you respond to Liya's statement about her *qi*?
2 What additional information should you seek from her?
3 If Liya reveals that she is being treated by a traditional Chinese doctor, what information will you need to give her? To the physician? Identify an approach that you might use as you interact with Liya.

3 Exploring Perspectives in Teams

Perspective involves the discipline of examining how ideas look from different points of view and recognizing that there are often multiple "answers" to complex questions. In small groups or on your own, reflect on possible alternative views or answers and summarize your findings.

1 Consider the changes discussed in the chapter that will occur in healthcare during the twenty-first century and discuss how they might affect the role of the medical assistant.
2 Review the mind-body and manual healing therapies presented in this chapter and identify the specific conditions that may potentially be successfully treated with each of the therapies. If you have had direct or indirect experience with a particular therapy, share that experience.
3 A patient with Parkinson's disease wants to try an acupuncture treatment that he learned about on the Internet. He would like a doctor's referral, but you know that his primary doctor is skeptical of alternative treatments in general. How would you advise the patient to approach the doctor? Specifically, what information should he have about the Internet site? What if the situation were reversed with the doctor recommending alternative treatment and the patient reluctant? How would you advise the patient?
4 Do you think traditional and alternative medicines primarily conflict with or complement one another? Think of three conditions supporting the view that they conflict and then three supporting the view that they complement each other.

Medical Assistant—Entry-Level Competencies

Administrative Competencies

Perform Clerical Functions
- Schedule and manage appointments
- Schedule inpatient and outpatient admissions and procedures
- Perform medical transcription
- Organize a patient's medical record
- File medical records

Perform Bookkeeping Procedures
- Prepare a bank deposit
- Reconcile a bank statement
- Post entries on a daysheet
- Perform accounts receivable procedures
- Perform accounts payable procedures
- Perform billing and collection procedures
- Prepare a check
- Establish and maintain a petty cash fund

Prepare Special Accounting Entries
- Post adjustments
- Process credit balance
- Process refunds
- Post NSF checks
- Post collection agency payments

Process Insurance Claims
- Apply managed care policies and procedures
- Apply third party guidelines
- Obtain managed care referrals and pre-certifications
- Perform procedural coding
- Perform diagnostic coding
- Complete insurance claim forms
- Use a physician's fee schedule

Clinical Competencies

Fundamental Principles
- Perform handwashing
- Wrap items for autoclaving
- Perform sterilization techniques
- Dispose of biohazardous materials
- Practice Standard Precautions

Specimen Collection
- Perform venipuncture
- Perform capillary puncture
- Obtain throat specimen for microbiological testing
- Perform wound collection procedure for microbiological testing
- Instruct patients in the collection of a clean-catch mid-stream urine specimen
- Instruct patients in the collection of fecal specimens

Diagnostic Testing
- Use methods of quality control
- Perform urinalysis
- Perform hematology testing
- Perform chemistry testing
- Perform immunology testing
- Perform microbiology testing
- Screen and follow-up test results
- Perform electrocardiograms
- Perform respiratory testing

Patient Care
- Perform telephone and in-person screening
- Obtain vital signs
- Obtain and record patient history
- Prepare and maintain examination and treatment areas
- Prepare patient for and assist with routine and specialty examinations
- Prepare patient for and assist with procedures, treatments, and minor office surgery
- Apply pharmacology principles to prepare and administer oral and parenteral medications
- Maintain medication and immunization records
- Obtain CPR certification and first aid training

Transdisciplinary Competencies

Communicate
- Respond to and initiate written communications
- Recognize and respond to verbal communications
- Recognize and respond to nonverbal communications
- Demonstrate telephone techniques

Legal Concepts
- Identify and respond to issues of confidentiality
- Perform within legal and ethical boundaries
- Establish and maintain the medical record
- Document appropriately
- Perform risk management procedures

Patient Instruction
- Explain general office policies
- Instruct individuals according to their needs
- Instruct and demonstrate the use and care of patient equipment
- Provide instruction for health maintenance and disease prevention
- Identify community resources

Operational Functions
- Perform an inventory of supplies and equipment
- Perform routine maintenance of administrative and clinical equipment
- Utilize computer software to maintain office systems

Source: From the 1999 Standards and Guidelines, developed by CAAHEP in conjunction with the Curriculum Review Board of the American Association of Medical Assistants' Endowment. Reprinted by permission.

Part II

ADMINISTRATIVE PROCEDURES

Systems and Solutions

Learning Outcomes

- Demonstrate efficient administrative systems and procedures.
- Explain and adhere to office opening, closing, and security procedures.
- Use and maintain various types of medical office equipment.
- Process and access medical information using computer systems and software.
- Identify decision-making factors in selecting office computer systems.
- Identify leasing versus buying options for office equipment.
- Establish and maintain equipment and supply inventories.
- Manage vendors and outside service contracts.

Performance Objectives

- Select an efficient computer system for a medical office.
- Demonstrate the correct procedures for using office machines.
- Demonstrate the correct procedure for storing scheduled drugs.

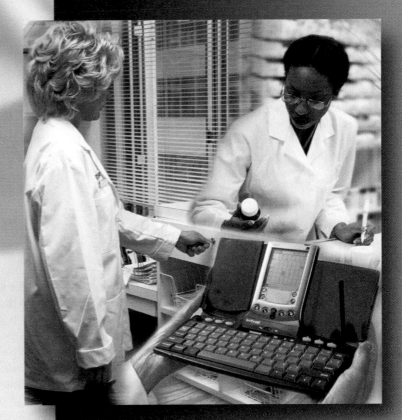

Within the practice of *medical assisting, you will be expected to master and demonstrate administrative skills. You may be required to maintain the administrative and reception areas, participate in purchasing office equipment, hire outside service providers, inventory and track supplies, select pharmaceutical and other product vendors, understand equipment leasing, and oversee office security. You also will be expected to understand computers, including hardware and software products appropriate for the medical office.*

Managing Administrative Procedures

Patient Concerns

*P*atients expect the best medical care possible from their physicians at a reasonable cost in an environment that is pleasant, orderly, and efficiently managed. The medical assistant plays a significant role in satisfying these expectations by maintaining the reception area and administrative workspace, making sure that needed supplies are on hand, and keeping equipment in good working order. Wise purchasing decisions and proper care and use of equipment help to control costs. The use of computers provides access to the latest healthcare research and medical developments and lets the physician communicate with medical experts anywhere in the world.

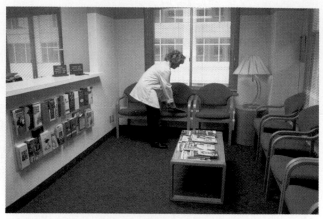

Maintaining the reception area so that it is clean, neat, and meets patients' needs is an important part of the medical assistant's work.

Managing the Administrative Workspace and Reception Area

The medical office environment can have as great an impact on patients as any other aspect of the practice, including the quality of the care. Patients are influenced by the atmosphere in all office areas. For example, if the reception area is shabby and untidy, patients may conclude that the care they receive in the examination areas will be less than adequate.

As a medical assistant, it is your responsibility to maintain the office so it demonstrates that patient comfort and care are top priorities. The entire office area must be attractive, neat, and clean. The way the office is maintained can make the difference between a successful practice and an unsuccessful one.

Administrative Workspace

The administrative area is reserved for secretaries, receptionists, other office workers, and authorized medical personnel. Many activities taking place in this area can be seen clearly by waiting patients. While a large divider may separate the administrative area from the reception room, it is still part of the "public area." Therefore, it is essential that activities in this area run smoothly and be handled in a professional manner. This includes careful monitoring of how patients are greeted upon arrival, how nurses or assistants tell patients the doctor is ready to see them, how phone calls are handled, and how office personnel talk to one another. Any sign of disorder, unpleasantness, or rudeness is easily observed by waiting patients. Negative observations can be very detrimental to the medical practice.

Reception Area

Patient comfort should be the primary concern in the reception area. This means keeping it neat, clean, and attractive. During the day, you should check the reception area frequently and remove any trash or debris. Clean up spills, straighten magazines and other reading materials, and give any soiled areas a quick spot cleaning. Rearrange furniture that is out of place and remove any withered leaves from plants. Check glass and polished surfaces for fingerprints, and use a nonstreaking all-purpose cleaner to remove dirt. Replenish any supplies or materials designated for patient use, such as pens, pencils, writing paper, and tissues.

KEEPING THE AREA CLEAN The reception area should receive a thorough cleaning nightly, including dusting furniture and plants and vacuuming the carpet and upholstered furniture. Special attention should be given to magazine covers, walls, pictures, lamps, lighting fixtures, curtains or draperies, and accessories. Any of these items that become very soiled or worn should be replaced.

If a professional housekeeping staff is used, the medical assistant is responsible for educating its members about the office's cleaning requirements. For example, you must ask them to use only treated dust cloths and to avoid moving dust by shaking linens. The housekeeping staff usually vacuums carpeted areas, scrubs floors, dusts furniture, washes windows, and cleans blinds. It might also be contracted to clean window treatments and shampoo carpeting on a scheduled basis.

You also may be required to supervise the professional cleaning service. Evaluate the cleaning work frequently. Correct any problems as they arise to assure that the reception area is fresh and inviting.

RECEPTION AREA DÉCOR A primary factor in decorating the reception area is the physician's medical specialty. A pediatric reception area probably will have bright colors and a play area. A urologist's reception area, where most patients are male, may have a more masculine atmosphere, while a gynecologist's office will be designed with women's tastes in mind.

The area should have comfortable, attractive seating. Some medical office reception areas offer a small writing desk, stocked with attractive paper and pens, for waiting patients. Writing offers a welcome diversion and helps the time pass more quickly for some patients. A variety of magazines suited to the practice's clientele should also be on hand.

A pediatric reception area has very special requirements. Younger children relieve tension through play—and a visit to the doctor can be a tension-producing time. Older children may need opportunities for distraction to help alleviate their fears. The pediatric reception area must be arranged to provide both ample play opportunities for children of varying ages and quieter activities such as books, games, and puzzles for older children.

Any area that encourages physical activity should include a mat or thick pad on the floor to prevent injuries from falls. Make sure that all toys in the area are unbreakable and too large to fit in a small child's mouth. You will need to clean and straighten the children's play areas several times during the day. Remember that both adults and children can trip over out-of-place toys. Toys must be washed and scrubbed at least daily with a 10% bleach solution (1 part bleach to 10 parts water). Remove broken or worn toys or damaged play equipment immediately.

For all reception and back office areas, you will need to restock depleted supplies and empty garbage and laundry receptacles.

Opening the Medical Office

When you open the medical office, one of your first tasks may be to disarm the security system or reset it to a daytime mode. You need to turn on the lights and sound system, check that the temperature is comfort-able in both front and back office, and readjust the thermostat if necessary or open windows for fresh air.

Check all areas for cleanliness and safety. Inspect the reception area to see that the furniture is in order, wastebaskets have been emptied, magazines are straight, and the area appears warm and inviting. If coffee is provided for patients, you need to brew the first pot and make sure there are cups, cream substitute, sugar packets, and stir sticks. Inspect the examination area to ensure that sufficient medical supplies are available, noting particularly the supply of patient gowns, blankets, and drapes. When possible, test the examination equipment to see that it is working properly. In addition to checking for cleanliness, you should make sure the bathrooms are adequately stocked with paper towels, toilet paper, and soap.

Check the answering machine and/or answering service for messages and make certain that all messages are properly logged, recorded, and distributed. Turn on the office computers and other equipment. Check for faxes or e-mail messages that might have arrived since the previous work day, and log and file them.

Consult the schedule (or patient appointment list prepared the night before) to determine which charts need to be pulled from the files. Arrange them in the order in which they will be needed and put them in a convenient place. (Many offices use a standup file for this.) Check each pulled chart to see that it is current and contains recent laboratory results, x-rays reports, and correspondence. A last-minute search for a missing lab report while a patient waits in the treatment room is hardly conducive to a serene atmosphere or patient comfort. A number of chart sets should be assembled in advance and kept on hand for new patients. Put out the day's register for patients.

Once everything is ready, and well before the first patient is due to arrive, unlock the office entrance. Be sure that all coworkers are at their workstations. If an employee is unexpectedly out for the day, make plans to cover that position by either calling in a temporary employee or allocating the absentee's responsibilities to others.

Office opening should be detailed in the procedure manual. Follow the routine described there, and if your office does not have such a manual, look into establishing one. Procedure 6.1 provides a starting point for developing an opening procedure.

Closing the Medical Office

Do not begin closing procedures until all patients have left the office. Routines such as shutting down equipment and locking cabinets signal preparation for leaving and can make patients feel rushed.

Procedure 6.1

Opening the Medical Office

Purpose: To open the office at the start of the business day in a way that will facilitate efficient and successful operation of the practice throughout the day.

1 Disarm the alarm system or switch to daytime mode.
2 Unlock doors.
3 Turn on lights.
4 Check answering machines and/or answering service for messages. Deliver messages. Turn off the answering machine during normal business hours.
5 Check the fax machine for messages. Deliver messages as needed.
6 Unlock drawers, desks, cabinets, and filing cabinets that are routinely unlocked during operating hours.
7 Turn on office equipment such as computers, printer, copier, etc.
8 Check temperature and adjust as necessary.
9 Check e-mail messages. Deliver messages as needed.
10 Make sure the reception area is neat, clean, and ready for patients and visitors.
11 Check exam rooms for readiness.
12 Check bathrooms to make sure they are adequately stocked.
13 Check and/or restock daily supplies (pens, pencils, note pads, paper clips, stapler, etc.).
14 Pull charts and put them in order of appointments scheduled.
15 Put out the day's register for patient use and fill in the date.
16 Check that all coworkers are at their workstations.
17 Unlock the patient entrance.

At the end of the business day, all office areas should be straightened, and equipment, files, and other items should be put in order. Trash baskets should be emptied. Daily accounts should be balanced or prepared for balancing. Place receipts that have not been deposited into a safe or other secure area. File cabinets, doors, and drawers should be locked, and all drugs secured. Equipment that will not be needed immediately upon opening should be turned off, including autoclaves, diagnostic equipment, and office equipment. Confirm that the fax machine is stocked with paper and is on standby. Answering machines should be turned on and/or a message left with the answering service. Turn off all lights unless local security or law enforcement officials advise against this. Arm the security system or switch into the nighttime mode.

As with opening procedures, office closing routines should be described in the procedure manual. Procedure 6.2 outlines the steps to follow when closing the office at the end of the day.

Procedure 6.2

Closing the Medical Office

Purpose: To close the office at the end of the business day in a safe and orderly manner.

1 Straighten the reception area and all exam areas. Empty trash baskets and attend to aquarium, live plants, etc. Turn off TV/VCR and any other equipment.
2 File all charts and other information or place them in a holder for filing.
3 Balance daily accounts or prepare accounts for balancing.
4 Lock receipts in a safe or other secure area.
5 Turn off office equipment such as computers, copier, and paper shredder. Leave fax machine on for overnight messages. Confirm that fax machine is loaded with paper.
6 Lock drawers, desks, and cabinets, including filing cabinets.
7 Leave closing message with the answering service and/or turn on the answering machine. Notify building security, if appropriate.
8 Wash hands. *Washing hands before leaving the medical office will help prevent the spread of infection.*
9 Turn off lights and activate the alarm system.
10 Leave and lock the door.

and drugs also must be secured. Usually, these materials are stored in locked cabinets that only staff members who need access have keys to. Entrance keys to the office are usually given to all staff members. Be sure to ask departing employees to return their keys.

Office Security Systems

Even in an office building with a security patrol, many medical offices have their own security system. A medical office is vulnerable to vandalism, burglars seeking money or drugs, and even those wishing to gather private information on individual patients. A good security system provides protection against a number of situations that could lead to disaster. The last person leaving the office at night must arm the system, and the staff member opening the office in the morning must disarm it. Staff members should receive adequate training in use of the security system to avoid problems arming, disarming, and using it.

Emergency Plans

To promote patient and healthcare team safety, the medical assistant needs to keep the front office and examination areas free of clutter. All items not in use should be appropriately stored. Closet doors and cabinet drawers should be kept closed unless in use. Furniture should be examined for rough and sharp edges. Make sure to replace torn cushions or broken parts. Floors must be clean and free of unnecessary clutter; carpeting must be tacked down securely. Check for frayed cords on lamps and all electrical equipment. You or another assistant assigned this responsibility should conduct routine weekly safety inspections of the entire facility. Such inspections should be documented, showing the date of the inspection and the assistant's signature.

The presence of combustible equipment and supplies requires that fire safety be a major concern for medical personnel. Electrocardiogram machines and radiologic devices in the examination area can start electrical fires. Patient gowns and blankets can ignite. Combustible materials must be labeled and appropriately stored. "No Smoking" signs should be posted. Fire extinguishers should be placed throughout the examination areas and checked frequently to ensure that they are operational.

A medical office should have at least two exit doors marked with illuminated "Exit" signs using a backup power system. Check the signs routinely to confirm that they are illuminated. Most local building codes dictate the number and location of exit doors, stairways, and other emergency exits. Staff members should be thoroughly familiar with the exit routes to use in an

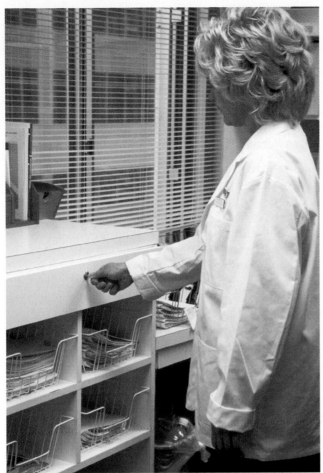

Drawers, desks, and cabinets containing files or drugs should be kept locked when not in use to prevent access by unauthorized persons.

Managing Office Security

Safety and security issues include such diverse concerns as limiting access, drug security, burglary protection, and fire safety.

Limiting Access

Records and medicines must be protected from theft or use by unauthorized persons. Computer security is discussed later in this chapter. However, paper files

Dangerous Situation
Locks should be changed periodically or when there has been significant employee turnover.

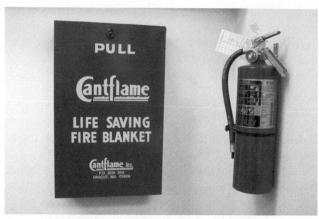

Fire extinguishers should be readily available for use in case of an emergency. This medical office also has a fire blanket.

emergency, and should be prepared to direct patients and visitors to the appropriate exit. The office, or building, should have a fire escape plan that addresses alternatives to blocked exits.

Most offices have a disaster plan manual that includes contingencies for fire, flood, dangerous weather, intruders, and other hazards. It should list steps for staff members to take to ensure their own safety and that of patients and visitors. All office personnel should become familiar with the manual. If your office does not have such a manual, offer to help develop one.

Smoke detectors are essential in a medical office. Most communities require them in both public and private buildings. Remember to check them frequently to see that they are working. Staff members should be trained in implementing emergency procedures whenever smoke alarms are triggered.

Many buildings also are equipped with sprinkler systems required by local building codes that are triggered by the presence of heat or smoke.

All staff members should know when to dial 911 for assistance. If the office must be evacuated, it is essential to make sure no one is left in a bathroom or examination room. Be prepared to help those who have difficulty walking and those with small children.

Working Smart
Always be on the lookout for ways to improve office safety.

Managing Office Equipment

Today's technology provides many tools to help organize the medical office. A variety of machines and equipment are available that require minimal skill to operate and have both a precision and a range of capabilities that human labor cannot match. Their primary advantage, however, is speed. Automation can speed up routine office tasks to make workers more productive. One reported estimate is that automation has reduced the total number of office workers by 75% in the past 30 years. The medical assistant must be proficient in the use of all medical office equipment and must be able to properly select and maintain these devices for maximum efficiency.

Adding Machines and Calculators

Adding machines and calculators are useful for tasks that require simple mathematical functions such as addition, subtraction, multiplication, or division. Preparing patient bills, reconciling bank statements, and computing payrolls are examples of tasks for which numerical accuracy is essential and the use of calculating equipment helpful.

Adding machines typically run on electricity and print a copy of the calculations on a paper tape. Calculators are usually battery- or solar-powered, and some are small enough to fit in the palm of your hand.

When using an adding machine or a calculator, it is important to double-check your work. Cross-check the figures on the paper tape against the numbers you are working with or, if there is no paper copy, run the numbers at least twice to make sure you get the same results.

Transcription Equipment

Transcription equipment is used to convert recorded spoken words into written text. A busy physician can record correspondence, memos, or reports with a portable dictation device. The medical assistant then uses the transcription machine to listen to the tape while working at a computer. Foot pedals on the transcription machine are used to start, stop,

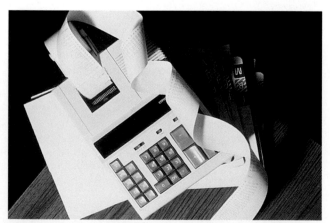

Even though a calculator will not make a mathematical error, always double-check your work to make sure you input the correct numbers.

Table 6.1 Tips for Dictation

- State date, type of document, and any specific instructions.
- Spell out all names, addresses, and unfamiliar terms.
- Dictate desired punctuation, such as "new paragraph" or "quotation marks."
- Speak clearly and slowly.
- Avoid dictating in an area with loud background noise.
- Refrain from eating or drinking while dictating.
- Clearly indicate when finished.

and rewind the tape. Other features of the machine include speed settings and volume and tone controls. Table 6.1 lists tips for dictating clearly for transcription. Share these tips with the physician doing the dictation to help make your transcription as accurate and efficient as possible.

Voice recognition is a developing technology that lets a user issue commands to a computer by speaking into an attached microphone. Although it is used more widely with larger systems than with desktop machines, voice recognition software may soon replace some types of transcription equipment.

Paper Shredders

It is sometimes necessary in the medical office to throw out old medical records, expired documents with personal information, or first drafts of confidential memos and letters. Paper shredders are used to quickly and thoroughly destroy any documents containing sensitive information. Once the paper is fed into the shredder, it is sliced into hundreds of tiny pieces and then emptied into an attached wastebasket. Most paper shredders have an electric eye that starts the machine when paper is placed into the feeder. Be extra careful when opting to use the shredder to discard a document. Once something is fed into the machine, it is irreversibly destroyed.

Microfilm and Microfiche

A medical office needs access to a vast amount of medical information and literature. One space-saving strategy is to have medical documents and manuscripts duplicated onto microfilm and microfiche. Information that would take up an entire storage room in its original form can be condensed into this much smaller form. Although data is now more commonly stored on computer disks, many medical records and back issues of medical journals and other publications are archived on microfilm and microfiche.

Microfilm has information printed onto reels or cartridges of film, which are then fed into a microfilm reader for viewing. Microfiche has the information condensed and printed onto special sheets that are placed on the glass surface of a microfiche machine to be read.

Microfilm and microfiche readers are generally equipped with features for focus adjustment, fast-forwarding, zoom lens, and printing capability.

Photocopiers

Photocopiers, sometimes called just "copiers," are used to reproduce office documents. When a document is entered into the machine for duplicating, the equipment makes a photograph of it, then uses either liquid or powdered toner (a type of ink) to transfer the photograph image to ordinary paper. The page is then exposed to heat to set the toner and make the copy permanent. Photocopiers can make an unlimited number of copies and can handle a variety of sizes of originals and copies. They also can reproduce on colored paper, cardstock (a thick type of paper), or sheets of acetate (a transparent material) to produce overhead transparencies.

Photocopiers range in size from small, desktop models that can handle only a limited number of reproductions to huge, industrial, high-capacity machines that can produce thousands of copies in a single run. Most copiers reproduce documents in black ink, although color copiers are available at a higher cost. Copying features include size options, the ability to change the orientation of the document on the paper, contrast adjustment, and production of double-sided copies. Some copiers also have a scanning feature that lets them send information to and receive it from a computer.

Processing features include collating (arranging multiple-page copies in sets to match an original set), stapling, or hole punching. Some of the newest copiers offer an additional range of binding options, including spiral binding and saddle-stitching. Many copiers have a microprocessor chip that directs copy functions and offers assistance to the user through a "help" menu. Procedure 6.3 details the steps to follow for using a photocopier.

Fax Machines

Fax machines scan a document and transmit it via telephone lines to a distant location, where it is received by another fax machine and printed as an exact duplicate of the original. Fax machines make it possible to instantly transfer documents across huge distances, eliminating information delays associated with mail. The cost for sending a local fax is virtually nothing, since local calls are not charged an extra fee; however, faxing to a distant location costs the same as a long-distance telephone call. An office fax machine should have a telephone line dedicated to its use because faxing or receiving multiple documents can tie up a

Procedure 6.3

Using a Photocopier

Purpose: To make an exact duplicate of a document.

Equipment/Supplies: Document to be copied, staple remover, photocopier.

1 Check that the machine is on and warmed up. Look for the indicator light showing when the machine is ready.
2 Prepare the material you want to copy by removing all staples, paper clips, self-adhesive notes, and other items that may jam the machine.
3 Place an original page face down on the glass, or place multiple pages into the document feeder.
4 Select the paper size and number of copies you want.
5 Press start.
6 Remove your original as well as your duplicate copies from the machine.
7 Press clear or reset.

phone line for a long time. The use of a fax machine is outlined in Procedure 6.4.

Higher-end models offer faster speed, better quality paper, and extra capabilities such as high-resolution scanning. Additional fax machine functions may offer the ability to photocopy, produce specialized reports of faxing functions, and permanently store fax telephone numbers for automatic dialing.

Fax machines use either plain paper—the same as in a copier or laser printer—or thermal paper. Thermal paper is treated with chemicals to react to heat and electricity, and looks and feels different from regular paper. It also has a major disadvantage in that the images on it can fade over time, especially when repeatedly exposed to light. These faxes must be photocopied for long-term storage. Plain paper machines are usually more expensive to buy but may be cheaper to operate, since thermal paper costs more. Newer fax machines eliminate the thermal paper vs. plain paper debate by using only plain paper.

Buying Equipment for the Medical Office

Choosing the right equipment for the medical office is extremely important. As a medical assistant, you may be involved in these purchase decisions. You also may need to evaluate and understand equipment warranties, consider the pros and cons of leasing vs. buying, and actually purchase a computer or other office equipment.

Procedure 6.4

Using a Fax Machine

Purpose: To transmit a document's image instantly to a different location.

Equipment/Supplies: Document to be transmitted, fax number, fax machine.

1 Prepare a cover sheet to provide information about the transmission. Include the name, address, telephone number, and fax number of both the sender and receiver; number of pages (specifying whether the cover sheet is included or not); date; and whether the information is confidential.
2 Insert the original. Most machines require that the document be face down.
3 Enter the telephone number of the fax machine you are sending to.
4 Press the "start" button. The remainder of the process is automatic, and the machine will stack the originals in a bin for you to retrieve. Faxed pages are not to be destroyed or damaged in any way and should be retained for filing or other requirements.
5 Look for a confirmation message to make sure your fax was transmitted successfully. The machine will print an error message if it was not.

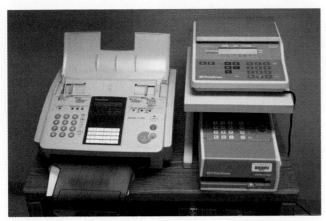

The fax machine makes possible instantaneous transmission of documents to distant locations.

The Decision-Making Process

Certain steps must be followed to reach a decision. You will need to understand the basics of the equipment involved and determine the functions it will perform and the features required. Product catalogs will give you a general idea of what is available.

Next, you must establish a budget or price range, shop for specific models, and evaluate vendors. Finally, consider all the information you have gathered—this may include changing or modifying some of your ideas or opinions—and make your final decision.

Warranties

Most new equipment comes with a warranty contract that guarantees free service and replacement parts for a limited time. It is sometimes possible to extend a warranty by paying more. Warranty coverage can be an important consideration when comparing different models of equipment. Be sure to fill out the warranty card and mail it to the manufacturer after any purchase. The receipt and the warranty information should be filed for future reference.

Leasing vs. Buying Equipment

In recent years, equipment leasing has become an increasingly popular alternative to buying, and it is an option that many medical offices consider. If you purchase a piece of equipment, you own it—with all the rights and responsibilities of ownership. If you lease it, the owner of the equipment makes it available for your use but retains ownership, and may assume some of the responsibility for maintaining it. A lease agreement usually calls for a large initial payment and small monthly payments for the length of the lease. The agreement specifies the length of time the equipment

will be leased and what will happen to it at the end of the lease.

If you are responsible for gathering leasing information or deciding on equipment leasing, there are several important points to consider:

- Leasing can markedly reduce the amount of money required to start a medical office or acquire an expensive piece of new equipment for an existing office. The initial payment is usually only a small fraction of what the equipment would cost if purchased outright, and monthly lease payments are generally much smaller than payments on a purchase.
- Leases usually provide for new or upgraded equipment every few years, resulting in newer equipment at a lower cost.
- Companies that lease equipment are often responsible for its maintenance and repairs—a convenience for routine maintenance and a considerable advantage if there is a major breakdown.

You should collect leasing information and make vendor choices as carefully as if you were buying equipment or supplies—perhaps even more carefully, since the leasing contract will establish a relationship that may last several years. Questions to ask include:

- Is there a discount on lease rates if you lease more items?
- Who is responsible for routine maintenance and repairs? Is a service contract required?
- Is there an option to buy the equipment at a greatly reduced cost after the lease ends?
- Is there a delivery and/or setup fee?
- Who insures the equipment?

Ask for price quotes, vendor background information, and information on policies and customer service. Get quotes from several companies and consider all the information you gather before making a decision. Be sure you understand the lease agreement completely. It may be a good idea to have an attorney who specializes in medical office matters review the agreement before anything is signed. Once the lease is signed, note the important points for reference and put the original lease in a safe place.

Buying a Computer System

A computer system is probably the most important, complex, and expensive purchase for a medical office, and has its own particular considerations. You need to carefully consider the needs and uses in your office. You may have to arrange to have it installed, unless you or someone else in the office is proficient with installation. You also must consider training needs. Even workers who are very familiar with a computer system can use a few tips to help them adapt to a new system. Those who are completely unfamiliar with computers will require extensive training to make them efficient users of the computer system. Some vendors offer training, either free or at a reduced cost, with the purchase of hardware and software.

For such a major purchase, it may pay to use the expertise of a professional computer consultant. Such a consultant can help with the entire process, from selection to purchase to installation to training. Computer consultants are located in all major cities and many smaller towns. They can be located through the local chamber of commerce, merchants' association, or telephone book advertising section. If you decide to hire a consultant, check references and credentials. Make sure there are no misunderstandings about services, fees, and associated items, and put the agreement in writing. Because you will have to open your office and your files to the consultant, you should also request a confidentiality agreement before the consultant begins his work.

Maintaining the Equipment

Maintaining equipment in the medical office involves keeping an inventory of what your office has and establishing equipment service contracts for routine maintenance and repair.

Equipment Inventories

It is important to keep an **inventory** of the medical office's equipment, a simple count of all the items on hand. Equipment inventories can be established in a computer spreadsheet, a database, or even a word processing program. A simple alternative for a smaller office is to keep an equipment inventory on index cards.

Record the type of equipment, the brand name, model, serial number, and other identifying information. Also note the date of purchase and whether the equipment was new or used. Record the purchase price and any additional information on current value, such as a recent appraisal. Include the name, address, and telephone number of the vendor and repair shop, and add the date and a brief note each time a piece of equipment is serviced or repaired.

It is a good idea to inventory all equipment at regular, established intervals. The office procedure manual should state when inventories will be performed and by whom. Each piece of equipment's condition should be noted at the time of the inventory. Be sure

> ### Working Smart
> Inventory information is especially valuable for tax purposes and to establish an insurance claim. It is important to keep the inventory record accurate and up-to-date.

to keep equipment inventories current and stored in a safe place.

Equipment Service Contracts

Equipment service contracts, sometimes called maintenance agreements, provide for routine maintenance and most repairs of the covered equipment. Service contracts usually provide for routine maintenance at no charge or a substantially reduced cost. Routine maintenance is usually required to keep the agreement in force. The office pays an upfront amount for the service contract and agrees to pay a small monthly or yearly fee. Needed repairs are performed at no charge or for a small fee. Some service contracts provide for only labor and bill the office for any parts required; other agreements cover both labor and parts. Some service contracts cover all costs up to a maximum stated in the agreement and charge the office for work over that amount.

As with lease agreements, service contracts can vary significantly. Make sure you fully understand all aspects of a service contract before you agree to it. File all documents related to the contract in a safe place.

Using Computers to Process Information

Computers are an essential part of any office, and a medical office, in particular, relies on them heavily to perform functions from scheduling to Internet research. In recent years, computers have dramatically changed the way medical office personnel perform routine activities. Thus, it is essential that a medical assistant be thoroughly familiar with computer concepts and functions. Some medical office computer activities are:

- creating and maintaining a database of patient demographic information
- accounting, billing, coding, and collections
- patient scheduling
- e-mailing, faxing, and online communication

- transcribing and preparing medical documents and correspondence
- creating and maintaining databases of supply and equipment inventories
- researching medical conditions, treatment protocols, and resources for patients

A medical office computer system may be made up of any number of components, selected and linked to provide a custom package to suit the medical office's needs. While computer systems differ because they are designed to meet specific needs, they all have some things in common. The system is built around a mainframe, minicomputer, or microcomputer, and other **hardware** components such as a keyboard, mouse, and printer. Each system includes processing and storage devices as part of the main component and peripherals that are designated as input and output devices. **Software** programs instruct the computer on how to process data and guide it in performing tasks.

Types of Computers

Computers are generally one of three main types: mainframe, minicomputer, or microcomputer (including portable models). These names indicate the computers' capabilities and how they might be used in a system.

MAINFRAME A mainframe computer is very large and can store and process vast amounts of data. It generally is used by government agencies, universities, and very large businesses to provide multiple capabilities at several locations. Medical office microcomputers may be able to access a mainframe to share information or for electronic mail capabilities.

MINICOMPUTER A minicomputer is smaller and less powerful than a mainframe but larger, and with more capabilities, than a microcomputer. Several minicomputers may be linked to form a network, and one of them may be designated as a "server." Servers collect and store information for the entire group, and make it available to others on the network. They also handle functions such as printing and communication among the group. More information on networks is offered later in this chapter.

MICROCOMPUTER A microcomputer is a small, self-contained unit that is ideally suited to homes, small offices, and some schools. Microcomputers—sometimes called personal computers or desktop computers—are less powerful than minicomputers, but changes in technology are rapidly shrinking the gap in capability between them. Microcomputers may be

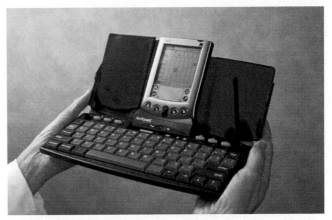

As technology advances, computer equipment becomes both smaller and more powerful.

linked in a network but also function well as stand-alone units.

A portable computer is a type of microcomputer. It is a personal computer that can be easily moved from one location to another. Portable computers are sometimes called laptop, notebook, or palmtop computers, and range from the size of a large textbook to something smaller than a standard No. 10 envelope. Portable computers have less power and storage capacity than other computers but offer obvious advantages that the others cannot match.

Computer Hardware

Computer hardware includes devices to put information into the computer and process, store, and output it. Some examples of hardware are the central processing unit or CPU, the monitor, keyboard, mouse, and various drives. **Computer peripherals** are equipment that is connected to the main unit, such as scanners and printers.

INPUT DEVICES Input devices allow information, or data, to be entered into the computer and let users communicate with the machine. Input devices include scanners, modems, keyboards, mice, or pointing devices. Some hardware items, such as modems and disk drives, can be used as either input or output devices.

The most common means for inputting data is the keyboard. The standard keyboard contains letter, number, symbol, and punctuation keys; arrow keys to move the cursor; a numeric keypad; and function keys used to perform processing or formatting functions.

Pointing devices enter data into the computer or direct the computer in certain processing functions. There are four types: a mouse, a trackball, a pen, and a touchpad.

- A mouse is probably the most familiar pointing device. It consists of a movable unit that fits easily under the hand and includes keys for directing functions. When you move the mouse, an indicator—called a cursor—moves on the screen, directed by your hand on the mouse. You can click or press mouse buttons to select or alter items displayed on the screen.
- A trackball works much like a mouse. It is a fixed-position ball that turns on an axis to move the cursor on the screen.
- A pen is a device that is used to point to, or select, items displayed on the monitor. Pens are often used in healthcare settings because they can be covered by a disposable plastic pouch to prevent contamination.
- A touchpad is a small, flat, sensitive pad that lets you move the cursor by simply moving your finger over the surface of the pad. Touchpads also have buttons that provide the same functions as the buttons on a mouse.

A **modem** is a device that transmits data electronically through a telephone line. This lets a computer communicate with other computers in distant locations. Modems are designated in terms of their speed, or baud rate. A higher baud rate means the modem can send information faster.

A **scanner** is another type of input device that is often found in a medical office. A scanner inputs graphics (pictures) or text (printed material) rapidly, in a format that the computer can use. Each scanned item is stored in the computer as a file. There are three primary types of scanners: hand-held, single sheet, and flatbed. Hand-held scanners are relatively inexpensive but difficult to use. They produce a poor-quality result. Single sheet scanners require that one sheet at a time be placed in the scanner. Their cost is moderate, and results are usually quite good. Flatbed, multisheet scanners are the most expensive and easiest to use, and produce a high-quality computer file. If your office requires the scanning of documents, buying a fax machine with scanning ability may be more practical than purchasing a separate piece of equipment.

PROCESSING DEVICES Processing devices are usually inside the computer cabinet, included as part of the main unit. These devices calculate, format, sort, and manipulate data. Processing devices include the motherboard and the CPU, or central processing unit, sometimes called a microprocessor.

The **motherboard** is the foundation of the computer system. It is the primary circuit board that holds or has connections for all the other computer components. It allows for control and communication among the components. Different sizes and types of motherboards permit faster processing and expandability.

The **central processing unit** (**CPU**) is the main chip that runs the computer and directs the processing of data. The CPU is also responsible for interpreting and carrying out instructions in the software. The type of CPU determines the speed and capabilities of the computer. Various microprocessors have different names, some designated by a number, such as 486, and others by a name, such as Pentium or Celeron. Different processor chips have somewhat different capabilities, but all microprocessors are rated for their speed, measured in megahertz (abbreviated MHz). The higher the number of MHz, the faster the microprocessor works.

STORAGE DEVICES Storage devices are necessary to store and retrieve data in the computer system. Computers use memory, along with the storage devices, to temporarily or permanently store information. **Read only memory** (**ROM**) stores information permanently, while **random access memory** (**RAM**) is temporary storage. The ROM is a part of the computer system that is inaccessible to the average user, and is responsible for starting, or "booting up," the computer. The RAM is usable only if the computer is running. If it is turned off, or electricity is interrupted, data in the RAM that has not been saved to a permanent storage device such as a drive will be lost. The RAM is measured in megabytes (MB). The larger the number of megabytes or gigabytes (1,000 megabytes equals one gigabyte), the greater the storage capacity. Many popular software programs require large amounts of RAM.

The computer's main drive, called a **hard disk or hard drive**, is housed in the main computer case and offers a large amount of permanent storage. Hard drive storage capacity is measured in megabytes or gigabytes, and, like other computer components, the larger the number, the greater the capacity. The programs or applications that give the computer its capabilities are usually stored on the hard drive, along with other important data that need to be readily accessed. Today's computers commonly need hard drives with many gigabytes of capacity to store popular software programs.

Diskette drives are additional drives that write or store information on **diskettes**, commonly known as disks. The information then can be read or retrieved from the diskette. The diskette itself is composed of a small circle of magnetized material housed in a plastic casing. This system provides for permanent data storage. The most common diskette size is 3.5 inches. Table 6.2 lists things to consider when using and storing disks.

Table 6.2 Diskette Care and Storage

- Never expose the diskette to extremely hot temperatures. Disks left on the dashboard of a car in summer have melted, and extreme heat also can cause loss of data.
- Always make sure the diskette is protected with a plastic sleeve or a diskette holder. Disks can be damaged by bending, breaking, or having liquids or particles spilled on them.
- Keep diskettes away from strong magnetic fields. This includes refrigerator or filing cabinet magnets, stereo speakers, telephones, and microwave ovens. Exposure to magnetic fields can result in loss of data.
- Never touch the magnetic surface of the diskette with your fingers. Fingerprints can destroy data or make it impossible for files to be copied onto the disk.
- Never insert a damaged diskette into a disk drive. Damaged diskettes can become stuck in the drive, damaging the drive.

CD-ROM drives use a small, flat object called a compact disk, or CD, which looks very much like a music CD. The CD is inserted into the CD-ROM drive, which then reads information from the disk. CDs can hold very large amounts of data, much more than diskettes, and offer longer-lasting storage. Many software programs are stored on CDs and loaded into a computer through the CD-ROM drive. CDs can produce high-quality graphics, animation, and sound—a combination called multimedia. Table 6.3 describes the proper care and storage of compact disks.

A good way to save storage memory space when sending several files over the Internet is to use a compressed file. Instead of downloading several files individually, a user can compress them all into a single file in one step. Later, the files can be retrieved and decompressed back to their original state. The software used to create these files is called a compression utility.

Technology Tip

WinZip, a common compression utility is available at www.winzip.com. Evaluation versions are available at no cost.

Working Smart

When selecting a printer for the office, consider the cost of toner cartridges as you assess each model's price and features.

Table 6.3 Compact Disk Care and Storage

- Keep compact disks in a plastic sleeve or storage container to protect them from scratches. Scratches can make a CD unreadable.
- Periodically blow dust off CDs with a can of compressed air, or wipe them gently with special cloths designed for cleaning CDs. Never insert a dirty CD into your computer's CD-ROM drive.
- Do not expose CDs to extremely hot environments. CDs are made of plastic and can warp or melt under extreme conditions.

Tape drives are usually external drives (outside the main computer cabinet) that are used to store, or "back up," the entire contents of the hard drive for protection against data loss. Tape drives can be bulky and slow, and are being replaced, at least partially, by Zip® disks that offer a much more compact solution to storage problems.

OUTPUT DEVICES Output devices let the computer display or give out information that has been received or processed. Monitors and printers are examples of output devices.

A monitor works like a television screen to display information the computer has processed. Monitors are judged by their resolution and screen size, and come in monochrome (single color) and color versions. Many popular software programs require a color monitor.

Resolution describes the sharpness of the image the monitor displays. It is measured in pixels—the greater the number of pixels, the higher the resolution and the sharper the image. Monitor screen size is measured diagonally, in inches, from one corner to another. Common screen sizes range from 14 to 16 inches, or larger. Programs that display a lot of graphics generally require a larger screen, while word processing programs can generally use a smaller screen. If your office uses scheduling and accounting software, the larger screen will be more useful.

A printer is essential in a medical office to produce printed material, or "hard copy," from a computer. Printer technology is advancing and resulting in lower prices. Resolution and speed are the primary means of evaluating and comparing printers. Resolution is measured in dots per inch, or dpi. A higher-dpi printer produces higher-resolution output, or sharper letters and pictures.

Printer types include dot matrix, inkjet, and laser. Dot matrix printers are an older type and usually print on continuous-feed paper. They are quite inexpensive but produce low-resolution output. Other major disadvantage are that they are noisy, incapable of color printing, and much slower than other types of printers.

Inkjet printers use a fine spray of liquid ink to transfer images to the paper. They are quiet, relatively inexpensive, and produce high quality output. Inkjet printers can produce color images by using different color inks, so they are very versatile. They are generally much faster than dot matrix printers but often slower than laser printers. A disadvantage is that they cannot produce high-resolution images as well as laser printers.

Laser printers use micro-fine powdered toner to transfer images to paper. The toner is made to penetrate the paper when heat is applied. The heat melts the toner powder and bonds it to the paper. Laser printers are very quiet and quickly produce printed pages. Color laser printers are also available. While they are the most expensive, they also offer the highest resolution of any generally available office printer.

Software

Software (also called "applications" or "programs") is the set of instructions that tells the computer how to process data. Software available for today's medical office lets you perform a tremendous variety of functions with speed and accuracy. These include word processing, spreadsheets, database use, desktop publishing, presentations, virus protection, and security management; there are also integrated software packages that combine these functions. Software programs are continually being improved, or **upgraded**. Table 6.4 lists issues to consider when investigating a software upgrade.

Computer software programs are licensed by the company that wrote and trademarked them. When you buy the software, you also purchase a limited right to

Legal Issue
Violations of software licensure laws can result in fines or imprisonment.

install it on a computer and use it. **Licensure** is governed by federal law.

If the software license only permits the user to install the software on one computer, you may need to purchase additional licenses if you have several computers. These can be bought from the dealer where the software was purchased or the company that produced it, without buying additional copies of the software.

The software program will be written on a compact disk or a series of diskettes and will typically be packaged in a box along with the licensure information and instruction manuals for installing and using the program. It is important to read the instruction manuals (often called "documentation") and keep them in a safe but convenient place. The manuals may also contain important information on how to get information and help with the installation and use of the software. With newer programs, documentation and support are available online.

Technology Tip
Many software companies have experts who give help and advice about their software. This is called "technical support" and is often available through a toll-free number, online, or by fax.

WORD PROCESSING SOFTWARE Word processing software lets you enter text into the computer and format, edit, and manipulate that text in various ways. These programs may include the ability to use pictures or figures (called "graphics"), and also may include elements of other software types. For example, some word processing programs have limited spreadsheet or database capabilities. In a medical office, word processing programs can be used to produce letters, memos, and reports. These programs also can be used to transcribe the physician's dictated notes, patient progress reports, and other medical record documents. Examples of popular word processing software are WordPerfect® and Microsoft Word®.

DESKTOP PUBLISHING SOFTWARE Desktop publishing is the production of text and images so that the result is suitable for high-volume reproduction. Desktop publishing software lets a computer user create a finished product that is comparable to the result formerly achieved only by sophisticated printing processes. In the medical office, desktop publishing

Table 6.4 Software Upgrades

- Before making a purchase decision, consider whether upgrading is right for your office. If you are planning to install a new computer system soon, upgrading existing software would waste time and money, or your office simply may not need an upgraded version of its software.
- When buying new versions of software, look for special upgrade packages designed for current users of the software. These let you install files that bring software already on your computer up to date, giving you the newest version of the software. Upgrade packages are much less expensive than buying the entire new version of the software, and they can be installed faster.
- Consider licensure. You will need to purchase an upgrade package for each computer on which software will be upgraded unless you buy a special site license for the upgrading.
- Read all directions and instructions before you install the upgrade software. Most software producers offer a technical support number you can call for assistance with upgrading. Note that there may be a charge for using the technical support service.

software is used to produce brochures, newsletters, fliers, signs, and other items without having to use a print shop. QuarkXPress® and Pagemaker® are two well-known examples of desktop publishing software. However, many functions of desktop publishing software can be handled by word processing programs such as Microsoft Word®.

SPREADSHEET PROGRAMS Spreadsheets are programs used for accounting purposes that let you enter numerical data and manipulate it in various ways, including performing mathematical calculations. Many spreadsheet programs also can handle word processing and graphics. Spreadsheet programs are used for expense sheets, tax calculations and reporting, and other financial matters. A spreadsheet program may be part of a medical billing software package. Microsoft Excel® is an example of a commonly available spreadsheet.

DATABASE PROGRAMS Database applications let you enter components of related data and manipulate them as blocks or individual components. Database software has a variety of uses in the medical office, including:

■ managing employee information for communication, payroll, and other purposes
■ handling patient demographic information such as names, addresses, identification numbers, and insurance information for billing and communication
■ compiling lists of vendors or suppliers

Databases can sort and rearrange the information in various ways, as well as manage database files. Microsoft Access® is an example of a database.

PRESENTATION PROGRAMS Presentation software is designed to produce high quality graphics with limited amounts of text in a format suitable for displaying on a computer monitor's screen or projecting onto a larger screen. It is used to present ideas using primarily images, and often involves animation. In the medical office, presentation software may be used for patient and staff teaching. PowerPoint® is an example of presentation software.

VIRUS PROTECTION AND SECURITY SOFTWARE Antivirus software is essential for any computer system. It protects a computer against being infected by a range of viruses and cleans any existing viruses from files. Any computer is susceptible to viruses, especially computers that download files from the Internet or similar sources. Antivirus software can literally save a computer system (and associated electronic files) from destruction. In a medical office, this might include medical records, patient billing files, financial and tax

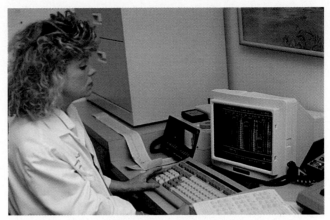

Medical assistants use computers for scheduling, billing, maintaining patient records, and many other functions.

records, and all the information required to successfully manage a practice. Antivirus software should be considered as very reasonably priced insurance for electronic data. Norton AntiVirus® and McAfee VirusScan® are examples of virus protection software.

INTEGRATED SOFTWARE Integrated software packages offer several types of software in a single program or package. Medical management packages, such as Computer Solutions' MEDWARE®, have been designed specifically with the medical office in mind. They contain software that facilitates appointment scheduling, insurance processing, inputting of diagnosis codes, tracking patient treatment and history, maintaining patient charts, and compiling mailing lists. Integrated software packages can solve many of a medical office's information needs and offer the advantage of being able to transfer data smoothly from one part of the application to another.

Computer Networks

A series of minicomputers or microcomputers linked together form a network. Some networks have one computer, called a server, that acts as a central storage unit or processor. Networked computers can share information rapidly and easily, and permit almost instant communication among the network locations. Computer networks can be quite flexible and can have their components in a small area, such as a single room or building, or in very remote locations. Arranging or configuring a computer network usually requires the knowledge and experience of someone familiar with network hardware and software.

LOCAL AREA NETWORKS A local area network (LAN) connects computers that are close to one another, such as on the same floor or in the same building. Typically, they share one or more printers and a storage device. In a medical office with a LAN, one user can work on a patient's insurance claim while another is simultaneously accessing the same file to update the patient's history. Office staff members can also communicate with each other without leaving their desks by sending e-mail.

WIDE AREA NETWORKS A wide area network (WAN) spans a vast distance and connects two or more LANs. For example, many governments and universities use WANs to share data among networks.

Special Uses of the Computer in the Medical Office

Computers can be used to simplify and speed up the day-to-day work in a medical office. They offer many advantages in areas that require manipulation of data, simplified data storage, or highly repetitious work involving information. A computer with online capabilities can significantly streamline communication. In a medical office, computers are used to create templates, provide instant local and long-distance communication, transfer information, do research, share medical records instantly among healthcare providers, and submit medical insurance claims.

CREATING FORM LETTERS AND OTHER TEMPLATES
Templates are basic files that are used repeatedly to speed up work. Unique data can be added to each of a series of templates to produce a set of originals that have a basic format in common. Templates are used extensively in any office and may be as simple as a memo or fax cover sheet or as complex as an entire presentation format. Computers allow the basic template to be produced and stored electronically, then retrieved and modified by the addition of selected data. Creating and using templates requires no additional equipment beyond the usual computer components but may demand larger-than-usual electronic storage capabilities.

COMMUNICATING VIA E-MAIL AND FAX E-mail, or electronic mail, has revolutionized communication in the past few years. Computers connected to a large network make this possible. In addition to using e-mail, a computer with an online connection can fax large amounts of data across tremendous distances almost instantly. Data can be input in one location and printed out in another thousands of miles away. This means that communication and data transfer can be accomplished without leaving the office—activities that previously required a great deal of effort and expense. E-mailing and faxing require that the computer have a modem and access to a telephone line.

RESEARCHING VIA THE INTERNET Internet capabilities provide a large variety of information resources for a medical office. An Internet connection is the equivalent of having a huge library at the fingertips of the computer operator. Internet access permits rapid searching and retrieval of information. Like e-mail and faxing, Internet research requires a modem and access to a telephone line and a connection with an Internet service. America Online® is an example of an Internet service provider.

SHARING MEDICAL RECORDS In the past, healthcare has been limited by the fact that the healthcare provider and the patient had to be in the same physical location. Computers and the Internet have changed all that. By using **telemedicine,** the transmission of video images for medical purposes, patients can be routinely diagnosed and even treated by physicians many miles away. Computers allow information to be shared instantly so that medical care can be provided to almost anyone, anywhere.

For example, a home healthcare nurse in a remote mountain location can share information with a physician specialist in a metropolitan area via computer. The doctor can see the patient's appearance, and the nurse can transmit sophisticated information, such as an ECG tracing, to the physician. The nurse can then receive an instant diagnosis and orders for treatment of the patient.

Information sharing may require a modem, Internet access, a phone line, or other specialized equipment—depending on specific activities—in addition to a basic computer system.

Legal Issue

Telemedicine is an exciting development in healthcare that is certain to grow rapidly in the coming years. However, the advances in telemedicine also raise complicated legal issues:

- How can physicians assure privacy for personal medical records that are sent via telecommunication?
- If the parties are in different states, which state's malpractice laws would be in effect?
- Considering that doctors can only practice in the state in which they are licensed, are they crossing state lines when they practice telemedicine?

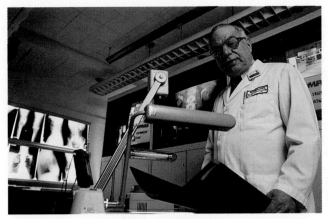

Telemedicine makes this doctor's knowledge and experience available to help patients many miles away.

Table 6.4 Getting the Most Out of Your Computer System

- **Have at least a basic working knowledge of how your computer functions.**
- **Make good use of hardware and software manuals that come with your computer.** These are written by the people who know the most about your computer. Keep all manuals, instruction cards, and documents supplied with the computer and/or software. Refer to them when you have a question or have problems with the computer. Be sure to keep manuals in a safe place, where they are accessible but protected.
- **Use reference materials.** Most bookstores sell a variety of reference books on computers, including ones dealing with popular software. These books are often written in a very readable style and are designed to help novices become acquainted with software products. Bookstore personnel can sometimes recommend a particular type of reference book.
- **Get adequate training on new software.** Training classes are available through computer consulting firms in most cities. Classes are also taught through universities, as non-credit courses, and through community colleges. Some software producers offer training videos to help users get the most out of their products. The Internet can also be an important source for training and training materials.
- **Use technical support when appropriate.** Many software companies offer technical help for users of their software. Usually, you can call a toll-free number for direct assistance from trained personnel. Be aware, however, that there may be a charge for the assistance and call. If you use a fee-based technical support service, make sure you outline your questions in writing first.
- **Online help may be the answer.** You may be able to get technical assistance directly from the software producer through the company's website. This online help is often free and can provide a quick, efficient way to get your questions answered. Make sure you know the extent of the services offered and whether there is a charge.

SUBMITTING CLAIMS Computers are used to submit medical insurance claims almost instantly, a process that previously required several days. Computers can associate required billing codes with diagnoses and procedures, insert data appropriately into billing form templates, and transmit the information to the claim processor instantly. These activities require a modem, telephone line, and careful coordination between the parties involved in submitting, receiving, and processing medical claims.

Managing the Computer

The computer is only as good as its user. You will want to become educated in the use and care of your computer. Learn how to create and organize files to best suit your office's needs. It will be important to periodically clean up the hard drive, discarding unneeded files, and to make backups of essential information. It is also important to understand and avoid physical problems that may be associated with computer use. Table 6.4 offers suggestions for learning about your computer system.

MANAGING THE HARD DRIVE The hard drive is the primary storage unit used with most computers. The large storage capacity houses operating systems, applications programs, and data files. When setting up a hard drive, be sure to follow the manufacturer's guidelines for installing and formatting. Load operating systems first, then fonts, applications programs, and data files, in that order. Be aware that if less than 10% to 15% of the computer's capacity is left unused, it may develop problems that slow its functioning or cause printing errors.

ORGANIZING FILES Any software application can be used to create files. For example, document files are created by word processing programs, spreadsheet files by spreadsheet programs, and database files by database programs. Each file is given a file name so that it can be saved and retrieved for later use. A file name is generally eight characters or fewer, and does not have spaces or special characters such as "&" or "#."

To keep files straight, the user should organize them into directories and subdirectories (DOS operating system) or into folders (Macintosh and Windows operating systems). Some people create separate directories or folders for applications (such as Word or Excel) so that all Word files are stored in one folder. Others create directories for separate projects or topics. For example, you might create a folder on your hard drive that is called "templates." Within the templates folder, you might have a subfolder or subdirectory called "letters." Within this folder, you might save standard form letters that you will call up and adapt for each situation. One such document might be a Word form letter to use when submitting an invoice to a patient, called "inv.doc." By organizing information in folders and

Figure 6.1
Organizing Folders and
Files on the Hard Drive

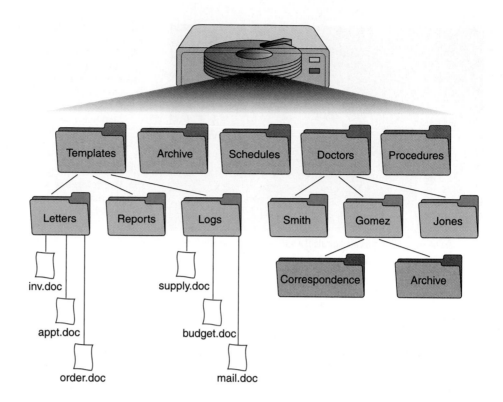

subfolders, the computer user develops a hierarchical structure like the one shown in Figure 6.1.

There is no one correct way to organize your hard drive, but as hard drives get larger, keeping your folders and files organized is essential. Experienced computer users typically create separate folders representing each main area of their job. This could include different folders for individual projects; separate folders for business documents and personal documents; different folders for each physician, physician's assistant, or nurse practitioner; and different folders for archived files versus works-in-progress.

BACKING UP FILES It will be necessary to copy vital data at regular intervals. Tax records, invoices, reports,

> **Working smart**
> Do not store backup files near the original files; keep them in a secure storage area away from the office. This will protect the data in case of fire or a natural disaster.

and other essential data need to be backed up in case of natural disaster or storage device failure. Duplicate files can be saved on diskettes. If your computer is on a network, you can make one copy on your own hard drive and another on the central server. Periodically, the entire network can be backed up and the copy taken to a secure storage area. Some computers automatically back up data to a high-capacity storage site during low-usage hours.

UNDERSTANDING ERGONOMICS Ergonomics is the science of interactions between people and their work environment. Computers present a number of ergonomic concerns. Health risks associated with computers include eyestrain, backaches, and repetitive motion disorders such as carpal tunnel syndrome, in which nerves in the arm become pinched. There is also the psychological stress that can result from prolonged, repetitive activity that is monotonous and yet

> **Legal Issue**
> Maintaining the security of computer files is essential. In some offices, each employee with access to the computer system is given a password. This password should never be shared with anyone except the office manager. If an employee quits or is fired, that password should be deleted from the system.

requires constant attention. To avoid physical and psychological problems from computer use, keep these tips in mind:

- Take regular breaks.
- Type at a keyboard lower than your elbows.
- Use a wrist pad.
- Sit in an ergonomically designed chair, resting your feet squarely on the floor, with thighs parallel to the floor.
- Use an antiglare screen, or position the monitor to avoid glare.
- Keep your eyes at least 18 inches from the monitor, and use a large screen, if possible.
- Avoid small type.

Overseeing Supplies for the Medical Office

Every medical office needs a system for managing the hundreds or thousands of items it must have to operate efficiently. You will need to identify the supplies that are needed. They should be inventoried periodically and restocked when necessary. A good supply tracking system will tell you the name and quantity of items you should have on hand, what you actually have at any given moment, and how many of each item you should order. The system also should provide for correct storage of individual items, including temperature control, security of drug supplies, and a labeling method for storage areas.

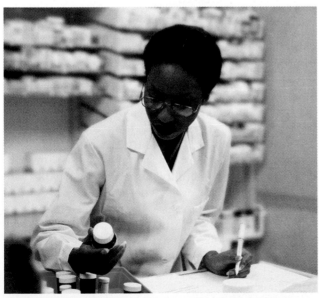

Maintaining medical supplies requires careful attention to detail and accurate documentation.

In an established office, an efficient supply management system should already be in place. In that case, your job will be to use and maintain the system. Some medical assistants, however, will be called upon to establish a supply management system in an office where none exists or to correct an inadequate system. In any event, you will need to understand the basics of supply management so that you can establish, use, and maintain a functional system.

Identifying Necessary Supplies

The first step in creating a supply management system is to identify necessary supplies. If you are working in an established office, you may only need to inventory existing supplies and identify items that are needed but missing. If you are managing supplies for a new office, you need to list all items the office will need.

The system will work best if you make separate lists for front office and back office supplies. Some supplies, such as pens, notepads, and tape, are used in both places.

Supplies for the front office will include everything an administrative office requires for day-to-day functioning. Examples are desk items such as paper clips and staples, copier and printer toner or toner cartridges, paper and envelopes, various forms, file folders and filing materials, appointment books, reference books, equipment cleaning supplies, and computer disks. Back office supplies will include needles, syringes, wound care and dressing supplies, items used in minor surgery, suture removal kits, autoclaving and sterilization supplies, sterile and non-sterile gloves, solutions and medications, and other items required for direct patient care.

Supply items should be clearly labeled, and each type of item should have its own storage area. The area should be identified with the names and quantity of each item. You may find it helpful to use label-making equipment and create permanent labels identifying the general contents of individual storage areas. Then, tape a paper list or computer printout of the exact contents and quantity of each item inside the cabinet or drawer. This method will help you and your coworkers quickly identify where supplies are stored, and it can help alert you to items that may need to be reordered.

Establishing a Supply Tracking System

If your office is new and you are ordering supplies for the first time, it is easy to key them into a computer database or inventory control program as you make out order forms. If you are working with an existing office, you can use your inventory list. Either way, you will need to have a method that lets you see instantly what you have on hand, what you should have, and what needs to be ordered.

A very good computerized supply tracking system will tell you the last time an item was ordered, the name and address of the supplier, and the price. It also may have an option that allows you to compile an order list. Stores selling office supplies or computer software may be able to provide a simple system that meets your needs. Or you may want to get a high-end system designed just for tracking inventories. Shop around to see what types of systems are available and which best meets the needs of your office.

If you cannot use a computerized system to oversee supplies, the job of tracking them will be more difficult and time-consuming. However, a manual or paper-based supply tracking system can be almost as efficient if used correctly. Some manual systems use formatted cards to note the name of the item, quantity on hand, date of last order, quantity received, cost of the item, and ordering information. The cards are kept in a filing box with a metal or plastic marker that flags the card of each item that is to be reordered. Supply items can be inventoried on formatted cards kept in a filing box or simply listed on paper, with rows for supply item names and columns for quantity, cost, ordering information, etc.

Once you have an established supply tracking system, you will need to use it correctly. Be sure to conduct inventories at times specified by the system, and to count all items. Keep pricing and ordering information updated by immediately entering all items received into the tracking system. The tracking/inventory system is only a tool—how well it serves your office depends on how well the tool is used and maintained.

Ordering Supplies

The way you order supplies will be determined, at least in part, by the requirements of **vendors** (companies that sell supplies). You will need to start with a list of the supplies and quantities you need, extracted from your supply management system. The system should also tell you where and how to order, and provide current prices. Some vendors may provide you with order forms, while others may expect you to send a printed list of items and quantities. Many vendors accept fax or e-mail orders.

Make sure any orders you submit are complete and correct. Include the full name of each item, any reference numbers, size or type, quantity, and price. Some vendors may want you to refer to a catalog or brochure

> ### Working Smart
> In deciding when to reorder, consider how much of the stock will be used while waiting for the new order to arrive. You don't want to be caught short, and rush orders can be very expensive.

number. Make sure your order is legible and that all information has been included. Be sure to indicate if payment is enclosed or if the order is being charged to an account.

Keep a copy of each order you place. File the copy and make an entry in a tickler, or pending, file on the date you expect to receive the shipment. If an order doesn't arrive when you expect it, call the vendor to ask why. Be sure to have a copy of the order and any other pertinent information at hand. If an order or shipment has been lost or misdirected, the vendor will not know until you call.

> ### Working Smart
> When storing supplies, place the newest stock in back so the older supplies are used first. This is especially important when dealing with medications or anything with an expiration date.

Receiving and Storing Supplies

When you receive a supply order, check it carefully for problems. Make sure the shipment matches the order, that all items are included and in good condition, and that quantities are correct. The vendor will probably include a copy of your order or a shipping invoice that notes what you ordered.

If you find a problem, first check the ordering information and shipping invoice to see if any items were back-ordered or substituted. Notify the vendor of problems immediately, and ask that missing items be sent as soon as possible. If the vendor substituted an item for one you ordered and you find the substitute unacceptable, let the vendor know so that the correct item can be sent or the charge can be removed. Broken or damaged items also need to be replaced or have their charges removed—if the vendor accepts responsibility for shipping. If the vendor's responsibility ends when the order is turned over to a shipping company, you will need to indicate if the damage occurred before you received it. Any merchandise sent in a damaged condition is the responsibility of the vendor. If items were broken or damaged during shipping, you should file a claim with the shipper.

Supplies should be entered into the inventory/tracking system as they are received. However, do not

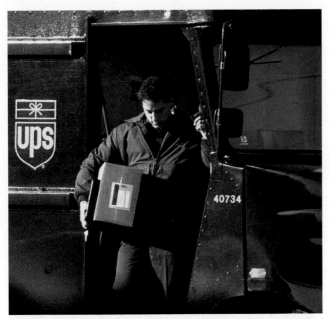

When a shipment from a vendor comes in, you must make sure it matches the original order and that all items are in good condition.

include broken, damaged, or otherwise unacceptable items from a shipment.

Make sure that all items are stored properly. Some (such as blood-agar plates for cultures or certain drugs or solutions) may need to be kept refrigerated. If the need for refrigeration, or other special handling, is noted on the shipping label or outside of the container, it is the shipper's responsibility to provide the special handling. Items that require cold temperatures must be refrigerated immediately when they are received. You may need to tell coworkers when you are expecting a shipment that requires special handling so someone else can see that it receives proper care if you are not available.

Storing Drugs

Any drugs in a shipment should be included in a special drug inventory and stored in a safe place. **Scheduled drugs**, in particular, must be carefully inventoried and stored in a locked drawer or cabinet with limited access. (In many offices, only the physician has a key.) These drugs, referred to as controlled substances, are dangerous and have the potential for abuse or addiction. Their distribution and use is controlled by the Drug Enforcement Administration (DEA) of the Department of Justice. These drugs are separated into five categories called "schedules," and are strictly regulated by federal law. In addition to your regular office drug inventory, any scheduled drugs received must be entered on DEA drug inventory forms. Two people should always sign when scheduled drugs are added to

or removed from the inventory. If a drug order is short, notify the physician at once. If the shortage includes scheduled drugs, the DEA and local law enforcement officials must be informed. It is a good idea to keep all drugs—even non-scheduled ones—in a locked storage area.

Selecting Sources for Supplies and Services

As a medical assistant, it is your responsibility to make wise purchasing decisions for the medical office. Whether you are ordering supplies, buying new equipment, or investigating the use of an outside service, you must be sure you are getting the most for your money. Explore the various sources available, and do "comparison shopping."

Vendors

Choose supply and equipment vendors carefully. Keep in mind that you will be establishing a long-term relationship (provided the vendor gives you good service), one that can impact the economic status of your office. Price is not the only concern when selecting a vendor. You also need to consider service, warranties, shipping, and payment terms. When you evaluate potential vendors:

- Ask for bids on certain common items that you order frequently. Check prices to see who is lowest, but also ask about ordering requirements. Some vendors offer lower prices only if you order very large quantities.
- Check shipping and/or delivery times. If you have to wait three weeks, a month, or more for your order, a lower price may not be much of a bargain.
- Ask potential vendors to submit their payment terms. You may find that some supply houses have such stringent payment requirements that your accounting systems cannot accommodate them, or that vendors who give discounts for prompt payment have a payment schedule that makes it impossible to actually get the discounts.
- Ask if the vendor pays for shipping, or if you must add that cost to your order.
- Find out about service. Does the vendor offer a toll-free number you can call to resolve problems? Are customer service representatives friendly and courteous? Can they answer your questions? How are returns handled?

If you do not like the answers you get from a potential supplier, seek out another or ask the supplier to accommodate your needs. You may want to quote prices, terms, or services of another potential supplier and negotiate for similar arrangements. Some vendors may offer a contract, specifying prices, terms, and service for a given amount of time. A contract may require you to order exclusively from one vendor for the length of the contract, or may specify that you will pay for a certain quantity whether or not you can use it. These arrangements may not serve your needs, so make sure you understand all the terms and conditions before you enter into any agreement.

Some offices routinely review all vendors once a year and decide whether to continue using each vendor or to shop for another. If you are placing an order with a vendor for the first time, it is a good idea to contact a representative of the vendor—even if your order seems small. The contact gives you an opportunity to ask questions and clarify ordering and payment procedures, discounts, and related issues.

Sales Representatives

Many supply houses have sales representatives who visit physicians' offices periodically. These representatives can be valuable sources of information and can help you establish a relationship with their organization. They can explain their ordering process and methods of handling problems. They also keep you informed about new products and services and often provide samples for you to evaluate before you commit to an order.

Catalogs

Your office will probably receive catalogs from potential suppliers in each day's mail. If you would like to see more, you can call supply houses and ask them to send their current catalogs. Some suppliers also provide information by fax or through the Internet. You may want to create a special file for these catalogs and review them when you make decisions on vendors.

Catalogs include important information on the supply house's ordering, shipping, and payment policies. Some catalogs have an order form bound into the book, with adjacent pages containing policy information. Read this carefully. After comparing policies on returns, billing, special orders, and other items important to your office, select a supplier that offers the type of service you want. If you cannot find answers to your

questions in the catalog, most supply houses have a toll-free customer service number.

Outside Service Providers

Your office may need to use outside services in addition to those the regular staff provides. This may be temporary, to cope with unusually heavy demands, or permanent, to manage the daily work flow. Services provided by outside contractors include diagnostic services, equipment maintenance and repair, office cleaning, transcription, billing, accounting, payroll, human resources, security, and waste and hazardous material removal.

Advantages of using outside service providers include:

- Cost efficiency—It may be more cost-effective to use outside services, as opposed to hiring office staff to manage the workload. Using outside service providers can eliminate the need to recruit, screen, hire, and train employees. In addition, workers supplied by an outside provider don't have to be retained when work volume is low or the office is closed for an extended time.
- Convenience—For example, instead of managing payroll and taxes for six transcriptionists, the office manager pays the transcription service provider with a single check.
- Expertise—Often, a physician's office will use outside contractors because it needs specialty work beyond the experience of the office staff.
- Legality—Most state and local laws require that certain products be recycled. A waste management contractor can assist you with recycling paper, plastic, aluminum, and glass products.
- Safety—Hazardous materials such as contaminated needles and surgical waste require specific disposal methods. Your office can contract with an organization that specializes in disposing of hazardous medical waste. The contractor provides your office with containers for disposing of these materials and removes them periodically.

NEGOTIATING PRICES AND CONTRACTS When you are looking for providers of outside services, always check with several providers and ask for bids. The bidding process can be as formal or informal as you like, but you should never contract with one provider— even for a small job—without first considering all the options available. Ask suppliers to put their bids in

> **Technology Tip**
> Many vendors provide up-to-date product information on their websites. Use the Internet rather than cluttering the office with old catalogs.

writing, especially if large sums of money are involved. Keep records to show how and why you selected the provider, and include all bids that were submitted. Notify the provider you select in writing, and refer to the bid so there is no misunderstanding.

If you do not seek bids, you may want to choose one supplier or service provider that offers the services or equipment you want and then negotiate for the best overall agreement. This may include substituting some services or equipment, reducing lease rates or purchase prices, or providing additional supplies, equipment, or services as part of the agreement.

Never hesitate to ask for a lower rate or price if you believe the original rate you were quoted is excessive. While negotiation may not be the norm in everyday transactions between individuals, it is quite common in business. Become aware of how business transactions are managed to ensure that your office secures the most advantageous agreements.

EVALUATING SERVICES Periodically evaluate the quality, quantity, and cost of all services. Use your evaluations to decide if you should continue using the same provider, seek a different one, or discontinue purchasing the service altogether.

You will probably find it efficient and effective to use the same criteria you use for identifying vendors and suppliers in evaluating existing providers. Consider cost, quality of service or product, reliability, provider policies, and other factors. After comparing your office's current arrangements with those offered by new providers or suppliers, negotiate for the best agreements. If you find that a new vendor can offer a better deal but you like working with an existing vendor, approach your sales representative about negotiating a new contract. As always, make sure agreements are in writing and that all your questions are answered. Keep records of your negotiations, decisions, and agreements.

Challenging Situations

*T*he front office of a medical practice may be clearly visible to patients in the waiting room. Keep in mind that nothing going on in the front office will go unobserved. You will want to convey the impression of a well-organized, professional office. Monitor your interactions with coworkers. Loud joking or angry exchanges do not convey a businesslike atmosphere. Be careful to keep any confidential information you may be discussing in the office out of earshot of waiting patients. You may be handling both patients entering the office and administrative duties at the same time, but be certain you never give the patients the impression that they are interrupting your work. Let them know that their needs come first.

Signing up with a service provider, getting into a lease program, or hiring a consultant are long-term commitments that require careful scrutiny. You will want to make sure that the individuals or organizations you are dealing with are reputable. Ask for and call references. Contact the local Better Business Bureau to check on their record. Past history goes a long way in determining future performance.

Clinical Summary

- A medical assistant may be required to perform a number of non-clinical tasks relating to the administrative functions of the medical office.
- Administrative and reception areas of the office should be kept attractive, clean, and uncluttered.
- Medical office décor usually reflects the physician's medical specialty.
- Following correct procedure in opening and closing the office is absolutely essential.
- Security issues involve securing drugs and records from unauthorized use and providing for burglary protection when the office is closed.
- Safety of patients and staff is paramount. An emergency plan should be documented in the office's safety manual. All staff members must be familiar with the procedures in the manual.
- Medical offices are using technology with increasing frequency, and medical assistants must be able to manage and efficiently use the most up-to-date equipment, including computers.
- The medical assistant should understand the features and uses of basic office equipment, and should be aware of decision-making points in regard to its purchase.
- A computer system consists of both hardware (equipment) and software (instructions that let users interact with the hardware) selected for a particular use.

- A computer system's primary hardware components include processing, storage, input, and output devices. Software, sometimes called programs or applications, is usually one of several types: word processing, spreadsheet, database, desktop publishing, presentation, virus protection and security, or integrated packages.
- Software licensure is an important legal aspect of computer purchase and use in any office. The medical assistant should be aware of and adhere to licensing agreements.
- Computer networks consist of several computers linked together so they can share information, including software, available on the network.
- Computers have a variety of uses in the medical office. These include preparing letters, memos, and reports; accounting and record-keeping functions; e-mail and faxing; Internet research; and communication. Less-recognized uses include creating form letters and other templates, sharing electronic medical records, and submitting insurance claims electronically.
- Medical office equipment should be inventoried regularly. A responsible medical assistant keeps careful records on equipment inventories, maintenance, and repairs.
- Decisions about the medical office include whether to buy or lease equipment, and whether to purchase a maintenance agreement or service contract on equipment.
- Overseeing supplies is important in any medical office. There should be a system that provides for consistency in ordering, receiving, storing, and maintaining supplies. Establishing the system begins with identifying necessary supplies and making a comprehensive list of all supplies.
- Identifying and working with vendors or suppliers is an important part of maintaining office supplies.
- Talking with sales representatives and reviewing catalogs can provide important information about vendors and make the process of selecting one easier. It is important to consider all aspects when selecting a vendor, including service, quality, and price.
- Many offices find it helpful to use outside services for some medical office functions. Common functions handled by outside service providers include billing, accounting, and payroll. Choosing an outside service provider is very much like choosing a vendor for supplies or equipment.
- Outside service providers, supply and equipment vendors, and service contracts should be reviewed periodically and evaluated in terms of cost, quality, and effectiveness. New agreements should be sought if doing so would be advantageous for the office. Negotiation is an important part of establishing any agreement for products or services purchased for a medical office.

The Language of Medicine

central processing unit (CPU) The main chip that runs a computer and directs its processing of data.

computer peripherals Equipment connected to the main unit of the computer, such as scanners or printers.

diskette A small circle of magnetized material, housed in a plastic casing, that provides for permanent data storage; often called a "disk."

diskette drives Drives that write or store information on a diskette.

hard disk or hard drive The computer's main drive, offering a large amount of permanent storage.

hardware The physical parts, or machinery, that make up a computer system.

inventory A count of all items on hand.

licensure Limited legal permission to use a product such as a computer software program.

modem A device that transmits data electronically through a telephone line.

motherboard The primary circuit board of the computer that holds or has connections for all other computer components.

random access memory (RAM) A part of the computer that stores information temporarily.

read only memory (ROM) A part of the computer that stores information permanently.

scanner A device that inputs text or graphics into the computer.

scheduled drugs Drugs that have been designated by the DEA as having potential for addiction or abuse; also called controlled substances.

software Instructions that tell a computer how to process information; also called "applications" or "programs."

telemedicine The transmission of video images for medical purposes.

templates Basic files that are used repeatedly to speed up work.

upgraded Enhanced or improved computer software programs.

vendor A company that sells supplies.

Signs/Symptoms of Progress

Recall, Question, Connect

Recall

List six ways computer software applications are being used in a medical office.

Question

What types of questions do you have about computer use in the medical office? Consider such areas as file sharing, privacy, security, ethics, or information flow.

Connect

Identify two ways a physician might use a laptop computer away from the office. Jot down two ways data might be transferred from the laptop to the office computer or from the office computer to the laptop.

Educating the Patient

As a medical assistant/office manager, you have purchased a new computer system for the office. Technicians install the machines and train your office staff on the new system. Everyone feels confident that she or he can use the system, but one staff member raises an important point: "The other day, my patient needed an inactive file. What do we do if we need an inactive patient file? On the old system, we could access those. Where are they on the new system?" You realize that inactive files were not transferred from the old computers to the new ones.

1 What should you do to correct the problem?
2 What is your immediate response to the staff member's question?

Exploring Perspectives in Teams

Perspective involves the discipline of examining how ideas look from different points of view and recognizing that there are often multiple "answers" to complex questions. In small groups or on your own, reflect on possible alternative views or answers and summarize your findings.

1 Your supervisor insists that you use his son-in-law's company as one of your supply vendors. The product prices are slightly higher than those of the competitors, but the real problem is that no one likes working with the son-in-law. In addition, he promises delivery dates he does not meet and takes too long to present product information. How would you approach this problem with your supervisor? How would you approach it if his son-in-law's prices were lower than the competitors'?
2 Think about the type of medical work you are planning to do. Plan the ideal computer system for your workstation. Specify the computer components, software applications, and networking features you want at your disposal.
3 Create a chart comparing the disadvantages and advantages of leasing versus buying equipment for the office. Identify the global factors that will affect your decision: size of office, frequency of use, etc.

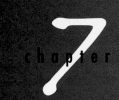
Learning Outcomes

- Plan medical office communication systems.
- Select communication equipment for efficiency and cost effectiveness.
- Use efficient, professional communication techniques.
- Maintain confidentiality in communicating patient information.
- Manage incoming and outgoing calls, including telephone referrals.
- Manage incoming and outgoing mail.
- Compose and prepare written communication.

Performance Objectives

- Project a professional manner and image in all written and oral communication.
- Treat all patients with compassion, empathy, and respect.
- Use professional telephone technique.
- Use effective and correct oral and written communications.
- Receive, organize, prioritize, and transmit information.
- Ensure the security of all confidential information.

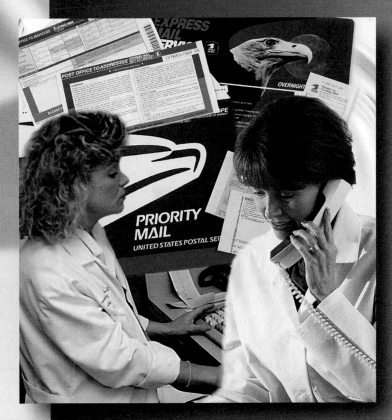

Communication is a crucial part of the medical assistant's daily responsibilities. Adequate, efficient communication can enhance a medical practice and help provide high quality healthcare for patients, while poor communication can cause irreparable harm to a physician's practice—including legal difficulties and loss of revenue. An effective medical assistant answers the telephones, makes outgoing calls, handles the mail, and composes letters in a manner that projects professionalism and adheres to office policies and procedures.

Managing Communications: Telephones, Mail, and Correspondence

Patient Concerns

A family practice medical office installed an automated answering system after the office manager submitted a proposal showing that the new high-tech system could save over $10,000 the first year by eliminating a receptionist position. The automated system had many advantages and could be customized to meet the office's specific needs. However, the person who set up the system did not include an option allowing a patient to talk directly with a medical assistant. Callers who had difficulty understanding the recording, for example someone not fluent in English or an elderly patient uncomfortable with the technology, could not speak with a person. Patients did not continue the phone call, even when their health was involved, and tried another office with a more patient-friendly phone system.

Patients need to be able to express their concerns, ask questions about their appointments, and discuss their healthcare comfortably on the medical office's phone system. Automation, though in some ways more efficient, cannot always address a caller's individual needs.

Planning Telephone Systems

Studies of medical practices around the country have shown that 85% to 90% of patient appointments are made by telephone, and that the phone provides the initial contact for most new patients. The telephone is a powerful tool for public relations and productivity. As a medical assistant, you will use it to welcome prospective patients, reassure current patients, request assistance, order services and supplies, and deal with emergencies. Because the telephone is often the first point of contact for anyone dealing with the medical office, the medical assistant must have the telephone skills to make that first impression a positive one.

Basic Telephone Features and Options

Today's technology provides a wide range of telephone equipment and services to meet the needs of any office. The standard individual telephone is a touch-tone desk style phone capable of connecting with at least three lines. The telephone may include a button to place a caller on hold and an intercom feature to facilitate communication among different areas of the office. A number of other options, including call forwarding, voice mail, and caller ID, can be purchased.

CALL FORWARDING Call forwarding automatically directs a call to another specified telephone number when it is not answered at the initial number. For example, if a department closes early, all of its calls could be forwarded to a department that is still open.

VOICE MAIL **Voice mail** provides a recorded message for callers and records messages from them when a telephone line is not answered. The messages can be retrieved from any phone, even one outside the office.

CALLER ID Caller ID displays the identification and phone number of the caller in a small panel on the telephone. This can help if you need to return a call and failed to ask for the patient's number, or if a patient with an emergency is unable to give you that information. Caller ID is only available in certain areas.

Phone Lines

The number of phone lines a medical office needs depends on the number of physicians in the office and the number of patients served. Most offices have dedicated phone lines for a fax machine and computer modem so that voice lines are not blocked when a fax or e-mail message is being transmitted or someone is doing Internet research.

Customer Service

While some offices provide a telephone in the reception area that patients can use to make local calls, many medical office managers have found this an unwarranted expense. Making a phone readily available to patients, however, can eliminate interruptions and busy phone lines when patients ask to use the office phone for personal calls.

Systems to Direct Incoming Calls

There are several ways to transfer calls that come into an office. The size of the office determines which type of system will be most efficient.

CALL-DIRECTOR A **call-director** is a touch-tone phone with up to thirty buttons. The person answering the phone at the reception desk directs incoming calls to the desired party by pushing the appropriate button.

SWITCHBOARD A larger medical office with many departments may use a switchboard set up in a centrally located area and attended by an operator whose sole purpose is to direct calls.

AUTOMATED ROUTING UNIT A system that frees up personnel for other duties is the Automated Routing Unit (ARU). The ARU answers the phone with a recorded voice and offers the caller a menu of departments or services. The caller then accesses menu choices by pressing buttons on her phone that correspond to the listed items. This system does not work for callers without a touch-tone phone and transfers those callers to an operator or receptionist. More advanced systems will let callers select an option by speaking the option's number into the phone. Patients who have difficulty navigating through the ARU should be given the option of routing directly to a receptionist or an after-hours answering service. You can program the system to provide sub-menus for any of the numbered choices on the original menu so that callers can browse among the menu selections without having to hang up and call again. Table 7.1 lists the advantages and disadvantages of ARUs.

If your office uses an ARU, make sure patients are given adequate information about how to use the system and how to contact the office in an emergency. You may want to provide printed cards to make calling easier, and may find that including them in new-patient information packets helps patients become accustomed to the system. In addition, many medical offices give detailed instructions in the ARU's greeting message.

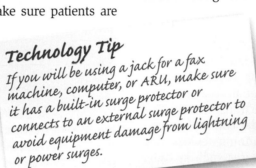

Technology Tip

If you will be using a jack for a fax machine, computer, or ARU, make sure it has a built-in surge protector or connects to an external surge protector to avoid equipment damage from lightning or power surges.

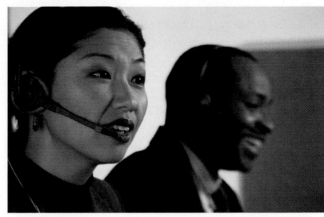

A medical office may contract with an answering service to pick up calls when the office is closed.

Systems for Answering Calls after Hours

A system must be provided to answer all calls that come in when the office is closed. This can be either an answering machine or an answering service.

ANSWERING MACHINES An answering machine collects all incoming messages on an analog recording, such as a tape, or in a digital format. The outgoing message should give either a telephone number where the physician can be reached or a number to call in an emergency. The messages must be checked frequently to ensure that essential calls are answered in a timely fashion.

ANSWERING SERVICES A more flexible, but more expensive, option is the answering service. An answering service is an outside company that has live operators handling calls. A live voice can be very reassuring to a patient. Another advantage is that operators can screen and route calls and can locate the physician when necessary. The answering service may also have a direct connection to the office and be able to pick up any call that is not answered within a certain number of rings.

COMBINED SYSTEMS Many offices use both answering machines and answering services to reduce expenses while providing a high level of urgent service to patients. In these offices, after-hours calls are answered by a machine that takes messages for non-urgent calls but transfers the call to an answering service if a physician is needed urgently. The operator at the answering service then calls or pages the physician, who returns the patient's call.

Table 7.1 Advantages and Disadvantages of the Automated Routing Unit

Advantages	Disadvantages
■ Personnel are freed up from answering the telephone.	■ Some callers may have difficulty hearing the recorded message.
■ Programming can be revised to accommodate changes in office practices.	■ Some callers may not understand the menu choices or how to use the buttons on their phone to access menu choices.
■ Information can be provided to answer routine patient questions such as calls about office hours, services available, prescription refills, and directions to the office.	■ Many patients may prefer a live voice.

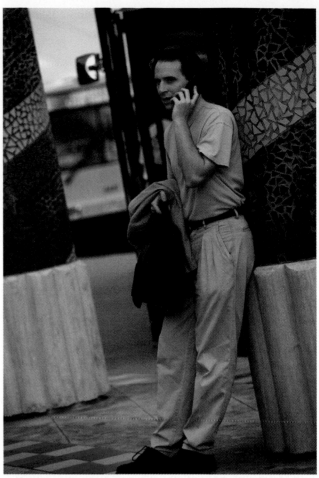

Physicians who are on call can be reached by cellular phone or pager. These devices keep the doctor accessible to the medical office without being restricted to one location.

Other Telephone Technology

Doctors and healthcare workers sometimes need to be accessible when they are not in the office. Fortunately, cellular phones and pagers make such communication possible.

CELLULAR PHONES Cellular phones offer true "wireless" communication, since they are not connected to a line or cable. A huge variety of cellular phones is on the market, and they are becoming increasingly compact. Their portability allows for immediate voice contact anywhere, anytime.

The original cellular phones used analog technology, which transmitted voice-modulated radio waves. Newer, more expensive, digital models break down the information into coded digital signals that must be decoded at the receiving end of the transmission. This results in a clearer conversation that cannot be intercepted by people listening with scanning devices. Digital phones offer a number of features such as caller identification, speed-dialing, and the ability to send faxes and e-mail.

PAGERS A **pager** offers the advantage of privacy at a relatively modest cost but provides only one-way communication. Each pager is assigned a telephone number. When the number is called, the pager is activated to beep, buzz, or vibrate. Most pagers display a number to call, and many can store several numbers in their memory. The person who is paged must make a phone call to retrieve the message, making the communication more cumbersome than using a cellular phone.

Evaluating Phone Systems and Communication Technology

The medical assistant will probably be asked for input when a new phone system is being considered for the office. Important factors to be considered include cost, efficiency, quality, time, and ease of use.

- Cost. How does the cost of a new system compare with that of the current system, including labor, service, and supplies? You will need to look at past bills and invoices to get that information about your current system, and compare it with advertisements and sales brochures containing pricing information on new systems.
- Efficiency. How does the efficiency of a telecommunications system compare with the current system? Are calls currently answered in a timely fashion? Do patients complain of being on hold or being cut off? Is it easy to transfer a call?
- Quality. How does the system rank in terms of usability and quality of transmission?
- Time. How quickly can calls be accessed and routed?
- Ease of Use. How long would it take office personnel to feel comfortable with a new system?

Managing Telephone Communications

When using the telephone for communication, you represent the entire office. It is important that you project a professional, competent image. Good telephone skills can help promote a positive impression of your office and will help you use your time productively. It is essential to pay careful attention to the voice you use and to follow the rules of telephone courtesy. You want to be prepared for all the types of calls and to be knowledgeable in transferring calls and arranging conference calls.

Telephone Techniques

Although the telephone is a common tool, it has some specific techniques and rules of protocol. To communicate effectively over the phone, it is important to learn these techniques and monitor their effectiveness with each call.

TELEPHONE PREPAREDNESS Taking a few minutes at the beginning of the day to prepare for incoming calls can make a big difference in how efficiently you manage phone calls during busy times. Before the office opens, make sure you have the necessary supplies beside each phone such as pen, note paper, and message pad. You need the schedule book or computerized scheduling program your office uses for managing appointments, and a list of extensions for transferring calls. Be sure to have a list of healthcare service and supply providers for referring callers and a telephone **triage** manual or a copy of your office's guidelines for dealing with emergency calls.

Before answering the phone, take a deep breath, slow down, and prepare yourself to focus on the caller's needs. Remember that it is your job to identify the needs of the caller and try to meet them as efficiently and courteously as possible.

YOUR TELEPHONE VOICE Because you cannot rely on facial expressions or body language to convey your message when speaking on the phone, you must strive to use a voice that communicates clearly and professionally. To make the most of your telephone voice, keep these suggestions in mind:

- Speak at a natural pace and in a normal conversational tone.
- Speak directly into the receiver so the equipment can pick up your voice without distortion.
- Visualize the person you are speaking with and try to project an attitude of respect, concern, and competence.
- Use words and phrases that you are certain the caller can understand, and avoid slang or medical/technical jargon.
- Avoid speaking in a monotone. Vary the pitch of your voice to make it more interesting and easier to listen to.

- Make sure you pronounce words correctly, especially proper names. Ask the caller how to correctly pronounce his name, if necessary.
- Be certain that you enunciate clearly. Avoid slurring words or phrases, and make sure each word you speak is crisp and easy to understand.
- Never chew gum or have food, candy, or any object in your mouth when you are talking on the phone. Not only does it make understanding your words more difficult, it also conveys the impression that the call is not important.

As with any conversation, always pay attention to how the caller is responding. Give her a chance to ask questions and to confirm that you understand each other.

TELEPHONE COURTESY Just as good manners demand certain behavior when you are speaking with someone in person, they also dictate conduct on the telephone. Too often, people are unknowingly rude during phone conversations because they simply don't know the rules. Make sure you follow these guidelines for courtesy on the phone:

- Aim to answer the telephone on the second ring. Answering sooner may be disconcerting to the

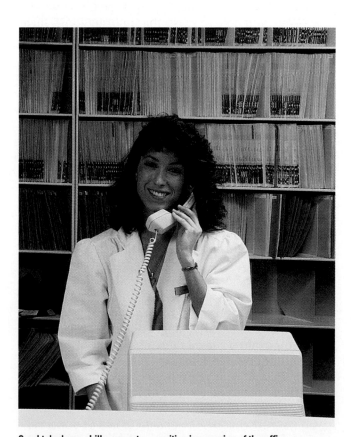

Good telephone skills promote a positive impression of the office.

caller, while answering later may cause the caller to think the office is closed.

- Identify yourself when you answer the phone and include a helpful phrase indicating your willingness to assist the caller. When you say something like, "Dr. Johnson's office. This is Janice. How may I be of assistance?" callers know immediately whom they have called, and that you are ready to help.

- Give the caller your undivided attention. Do not try to type, file, or converse with anyone else during a phone call. This is disrespectful to the caller and can lead to errors with serious consequences, both in the phone call and the other task you are trying to accomplish.

- Use the caller's name frequently during the conversation. This demonstrates concern and respect and gives the caller a sense of reassurance. If the caller does not identify herself at the beginning of the call, be tactful in asking for a name. A phrase such as "May I ask who's calling?", spoken with respect, will allow the caller to give you her name.

- Check to make sure the caller understands any information or instructions you provide, and phrase your inquiry in a way that puts the responsibility on you. Ask, "Did I explain that adequately?" or "Were my instructions clear?" Do not say, "Could you understand those directions?" or "Were you able to grasp that information?" since phrases that focus on the other person imply that a caller who missed some of the information is inadequate.

- Be cheerful. The person you're talking with can't see you, but he can hear the positive tone of your voice.

- Be respectful of the person you're talking with. If you need to leave the call, state how long you will be away and offer options. Say, "It may take me several minutes to collect that information. Would you prefer to hold, or shall I call you back?"

- End your call in a businesslike manner. First, summarize the important points of the call. Refer to your notes at this point to make sure you've covered everything. Then, bring the call to a close. This is the responsibility of the caller, although in some cases, it may be difficult. You might try some suggestive phrases such as, "Thanks for your help," "I've enjoyed talking with you," or "May I call you again if I need more information?"

- Avoid multiple callbacks, or "telephone tag." If you call someone who's not in, ask when you should call back. You may want to offer to call at a specific time, and if you do, make sure you call at the time you gave. If you ask the person to call you at a certain time, make sure you're available then.

- Leave efficient voice mail messages. Be sure to give your name, phone number, and the date and time of your call. Explain the purpose of your call completely but without excessive wordiness. Include information on the best times to call back, and end your call with a word of appreciation.

Following standard rules of etiquette will help you when speaking over the phone. Be patient, aware, and considerate in all interactions. Some callers may be difficult to communicate with because of physical, cultural, or language barriers. Table 7.2 provides some tips for overcoming these obstacles to effective telephone communication.

TAKING MESSAGES Never depend on your memory to relay a message about any call. You may want to use

Table 7.2 Overcoming Obstacles to High-Quality Telephone Communication

When communicating with callers with hearing loss:

- Persons who have a severe hearing loss that prevents them from using a regular telephone may use a TDD system. This requires both sending and receiving telephones that allow typed messages to be exchanged.

- A person with a hearing loss can also connect with a special operator who can relay messages to a non-TDD phone.

- A person with a hearing aid may receive interference from the telephone or other electronic equipment. Ask the caller what you can do to improve the quality of the call. You may need to speak louder or softer—or you may need to turn off office machines that cause background noise or interference. Enunciate clearly.

When communicating with a caller with a speech impairment or one using an electronic speaking aid:

- If you cannot understand the patient's speech, ask him to repeat the statement. With subsequent attempts, your understanding of the electronic or impaired speech may improve.

- Apologize to the caller if you must repeatedly ask that a statement be repeated and assure the caller that your primary concern is to provide assistance and meet her needs.

- At some point, you may want to ask if someone else is available who might be able to assist with communication.

When communicating with a caller from a cultural background very different from your own:

- Recognize that cultural differences may affect communication.

- Learn about customs and beliefs of different cultural groups in the community you serve.

- Understanding and sensitivity can alleviate many problems and make communication easier.

an ordinary spiral-bound notebook for calls, or your office may have preprinted telephone message pads. These come in individual pads or in spiral-bound books that automatically create a carbon copy of each message as you write. The carbon copies are useful for tracking messages and making sure each message was delivered or acted on properly. Never write phone messages on small scraps of paper that can easily be lost or mistaken for something unimportant. Be sure to put the date and time the call was received on each message and deliver messages or follow up on calls promptly. If you take a message for the physician and your office has established callback times, be sure to tell the caller approximately when to expect a call from the doctor. Procedure 7.1 provides general steps to follow when taking a phone message. Note that when taking messages, you may not be able to follow these steps in the indicated order, but all of them should be completed.

TRANSFERRING CALLS You will occasionally need to refer the caller to someone else or transfer the call. In these cases, you should always note the caller's name and phone number and the nature of the call. Follow Procedure 7.1 even if you are transferring the call. If the caller is cut off during the transfer, having her phone number will let you reestablish the call. If you refer the caller to another office, you may need to follow up later with that office or with the caller. In either event, it is important to have the name and phone number of the caller.

Working Smart
Do not rely on your memory. Write phone messages down and confirm the information with the caller before ending the call.

Customer Service
Never put a caller on hold without first asking permission to do so. Give the caller a chance to indicate if a call is an emergency or requires immediate attention. While on hold, callers should hear either music or a recorded message to let them know they have not been disconnected and that their needs will be addressed shortly.

Procedure 7.1

Taking a Phone Message

Purpose: To take a complete, accurate phone message.

Equipment/Supplies: Pen or pencil, carboned spiral message book, phone.

1 Answer the phone after the first ring but before the third ring.
2 Identify yourself and the medical office and ask how you can help the caller.
3 Determine the caller's basic needs. ✵**WARNING!** For emergency calls, follow the medical office's special procedures. These may include immediately putting the caller through to the physician or directing patients to call 911.
4 Ask for the caller's name, write it down, and confirm the spelling with the caller. Use the caller's name during the conversation.
5 Answer the caller's questions if you can and it is appropriate to do so.
6 If you cannot address all of the caller's needs, begin to

take a message by noting the time of the call in the message book.
7 Determine the callback phone number and confirm the number by reading it back.
8 Write down the name of the person to whom the message you are taking should be addressed.
9 Restate and summarize the content of the message as you write it down. Ask the caller to confirm that the information is correct.
10 Determine the level of urgency of the message. One way to do this is by asking the caller what follow-up action he wants. Note the follow-up request on the message. If the patient requests a callback by the physician, tell him when to expect the call based on the physician's callback schedule.
11 Ask the caller if there are any additional questions, comments, or concerns.
12 Thank the caller and hang up.
13 Deliver the message by following the appropriate office protocol. Keep the carbon for the office records.

Before you transfer a call, ask the caller's permission to place the call on hold while you transfer it. Say something like, "Do you mind holding while I transfer your call?" and wait for a response. Some callers would prefer not to hold and may want to have a phone number so they can call later. Only after you have received permission should you put the call on hold and transfer it. Table 7.3 provides guidelines for putting a caller on hold.

When the person to whom you are transferring a call answers, give the name of the caller and the nature of the call. This helps the person who receives the call to efficiently meet the caller's needs.

CONFERENCE CALLS As telephone technology has improved, **conference calling** has become increasingly available and a popular way for healthcare teams to communicate. Conference calls also offer an efficient way for families and physicians to communicate about the care of a family member. This can be especially important when decisions must be made quickly about the care of an elderly or incapacitated person.

If you are asked to arrange a long-distance conference call, tell this to the customer service department or the operator for your long-distance service. You will need to supply the name and phone number of each participant. The operator will establish the connections for the call. It usually helps to arrange the date and time of the call with all parties in advance to avoid last-minute confusion.

Conference calling can connect from three to fourteen phones at once, with each party able to both listen and speak. Charges are based on the number of

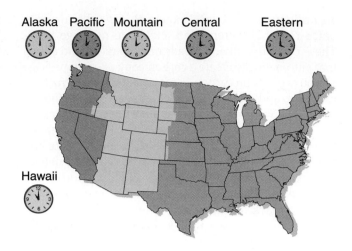

Figure 7.1
United States Time Zones

points connected, distance, and length of the call. Local conference calls can also be established by calling the local operator.

TIME ZONES There are four time zones in the continental United States: Eastern, Central, Mountain, and Pacific, with a three-hour time difference between the coasts. For example, when it is noon in California, it is 3:00 P.M. in Virginia. Figure 7.1 shows these time zones. When making a long-distance call, look at the clock and determine the corresponding time for the zone you are calling to make sure your timing is appropriate.

Customer Service
Avoid calling private homes before 9:00 o'clock in the morning.

Telephone Policies

Your office may have a policy manual that provides guidelines about telephone use in certain circumstances. It is important to be aware of office procedures regarding emergency calls, confidentiality, personal use of the telephone, sales calls, and calls from other healthcare providers.

EMERGENCY CALLS Emergency calls involve conditions that require immediate medical attention. Your office should have guidelines, developed by the physician, on how to handle emergency calls both when the doctor is in the office and when he is out.

Infrequently, a caller may tell you that a situation is an emergency but describe symptoms that do not seem to require urgent attention. If you are uncertain of

Table 7.3 Guidelines for Putting a Caller on Hold

- Before putting someone on hold, always let the caller state the nature of the call so that you do not put an emergency call on hold.
- Never leave the phone's receiver on the desk, where the caller can hear unrelated—and perhaps confidential—conversations if you have not pressed the hold button.
- Ask permission first. Say something like, "May I put your call on hold while I locate your lab reports?" then wait for a response. Some callers may not be able to hold.
- Do not leave a caller holding for more than a minute at a time. If you need longer to locate someone or gather information, return to the line each minute and let the caller know you are working on the request or problem.
- Always thank the caller for holding and offer the option of continuing to hold or having you return the call when you have a complete response to the caller's request. Say something like, "Thank you for holding. I've been unable to locate all the information you requested, and I may need several more minutes. Would you prefer to continue to hold, or shall I return your call when I have the information?"

whether a call is an emergency, always treat it as an emergency. It is generally better to err on the side of safety than to allow an emergency to go unattended.

In an emergency, the caller is often panic-stricken and may not be thinking clearly. It is essential that you remain calm to help the caller regain his composure so that you can effectively manage the call. Of course, once you have identified the call as an emergency, the objective is to get help to the person in distress as quickly as possible. Most offices specify that emergency calls be transferred to the physician immediately. Be sure to:

1 Obtain the name and phone number of the caller.
2 Obtain the name of the patient.
3 Inform the physician of the call, and put the call through to the physician as quickly as possible.
4 Pull the patient's chart and give it to the doctor. The chart may contain important information that will let the physician assess the problem and make recommendations more quickly.

If the physician is not in the office, you need to get the patient's name, age, and a complete description of the symptoms, then handle the call according to office policies. These may include instructing the caller to dial 911 and request assistance, transferring the call to a nurse practitioner or other medical personnel, or instructing the caller to go immediately to the nearest emergency room.

No matter what action you take, be sure to document both the call and your action in the patient's chart. Include:

■ all information you receive from the caller
■ any attempts you made to transfer the call
■ your instructions to the caller
■ the date and time of the call

If you receive an emergency call from an individual who is not a patient (and therefore does not have a chart), document the call and your response on paper and keep the report in a safe place for future reference.

ISSUES OF CONFIDENTIALITY By law, medical information is confidential and cannot be released without the patient's specific, written permission. It is critical to patients that their personal information not be shared with anyone they have not authorized to receive it.

Before releasing any information—by phone or otherwise—you must have the patient's permission. The telephone can present problems in regard to confidentiality because it is sometimes difficult to know to whom you are talking or who might be overhearing

the conversation. While it is best to avoid giving confidential information by phone, there are occasions when there is no other choice. If you must give confidential information to a caller—perhaps someone from another medical office or a lab handling a patient's tests—make sure the phone you use is out of the hearing range of patients and others who are not part of the medical office team. Always make certain you positively identify the person to whom you divulge confidential information, and do not release the information in a situation you believe is questionable. Remember also that faxed information may be confidential, and take precautions to make sure it is not read by unauthorized persons in your office. You can protect confidential telephone messages and faxes that are received by placing them in a folder marked "confidential" before leaving them on the physician's desk for a response.

You may not release any medical information without the patient's written consent, even to a close friend or relative of the patient. If you receive calls from

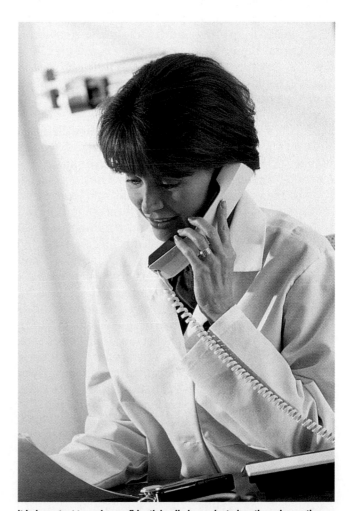

It is important to make confidential calls in a private location where other staff members or patients cannot overhear the conversation.

someone close to a patient, be courteous and respectful and explain that you cannot provide any information without the patient's written consent. Suggest that if the friend or relative will be a contact person, the patient may want to sign a release-of-information form on her next visit to the office.

> ## Legal Issue
>
> Be careful not to convey or repeat confidential patient information over the telephone where others may overhear the conversation. Also, take caution when delivering telephone messages or faxes containing confidential information. Ensure that they are not seen by unauthorized individuals.

PERSONAL CALLS Familiarize yourself with the office guidelines on handling personal calls for the physicians. Because an arduous schedule can keep a doctor away from family members during important times, she may encourage them to call the office to keep in touch. The doctor will want to know about the call as soon as possible but will most likely not appreciate interruption of a patient exam.

If you receive an incoming personal call for a coworker, route the call directly to that person, if office policies permit and it is appropriate. Never interrupt a coworker's interaction with a patient for a personal call. You may need to ask if the call is an emergency, and if not, ask the caller to leave a message. You will probably be given instructions on handling personal calls for the physician. If you are uncertain how to proceed with personal calls, refer to your office's policy manual or ask the office manager or physician.

You may be permitted to use the office phone for personal calls during lunch and break times. If this is the case, be sure to limit your personal calls to appropriate times and never make personal calls within the hearing of patients. Never charge personal calls, services, or merchandise to the office telephone. If you must make a long-distance call, use a telephone credit card or charge the call to your home phone.

CALLS FROM PHARMACEUTICAL SALESPERSONS As a medical assistant, you may be the primary contact for salespersons calling the office. You should be familiar with office policies that address these calls and be prepared to handle them efficiently and politely. Often, the physician sets aside certain days and hours to see salespersons, and there may be specific routines for

these times. The salesperson may be required to schedule an appointment, or the physician may see callers on a first-come basis. You may want to suggest that the salesperson send information that the physician can review before the meeting.

CALLS FROM OTHER HEALTHCARE PROFESSIONALS Often, a large team of healthcare workers is needed to treat complex patient problems, and communication is important to the team's efficient functioning. Physicians, therapists, home healthcare nurses, social workers, medical equipment suppliers, and other healthcare workers may occasionally call your office with important communication about patient-related matters. As a general rule, you will need to route those calls directly to the physician.

CALLS FROM ATTORNEYS Some medical offices retain the services of an attorney on an ongoing basis to advise the physician and office personnel on routine matters involving the practice. If this is the case, you may receive calls from the attorney or someone at the attorney's office. However, if you receive a call from any other attorney, you should handle it with caution. Be sure you are familiar with office policies regarding attorney contacts, and do not deviate from the guidelines. If a call does not seem to fall within the guidelines, do not provide any information, and ask the office manager or physician how you should proceed.

Managing Incoming Calls

Your initial task with any incoming call is to determine its nature so you can respond appropriately and in the most helpful manner. Most calls coming into the office will involve a request for an appointment. How to handle these is discussed in detail in Chapter 8, "Scheduling Appointments and Managing Time." Other calls, however, will be more complex, presenting requests for medical advice or prescription refills, inquiries about progress reports and test results, complaints, and billing and insurance questions.

MEDICAL ADVICE As a medical assistant, you are not licensed to diagnose or to prescribe medication, and you are not trained to give medical advice. You need to explain this to a caller and emphasize that the patient must see the physician. If the patient is unable to come into the office, say that you will relay the information and request. Ask for permission to call back with the doctor's response. Sometimes, the physician may not be able to respond adequately by phone and may urge the patient to come to the office. Always document the call in the patient's chart—including your actions, the physician's recommendations, and the patient's response. If the patient refuses to come to the office, recommend that he go to the nearest emergency room.

Some offices establish certain times of the day when the physician returns non-emergency calls. If this is the case in your office, be sure to tell callers approximately

Legal Issue

Remember that your employer is legally responsible for your actions—including any advice or information you give by phone—so use caution when handling calls that request advice or involve emergency situations.

when they can expect the doctor to call. Remind the patient to have all the pertinent information available.

PRESCRIPTION REFILLS A request for a prescription refill may come from the patient or from a pharmacist. A medical assistant needs to be familiar with office policies and state laws concerning prescription refills. In general, a medical assistant can call a pharmacy to order or refill a prescription only if directed to do so by the physician.

When a patient calls, be sure to obtain the patient's name and phone number, the phone number of the pharmacy, and the name and strength of the medication. Pull the patient's chart, note the request in the chart, and pass the chart and message to the physician for review and approval.

If a patient asks a pharmacist to refill a prescription that is over a year old, the pharmacist will often call the medical office. The pharmacist will also call if refills were not authorized on the original prescription or if there are any unusual circumstances such as a possible allergy or drug interaction. Respond to these requests by obtaining the patient's name as well as information about the prescription. As with the patient's request for a prescription, pull the patient's chart, note the information in the chart, and pass the chart and phone message along to the physician for review and approval.

Working Smart

Document all calls about prescription requests in the patient's chart.

Sometimes, the physician will decline to refill a prescription until the patient comes in for another appointment. In these circumstances, it may be your responsibility to call the patient to schedule such an appointment.

PROGRESS REPORTS AND TEST RESULTS Occasionally, the physician may ask a patient to phone the office with a report of progress or response to treatment. When a patient calls with a progress report, note the information in the patient's chart and inform the physician of the call. Before hanging up, ask if the patient has any additional concerns or questions that you should bring to the physician's attention.

When a patient calls requesting test results, check the chart first to determine whether the results have been received. If there is no report, you may need to call the lab or other service provider to request the report and suggest a time when the patient can call back to learn the results.

Some offices may permit the medical assistant to report test results to patients if they are negative or within normal limits. Always note in the patient's chart any requests for test results and any information you give the patient. In most offices, the physician will report any abnormal results to the patient. If the results the patient calls about are abnormal, tell him the report has been received and that the physician will call back with the results; do not reveal the test results. Note the call and place the notation with the patient's chart on the physician's desk.

COMPLAINTS Complaints are not uncommon in a medical office, even when the highest quality of care is provided. Sometimes, you only need to listen and provide an empathetic response. On occasion, however, a patient may have a valid complaint, and listening and empathy are simply not enough. A problem may have arisen that demands attention and correction.

When a patient in your office complains, give her your complete concentration and listen carefully to what she is saying. It may help to discuss this in a private area to avoid upsetting or disturbing others in the waiting area. Follow these tips for handling a complaint:

- Try to understand the problem from the patient's point of view, and acknowledge any anger or other negative feelings. This can help to diffuse the emotions so that you and the patient can concentrate on resolving the problem.
- Always be respectful and speak gently.
- Do not communicate defensiveness or anger in response to the complaint.
- Under no circumstances, should you attempt to place blame or make accusations.
- Never interrupt the patient. Permit him to speak openly, and do not react to statements with

obvious emotion, but do not let the patient use inappropriate language or become verbally abusive.

- When talking with an abusive complainer, you may need to say, "I will try my best to help you, but there is nothing I can do if you continue to use inappropriate language."
- Be an empathetic listener and demonstrate by your body language and facial expressions that you are concentrating on the complaint. Let the patient know that you care, will thoroughly investigate the complaint, and will take appropriate action.
- If it is readily apparent that the office made an error, apologize immediately and offer an explanation if appropriate.
- Tell the patient you will correct the mistake immediately.
- Do not make promises that you cannot keep. You may need to explain office policies to the patient, but do so in a calm, respectful manner, and check to make sure the patient understands.
- Thank the patient for bringing the complaint to your attention and for discussing it with you.

If the patient remains dissatisfied, you may need to refer him to the physician. Notify the physician immediately if a patient threatens to take legal action. Most offices have access to legal counsel on an as-needed basis, and if your office does, you may need to request advice from the attorney on how to handle certain complaints. Always document complaints and your action, but keep such documentation in a secure place, separate from the patient's chart. Do not refer in the patient's medical chart to any complaints that do not apply to treatment.

If a patient's complaint is about treatment or care, it should be documented in her medical record along with all follow-up or resolution details. A patient who complains about a course of treatment may later claim nothing was done to resolve the complaint. A complaint about treatment, properly documented in the medical record, could show negligence and culpability by the patient if he failed to follow the physician's recommendations.

BILLING AND INSURANCE QUESTIONS   When a patient calls to inquire about insurance or billing, you need to get the patient's full name and the date of the last office visit. Pull the patient's chart and financial information to make sure the billing was accurate.

If the patient complains that she was overcharged, and you find that is the case, apologize immediately and tell her you will send a corrected statement at once. Let her know you will investigate and correct the problem to prevent future billing errors.

If a patient believes he was overcharged but you determine that the bill is accurate, you may want to

discuss the matter with the physician before responding to the patient. There may have been unusual circumstances that resulted in a higher-than-expected fee, or the physician may be able to otherwise clarify the bill. Most offices will accept partial payments on a large bill if special circumstances affect the patient's ability to pay.

If the patient is still dissatisfied, direct the call to the physician or the office manager, and document all the information you obtained.

Managing Outgoing Calls

There are a few types of outgoing calls a medical assistant will make repeatedly: scheduling admissions, arranging referrals, requesting home care services, and ordering medical equipment. Each of these requires different information and a slightly different approach.

SCHEDULING ADMISSIONS OR TESTS   Advance preparation will help when you schedule surgery, tests, or admissions for patients. Before calling, make sure you have the following information:

- a release of information form completed and signed by the patient that allows you to transfer information to the hospital or other facility (A sample of a form used to approve the release of information was presented in Chapter 3, "Understanding Legal and Ethical Issues.")
- the patient's full name, address, and phone number
- the patient's social security number or other identification number
- insurance information
- days or times when the patient is not available
- a complete description of any special needs or circumstances (such as a wheelchair, prostheses, speech or hearing difficulty, assistance animal, religious convictions that affect healthcare, etc.)

Much of this information is also required when arranging a referral to another practice, such as a specialist's office.

Have the patient's chart beside the phone for easy reference, and make sure you have complete orders from the physician stating the type of test or admission, the current diagnosis, other relevant diagnoses, brief history of the illness, and any other pertinent information. Be sure you know which facility to use. In some cases, there may be only one facility in your area that performs the needed test or procedure. In other instances, several options may be available, but the physician or the patient may have a strong preference.

When you make the call, be sure to address all items of information requested by the admitting or testing facility. If the request includes a copy of the patient's chart, confirm that a signed medical information release form is on file, copy the chart, and have it at the facility before the scheduled admission. Find out if the facility will call the patient to confirm the appointment and give special instructions. If not, you need to call the patient to inform him of the schedule. When you talk with the patient, be sure to ask if there are any questions about the procedure. If the patient has questions, attempt to answer them as completely as possible. If you do not have complete answers, offer to call the facility that will be doing the procedure to get answers or ask that someone from the facility call the patient before the appointment. In some cases, you may need to transfer the patient's call to the physician.

REQUESTING HOME CARE SERVICES Home healthcare is rapidly becoming a viable alternative to some types of hospitalization. Often, a patient can receive skilled nursing care or therapy at home and avoid going into a nursing home or rehabilitation facility. Generally, home healthcare is paid for either by an insurance plan such as Medicare or Medicaid or by the patient. You may need to arrange appropriate home care service to meet a patient's specific needs.

If the patient pays privately, there are virtually no restrictions on the type of care other than the doctor's order. Services may include anything from around-the-clock skilled care by a registered nurse to weekly visits from a nurse. Most home care organizations offer personal care services (bathing, shampoos, nail care, etc.) and some type of housekeeping services. Many also provide live-in companions who are not nurses but are with the patient twenty-four hours a day to assist with medications, personal care, errands, housekeeping, and other duties.

If services are paid for by insurance, there probably will be restrictions on both the type and length of service. Generally, there is a requirement that the patient need **skilled nursing care** (provided by a registered nurse) and be **homebound** (unable to walk without assistance or requiring a device to aid with walking, moving, breathing, etc.). If a patient's condition changes so that she no longer fits the home care categories, services will have to be discontinued.

Most home care organizations handle billing for the patient. The physician does not necessarily have to specify the length or frequency of service, since that is often determined by Medicare, Medicaid, or other insurance guidelines.

ORDERING MEDICAL EQUIPMENT Medical equipment used by patients at home is usually referred to as **DME**, or durable medical equipment. It includes hospital beds, bedside commodes, patient lifts, oxygen, special bathing equipment, wheelchairs, walkers,

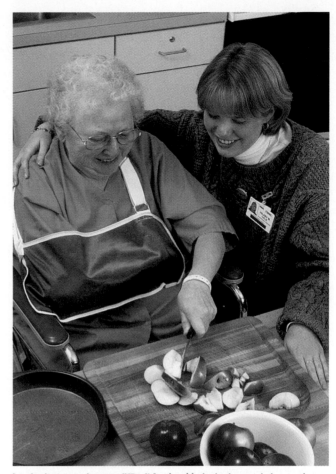

Leaving home can be very difficult for the elderly. As the population continues to age, the demand for home care services will continue to increase. Such services allow the elderly to stay at home longer and more safely.

crutches, canes, and a variety of other items for safety, therapy, assistance, and convenience. This equipment is usually available for rental or purchase and is often paid for by Medicare, Medicaid, or other insurance, with a doctor's prescription. As with other types of healthcare, check the patient's insurance to determine if you need to choose a provider from a preselected list.

When you call to order the equipment, you will need generally the same information as for scheduling admissions or tests or ordering home care. The DME company will deliver and set up the equipment and instruct the patient, caregiver, or both in its use. The DME company will also maintain rented equipment at no extra charge. Most suppliers of DME will also bill Medicare, Medicaid, and insurance carriers for the equipment and services at no extra charge. DME companies usually do not provide progress reports to the physician as a matter of routine, so if the doctor requires some type of reporting, you will need to tell the company when you place the order.

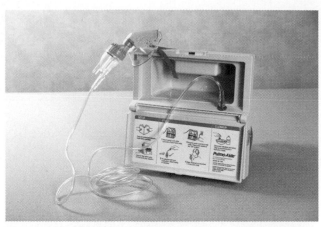

Medical assistants may help patients order and learn to use specialized equipment such as this nebulizer.

Managing Postal Correspondence

Much of the business conducted by a medical office has traditionally involved written communication through the U.S. Postal Service, a parcel delivery service, or—in some areas—a special courier/delivery service. The medical assistant needs to be aware of all aspects of preparing and sending written and electronic communications to make the best decisions about a particular communication need in the medical office environment. Use of electronic communication by fax machines and computers with modems was discussed in Chapter 6, "Managing Administrative Procedures."

Incoming Mail

Attending to incoming mail is part of the routine in any medical office. This mail may include personal correspondence for the physician; payments by patients and insurance companies; laboratory, x-ray, consultation, hospital, and test reports to be included in patients' charts; magazines, professional journals, and advertisements; accounts payable statements; and a variety of other correspondence. The first step in managing incoming mail is to sort, open, mark with the date received, and prioritize each piece. Then, the mail is logged and distributed.

SORTING MAIL You may be able to sort some pieces of mail without opening them. The appearance of the envelope often indicates whether it contains an advertisement, a statement or bill, a payment, or another type of communication.

Priority mail should be given immediate attention. This applies to:

- overnight mail or packages

- certified mail
- registered mail
- special delivery mail or packages

Other mail-related tasks should be temporarily set aside until mail in these categories is distributed. If you cannot deliver these types of mail to the person to whom they are addressed, notify the office manager or the physician at once.

> ### Working Smart
>
> You will quickly learn to distinguish "junk" mail from important office correspondence. Junk mail often includes unsolicited or inapplicable advertisements. These mailings can quickly clutter up an office and should be discarded.

THE MAIL LOG Many medical offices keep a mail log, a list of mail received each day. It is an important tool for tracing lost items and keeping current with correspondence. A notation in the log should indicate what type of follow-up is required and the deadline for follow-up. Most administrators believe mail logs should be retained for a minimum of six months or up to three years. Figure 7.2 provides a sample of a mail log that you can adapt for use in your medical office.

As you open mail and prepare to log it, confirm that all the items listed on the cover sheet, if there is one, are, in fact, enclosed. If a cover letter indicates that enclosures have been sent, confirm that the items are there, and staple or paper clip them to the cover letter. If something appears to be missing, you may have to contact the sender to find out its status. Document the results of your inquiry on the cover letter.

To log non-confidential material properly, you will have to read the cover letter or correspondence first. Depending on the policies of your office, you may be asked to highlight key information on letters or documents received in the mail. When doing this, review the document for important information, such as dates and names. If it needs the attention of more than one person, you may need to make copies or indicate that it should be passed along after being read by each person listed.

DISTRIBUTING MAIL If your office has mailboxes where employees collect mail or messages several times a day, place non-priority mail there. If not, you

	Time Received	To	From	Delivery Type	Description	Follow-Up Needed No/Yes: Description	Follow-Up Deadline	Task Completed
1								
2								
3								
4								
5								
6								
7								
8								

Figure 7.2
Incoming Mail Log Template

may need to deliver it to each addressee. In some offices, a courier or designated worker routinely delivers mail to each workstation. Priority mail should be handled so that it reaches the addressee within an hour of its arrival in the office. Make sure you know your office's mail routines and policies, and follow them to avoid confusion in mail routing and delivery.

PHYSICIAN'S PERSONAL MAIL When mail for the physician marked "personal" or "confidential" on the envelope arrives at the office, deliver it unopened. The physician also may provide names or addresses to help you identify personal mail from the return address. If you are unsure whether mail is personal, it is usually best to place it on the physician's desk unopened for review. If you open a personal communication by mistake, return it immediately to the envelope without reading it and apply a small piece of tape to hold the envelope closed. Place the envelope on the physician's desk with a note stating that it was opened by mistake.

Remaining mail should be sorted by type, and any item that requires an immediate response should be separated for prompt attention. As you open each piece of mail, paper clip any loose pages together. If you receive returned mail, it should also be stamped and set aside for separate attention. Depending on the office's policies, you may place each category of mail in a separate folder, tray, or bin to be attended to at a later time.

PRODUCT AND DRUG SAMPLES Samples of drugs and other products that arrive by mail or overnight delivery

> **Working Smart**
> Priority mail should get to the person to whom it is addressed within an hour of delivery.

service must be handled separately from the regular mail. Most offices have policies specifying how such samples will be handled.

Often, small, sample-size, non-prescription products such as skin cream, lip balm, hand soap, or cough drops are placed in small baskets in the patient treatment area for patients to take and use as they desire. Samples of new prescription drugs should be placed on the physician's desk for review. After the physician's review, sort drug samples by standard drug classifications (antibiotics, NSAIDs, antiemetics, etc.) and store them in a locked cabinet or safe area specifically designated for drug storage. A running inventory of the drug sample storage area should be kept, with new drugs added to it as they arrive.

Outgoing Mail

Most medical offices send out a variety of mail each day by way of the U.S. Postal Service and various delivery services. Correspondence is also commonly sent by fax machine and e-mail.

It is a good idea to establish an outgoing mail log so that you can track each item mailed. It should include the name and address of the intended recipient, the type of mail or delivery service, and the date of mailing. Figure 7.3 provides an example of an outgoing log template. Some offices contract or have special arrangements with a specific delivery service that they use exclusively because of service or financial considerations. It is essential that you follow established policies to maintain these contracts and arrangements in good standing. In the absence of any specific policies

Procedure 7.2

Handling Incoming Mail

Purpose: To open, sort, annotate, and distribute incoming mail in an efficient manner.

Equipment/Supplies: Letter opener, date and time stamp, stapler, paper clips, pencil.

1 Check addresses to make sure all the mail received has been delivered to the correct location.
2 Separate all priority items and handle them immediately.
3 Remove all items marked "Personal" or "Confidential" and route them to the proper recipient.
4 Stack all envelopes in the same direction.
5 After giving the stack a quick tap to shift contents downward, slice open the tops of the envelopes with a letter opener.
6 Sort into piles: mail from patients; mail from other physicians; mail from insurance companies; miscellaneous; magazines, newspapers; drug samples and advertisements.
7 Remove the contents of each envelope. If there is no return address on the contents or one differing from the address on the envelope, cut the address off the envelope and staple it to the letter. **ATTENTION!** Be careful not to staple x-rays or other items that need to remain unblemished.
8 Compare the date of the letter with the postmark on the envelope. If there is a significant gap, clip the envelope to the letter. You may want to keep the postmark on file for legal reasons.
9 Note the enclosures. If there is a discrepancy between what the letter says is included and what is actually in the envelope, mark the item "Missing" and make a note to yourself to contact the sender.
10 Discard all other envelopes.
11 Date and time stamp each item in the upper right-hand corner.
12 Read all mail and annotate important points or actions to be undertaken in pencil to alert the recipient.
13 If the letter refers to a document or file, clip it to the letter.
14 Enter each piece of mail in the incoming mail log, noting the sender, recipient, date, type of follow-up required, and the deadline for follow-up.
15 Route the mail to the intended recipients.

	Date/Time Sent	To	From	Delivery Method and Tracking Information
1				
2				
3				
4				
5				
6				
7				
8				

Figure 7.3
Outgoing Mail Log Template

or instructions, you should select the type of service that offers efficiency at the lowest cost.

Almost all correspondence produced in the office will be sent in an envelope. Exceptions are self-fold items, such as fliers or brochures, and postcards. You should keep a selection of the following on hand:

- business-size, No. 10 envelopes for correspondence (These measure $4\frac{1}{8} \times 9\frac{1}{2}$ inches and should be matched to the office's letterhead stationery in both printing and paper.)
- envelopes for statements and invoices (These may be smaller and have a transparent window so that the

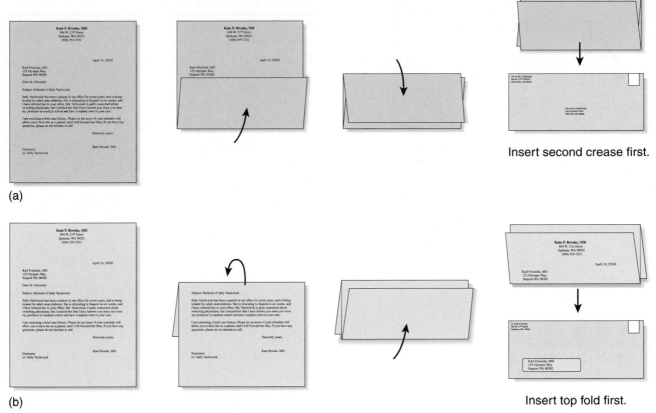

Insert second crease first.

(a)

Insert top fold first.

(b)

Figure 7.4
Folding a Document for Insertion in an Envelope

(a) Folding an 8½ x 11 sheet for a No. 10 envelope. (b) Folding an 8½ x 11 sheet accordion style for a No. 10 window envelope. Always confirm that the address shows through the envelope's window before sealing.

name and address on the statement or invoice shows through. You may include smaller envelopes for patients to use in sending payments. These are often included with invoices or statements, and usually have the address of the medical office preprinted.)

- large clasp-style envelopes in white, manila, or kraft-type paper for large, heavy, or bulky documents (Stock these in a variety of sizes to accommodate various types of mailings.)
- padded envelopes and mailing tubes for sending special materials that require extra protection

You will want to fold correspondence and insert it into the proper envelope in a way that maintains a professional look. For 8½ x 11 sheets in a No. 10 envelope, fold the page or pages in thirds before inserting them. If the envelope and letterhead are smaller, a single horizontal fold is sufficient. When using a window envelope, an accordion fold is necessary. These steps are illustrated in Figure 7.4.

Enclosures should be securely attached behind the letter before folding. Page-size enclosures that are not attached should be placed under the letter and folded with it. Smaller enclosures can be tucked inside the letter after it is folded.

Labels come in a variety of types and an enormous array of sizes to meet the needs of the individual office. If you use them in your office, select labels that are right for your printer to avoid jamming. The easiest-to-use labels come in 8½ x 11 sheets that simply load into your printer's paper tray. Most computer word processing software can arrange information to be printed on labels, using preset formats for label size and type. Most computer printers also will print address information

Working Smart

Before you seal the envelope, check to make sure the letter has been signed and that any attachments or enclosures are included, and make sure the address on the letter is the same as the one on the envelope.

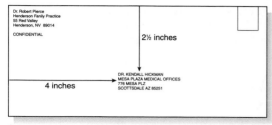

(a)

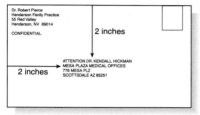

(b)

Figure 7.5
Address Placement for Standard Envelopes

(a) The correct placement for an address on a No. 10 business envelope. Note the position of the "confidential" direction. (b) The correct placement for an address on a No. 6 envelope. Note that the attention line is the first line of the address.

directly on standard-size envelopes. Figure 7.5 shows the correct position for placement of addresses on common letter-size envelopes.

U.S. POSTAL SERVICE (USPS) The USPS offers two types of service: regular mail and special delivery services. Regular mail includes first class, fourth class, priority, and express mail. Special delivery services include certified mail (with or without return receipt), registered mail, and special delivery. These services are outlined in Table 7.4.

In addition, the USPS offers two specialized types of mailing services: certified mail and registered mail. Certified mail service guarantees that a piece of mail is delivered at the right place. The customer receives a receipt showing when the item was sent, and for an extra charge can receive a "return receipt" proving that the item arrived at its destination. Registered mail should be used when sending valuable items. The package is carefully tracked as it moves through the postal system. Upon delivery, the person accepting it will sign a receipt.

Special mailing supplies for USPS services, including priority and express envelopes and labels, forms for registered and certified mail, and other items, can be

Working smart

While labels are acceptable for use with manila envelopes, packages, and some types of mass mailings, they should never be used for business letters.

Table 7.4 USPS Mailing Classes

First Class Mail—for letters, postcards, invoices, and payments.
- Items must weigh 11 ounces or less.
- Items must also be no larger than 6⅛ x 11½ inches. Postcards must be no larger than 4½ x 6 inches and no smaller than 3½ x 5 inches.
- Mail that is larger or heavier is charged extra.
- Postcards are charged at a lower rate.

Fourth Class Mail (Parcel Post)—for items weighing from one pound to 70 pounds.
- Do not use for mail that requires rapid delivery, since items in this category may not be delivered for a week or more.
- Charges are based on weight and distance. Some books and manuscripts may be eligible for a lower rate.

Priority Mail—for items of various sizes and weights that require rapid delivery.
- Delivery is usually completed within three days anywhere in the continental United States.
- Rates vary with the weight of the item and the distance it travels.
- A special flat rate is offered for any items that can fit into the standard Priority Mail envelope.

Express Mail—for the fastest delivery in the USPS system.
- For items up to 70 pounds and 108 inches combined length and girth.
- Overnight, second-day, and Saturday delivery options are available.
- Rates vary with weight, distance, and delivery options.
- A special flat-rate Express Mail envelope is also available for smaller, lighter items.
- This rate includes insurance against loss or damage.
- A pickup service is available for Express Mail items.

Special Delivery—for direct delivery of an item as soon as it arrives at the local post office, even before regular mail.
- There are limitations on distance and hours.
- Rates vary by weight and distance.

obtained at local post offices. It is a good idea to keep a supply of these in the office.

All outgoing mail should be weighed to determine the type of mail or delivery service it qualifies for and the amount of the postage or fees. A postage scale is the most accurate and convenient way to do this, but you can also use any scale calibrated to weigh in ounces. Charts of per-ounce postage rates are available at post offices, along with a variety of materials

Table 7.5 USPS Abbreviations

Avenue	AVE	Highway	HWY
Boulevard	BLVD	Junction	JCT
Center	CTR	Lane	LN
Circle	CIR	North	N
Corner	COR	Parkway	PKY
Court	CT	Place	PL
Drive	DR	Plaza	PLZ
East	E	South	S
Expressway	EXPY	West	W

Table 7.6 USPS State Abbreviations

Alabama	AL	Montana	MT
Alaska	AK	Nebraska	NE
Arizona	AZ	Nevada	NV
Arkansas	AR	New Hampshire	NH
California	CA	New Jersey	NJ
Colorado	CO	New Mexico	NM
Connecticut	CT	New York	NY
Delaware	DE	North Carolina	NC
District of Columbia	DC	North Dakota	ND
Florida	FL	Ohio	OH
Georgia	GA	Oklahoma	OK
Hawaii	HI	Oregon	OR
Idaho	ID	Pennsylvania	PA
Illinois	IL	Rhode Island	RI
Indiana	IN	South Carolina	SC
Iowa	IA	South Dakota	SD
Kansas	KS	Tennessee	TN
Kentucky	KY	Texas	TX
Louisiana	LA	Utah	UT
Maine	ME	Vermont	VT
Maryland	MD	Virginia	VA
Massachusetts	MA	Washington	WA
Michigan	MI	West Virginia	WV
Minnesota	MN	Wisconsin	WI
Mississippi	MS	Wyoming	WY
Missouri	MO		

on rates and services, and information on efficient use of the postal service.

Many offices apply postage with a postage meter, a machine that stamps the correct postage on an envelope or package and may even seal the envelope. A postal management account must be established with an amount of postage prepaid. As a convenient alternative, stamps can be ordered by phone or from the Postal Service's website. Delivery usually takes five to seven business days.

The USPS uses electronic scanners called Optical Character Readers (OCRs) to sort mail speedily and efficiently. The OCR reads the last two lines on an address. When preparing an item for the USPS, be sure to use the approved USPS abbreviations for states and addresses (see Tables 7.5 and 7.6) and double-check the zip code you are using. Use all capital letters and do not punctuate within shipping addresses.

DELIVERY SERVICES A number of companies provide letter and package delivery for a variety of fees. Types of delivery services vary, depending on locale. Information is available by calling businesses listed under "delivery services" in your local phone book. Some nationwide delivery services are United Parcel Service (UPS), FedEx, and Airborne Express, although not all of these offer service in all areas. Local businesses may also provide similar services in limited regions.

In general, you may take packages to a central location or have them picked up at your office. Some services have drop boxes in convenient locations that often contain materials to prepare packages for shipping via the service. Rates depend on weight, distance,

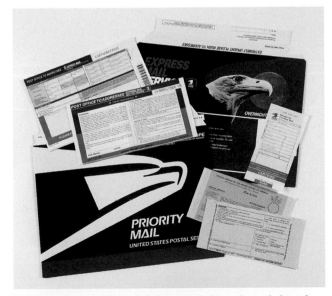

The USPS provides mailing supplies for categories such as priority and express mail.

type of delivery (overnight, second-day, Saturday, etc.), and whether the package goes by air or ground transportation. Not all services are offered at all times of day or all days of the week. Most services automatically insure packages against loss or damage.

Many cities and larger towns have messenger services that provide an option for local, same-day deliveries. Rates vary and can be quite reasonable. Some services will contract with an office to make deliveries at a reduced rate. Messenger services are listed in the yellow pages of your local telephone directory.

FAX MESSAGES Communication by fax has revolutionized the medical office by enabling it to send and receive all types of messages faster. Anything that can be scanned by a fax machine can be transmitted through telephone connections to another location—across town or across the country. You can fax printed text or any image such as photographs, drawings, charts, graphs, and forms. If you are not faxing though a computer modem, make sure all the pages

you are sending are a size and type that will not jam the machine.

All fax transmissions should start with a cover page or fax transmittal form. The cover page should include the name of the person to whom the fax is directed, the number to which you are faxing, the name of the person who wrote or originated the fax, the date, and the number of pages in the document (specifying whether the cover sheet is included). A good fax cover page will also offer a space for comments and should specify a return fax number or a phone number to call if there are problems with the transmission. Develop a fax cover sheet template to meet your office's needs following the sample in Figure 7.6.

Use the comment section of the fax cover sheet to briefly and clearly state the content and purpose of the fax. Details that should be included in this section might be the response requested from the recipient and how soon the response is expected.

You must take great care when sending confidential medical information by fax to make sure that it does

Figure 7.6
Fax Cover Sheet Template

FAX COVER SHEET

To: _____

Attention: _____

Fax number: _____

Urgent: __ Yes __ No
Confidential: __ Yes __ No

From:
　　Physician Name _____
　　Clinic Name _____
　　Address _____
　　Phone _____
　　Fax _____

Faxed by: _____

Number to call if problems receiving fax: _____

Number of pages, including cover sheet: _____

Comments: _____
_____
_____

not end up in the hands of someone not authorized to receive it. If it is necessary to send a confidential fax, make sure the cover sheet clearly indicates that. Be sure that the patient who is the subject of the medical information has completed and signed a release form. Ask the recipient of the fax to phone you when it is received. Fax confidential information only to a machine in a secure area, such as a private office or nursing station. Never fax it to mail rooms, office lobbies, or other open areas, and never fax financial information. If your fax machine prints a copy of the transmission as verification that it was sent, either destroy the copy or file it with the patient's chart.

E-MAIL E-mail, or electronic computer mail, is much like faxing because there is a risk that it can be misdirected and confidential information can be inadvertently revealed to people who have no right to it. The same considerations that apply to faxing apply to e-mail, with even more stringent precautions.

You should only send e-mails that contain confidential medical information through a secure, internal network. The messages should be encrypted, or converted to a code, to give maximum privacy. Make certain that you note the message as being confidential and that you take all precautions for privacy. Never send confidential medical information by regular Internet e-mail.

E-mail is one of the most common methods of communication, but because it is easy and quick to use, there has been a tendency not to apply the same standards to e-mail that we apply to other forms of written communication. To write an effective e-mail message, be sure to:

- include a clear subject line
- start with a greeting
- write clearly and as concisely as possible
- include a clear request for action
- check for correct grammar and spelling
- send copies to only the necessary recipients
- end with a sign-off

It is important to remember that all outgoing correspondence will reflect on the professionalism of the medical office. Do your part to ensure that all materials, even e-mails, are prepared with this in mind.

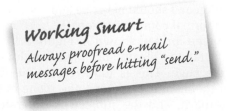

Working Smart
Always proofread e-mail messages before hitting "send."

Preparing Documents and Correspondence

Correspondence is an important part of any medical office and demands careful attention by the medical assistant. Because written communication can present a professional image for the office while conveying vital information, it is crucial that your correspondence reflect skill and efficiency.

Most correspondence consists of letters and e-mails intended to inform or inquire. Letters may go to other healthcare professionals, hospitals, patients, patients' family members, suppliers, insurance companies, or others connected with the medical practice. Correspondence may also include memos, proposals, and recommendations. It is essential for the medical assistant to be proficient in handling all types of written communication.

Elements of the Business Letter

Presenting information in a standard format lets the reader find pertinent information quickly without searching through the document. The elements of a business letter are the heading, the opening, the body, and the closing. Within this structure, the letter should communicate information in a formal manner and use a professional tone. Other methods of written communication, such as faxes and e-mails, also have standard formats that evolved from the traditional business letter format. Figure 7.7 illustrates the elements of the business letter.

THE HEADING The heading consists of the letterhead and date line. The letterhead contains all the basic information about the sender, such as the name of the physician or practice, the office address, and the phone number. It may include medical specialties, fax or voice mail numbers, and other information.

The date line should have the month spelled out, and the year should contain all four digits.

THE OPENING The opening contains the name and address of the recipient, the salutation, and the attention line or reference line. The first line is always the recipient's full name, including any professional notations and/or academic degrees. Use either a courtesy title such as "Dr.," "Rev.," "Mr.," or "Ms." in front of the name, or a professional or academic notation such as "M.D." or "Ph.D." after it. Do not use both. The salutation should use a courtesy title only.

The address lines should have the street address, with the suite or apartment number, on the second line. The city, state, and ZIP code go on the last line.

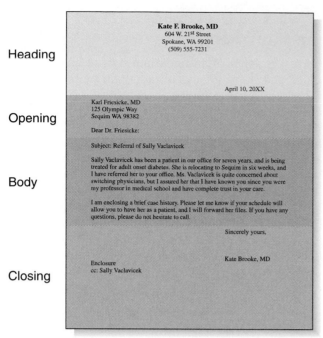

Figure 7.7
Elements of a Business Letter

The standard elements of a formal business letter are the heading, the opening, the body, and the closing.

THE BODY The body contains the message, or the main part of the letter, and the subject line. The subject line should begin with "Re" (short for "*in re*," Latin for "in the matter of") followed by a colon. If the subject involves a patient, it is best to avoid simply typing the patient's name. Try to be more specific, such as "Mary Johnson Surgery Consent Form" or "Michael Witherspoon Tonsillectomy." You may leave out the subject line when communicating with a patient, but it is very useful in correspondence with medical professionals.

Working Smart
Be careful when writing the subject line. Make sure it accurately and succinctly describes the content of the letter. Professionals rely on subject lines when reading correspondence.

THE CLOSING The closing includes the complimentary closing, the signature line, the reference initials, and any special notations. The complimentary closing is a pleasant way of ending the letter, such as "Sincerely" or "Very truly yours."

The signature line is the typewritten name of the sender, and the reference initials include both the initials of the person who dictated the letter and the person who transcribed it. A slash separates the initials.

Special notations include "Enclosure," "Attachments," or other information about items accompanying the letter. If there is more than one enclosure or attachment, specify the number in parentheses immediately after the notation.

Another example of a special notation is the note that a copy of the letter has been sent to another party or other parties. This is indicated by lower case "cc," followed by a colon and the names of the persons receiving a copy.

The Letter Format

The arrangement of the letter's elements on the page is called the letter format. While still following the rules and order established by the business letter elements, there are a number of different ways of arranging a letter on a page—some designed only for informal communication and some specifically for business use. The format dictates the placement of margins, indentations, and other elements in the letter. The samples provided in Figure 7.8 are all appropriate for use in the medical office.

The four types of business letter formats are as follows:

Block: All lines begin flush with the left margin, as in Figure 7.8(a).

Modified Block: All lines begin flush with the left margin except the date, complimentary closing, and the signature line, as in Figure 7.8(b).

Modified Block with Indentations: Identical to the Modified Block, except that all paragraphs are indented five spaces.

Simplified: Block format, but the salutation and complimentary closing are omitted. The body of the letter begins two lines after the subject line, as in Figure 7.8(c).

When typing letters of more than one page, always include the name of the addressee, the date, and the page number on pages following the first. Figure 7.9 shows two formats for these subsequent-page headings.

MEMOS A memo uses an informal format for conveying information to coworkers or close associates. It should be used only for communication within an organization and should never be substituted for letter format in formal communications.

The memo format, shown in Figure 7.10, usually has the notation "Memo" or "Memorandum" at the top of the page. This is followed by the date, the name of the memo's recipient, the name of the person sending it, and the subject. A separate line is

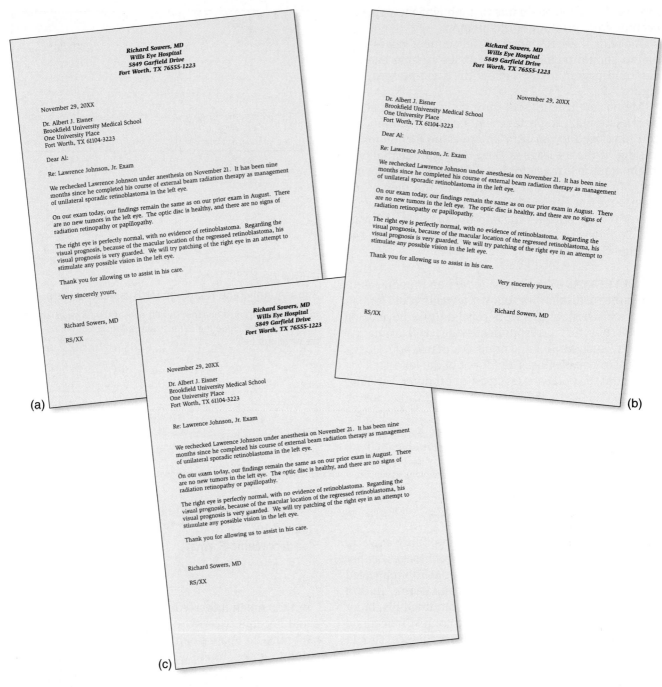

Figure 7.8
Business Letter Formats

(a) Block style sets all lines flush with the left margin. (b) Modified block shows all lines beginning flush with the left margin except the date, complimentary closing, and the signature line. (c) The simplified block format follows the block style but drops the salutation and the closing.

used for each of these. It is customary for the person sending the memo to either initial or sign it beside his name.

The body of the memo contains the message and should conform to the same standards as a business letter in format, style, and content. Paragraphs may or may not be indented. There is no complimentary closing and no signature, but the memo may have notations for enclosures (the abbreviation "enc." is often used) or copies (use the standard "cc:" as in a letter).

If the memo is intended to go to more than one person and the names are listed on it, mark a check next to the recipient's name or highlight the name on each original printout of the memo.

As with the letter format, subsequent pages of a memo should include the addressee's name and the date and page number. Follow the style presented in Figure 7.9.

Memos are usually sent through interoffice mail, or by fax or e-mail, so postage is not a consideration, but you may need to put it in an envelope for interoffice routing. If the message is extremely confidential, you might want to arrange for hand delivery to ensure privacy. In that case, you should place the memo in a plain envelope with the name of the recipient typed neatly on the outside. Include the notation, "Private and Confidential" on the outside of the envelope, and seal the flap.

FORM LETTERS Since many letters and memos written in the medical office follow the same basic format, a medical assistant can work efficiently by developing form letters for correspondence that will occur frequently, such as billing inquiries, thank you letters, and interoffice memos. The format of the letter and the content of the body are saved on a computer. Variables such as the date, address, and salutation can be merged with them or added to create a personalized version of the letter. Maintaining office form letters is usually part of the medical assistant's job. Keep a hard copy and electronic copies filed for easy reference and access by the staff.

Guidelines for Writing Quality Correspondence

As a medical assistant, you will probably have to compose letters, memos, or e-mail messages, either for your own signature or the doctor's. You may need to write letters to report on consultations, inform patients of test results, collect outstanding bills, order office equipment and supplies, or contest inaccurate bills from a supplier. Your correspondence should project a professional image of the medical office. Each written document should have a clear purpose and appropriate style. It is important to carefully proofread and edit the text before the final step of printing the document.

COMPOSING THE DOCUMENT Composing an effective, professional letter takes planning and adherence to rules of grammar, spelling, and punctuation. It is important to tailor the style of writing to best suit the reader and the purpose of the letter. The following guidelines can help in composing your correspondence.

- Determine the main purpose of the letter. A letter should cover no more than three items. If you try to

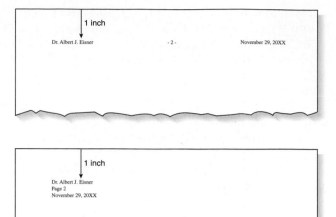

Figure 7.9
Subsequent-Page Headings for Business Letters

In business letters, a heading should appear on all pages after the first. It should include the name of the addressee, the date, and the page number.

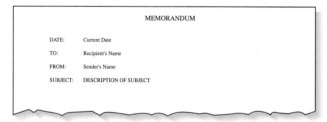

Figure 7.10
Standard Memo Format

put too much into a letter, it can confuse the reader and become so lengthy that it is tiresome to read.
- Identify the main points you want the communication to make. You may want to note several minor points under each major heading. Note any questions you need to answer or items in previous correspondence that require a response.
- Place the items in a logical order. The beginning should introduce the reader to the topic or topics to be covered. The middle should contain all the information pertinent to the main purpose. The conclusion should include any action that is to be taken by either the writer or the reader.
- Avoid jargon. Use words the reader will readily understand, and reserve highly technical words and phrases for those who work in the medical field. Make sure you fully understand the meaning of any medical terms you use. The wrong term can

communicate something very different from what you intend.

- Try to avoid pitfalls such as trite or often-used phrases and excessive wordiness. For example, use "now" instead of "at this point in time," "here" instead of "at this juncture," and "meanwhile" instead of "in the interim."
- Keep sentences short and to the point, and try to vary the rhythm of your sentences. A pattern of several very short sentences followed by one longer one tends to carry the reader along with the rhythm and breaks the monotony that can accompany a series of staccato-like sentences.
- A sentence should contain no more than one idea. You may need to use several sentences to adequately develop a particular thought. A new topic requires a new paragraph. Watch paragraph endings.
- Try to avoid using the same words or phrases repeatedly. Use a thesaurus to look up synonyms, and vary the wording of your sentences to keep your writing fresh and interesting.

Communication Challenge

It is important to use gender-neutral terms in professional correspondence to avoid unintentionally offending your reader. Today, one can never assume that a doctor is male, for example, or that a nurse is female.

EDITING Review your document carefully after it has been written. Read it with a critical eye, as you would expect the reader to do. Pay attention to the organization of the message, and make sure it clearly presents the points you want to make. Next, look for errors in spelling, grammar, and punctuation. While computer tools, such as a spelling checker, thesaurus, or grammar checker can be useful, your best devices for finding errors are knowledge, research, and careful reading. Your office should have a good set of reference books available, and you should not hesitate to use them when you are uncertain about the technical correctness of your writing. Read your letter or document from beginning to end several times. It is easy to overlook mistakes in a single quick glance.

If you have done your editing and revising to this point on a computer screen, it is time to print. You may want to use a lower quality, cheaper grade of paper for

first drafts and save the expensive letterhead paper for the final printing, after errors are corrected. After you print out your letter, read it several more times, paying particular attention to errors in spelling, grammar, punctuation, and abbreviations. The best insurance against errors is to ask a coworker to proofread your letter. It is often extremely difficult to see your own mistakes, even with repeated proofreading, but someone else may spot them instantly.

PRINTING THE FINAL DOCUMENT When you print your document, make sure the printer is clean and in good working order. Letters with toner streaks, smudged printing, or faded areas are hard to read and unprofessional in appearance.

If you are printing a formal letter, use the office letterhead stationery with the name, address, and phone number of the physician or the practice preprinted in an attractive format. The purpose of the letterhead is to present a professional image and convey important information about the sender. A letterhead sheet is used for the first page of most formal correspondence, and plain paper of like quality for subsequent pages. The quality of the paper and the skill and design of the printing determine the quality of letterhead. It is a good idea to print an envelope at the same time as the letter to save time later.

After the document has been printed, check it one last time for errors in composition, spelling, punctuation, grammar, and printing. Make sure that all pages have been printed and are in the correct order. Check to see that headings have printed on the correct page and that paragraphs are not split to leave just one line on a page. If you find mistakes, correct them immediately and reprint the letter.

Most word processing programs will let you print a business envelope directly from the address in the document. Make sure the format follows the style presented in Figure 7.5.

References for Quality Correspondence

Every medical office needs a good set of reference books, including non-medical references. Use an English language dictionary or a good medical dictionary to determine spelling and context for words. Refer to a thesaurus for synonyms and alternate words so that words are not repeated. A style manual can guide you in punctuation, grammar, and format. You may also want a drug reference book, anatomy book, and physiology book. Collect a good set of reference books, familiarize yourself with them, and use them often to ensure that your correspondence meets professional standards. Table 7.7 provides a sample listing of reference books for the medical office.

Procedure 7.3

Writing a Business Letter

Purpose: To compose, proofread, and print a professional document.

Equipment/Supplies: Computer, letterhead stationery and plain second sheets, reference books such as a dictionary, thesaurus, medical dictionary, and style manual.

1 Write down the ideas you want to present in the letter and put them in order.
2 Select the letter format you will use. Follow the examples in Figure 7.8.
3 From that rough draft, compose the letter following the guidelines offered in this section.
4 Proofread the letter on the computer. Use the computer's spell check, but also use your reference books to check for correct meaning or usage. Double-check grammar and look for words that are incorrect but spelled correctly.
5 Print a hard copy and proofread the letter again. Make any necessary corrections.
6 Print the original to be sent and a copy to be filed. Clip the envelope and any attachments to the letter, and present it to the physician to review and sign.

Table 7.7 Resources and References for the Medical Office

- *Roget's International Thesaurus*, edited by Robert L. Chapman, published by HarperCollins
- *Webster's School and Office Dictionary*, published by Random House, Inc.
- *Miller-Keane Encyclopedia and Dictionary of Medicine, Nursing, and Allied Health*, edited by Marie T. O'Toole, published by W. B. Saunders Company
- *Physician's Desk Reference*, published by Medical Economics Company
- *Chicago Manual of Style*, published by the University of Chicago Press
- *Merriam Webster Secretarial Handbook*, published by Merriam Webster, Inc.

Challenging Situations

*W*hen sorting and distributing mail, you may inadvertently open a confidential letter. Even though the envelope wasn't marked "personal" or "confidential," a quick glance at the contents will immediately reveal it as such. Place the contents back in the envelope, seal it with tape, make the notation "opened in error" on the envelope, and sign your name before routing it to the recipient.

On occasion, an e-mail, letter, or document may be sent that later is found to contain an error. You will need to determine the extent of the error and the impact it would have. For example, if it is just a small typo, you would only need to make a note to yourself to be more careful in the future. However, if the error could impact medical care or become a liability issue, you must discuss with the physician the best way to resolve the problem. Be sure to note in the file what action is taken.

Clinical Summary

- When selecting communication equipment and/or services for the medical office, consider the office's needs and how the equipment or services will be used. Plan communication systems for maximum efficiency and cost-effectiveness.
- Keep oral, written, and electronic communications professional. Use appropriate and effective techniques for accuracy. Good communication techniques are essential in the medical office.
- Maintaining privacy is a major concern in selecting and using communication equipment. Electronic communications (voice mail, e-mail, and fax) can offer numerous pitfalls in keeping patient information confidential.
- Never release patient information without proper, written authorization. Be careful that you do not inadvertently reveal confidential information.
- Be aware of office policies and procedures for handling incoming calls, and follow the guidelines. Use courtesy and patience in dealing with difficult callers.
- Make special allowances for callers with disabilities.
- Plan outgoing calls carefully to maximize effectiveness and minimize the possibility of errors.
- Follow accepted procedures for managing incoming and outgoing mail. Be aware of office policies regarding mail handling, and follow guidelines.
- Make full use of accepted reference materials when preparing written communication. Consult a dictionary, style manual, or other references to make sure letters, memos, and other communications are professional in content and appearance.
- Be aware of possible legal pitfalls in managing correspondence in the medical office.

The Language of Medicine

call-director A touch-tone phone with up to thirty buttons that is used to direct incoming calls.

conference calling A telephone conversation linking three to fourteen phones in which all parties can fully participate simultaneously.

DME Durable medical equipment used by patients at home such as hospital beds, commodes, oxygen, and wheelchairs.

E-mail Electronic mail sent and received by computer.

homebound Describing a patient who cannot walk without assistance or requires a device to aid with walking, moving, or breathing.

pager A messaging device that displays a phone number for the recipient to call.

skilled nursing care Home healthcare that requires the services of a registered nurse.

triage Screening of patients to determine priority needs in an emergency.

voice mail A messaging system that provides a recorded greeting for callers and records their messages to be retrieved later.

Signs/Symptoms of Progress

1 Recall, Question, Connect

Recall
Review the various ways correspondence can be transmitted in a medical office.

Question
What questions do you have about correspondence using these methods?

Connect
Briefly explain how you would decide on each method of correspondence. Consider confidentiality, time, and expense.

2 Educating the Patient

Sue Martin is a patient who visits your office regularly. She has a diagnosis of hypertension, and her high blood pressure has been treated by the doctor for several years. She sometimes forgets to take her medication and needs a reminder. At her last visit, her blood pressure was $^{200}/_{110}$. She was given additional instruction about her medication and is due to return to the office for a recheck tomorrow. Sue's neighbor, Marilyn Jones, calls you to ask about Sue's hypertension. She says, "I just wonder if Sue has been having trouble with her blood pressure."

1 Should you give information to Marilyn?
2 What should you say to her?
3 Marilyn mentions that Sue is complaining of a severe headache today and seems to have weakness on the left side of her body. How would you respond to this information?

3 Exploring Perspectives in Teams

Perspective involves the discipline of examining how ideas look from different points of view and recognizing that there are often multiple "answers" to complex questions. In small groups or on your own, reflect on possible alternative views or answers and summarize your findings.

1 Do you recommend writing a letter, e-mail, or memo when you are angry? Explain the reasons for your answer. What terms convey abrasiveness?
2 When should you use a conversational tone in letters and when is a more formal, even "stuffy," tone appropriate?
3 Rewrite the following letter body to make it more conversational and clear.

> It has come to our attention that the subscription for *Technological Advancements in Medicine* has been duplicated and is unnecessarily arriving twice at our office. We do not have any intention or desire to have more than one copy of your magazine in our office and respectfully request that you cancel or otherwise eliminate the double mailing and double billing.

4 Read the following e-mail message and rewrite it to follow a more appropriate style.

> Can you confirm that the physician is coming to the brunch on that Thursday? We need to know ASAP.

5 Discuss the advantages and disadvantages of using e-mail, fax machines, and more traditional mail delivery systems. Consider personnel costs, technical costs, privacy, speed of transmission, and level of frustration versus effectiveness.

Learning Outcomes

- List the objectives of time management in a medical office.
- Use appointment/scheduling tools and systems in a medical office.
- Identify patient status, and manage and appropriately schedule a variety of appointment types.
- Identify the legal implications of scheduling.
- Identify and resolve scheduling conflicts.
- Manage schedules for sales representatives, consultations, and other special circumstances.
- Understand the basics of planning and scheduling travel, meetings, and other engagements.

Performance Objectives

- Select and use a medical office appointment book or computerized scheduling system.
- Construct a scheduling matrix for a medical office.
- Arrange and coordinate physician travel, meetings, and speaking engagements.

Time management in a medical office revolves around planning work and scheduling appointments. Wise use of time will ensure that patients have a brief but pleasant wait before receiving personalized attention and a high quality of care, while also making maximum use of the physician's workday.

chapter **8**

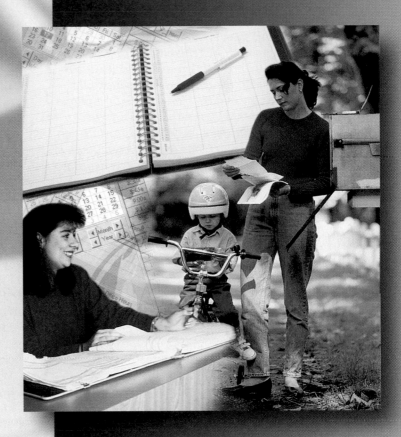

Scheduling Appointments and Managing Time

Patient Concerns

*M*any people view a trip to the doctor with anxiety, and a wait longer than fifteen minutes can compound the discomfort. The medical assistant can create a more relaxed atmosphere in the waiting room by providing a wide variety of current reading material, educational pamphlets and videos, toys to occupy children, and perhaps a phone for patient use. Plants, pleasant pictures on the walls, or even the calming effect of an aquarium can make a difference for a nervous or delayed patient.

Keeping patients informed of anticipated waiting times, explaining the reason behind a backlog in the schedule, and offering to reschedule if the patient becomes too inconvenienced will also help avoid tension in the waiting room on days when the schedule is not running as smoothly as it should.

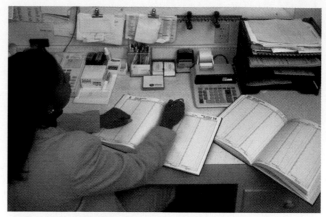

The appointment book should be able to schedule patients for the time span you choose on two facing pages.

Appointment Tools and Scheduling Methods

A variety of tools and methods can facilitate appointment scheduling. Understanding the characteristics and advantages of manual appointment books, computer scheduling programs, and the various scheduling methods will help you tailor your system to best meet the needs of your office. You will want to periodically evaluate whether these choices are working for your office or if changes should be made to improve the appointment scheduling system.

Appointment Scheduling Systems

The appointment scheduling system should be customized to suit the exact needs of your office. An appointment book that is handled manually might be appropriate for a small office, while the complexities of a larger medical group may call for a computerized scheduling system. The scheduling system should help you organize a smooth flow of patients, make efficient use of physician time, and maintain a clear record of the schedule. If there is more than one physician in the office, the system will have to provide for an easy, accurate way to track more than one schedule.

APPOINTMENT BOOKS There are many varieties of appointment books, and most are readily available in office supply or stationery stores and catalogs. To select the right appointment book for your office, you may want to shop around, or even try out different

types of books. Vendors who sell appointment books usually have sales representatives who come to your office with samples of books for you to review. Many even offer a few complimentary pages that you can use for a week or two to see if the system meets your needs. If you find that none of the preprinted appointment books are suitable, you can have an appointment book printed especially for your office.

Whatever type of book you select will need to be divided into sections appropriate for your office. Some appointment books have one day's schedule on two facing pages while others have an entire week there. You will need one column in each daily or weekly section for each physician in the office. Some offices will need additional columns for scheduling a nurse practitioner, dietitian, physical therapist, or other healthcare provider. The appointment book should be divided into five-, ten-, or fifteen-minute segments with room to write at least a name and phone number in each segment. Most books also note hourly segments. You will want to make certain that the various divisions and lines allow ample space for scheduling entries.

COMPUTERIZED SCHEDULING PROGRAMS Computerized scheduling programs offer speed and versatility. With the click of a mouse, you can change the view from day to week to month, or choose between single- or multiple-physician schedules. You can color code types of appointments, print out the day's schedule, and create no-show lists. Some scheduling programs come as part of an integrated software package that also includes accounts receivable tracking, insurance claim filing, and other management features specific to the medical office.

One disadvantage of computerized scheduling is cost. Software packages can range from several hundred

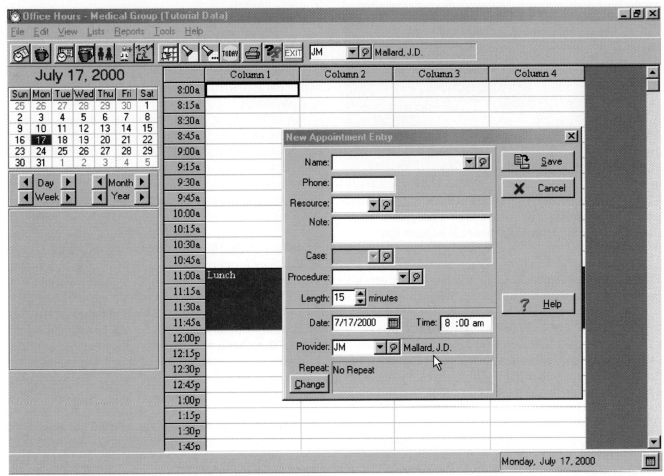

Computerized scheduling software such as Office Hours® Professional by MediSoft allows you to view scheduled appointments by day, week, or month, by multiple providers, or even by equipment or treatment areas.

up to $1,000, plus the necessary computer hardware. However, less expensive, user-friendly programs are available for smaller offices. Regardless of the software program, all users must be trained in how to use the software.

If your office chooses a computerized scheduling program, you may want to back it up with a paper appointment book so the information is available if a computer breaks down. If you do this, you must make sure both systems are updated simultaneously and follow a consistent procedure.

Scheduling Methods

A number of scheduling methods can be used to meet the needs of various types of offices and medical practices. The method you use will depend on your office's goals and location, the physicians' specialties, and the preferences of the physicians and other staff members.

In a practice with **open office hours**, all patients are walk-ins and are generally seen in the order in which they arrive. No appointment book is kept, but there is a **log** of patients who arrive to be seen by the physician. Because this can result in long patient waiting times and a heavy workload for the staff, it is commonly used only in urgent care facilities.

With **time-specific scheduling**, each patient is given an appointment. There are, however, several modifications to meet different office requirements. Time-specific scheduling allows an office to maintain a smooth flow of patients and a more even work distribution for the staff. Variations include stream, wave, modified wave, and cluster scheduling.

STREAM SCHEDULING With **stream scheduling**, each patient is given a time slot based on his status and need. For example, a new patient or one coming in for a complete physical would be booked for one hour, while a patient coming in for a follow-up visit is booked for only

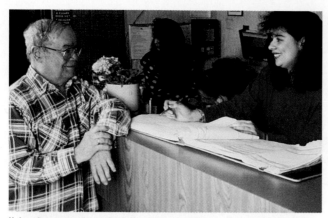

Using the appropriate scheduling method will help reduce patients' waiting time and ensure an efficient use of healthcare staff members' time.

fifteen minutes. The resulting schedule would provide each physician with a steady stream of patients.

WAVE SCHEDULING **Wave scheduling** is a type of time-specific scheduling that assumes that some patients will arrive late and others will require more or less time than scheduled. The objective is to begin each hour with the schedule on time. As the hour progresses, some patients will have minimal waiting times while others may have a longer wait. To put wave scheduling into effect, you determine how many patients can be seen in an hour, then schedule all the patients for a given hour to arrive at the beginning of that hour. They are seen in the order that they arrive, and by the end of the hour, all patients have been seen.

Although wave scheduling keeps the office schedule on track each hour, it can aggravate patients who have a longer wait or those who become aware that others were booked for the same time slot.

MODIFIED WAVE SCHEDULING One way to modify the wave system is to schedule patients in given increments, such as every fifteen minutes. Another modification involves scheduling four patients to arrive at intervals during the first half of the hour, with no patients arriving during the last half of the hour. Modified wave scheduling often results in less waiting time for patients and does not risk incurring the anger of patients who believe they have been "double-booked." This type of scheduling can also be easier for the front and back office staffs.

DOUBLE-BOOKING **Double-booking** is scheduling more than one patient for the same time block. It differs from wave scheduling in that wave scheduling has multiple patients arriving at the same time, but allows ample time for those patients to be seen.

Double-booking does not permit sufficient time for the physician and staff to attend to all patients.

Double-booking can work when patients scheduled for the same time have needs that dovetail. For example, if one patient needs lab work done first, the other patient with the same time slot can be in with the physician.

An office using double-booking will have to carefully monitor how well the system is working for staff members and patients, because it can often lead to long delays, a schedule that is backed up, and irritated patients. However, double-booking is commonly used because it ensures that the physician will always have a patient to see.

CLUSTER SCHEDULING **Cluster scheduling** groups similar appointments together at an established time of the day or day of the week. Also called categorization, this type of scheduling allows all patients who require a similar type of procedure to be scheduled around the same time. It is an efficient means of scheduling for offices that have specialized equipment or services available only at certain limited times. For example, all patients who require ECGs would be scheduled between 9:00 and 10:30 A.M.

ADVANCE SCHEDULING Advance scheduling is used when appointments must be arranged a considerable time—usually weeks or months—in advance. This type of scheduling is common in medical practices where annual exams are often booked well in advance. If your office uses advance scheduling, you will need to leave some time slots open each day for emergency visits.

COMBINATION SCHEDULING Many offices combine two or more scheduling systems. For example, patients may routinely be scheduled every fifteen minutes, with similar procedures grouped on certain days of the week. In addition, some appointments may be booked months in advance. Combination scheduling methods are often the most successful, resulting in higher satisfaction rates for patients and staff.

Evaluating the Scheduling System

You will need to review overall scheduling periodically to determine if the system is working properly or if changes are needed. The main goal in scheduling is to achieve a steady flow of patients that will make efficient use of the physician's day. You also want to be flexible enough to accommodate acutely ill patients and to adjust for scheduling disruptions or changes.

If you find that your office's scheduling does not accomplish these objectives, you may want to adjust

Date: Tuesday, April 18, 20XX

Patient	Appt. Type	Allotted Time	Appt. Time	Arrival Time	Escorted Back	Saw Physician	Appt. Ended	Remarks
Dr. David Campbell	Cons	20 min.	9:00	8:50	9:00	9:00	9:15 (15 min.)	
Jay Vanini	Ill	15 min.	9:20	9:15	9:20	9:21	9:45 (24 min.)	
Patrick Glover	NP	60 min.	9:35	9:40	9:45	9:50	10:45 (55 min.)	
Vicki Anthony	Re	15 min.	10:35					NS
Marissa Sorrei	Pap	30 min.	11:05	11:10	11:15	11:17	11:52 (35 min.)	
Kareem Nasser	Ill	15 min.	11:05	11:00	11:45	11:55	12:10 (15 min.)	Waited 50 min.
Florian Busching	Re	15 min.	11:20					Can

Figure 8.1
Sample Time Study

the mix, switch to another scheduling method, or make other changes to better tailor the schedule to meet the office's needs.

A time study may help determine what changes need to be made. Figure 8.1 shows an example of a time study chart. Such a chart tracks patients' arrival times, waits for the physician, and length of visit with the physician over a period of time, say one to two weeks. A time study also records the number of cancellations and no-shows during that period. Analyzing

Working Smart

Monitor the effectiveness of your office's scheduling system. Assess patients' waiting times and the downtimes of office staff members due to patient cancellations or no-shows. Determine if there are patterns indicating a need to change the system.

Procedure 8.1

Conducting a Time Study

Purpose: To collect data to analyze patient waiting times and appointment durations.

1 Make a chart with the following categories:
   - patient name
   - time of appointment
   - time patient arrived
   - time patient was escorted to the back office
   - time patient saw the physician
   - diagnosis or patient classification
   - time appointment was completed
   - special remarks (no-show, cancellation, walk-in, etc.)
2 Determine the length of the time study and make a chart for each day.
3 As each patient comes in, carefully mark the appropriate data in the chart.
4 At the conclusion of the study, review the charts and ask these questions:

   - How often do patients arrive on time?
   - How long do patients wait before seeing a physician?
   - Are we allotting enough time for each appointment type?
   - Is there a time of day or week when there are more no-shows or cancellations than other times? If there are, for example, a multitude of no-shows on Fridays, you may want to try double-booking or scheduling shorter appointment time blocks on those days.
   - Are the office hours appropriate? In other words, are patients still waiting long after office hours end? Is the office open so early that no one books appointments for the first hour of the day?
5 Consider the answers to these questions. Conducting a time study should help the medical office have realistic expectations for the schedule and adapt it appropriately.

the data will help you make adjustments based on realistic expectations. Procedure 8.1 outlines the steps to follow when conducting a time study.

Developing the Scheduling Matrix and Scheduling Appointments

You will use the basic information about office hours and physician availability to develop a scheduling matrix. To construct the matrix, block out all times when patients should not be scheduled for appointments. Procedure 8.2 details the steps in establishing a scheduling matrix. With an accurate matrix, you will have a clear picture of when you can schedule appointments. Most appointments will be made for patients, but on occasion, you will be scheduling appointments for other healthcare professionals and pharmaceutical representatives or other salespeople.

Establishing Office Days and Hours

Most offices will have established office hours before you join the staff. However, if you are involved with establishing office hours, factors to consider include the type of practice, the community in which the office is located, and prevailing customs regarding medical office hours. The type of practice will have a direct impact on your days and hours. For example, an orthopedic surgeon with a heavy surgery schedule will have limited hours available for office appointments, whereas a family practice specialist will want to offer a variety of office hours to accommodate working parents, children in school, and other family concerns.

A medical office in a rural area may be located in a storefront and have very different office days and hours than one in an urban office building. Some offices are open on weekend days while others are only open Monday through Friday. Medical offices in some areas may be customarily closed on a certain day of the week. Scheduling concerns related to local customs will need to be considered along with individual concerns.

The established office hours should be posted in a conspicuous place on or near the front door as well as near the check-in counter so that the information is easily visible to patients. Make certain it is in type large enough for visually impaired patients to read easily.

It is important that you schedule appointments within the posted hours, since failure to do so can confuse and frustrate patients and others. Start developing the schedule by blocking off all hours when the doctor is unavailable to patients, as detailed in Procedure 8.2.

> ### *Technology Tip*
> *Physicians may use small, computerized appointment devices, such as Palm Pilots, to keep track of their appointments. Because a Palm Pilot can be connected to the Internet, the physician can view or update her schedule away from the office.*

Once a schedule is blocked out and the times that a physician can see patients are clear, you can begin scheduling appointments. Procedure 8.3 shows the steps to follow in scheduling an appointment.

Marking Appointments on the Scheduling Matrix

When marking appointments, use ink and write clearly. Never erase or use liquid paper to cross out a name. Instead, write "can" for a cancellation or "DNA" for a no-show in front of the patient's name, and make a notation in the patient's chart. It may help to use different colored books for each physician. Remember to protect the confidentiality of the appointment book. Never leave it open where patients passing by can see it.

The appointment book is a permanent record of your office's schedule and is a legal document. For example, because it documents actual services provided and billed, the book could be vital in an audit by the IRS. Or if a patient makes a legal claim of medical abandonment, the appointment book could offer critical evidence that the patient canceled or did not keep appointments. Because appointment books are so important, all entries should be in ink, legible, and clear in meaning. Used appointment books should be filed in a safe place along with other important written and electronic files.

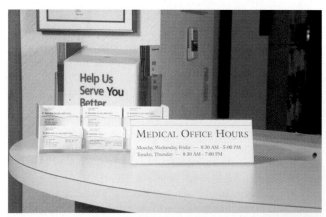

Clearly posting the clinic's office hours will tell patients when appointments can be made.

Procedure 8.2

Establishing a Scheduling Matrix

Purpose: To obtain an accurate picture of when appointments may be scheduled by blocking out in the appointment book all times unavailable to patients.

Equipment/Supplies: Appointment book, pen.

1 Block out all hours except those when the office is open. For example, if office hours are nine to five, everything before 9:00 A.M. and after 5:00 P.M. should be crossed out.
2 Block out all days when the office is closed. For example, holidays, weekends, and days set aside for workshops should be crossed out.
3 If there is more than one physician, you will need a

separate column or book for each of them. For each physician, block out all times that he or she is unable to see patients, such as personal or vacation days; days scheduled for meetings, seminars, or training; or times when the physician will be in surgery, making rounds, or at another clinic. Also block out any other times the physician has indicated a need for, such as time for returning phone calls or having lunch.

4 If any procedures need to be done at a special time, color code those blocks with highlighter. For example, if all well-child visits are to be scheduled between 1:00 and 4:00 P.M., highlight the schedule accordingly for the physician who handles those appointments.

Procedure 8.3

Scheduling an Appointment

Purpose: To schedule a time for a patient that accommodates his preference, allows for an appropriate amount of time with the physician, and maintains a flow of office visitors.

Equipment/Supplies: Appointment book and pen or computer program, appointment cards.

1 Obtain the patient's full name and telephone number.
2 Ask if the patient has seen the physician before. *It is important to determine if he is a new or established patient.*
3 Find out the purpose of the appointment, and ask for the patient's time preference.
4 Try to offer the patient a choice of at least two

appointments that will ensure adequate time with the physician without creating gaps in the schedule. For example, try to fill in the afternoon before scheduling appointments at the end of the day.

5 Note the patient's name, telephone number, and an abbreviation for the reason for the visit in the appointment book.
6 Repeat the agreed-upon time to the patient.
7 If the appointment is being made in person, offer an appointment card. If the appointment is being made over the phone, prepare an appointment card for mailing if appropriate.
8 Schedule reminder mailings or phone calls for the scheduled appointment, according to office policy.

Abbreviating common procedures and conditions will save time and space when you enter the appointment in the scheduling book. Table 8.1 lists common abbreviations. Use only those that are defined in your office manual. It is important that everyone use the same abbreviations and understand what each one means.

Determining Patient Status

When you respond to a request for an appointment, one of the first facts you need to determine is whether the person is an **established patient** (one who has seen the

physician in the past three years) or a **new patient** (one who has not). Your office will probably have guidelines on how much time to allow for each classification. For example, a new patient with cardiac symptoms who needs a physical examination will require more time than an established patient in for a follow-up appointment for an earache. Table 8.2 lists approximate times needed for various types of procedures.

NEW PATIENTS New patients require different scheduling management than established patients. You need to allow a few minutes for completion of the forms and

Table 8.1 Appointment Book Abbreviations

BP	Blood pressure check
Can	Cancellation
Cons	Consult
CPE	Complete physical exam
DNA	Did not answer (no-show)
ECG	Electrocardiogram
FU	Follow-up appointment
Ill	Illness
Inj	Injection
Lab	Laboratory
NP	New patient
Pap	Pap smear
Re	Recheck
Ref	Referral
RS	Reschedule
US	Ultrasound

Table 8.2 Estimated Appointment Duration

New patient visit	30 to 60 minutes
Detailed history and complete physical exam	30 to 60 minutes
Brief follow-up visit	10 to 15 minutes
Intermediate follow-up visit	15 to 20 minutes
Emergency visit	15 to 20 minutes
Routine prenatal visit	10 to 15 minutes
Pelvic exam and Pap smear	20 to 30 minutes
Well-child visit with immunization	10 to 20 minutes
Minor office surgery	20 to 45 minutes

questionnaires that are necessary before they see the physician. In addition, most doctors need extra time with new patients to become familiar with their history and medical concerns. Your office may ask the patient to arrive ten to fifteen minutes before her appointment or, since that can cause confusion, simply tell the patient the appointment is fifteen minutes earlier than the time you enter on the schedule. This will allow for completion of forms before seeing the physician.

When scheduling a new patient, you will need to offer certain information about your office and ask specific questions. Ask the patient:

- Who is financially responsible for the visit?
- What insurance will be used, if any?
- Who is the referring physician, if applicable?

Offer the patient information on:

- directions to the office
- any relevant office policies
- whether he needs to come in early to fill out paperwork

New patients may need additional time to become acquainted with the office. Some medical offices give new patients fliers and brochures on their policies and services, while others show new patients a video. Front office personnel will need time to create a chart for a new patient, and back office medical assistants will require time to collect patient history information and assess vital signs. Some physicians require that each new patient have a physical examination before any treatment is prescribed, while others simply address the presenting problem and prescribe treatment based on the individual's signs and symptoms. In either event, a new patient is more likely than an established patient to need diagnostic studies. These and other concerns will determine how much time you need to allow for the visit.

ESTABLISHED PATIENTS An established patient has seen the physician before, and the doctor is familiar with at least some aspects of the patient's history and medical conditions. This patient is less likely to need extra time for diagnosis. Therefore, established patients can be scheduled more easily.

Defining Appointment Type

The type of appointment the patient requests will have a major influence on how much time to allow and how soon you need to schedule the appointment. As a medical assistant, you will have to determine which appointment type a patient is requesting by gathering information from the patient.

Customer Service

When a patient calls for an appointment, give her your undivided attention. A calm, methodical approach and a courteous, matter-of-fact manner can help an apprehensive patient to communicate more clearly and will assist you in getting the information you need more efficiently.

EMERGENCIES **Emergency appointments** are the most time-critical. Since an emergency appointment in a physician's office may be very different from a trauma center's definition of an emergency, guidelines on what constitutes an emergency will help the medical assistant who does scheduling.

Emergency situations that are appropriately handled in a medical office involve a patient who has acute symptoms but does not need immediate care in a hospital emergency room. This would include, for example, rapidly worsening symptoms, symptoms of infection (including fever, pain, swelling, redness, and warmth), respiratory difficulties not of an emergency nature, patients whose prescribed treatment seems ineffective, and some patients with symptoms of a mild allergic reaction. An emergency patient should be scheduled to be seen the same day, if possible, and certainly within twenty-four hours. This patient will probably require a fifteen- to twenty-minute appointment.

Some physicians establish specific guidelines to help medical assistants determine what constitutes an emergency request for an office visit. A knowledgeable medical assistant will need to develop good telephone **triage** skills so she can adequately schedule or refer a caller.

Obviously, it is essential to discriminate between a caller who needs an appointment in the medical office and one who needs to go to a hospital emergency room immediately. A patient with cardiac symptoms, difficulty breathing, profuse bleeding, or serious injury will require the resources of a facility equipped to treat trauma cases. Having this type of patient come to the office can endanger the patient's life and place the office and the staff in an extremely difficult position. Your office should establish protocols for managing a patient whose care needs to be handled by a hospital emergency room or trauma center. These should be readily available to the medical assistant working in the front office, and all members of the healthcare team should be trained in these protocols.

FOLLOW-UPS **Follow-up appointments** are usually relatively brief and can be planned well in advance. The patient contact is established, and the physician is aware of the medical concerns involved. A follow-up visit is generally scheduled to check the patient's progress, determine the effectiveness of treatment, and/or discuss test results. A follow-up appointment should be made at the conclusion of the original appointment and usually requires ten to fifteen minutes.

TIME-SPECIFIC APPOINTMENTS **Time-specific appointments** require careful scheduling because the patient must be seen at an established time, or within a relatively narrow time range. These include patients who are fasting for lab work, those who must have blood drawn at a specific time, diabetics who must take insulin on a prescribed schedule, or anyone for whom the timing of exams or lab work is crucial from a medical point of view. Scheduling these patients requires an understanding of both the medical condition and the requirements for lab testing or exams. If the office routinely has time-specific appointments, the medical assistant should allocate slots in the appointment calendar to accommodate these patients. These should be scheduled first so that other types of appointments can be scheduled around them. Time-specific appointments will usually require fifteen to thirty minutes.

REFERRALS If you are scheduling appointments for a specialist, patients may be referred to your office for appointments. Patients referred by another physician usually are scheduled to be seen as soon as possible, depending on the patient's condition and the referring physician's request. Certainly, these patients should be scheduled within a few days, and within twenty-four hours if possible. They may be given the same scheduling considerations as an emergency patient or a new patient. A referral visit may also require extra time, since the patient will be new to your office, and the physician in your office will need to write a follow-up letter to the referring doctor. You should generally allow fifteen to forty-five minutes for a referral appointment, depending on your office's guidelines and the nature of the request.

Scheduling Time with Other Healthcare Professionals

Healthcare professionals who request meetings with a physician may include home health nurses, physical therapists, medical laboratory technicians, health information specialists, or members of the office staff. Each of these individuals has a problem or concern—usually regarding a particular patient—that he needs to discuss with the physician. While some offices set aside time each day or week for meetings with other healthcare professionals, many medical offices give these visits priority for the first available appointment. If another healthcare professional calls to request a meeting with the physician, you may want to ask about the subject of the meeting. This will not only let you be more helpful in scheduling the appointment but also will enable you to pull the patient's chart or have other information ready. If you are uncertain about the nature of the meeting, even after it has been described to you, consult the doctor before making the appointment.

Scheduling Sales Representatives

Pharmaceutical and other sales representatives can sometimes offer valuable assistance to the medical office. They can provide information on new products, drugs, and tools that may be useful for your office. Some sales representatives will offer physicians samples of the products they are selling. Therefore, you may want to reserve certain time slots one or two days a week for sales representatives whose products could be useful to the practice.

Any sales representative requesting an appointment for the first time should leave a business card and should be prepared to explain how his product could help the practice. Appointments for sales representatives are usually ten to twenty minutes. If you have a question about whether a particular sales representative should be scheduled, check with the physician first. Tell her about scheduled sales appointments so she can direct specific questions to the person meeting with the representative.

Maintaining the Appointment Schedule with Appointment Reminders

Maintaining a medical office schedule requires constant effort and attention to detail. Using patient reminder techniques and making necessary changes will result in a well-run office. Several methods can be used to encourage patients to keep or make appointments: giving out appointment cards, reminding them by phone or mail, or sending notices reminding patients to schedule a routine appointment. Using these methods to remind patients of appointments or the need to make a routine appointment will help keep the schedule running smoothly as well as provide a service to your patients.

Appointment Cards

Many offices give appointment cards to patients who schedule in person. The patient then has a written reminder that eliminates confusion and misunderstanding about appointment days and times. Some offices ask patients who schedule a follow-up appointment to self-address a reminder postcard, which then is mailed to the patient a few days before the appointment.

Appointment cards should include the patient's name and the appointment time as well as the office's location and phone number. Fill out the card and confirm it against the manual or computerized scheduling system before giving it to the patient. Also, if the patient needs any pre-appointment instructions, it may help to note them on the card. The appointment cards can also include a short statement of the office's policy on cancellations. Figure 8.2 shows an example of an appointment card.

Mail Reminders

Even if the office gave them an appointment card, patients who scheduled appointments more than a few weeks in advance will appreciate receiving a brief reminder. These notices should be sent so that patients

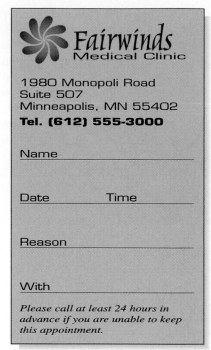

Figure 8.2
An Appointment Card

receive them three working days before the appointment. Include the same information that you put on appointment cards. Always mail appointment reminders in sealed envelopes to protect patient confidentiality.

Mail notices can be used to remind patients of appointments they have scheduled or that they should schedule an exam. For example, many gynecologic offices routinely send women reminders about their annual pelvic exam and Pap smear. This type of notice would ask the recipient to call to schedule an appointment.

Phone Reminders

A similar method involves calling the patient a day or two before an appointment as a reminder and confirmation. Some offices call all patients while others call only those who are prone to forgetting or arriving late. Call only a patient's home phone number for such a reminder, unless the patient has asked the office to call a different number. A statement like, "This is Dr. Edison's office reminding Kate of her 9:30 appointment on Tuesday, July 5." would be sufficient.

Responding to Scheduling Conflicts

The best planned schedule can be disrupted by patients who walk in unannounced or call at the last

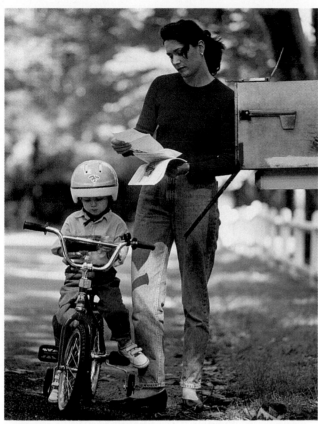

Giving patients appointment reminders is an important service for both the patients and the healthcare staff.

minute requesting immediate attention due to an urgent condition, or by those who arrive late, forget appointments, or cancel appointments at the last minute. A physician called away by an emergency or a patient whose concern turns out to be more complicated than originally assumed also can cause a back up in the schedule.

It is wise to review underbooking and overbooking periodically and adapt the schedule to avoid these problems. Be flexible and creative in dealing with the scheduling conflicts that can arise. Your goal is to get the schedule back on track, or to fill unexpected voids in the day.

Scheduling Walk-Ins and Last-Minute Callers Requesting Appointments

Occasionally, an office that uses time-specific scheduling will have a patient without an appointment walk in wanting to see a doctor. Or, a patient may call at the last minute and insist on seeing the physician that day. If it is an emergency, of course, it must be handled as such. If not, you may be able to work the person's appointment into a gap in the schedule or offer an appointment with another physician whose schedule has an opening. If that isn't possible, politely explain

that the doctor is completely booked and offer to schedule an appointment for a future date. You may want to create a daily waiting list so you can phone a patient if there has been a cancellation.

Managing Late Arrivals

If a patient arrives late, there are only two choices: arrange for the patient to be seen or ask the patient to reschedule. The choice you make will depend on your office's scheduling practices, its patient load for that day, and the patient's needs.

It may be helpful to schedule patients who are habitually late toward the end of the day so they would have less impact on the schedule by coming late again. Another tactic is to tell such a patient the appointment time is fifteen minutes earlier than what you enter in the appointment book.

Taking Advantage of Cancellations

When a patient cancels an appointment, you should indicate in the appointment book that the appointment has been canceled by drawing a single line through the name and writing "can." Then, note in the patient's chart that the appointment was canceled. Do not obliterate the patient's name in the appointment book, since the book is a permanent record of patient appointments. If that time slot is assigned to another patient, write in the name of the new patient without making the original appointment name unreadable. If a patient cancels an appointment, offer to reschedule at a later date.

You should try to fill the gap in the schedule created by the cancellation. Options are to have a waiting list of patients wanting to be called if something opens up, or to call a patient scheduled for the end of the day to see if he could come for the open time slot.

Handling No-Shows

No-shows are patients who do not show up at the scheduled time. You should note this in the appointment book by marking DNA for "did not answer." (In legal terms, the patient did not answer when called.) Some offices document this as NS for "no-show." Also indicate the no-show in the patient's chart. If the time slot is given to another patient, do not obliterate the name of the no-show in the appointment book. Some offices follow up by calling or sending a postcard asking the patient to reschedule.

For patients who may fail to hear their names called, post a sign at the reception desk asking anyone who has been waiting more than 20 minutes to notify office personnel. This avoids such a patient's being considered a no-show.

Dealing with Physician Considerations

Sometimes, the schedule can get backed up because of the physician in the office. Some physicians are habitually late, some are frequently called away for emergencies, and others may have meetings that run longer than planned. Sometimes, a patient whose appointment seemed routine turns out to be a more complicated case that requires more of the physician's time than allocated. If the physician is frequently the cause of scheduling difficulties, you may need to discuss how to better align the physician's schedule with the office schedule. Find out if longer appointments are needed, such as for thirty rather than twenty minutes each. If the physician is consistently late for the first appointment of the day, perhaps schedule that appointment ten minutes later to give the doctor time to settle in before seeing the first patient. You may find that you need to allow extra time after lunch or leave a fifteen-minute time slot free each afternoon for catchup. Building buffer times into the schedule can help keep the office running smoothly despite problems. However, always take steps like these only with the physician's approval since many doctors want to see the maximum possible number of patients each day.

Recognizing and Resolving Overbooking and Underbooking

Some offices find that they are unintentionally **overbooking** by not allowing enough time for individual appointments, double-booking too often, or beginning the day's schedule too early. By contrast, in some offices, **underbooking** occurs when too much time is assigned for individual appointments or the schedule is begun too late, resulting in large gaps in the schedule. These practices can result in inefficiencies and a schedule that does not work smoothly. Conducting periodic time studies can help identify patterns of overbooking and underbooking so that the problems can be resolved.

Scheduling Special Circumstances

From time to time, you may be called on to assist with types of planning and scheduling that do not directly involve the medical office. Some physicians use medical assistants as personal secretaries and expect them to help with a variety of tasks. If you are asked to plan meetings, arrange travel, or assist with preparations for a speaking engagement, you will want to make certain you understand what is being requested. Be sure you have complete information on dates, times, locations, and activities, as well as personal preferences. Write down all information before you attempt to make any arrangements. If the request is complex, you may need to organize the information into an outline, a time line, or another device to help you understand what needs to happen and in what order.

Keep careful records of everything you do, whom you contact, and dates, times, prices or fees you discuss. Of course, you should keep copies of all contracts, confirmations, and correspondence associated with the project.

Making Travel Arrangements

If you need to make arrangements for travel and/or accommodations, it is usually best to work with a travel agent. The services of most travel agents are usually free to the consumer, but confirm any fees prior to making arrangements. A travel agent can help you search for a particular flight, specific departure or arrival times, or the best fares. Travel agents also can assist with arrangements for ground transportation, hotel accommodations, sightseeing tours, cruises, and other recreational bookings. Keep careful notes on all arrangements you make, along with confirmation numbers, correspondence, brochures, contracts, and related materials. A few days before the trip, call to confirm all arrangements and type an itinerary for the physician that includes names, addresses, phone numbers, and confirmation numbers.

Meetings, Speaking Engagements, and Conferences

If you are planning a very complex event or one that a large number of people will attend, you may need assistance. Professional event planners are available in most large towns and cities. These individuals often work for a hotel, convention center, or chamber of commerce in the city where the event will take place, and their services are usually free. If you must plan a large or complex event without using a professional planner, you still may be able to get valuable help from a hotel sales staff, chamber of commerce, or tourism bureau.

As with travel arrangements, keep careful records and confirm all arrangements a few days before the event. The physician may want a list of all services to be provided, along with names, addresses, and phone and confirmation numbers—or may want you to give that information to an onsite coordinator for the event.

Keep in mind that if you or other members of the office staff will be away for more than a day or so, you may need to arrange for temporary help during your absence. You also may need to arrange for professional coverage for the physician during his absence, although some physicians prefer to handle this personally.

Challenging Situations

*T*he medical assistant will occasionally get a call from a patient who wants an appointment that day or week, even though the physician's schedule is full. It will be necessary to find out how urgent the situation is. If it is an emergency, it will need to be handled according to your office policy. If not, check the schedule for any cancellations or gaps where the patient could be worked into the schedule. Offer another physician, if possible. If you feel that an opening may come up, tell the patient he is welcome to wait in the waiting room for a possible vacancy in the schedule. You could also put the patient's name on a waiting list and offer to call if something becomes available. In a tactful way, let the patient know how far in advance appointments normally should be made.*

Some practices require that a patient make an annual or semi-annual appointment for a routine checkup. For example, patients in a gynecologic practice need yearly Pap smears and/or mammograms. If you are working in such a practice, you should have a clear idea of how far in advance a patient needs to

call to get an appointment at the appropriate time, and you should send timely reminders. For example, a clinic that is booking routine Pap smears three months in advance should send reminders to patients four months before the time they need to be seen.

Clinical Summary

- Good time management in a medical office will result in a smooth flow of patients and efficient use of the physician's time.
- An appointment book or computer program is necessary for scheduling in the medical office. A variety of appointment formats, either manual or computer-based, are available.
- Several types of scheduling methods are used in medical offices, including open office hours, wave, or time-specific scheduling. Stream, wave, modified wave, cluster scheduling, and advance scheduling are effective planning and scheduling tools, although combining two or more of them may be the most effective system. Double-booking must be used carefully to be effective.
- It is important to periodically evaluate scheduling and time management practices to make certain they allow for a smooth flow of patients through the front and back offices and that they are flexible enough to provide for emergency or unexpected situations.
- Before you can begin scheduling, you must establish the matrix—the days and times the physicians are available to see patients. This requires determining office days and hours and applying that information to the appointment book or program.
- An appointment book is a permanent record and should be maintained as such. Appointment books may be used in legal cases and to provide other historical information.
- When a patient requests an appointment, you will need to gather certain information, such as patient status and the type of appointment being requested. This information will help you determine how much time to allow for the appointment.
- Maintaining the appointment schedule may require giving patients reminder cards, sending out reminder notices, or making phone calls to confirm appointments.
- Even a well-planned schedule can be disrupted by unforeseen circumstances. It is important to be flexible and creative when dealing with scheduling conflicts.
- The medical assistant may occasionally be asked to assist with travel arrangements, meeting planning, speaking engagements, or other event planning. Travel agents and professional event planners may be helpful. The key to planning large or complex events is organization.

The Language of Medicine

cluster scheduling A method of scheduling in which similar appointments are grouped together at an established time of day or day of the week to allow for efficient use of personnel and equipment.

double-booking A method of scheduling in which more than one patient is given an appointment for the same time.

emergency appointments Appointments for patients with acute symptoms who need to be seen soon but do not require immediate care in a hospital emergency room.

established patient A patient who has seen the physician within the last three years.

follow-up appointments Appointments made for the physician to recheck the condition of an established patient.

log A book used to record the arrival of each patient.

matrix The basic format of an appointment book.

new patient A patient who has never seen the physician or has not seen the physician in the last three years.

no-shows Patients who do not show up for their appointments at the scheduled time.

open office hours A system in which appointments are not scheduled but the physician sees patients in the order in which they arrive.

overbooking Scheduling too many patients for the amount of time available, resulting in a day that is too crowded and a schedule that cannot be kept.

stream scheduling A system for scheduling patients based on their status and need.

time-specific appointments A system for scheduling appointments at an established time or within a relatively narrow range of time to meet specific medical requirements.

time-specific scheduling A system for scheduling each patient for a specific time slot.

triage A system of screening emergency patients to determine treatment priorities.

underbooking Scheduling that allows too much time for patients, resulting in large gaps in the schedule.

wave scheduling A system in which a given number of patients is scheduled for each hour and they are seen in the order of arrival.

Signs/Symptoms of Progress

1 Recall, Question, Connect

Recall
Describe exactly how you would perform a time study for a medical office.

Question
Write at least two questions you have about performing a time study.

Connect
How does the ability to perform a time study relate to the competencies of establishing office hours and constructing a scheduling matrix? How does it relate to the competency of identifying and handling scheduling conflicts?

2 Educating the Patient

You are working in the front office of a chiropractic practice answering phones and scheduling appointments. A woman calls to make an appointment for an adjustment. She has just moved to the city and has never been to the office before.

1 What type of patient is this? How would her status affect the appointment that you book?
2 After establishing an appointment time, what other information would you want to give to this woman?

3 Exploring Perspectives in Teams

Perspective involves the discipline of examining how ideas look from different points of view and recognizing that there are often multiple "answers" to complex questions. In small groups or on your own, reflect on possible alternative views or answers and summarize your findings.

1 Punctuality is not a universally shared value. One of your patients is habitually late for appointments, and the last time you talked to him about it, he accused you of being prejudiced and treating him differently from the other patients. He continues to arrive late for his appointments. Discuss how you would approach this situation.
2 Discuss which scheduling method would work best for a large urban clinic in which doctors are often off-schedule because of long surgeries. Which one would work best for a small clinic with a high number of "walk-in emergencies"?
3 Brainstorm ways of dealing with patients who arrive with a list of fifteen to twenty questions and monopolize the doctor's time far beyond the scheduled appointment. How would you handle this situation? How could the patient get answers to his questions? Keep in mind that the last time you spoke to the patient about this, he went home and faxed the questions to the doctor.
4 If a patient arrives late for a scheduled appointment and you cannot fit her in, what are the legal implications, if any?

Learning Outcomes

- Use, pronounce, and write medical terms correctly.
- Recognize and interpret different medical record formats.
- Identify the components of a medical record and record data in the medical record correctly.
- Establish charts for new patients.
- Recognize various types of medical record management systems.
- Identify the ethical and legal implications associated with medical records.
- Use effective transcription procedures.

Performance Objectives

- Use and read medical symbols and abbreviations correctly.
- Record information and data in medical records correctly.
- File documents correctly.
- Transcribe physician notes and reports accurately.

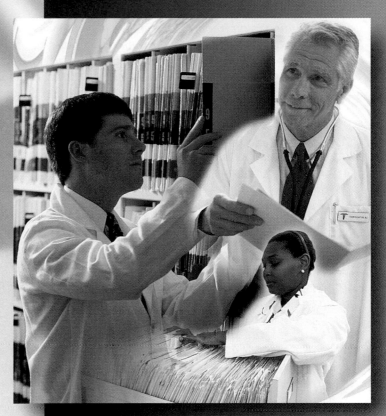

Managing Medical Records

Healthcare professionals *use medical records as tools to ensure quality patient care, communicate accurately and concisely, and preserve data for historical, statistical, and other analytical purposes. Complete, accurate healthcare records are essential for insurance billing and to document quality of care during audits. In addition, medical records are important in legal matters. For all of these reasons, medical records must be carefully managed and maintained.*

Using medical records demands a thorough knowledge of medical terminology and an ability to use that knowledge to both maintain the records and extract information from them. The medical assistant must understand different medical record formats and be able to identify the components of a medical record in the physician's office and other healthcare settings. The assistant must be able to establish a chart for a new patient as well as update and maintain existing records. Medical assistants are often responsible for arranging for the storage and protection of medical records. In addition, a medical assistant must understand the legal implications of medical record use and management.

Transcription is an important aspect of medical record management, and the medical assistant must understand transcription basics as well as be able to accurately and quickly transcribe the physician's notes.

Patient Concerns

A patient may be coming to the medical office for long-term treatment of a medical condition. Over the years, the patient may see more than one physician, specialists may be called in, numerous tests performed, insurance coverage may change, or there could be long gaps between visits. The patient's health depends on an accurate, up-to-date account in the medical record of her medical history and the care received. Additionally, the patient may count on the information in the medical record for use in a worker's compensation or other legal case. The patient trusts that the office staff will safeguard everything in her medical record and keep it confidential.

The Purpose of Medical Records

A patient's chart is a record of his medical symptoms, testing, diagnosis, treatment, and care. The primary purpose of a **medical record** is to document the physician's evaluation of a patient's condition and monitoring of his care, but it is a valuable tool in legal and other ways, too.

Evaluating the Patient's Condition and Monitoring Care

Medical records are an essential reference for physicians as they provide care to the patient. A record of the patient's personal and family history, lab tests, x-rays, and previous treatments help the doctor evaluate a patient's condition, make a diagnosis, and prescribe treatment. The patient's medical record also documents the physician's care throughout the course of treatment so that changes in the patient's condition can be monitored. From information in the record, the physician can decide whether treatment should be continued or altered.

Communication among Healthcare Professionals

A patient may be seen by a specialist or other physician, or be directed to a healthcare facility, during the course of her treatment. A clear medical record will give any

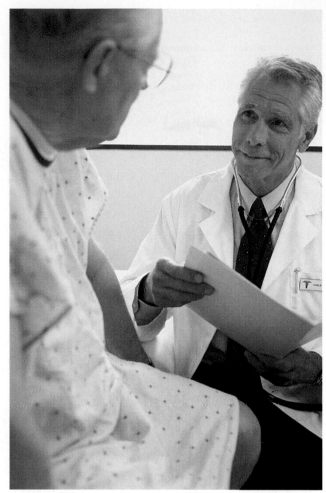

The information in the patient's medical record forms the basis of the physician's diagnosis and treatment decisions.

healthcare professional to whom the patient is referred an accurate picture of the patient's condition and needs.

Legal Documentation

An accurate medical record also provides a legal foundation for both the patient and physician in a court of law. A patient may ask a physician to appear on his behalf in court, and the medical record will back up the physician's testimony. The record is also vital as evidence in a defense against a medical malpractice lawsuit.

Legal Issue
The medical record may become evidence in a legal action. Falsifying information in a medical record is unwise and unethical.

Quality Assurance

Patient charts can be used to assess the quality of services provided by individual healthcare workers and/or healthcare providers such as physician offices, hospitals, laboratories, and clinics. Peer review organizations, the Joint Commission on Accreditation of Healthcare Organizations (JCAHO), or hospital or clinic quality assurance departments may review patient charts to determine whether services and fees meet accepted standards.

Education and Research

Patient education is also an important part of healthcare. Healthcare workers can use medical records to illustrate to a patient changes in her condition demonstrated by physical examinations or diagnostic studies and can relate the changes to following or not following the prescribed treatment plan.

In addition, patient records can be used in medical research projects to extract historical data on specific diagnoses or treatments, or demographic data for statistical purposes. Researchers use medical records to chronicle the effects of experimental treatments or procedures, to track side effects, and to determine the effectiveness of diagnostic measures. Medical records are often used in the education of healthcare students and professionals. Students may perform case studies on unusual diagnoses or conditions, the course of an illness or injury, effectiveness of treatment plans, or other aspects of care given to an individual patient or group of patients.

Medical records also have important public health implications. In the case of an epidemic, scientists may be able to determine the origin of the outbreak by researching the medical records of patients who became ill, and may be able to determine who else is at risk so that preventive measures can be taken.

Components of a Medical Record

The format—and sometimes the content—of medical records will generally vary according to the type of setting where care is provided. Physician offices have certain requirements for medical records that do not apply to hospitals, and hospitals need to include items that are unnecessary for medical offices. Figure 9.1

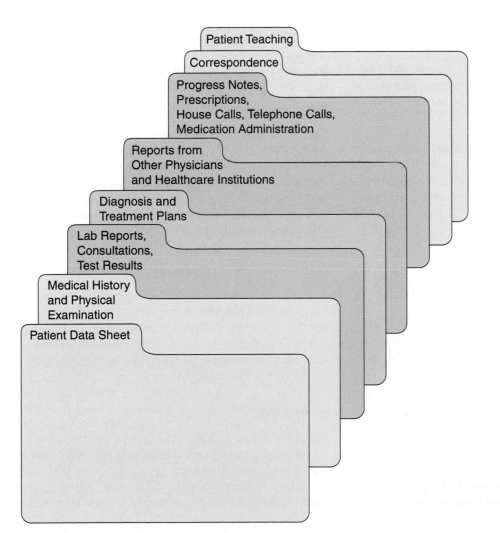

**Figure 9.1
The Components of a Medical Record**

Patient Teaching
Correspondence
Progress Notes, Prescriptions, House Calls, Telephone Calls, Medication Administration
Reports from Other Physicians and Healthcare Institutions
Diagnosis and Treatment Plans
Lab Reports, Consultations, Test Results
Medical History and Physical Examination
Patient Data Sheet

provides an overview of the important sections of a medical record.

The Patient Data Sheet

The **patient data sheet,** sometimes called the patient registration information sheet, contains demographic data about the patient. This may include full name, address, telephone number, birth date, marital status, employment information, social security number, insurance coverage information, and a section for release of information and assignment of benefits for insurance purposes. This form is usually placed in the front section of the chart.

The patient data or information sheet should be completed by the patient. If the patient cannot fill out the form, the medical assistant should gather the information from the patient and write it in the appropriate areas on the form and then make a note stating that the patient required assistance. The person receiving the completed form should make certain all necessary areas were filled out. The data sheet should be added to the chart immediately.

The Medical History and Physical Examination

Information on the patient's medical history and physical examination (H&P) can usually be found in a section following the data sheet, and often includes a questionnaire completed by the patient giving important health history information. Historical information may include past surgeries, diagnoses, and treatments; family history of illnesses; past injuries; pregnancies and outcomes; and other information that can offer clues to the patient's current health status. The history section may include a social history, giving information on the patient's lifestyle,

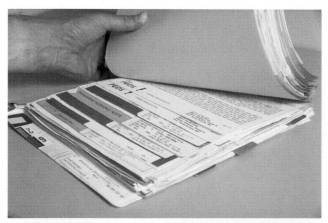

Your office's procedure may call for "shingling" certain types of documents, such as visit notes, to allow for easy review of a patient's treatment history.

and an occupational history that may provide clues to occupational exposures and health risks.

This section also includes the physician's written report of the initial physical examination. The report states the patient's chief complaint or the medical problem or concern responsible for the visit—in the patient's own words. The report includes the findings from the physical examination, results of diagnostic tests, the physician's diagnosis, recommendations for treatment, and the patient's prognosis, or expected outcome.

Lab Reports, Consultations, and Test Results

Although initial test results are included in the H&P section, later test results—including all diagnostic procedures—are often grouped together in a section of the chart that instantly identifies them. Test results include laboratory reports and results of x-rays, CT scans, MRIs, ultrasound examinations, ECGs, and other diagnostic procedures.

Each office will have a procedure for how to handle lab reports, such as placing them on the physician's desk for review when they come in and only including them in the chart after the physician has seen and initialed them. It is a good idea to keep a separate log of tests, consultations, and procedures ordered, and to note when the results arrive in the office.

Diagnoses and Treatment Plans

Diagnoses and treatment plans are statements of the physician's analysis of, and conclusions about, the patient's medical information, along with recommendations for addressing problems. The recommendations may include treatment for existing problems and plans for further diagnostic studies of problems not completely identified.

Reports from Other Physicians and Healthcare Institutions

Reports from other physicians and healthcare institutions may include consultation reports from specialists, operative reports, hospital charts, clinic records, and outpatient surgery records. Such reports are never entered into the medical record until they have been reviewed by the physician.

Progress Notes

Progress notes contain information provided by the patient and observations and examinations by healthcare personnel. Physician progress notes may also include a statement of the diagnosis and orders or recommendations for treatment. Entries by medical assistants may include, for example, notations that the patient was limping when he entered the office, had a blood-soaked towel wrapped around his left hand, or sobbed as he answered questions about his recently deceased wife. They may also include a patient's vital signs, a statement about why he came to the office today, or a description of the patient's diet and if he smokes or not.

PRESCRIPTIONS, HOUSE CALLS, AND TELEPHONE CALLS Notations on prescriptions, house calls, and telephone calls should be made in the progress notes, whether or not the patient actually comes to the office. Additionally, if a patient fails to keep a scheduled appointment or fails to make an appointment for a follow-up as instructed, the progress notes should reflect that. If the physician sees a hospitalized patient, that should be noted in the patient's office chart.

MEDICATION ADMINISTRATION The chart may have a separate section for recording medication administration, or the administration may be noted in the regular progress notes. Medication entries should receive special attention for accuracy. You should include the name of the medication, the dose, route by which it was administered, and time of administration. If the medication was injected, be sure to include the site. Note any apparent adverse effects, and include all relevant information for the particular medication. For example, respiration rates should be noted before administering morphine sulphate, and pulse rates should be assessed before giving digitalis preparations. Chart medication administration immediately to minimize errors and ensure that the record is kept up-to-date.

Correspondence

Correspondence may include letters of referral to other physicians, letters from patients to the physician's office, or letters from other healthcare providers about patients.

Patient Teaching

Any patient teaching regarding diagnosis, treatment plan, medications, tests, procedures, or other aspects of patient care should be well documented. Medicare, Medicaid, JCAHO, and most other auditors consider evidence of patient teaching an indicator of quality patient care.

It is frequently the medical assistant who conducts the teaching and who should make the chart entry. When you chart patient teaching, note the information provided and the medium (video, booklet or brochure, audiotape, illustrations or models, etc.) as well as the patient's response. If you are teaching a patient how to perform a procedure, the patient must demonstrate the procedure so you can be certain she will be able to do it at home. Make your entry immediately after the teaching, while the session is fresh in your mind, to increase accuracy.

Types of Medical Records

Different healthcare settings have requirements for medical records that may vary slightly from those of a physician's office. For example, a discharge summary is an important part of a hospital chart but is rarely included as a regular part of a medical office chart. Data on a patient's care in any one of the following facilities might be included in the patient's medical record that is maintained by the medical assistant.

HOSPITAL RECORDS Hospital records contain much of the same information and many of the same forms as physician office records, with a few exceptions. Requirements for hospital records differ because they reflect care provided in an institutional or residential setting, as opposed to an ambulatory care setting like a physician's office.

The first page of a patient's hospital chart is the **face sheet**. This is similar to the patient data sheet but is an abbreviated listing of demographic data. It often provides only the patient's name, hospital number, room number or location, attending physician's name, and admission date. The face sheet also may contain the logo of the hospital or healthcare institution. Since it does not contain sensitive information, it can help to cover and protect the pages that follow.

The **discharge summary** is another item that is specific to a hospital chart. It summarizes the course of the patient's stay in the hospital, including condition and diagnosis at admission; tests, procedures, and treatments; observations and progress (or lack of progress); and condition upon discharge. The discharge summary includes discharge medications and recommendations for further treatment, along with follow-up appointments and instructions.

Dangerous Situation
Always note information about a patient's allergies in the medical record.

Technology Tip
The American Health Information Management Association's website at www.ahima.org contains interesting information about patient records.

HOSPICE CARE RECORDS Hospice records are unique in that they address care provided to terminally ill patients. The records reveal the patient's concerns about and preparations for death. Hospice records also reflect the needs and concerns of the patient's family or other caregivers, as well as being a standard record of healthcare information like that found in any medical record. A patient receiving hospice care may be at home, with varying levels of care from hospice workers, or may be in an institutional setting. Hospice care requires certain records in the patient's chart to demonstrate that the care is desired by the patient and appropriate.

HOME HEALTHCARE RECORDS Home healthcare charts are unique in that they always demonstrate care given to a patient at home. These records usually reflect a case management approach in which one healthcare provider—often a registered nurse—assumes primary responsibility for coordinating the patient's care by practitioners from various disciplines (physical therapists, occupational therapists, medical social workers, home care aides, etc.). This care is provided under the orders of a physician. Home healthcare charts may have sections for progress notes by the various healthcare workers. There also will be a discharge summary if the patient is discharged from home healthcare. If the patient is a Medicare beneficiary, sections of the home health records will relate directly to Medicare requirements and will show that the patient meets Medicare requirements for care at home.

The facility responsible for the home healthcare will maintain the patient's medical records, which the personnel providing the care will update daily. In some limited circumstances, part of the patient's chart may be kept temporarily at the patient's home.

REHABILITATION FACILITIES RECORDS Rehabilitation facilities typically provide long-term care, since rehabilitation is usually a longer process than the short-term care a hospital offers. For the most part, these facilities are inpatient institutions, although some rehabilitation hospitals let patients go home on brief passes. In these facilities, sections of the medical records will record a patient's condition and instructions before leaving and upon returning. Charts in rehabilitation facilities also frequently reflect a case management approach similar to that of home healthcare, with sections for charting by practitioners of different disciplines. The chart will include a discharge summary for patients who leave the facility.

MENTAL HEALTH FACILITIES RECORDS The charts of mental health inpatient facilities include all or most of the sections you would find in any hospital chart but are handled differently. Because there is an even higher degree of confidentiality in mental health care, patients' charts may be maintained under stricter security than regular hospital charts. There will be sections for recording results of group and individual therapy sessions and sometimes areas noting progress in occupational therapy. Patients in an inpatient mental health facility are expected to carry out their own activities of daily living, and this will be reflected in the charting. Charts from a psychiatric hospital will have a face sheet and discharge summary, like those of other hospitals. Outpatient mental health charts will be similar but less detailed, since patients do not live at the facility during their treatment.

Medical Record Formats

There are a number of approaches to recording information in a patient's medical record. The two most commonly used are the narrative format and the Problem-Oriented Medical Record (POMR) format. Understanding the two basic approaches to organizing information in a patient's medical record will help you manage these important documents.

The Narrative Format, or Source-Oriented Medical Record (SOMR)

The narrative, or **Source-Oriented Medical Record (SOMR)**, format for making chart entries (also called the diary format) is traditional but sometimes difficult to follow. Information is organized chronologically according to its source (physicians, nurses, therapists, etc.). Specific data in these charts are difficult to locate quickly, and documents may contain much irrelevant information. Notes tend to ramble, depending on the author, and anyone reading them usually must go through the entire note to locate specific information. There is no specified format or structure to lend order to the chart entry.

The Problem-Oriented Medical Record (POMR)

The **Problem-Oriented Medical Record (POMR)** is a record-keeping method centered on the patient's specific health problems. It lends itself to the case management method of providing care and is widely favored because it provides for high quality care while meeting the requirements of third-party payers. POMR's problem-solving approach organizes data in a way that encourages ongoing evaluation and revision of the plan by any member of the healthcare team.

In the POMR method, each of a patient's problems is given a number. A concern the patient sees the physician with later is assigned another number. The POMR approach provides a logical, systematic analysis of relevant data and a highly effective means of communication among team members. The categories of information in a POMR include the database, the problem list, the plan, and progress notes.

Maintaining Medical Records and Other Files

Proper maintenance of medical records includes assembling the charts, making accurate entries, updating the record in a timely fashion, and following procedures for correcting any errors. Your office will have policies regarding how the files are classified and stored.

Assembling a New Chart

In an office that uses electronic medical records, establishing a chart for a new patient may be as simple as opening a computer file and typing in some information. Paper-based charting systems require a bit more planning. It is a good idea to keep an assembled supply of charts to avoid delays and confusion when a new patient arrives in the office. The office procedure manual should specify which forms are to be included in a new patient chart and in what order. The forms and chart holder can be gathered and assembled when the workload is light so the office is prepared for the arrival of new patients on busier days.

As long as a patient continues to receive care from the physician's office, her medical history continues to expand and the chart grows. Maintaining charts is often a matter of making entries on a timely basis and updating the charts as reports and other information arrive by mail or fax.

Customer Service

Preparing charts ahead of time will help reduce the time new patients will have to wait before receiving care.

Making Entries

Making concise, accurate entries in a patient's chart, or adding entries made by others to update a chart, are important aspects of the medical assistant's job. Only authorized medical personnel should be permitted to make chart entries. File clerks, maintenance and housekeeping personnel, and security guards should not be given access to medical chart contents. If one of these individuals has information related to patient care, he should relay it to a healthcare worker who can then add it to the chart, if appropriate. Only personnel with a direct responsibility for patient care should make chart entries or update a medical record.

All entries in a chart must be dated and signed by the person making the entry. If an entry is made about a time-sensitive issue, such as medication administration, it should note the time of day. Charting should be accurate and concise and should never include speculation or judgments by the healthcare worker, flippant comments, unsubstantiated information, or statements that could be libelous.

Working Smart

All entries should be clearly dated and signed by the individual making the entry. While some offices and healthcare facilities permit the use of initials instead of signatures in a chart, these should be used only if a prior entry includes a complete signature.

Financial or billing information should never be part of the medical record but should be kept in a separate file.

Correcting Errors

Charts should be updated as soon as information is available, and additions should be made carefully to reduce the possibility of error. Before you make an entry in a chart or add information that was prepared by someone else, always check the chart's label to make sure you are putting the information in the right chart. Many charting errors are made when a healthcare worker picks up the wrong chart by mistake.

Any record system is subject to mistakes, and it is essential that any errors in documenting patient care be corrected and clarified as soon as they are discovered. Although each mistake and correction must be considered individually, there are a few general rules.

■ Only the person who originally charted the material should correct it. An error in a handwritten or typed note should be corrected by drawing a single line through the incorrect information and writing the correction in the margin, beside, or immediately above the error. The notation "correction" (or the abbreviation "corr.") should be included, along with the date and the initials of the person making the correction.

■ For legal reasons, the use of correction fluid—or any method of changing information that obliterates the original—is completely unacceptable in medical records.

■ If an error involves several lines, the entry may need to be rewritten on a separate page and included in the chart.

Questions about acceptable methods of correcting errors in medical office charts may be directed to the physician or the practice's attorney.

Retaining and Protecting Files

Establishing a system for managing records involves decision-making about four main areas: how files will be classified and transferred among classifications; how long records will be retained, including consideration of legal issues; how active records will be protected and preserved; and how records will be stored long-term. In an established medical office, the policy and procedure manuals should describe the medical records management system; a new office will need to institute a records management system.

CLASSIFYING FILES One of the first steps in establishing a management system for medical records is determining how patient records will be filed—usually according to whether they are active, inactive, or closed. (See Figure 9.2.) **Active files** are those of patients currently receiving treatment and those

patients whose medical problem has been resolved recently; **inactive files** contain records of patients who have not been seen in the office for a specified period of time (usually six months or more) but who may be reasonably expected to return for care. Patient files are designated as closed when the patient terminates the relationship with the practice because of relocation or change of physician, or has not been seen for a longer period of time. (Some practices use three years as a guideline.) The records management system should specify how and when files will be transferred from one classification to another, and should define how records of hospitalized patients will be handled. A surgical practice may also want to provide for the charts of patients who are released from the physician's care. In some cases, these may be transferred to the inactive file. It is common practice to stamp or otherwise label the outside of the folder to indicate which classification applies to the chart inside.

DEVELOPING A RETENTION SCHEDULE The next step in establishing a medical records management system is to develop a retention schedule for the records. The Council on Ethical and Judicial Affairs of the AMA says a physician's office must retain patient records for as long as they can reasonably be expected to be of value to the patient, but there are no standard rules. Table 9.1 offers guidelines for the retention of medical records.

PRESERVING AND PROTECTING RECORDS The third step in establishing a medical records management system is to provide for protection of records in all three categories. Active records may be the most difficult

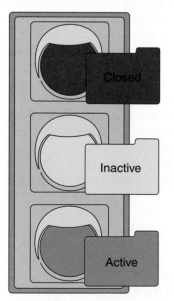

Figure 9.2
Classifying Files

Closed — Patients considered unlikely to return for care

Inactive — Patients expected to return for care in the future

Active — Patients currently receiving treatment

Table 9.1 Guidelines for Retaining Medical Records

■ Some states have laws governing the length of time medical records must be kept, with the time usually calculated from the date of the last professional contact.

■ Medical records should be kept, at a minimum, for the length of time of the state's statute of limitations on medical malpractice. This may be as little as one year, although certain circumstances can lengthen the time almost indefinitely.

■ Records of patients receiving benefits under Medicare or Medicaid must be retained for at least five years.

■ Medical considerations should be a strong determining factor in retention of patient records. For example, information on chronic conditions, operative reports, and cancer treatment records should always be retained.

■ A patient should be notified before any of his records are destroyed and should have an opportunity to claim them or have them transferred to another physician.

■ Old records should never be discarded but should be destroyed by shredding or incinerating. You will need to keep a list of all records destroyed, signed by the person destroying them.

to protect, since they are kept in an accessible area of the office and may be exposed to hazards if unexpected events, such as a fire or natural disaster, occur. Most offices routinely take precautions against fire by having smoke detectors, sprinkler systems, and fire alarms, although these may not protect against the water damage that often accompanies a fire. Inactive records may be protected by storing them in special containers or having them transferred to compact disks or microfilm which are more easily stored in protective devices. Storage of closed files is discussed in the next section.

All records should be protected against unauthorized viewing. Original documents should never be taken out of the office unless specifically subpoenaed by a court. If the information in them is needed outside the office, or if records are subpoenaed without originals being specified, photocopies should be made and the original records retained. If insurance companies, other physician offices, hospitals, or long-term care facilities request information, a summary should be prepared by the medical assistant and sent after physician approval to provide maximum privacy for the patient.

The records management system should provide for overnight storage of records in a manner that protects patients' right to privacy. Unfiled documents and charts that are left out of the regular storage area should be locked away in a designated file drawer. All regular records storage areas that have locks should be secured before the staff leaves for the evening.

LONG-TERM STORAGE OF FILES The final step in establishing a medical records management system is to provide for long-term storage of records. As mentioned previously, they may be transferred to microfilm or compact disk for storage. Paper often deteriorates and is usually more easily damaged by water, insects, or adverse conditions, so any paper records that are stored should be kept in protective containers designed especially for that purpose. There is no need to retain paper records that have been scanned into electronic files or microfilmed.

Filing Equipment

A variety of supplies and systems are used to organize files in the medical office including file storage units, guides, labels, and folders.

FILE STORAGE UNITS The three main types of file storage units are vertical filing cabinets, lateral file shelves, and movable file systems. The equipment and supplies your office uses for its document storage

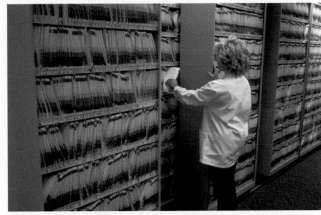

A movable filing system will allow you to store many files in a limited amount of space.

depend on its budget, the office layout, and the number of files to be stored.

- Vertical file cabinets have up to four stacked drawers that pull out. Within each drawer, files are organized from the front to the back. Inside each drawer, hanging folders with small metal arms are suspended on metal bars running along the sides of the drawer. These hanging folders can hold multiple files and make flipping through the file drawer easier.
- Lateral file shelves have doors that recess and shelves that slide out. Files are organized from left to right within a drawer. This type of cabinet uses more wall space than a vertical file cabinet but has much greater storage capacity.
- Movable file systems are more expensive but are very useful to store a large number of files in minimal space. File units move on tracks in the floor either manually or electronically, and shelves not being used are compressed together, leaving more space in the aisle around the files. Some movable file systems are computerized so that when a particular file is needed, the track moves until that file is in front.

LABELS Labels identify what is in the file. Medical records are usually labeled with the patient's name or a number assigned to her. Other files may be labeled "Invoices" or "Correspondence May 2007." Labels are also used to identify what files are in each drawer.

Date labels contain the last two digits of the current year and are usually color-coded. Many medical offices check the date label each time a patient visits the office to make sure it shows the current year and update it

> **Working Smart**
> All storage equipment and areas containing files should be locked securely before the staff leaves the office.

if necessary. That way, it is easy to see which patients have not been in for the length of time the practice requires to remove inactive files.

GUIDES Divider guides made of heavier cardboard or plastic are used to separate file drawers into sections to make files easier to locate. For example, a drawer containing files for patient numbers 000100 to 000500 may have guides separating the files at each unit of 100.

Out guides are usually a very bright color such as orange or red, and are used to mark the spot where a file has been removed. This indicates that the file is out and shows where it should go back in. Some out guides have pockets that hold a record of when the chart was removed and who has it now.

FOLDERS Folders house the documents within each file drawer or shelf. Folders generally come in 8½ x 11-inch or 8½ x 13-inch size, and are made of heavy manila paper. The back of the folder has a protruding tab which is used for labels. Folders come with tabs cut at spaced intervals, such as one-third cut or one-fourth cut, to make the labels easier to read.

Filing Procedures

Files need to be organized systematically so that everyone can locate and replace files accurately and efficiently. When you are filing, you will want to take great care to place the file in the right spot. The first step in filing is to make sure the document has been released by the physician. Next, determine the caption of the document: the name, number, or subject under which it should be filed. The caption should then be highlighted, underlined, or otherwise clearly marked on the document. Sorting everything you will be filing in a temporary storage unit will speed up the actual filing. It is important to double-check the file folder's label against the caption of each document you file. Place documents in the proper file face up with the most recent document on top. Procedure 9.1 details the steps for filing a document.

The filing system may be organized in alphabetical order, numerical order, or by subject matter. A tickler file organized in chronological order may be used to remind staff members of items needing action. Color-coded file folders can speed the filing process. It will also help to cross-reference any files that could logically be stored in more than one place.

ALPHABETICAL ORDER In this system, files are arranged according to the rules of alphabetical order.

> ### Dangerous Situation
> Use caution when filing to prevent accidents. Open only one drawer of a filing cabinet at a time. Opening more than one could cause the cabinet to become unbalanced and fall over, resulting in injury. Also, be sure to close a drawer when you are finished with it. Someone could easily trip over or walk into a drawer that is inadvertently left open.

Procedure 9.1

Filing Documents

Purpose: To correctly place documents in the appropriate files.

Equipment/Supplies: Documents to be filed, folders, file storage units, pen, highlighter.

1. Check to see that the physician has released the document for filing, usually indicated by initialing in the upper right-hand corner.
2. Index the document, deciding what caption will designate where it should be filed. Examples of captions are patient names, numbers, diseases, research projects, or procedures.
3. Code the document by underlining, circling, or highlighting the caption on it. If necessary, write the caption in the upper right-hand corner.
4. Sort the documents in filing order using a temporary storage unit such as an expandable alphabet file. This will speed up the filing later.
5. File the documents. Carefully check the caption against the folder. Place each document in the appropriate folder face up with the most recent document on top. Check that the folders are in good condition and that the labels are legible. If a file is becoming too crowded, divide the contents into two files. On the labels, type FILE 1 OF 2 and FILE 2 OF 2 to alert anyone using the file to the fact that it has more than one part.

The order is determined by looking at the first letter of the first word. If more than one item starts with that letter, base your filing on the second letter. For example, *Brooke* would come before *Bruckens*. When filing names, the last name is considered first, then the first name, and finally the middle name or initial. Though filing in alphabetical order seems as easy as ABC, you will need to learn the rules regarding alphabetizing prefixes, titles, abbreviations, and numbers. Table 9.2 lists some of these guidelines.

NUMERICAL ORDER In the numeric filing system, each file is assigned the same number of digits, starting with the lowest number and moving up. Files are then organized in numerical order. Many medical offices assign a number to each patient, with only the number and not the patient's name on the file's label. A master list of patient names and their corresponding numbers is then kept elsewhere. This system is very useful when patient information must be kept highly confidential, such as in a clinic that tests for sexually transmitted diseases.

Some hospitals and insurance companies identify patients by their nine-digit Social Security numbers. Another example of numerical filing may be a file drawer of invoices organized by invoice number.

FILING BY SUBJECT MATTER General files for correspondence, invoices, or research are often filed by subject matter. Within each file, documents are arranged either alphabetically or in chronological order, depending on the purpose of the file.

When filing by subject matter, you may come across a document that does not seem to belong anywhere. This would be placed in a file titled "Miscellaneous," but if you accumulate more than one item on a subject in the miscellaneous file, it is time to create a file for those documents.

COLOR CODING Color-coded files are used to ensure efficiency in locating and filing medical records. Colored labels and colored file folders can be used together or separately to create an organized filing system.

One way to color code files is to put colored labels on the tabs of manila file folders. Different categories of files can be assigned to certain colors. For example, each physician's files might be assigned a unique colored label. Or, files may be color coded to indicate different insurance carriers, which patients are covered by Medicare or Medicaid, or whether a patient has a particular condition such as diabetes or epilepsy.

Color coding also can be done by using colored folders for various file categories. Some offices use a different color folder for each letter of the alphabet. All patients with last names beginning with *A* might be in red folders, patients with last names beginning with *B* in green folders, etc. The labels can be laser-generated, either white or clear.

If you need to revise or reorganize the office files, ask your office products supplier to show you different

Table 9.2 Guidelines for Using Alphabetical Order

- Put the patient's last name first.
- When filing a hyphenated name, consider it as one unit.
- Consider a prefix, such as Mc, Van, or Von, as part of the last name and file alphabetically.
- File records with single-word names before those with two or more words, e.g., Fairview before Fairview Hospital.
- Take names word by word and file alphabetically. If the first names are identical, use the second name to determine alphabetical order.
- For a business whose name begins with *the*, place *the* at the end of the name for filing purposes.
- File names that consist only of capital letters according to whether those letters come before or after the letters that spell a name, e.g., CBS after Cabrini Medical Center.
- When a business name includes a number that is spelled out, such as First Ambulance Services, file it under the first letter of the spelled out number, e.g., *F* in this case.

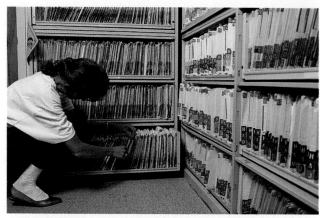

A color-coded system can help the medical assistant file and find records more efficiently.

types of filing systems and to help you determine which would be best for your office's needs.

TICKLER FILES A tickler file may be an expanding file, an index card file, or a file drawer that is set up with daily or monthly files to remind staff members of actions that need to be taken. For example, the tickler may hold reminders to pay taxes or annual license fees, send patients notices to make Pap smear or flu shot appointments, or renew memberships, licenses, or subscriptions. Tickler files can be used for anything your memory may need to be "tickled" about.

CROSS-REFERENCING A key to keeping your filing system working smoothly is to cross-reference any files that may present a question as to where they are located. Examples of files that should be cross-referenced are:

- a married woman who uses her maiden name professionally
- a patient who goes by a nickname as well as a full name (For example, John

> *Technology Tip*
> Research filing products on the Internet. Check out Smead Manufacturing Co. at www.smead.com and KARDEX Systems, Inc. at www.kardex.com.

> *Technology Tip*
> Many computer programs such as Microsoft Outlook have calendars and TaskPads for each day. You can use these TaskPads as you would a tickler file. But be sure to back them up to avoid losing data.

Throckmorton III may also be known as Trip Throckmorton.)

- children who have a different last name than the custodial parent
- a research article that could be filed under the disease it is discussing or the name of its author

To cross-reference, identify or select the primary name and create a file for all the medical records under that name. Then determine what other name or names may be used to identify that patient or topic. Using pieces of cardboard or a file folder cut in half, create and file cross-reference guides labeled with the alternative name(s) and the location of the primary file.

FINDING LOST FILES Despite all your precautions, a file may occasionally become temporarily misplaced or lost, but there are steps you can take to track it down. To minimize lost files, do not get behind on filing. Filing a stack of files can be an overwhelming task. Be careful not to rush when filing and pay close attention to the rules of your office's filing procedures. Nevertheless, on occasion, a file will get misplaced. To track down a file, try these suggestions:

- Look for clues on the out card.
- Check any cross-references.
- Check stacks of files waiting to be refiled.
- Check under the file drawer or in back of the shelf, in case the file slipped behind or under other files.
- Check in file drawers with names that sound like the one you are searching for, or in files that have alternative spellings of the name.
- Check for transposed numbers or letters. For example, 19 could be filed under 91.
- Look for folders that were pulled at the same time. For example, if the missing file was used for a research project, check near all the other files that were part of the project.
- Look on the physician's desk.
- Ask other staff members.

A missing file is a serious situation. If it is not found within two or three days, it may be declared lost. The physician will decide whether to tell the patient and what should be done to rectify the situation. It may be necessary to contact the insurance company, labs, or other providers to get duplicate copies of information.

Legal and Ethical Issues

Using and storing medical records raise some legal and ethical issues. Maintaining the confidentiality of medical

ical information without the informed, written consent of the patient. Since then, other legislation has been enacted to regulate who can have access to medical information and under what circumstances. Generally, however, even confidential information may be disclosed if a court finds the disclosure to be in the public interest.

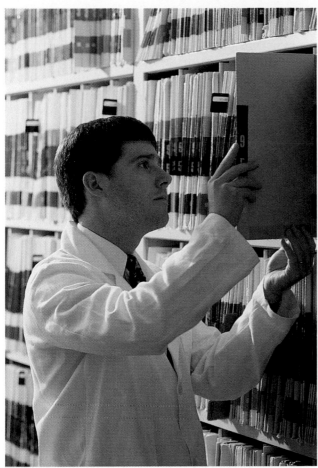

Use caution in handling any information you glean from a patient's chart. Make sure you do not discuss it with anyone who is not authorized to have the information, and

> ## Customer Service
> Demonstrating that you understand that records are private will help ensure patient confidence.

be sure your notes or other written material are not left where others can read them. It is impossible to stress too strongly the need for confidentiality in medical records, especially since violation of privacy through unauthorized release of records is rapidly becoming a major cause of litigation in the healthcare arena. Incorrectly or inappropriately released information can be extremely harmful to a patient and can result in a disastrous loss of trust by the patient. Ultimately, mishandled information harms the entire healthcare system, including workers who provide healthcare services and the patients who rely on them.

Misplacing of files can be reduced by staying on top of filing tasks and keeping a neat office.

The Release Form

While medical records are the property of the medical office, the patient owns the information contained in the records. This information is protected by law, and the unauthorized release or use of medical information is prohibited. As explained in Chapter 3, "Understanding Legal and Ethical Issues," before a medical record or any information it contains can be released, the patient or her legal guardian must sign a written consent form.

records, ensuring that release forms are signed before information is given out, and checking the credibility of faxed information are all important legal considerations. Ethically, it is important to keep financial and medical data separate to ensure that care is not compromised by the patient's financial position. Finally, a medical office that closes has legal and ethical responsibilities to its patients.

Confidentiality

Medical records are kept confidential through accepted ethical standards and state and federal laws. Medical ethics have long dictated that an individual's medical information be treated with respect and kept confidential, although ethicists have often debated the definitions of "medical information" and "confidential." The Family Privacy Act of 1974 was among the first pieces of legislation to establish laws governing the use and privacy of medical records. That legislation made it a violation of federal law to release confidential med-

> ## Legal Issue
> Violation of privacy through unauthorized release of records is rapidly becoming a major reason for litigation in the healthcare area.

This release form must specify which information is to be released, to whom, and for what purpose. The completed release of information form should be filed in the patient's chart, and a copy should go in the patient's financial record. The medical office should develop clear policies regarding the release of information from a patient's medical record. These policies must be based on state and federal laws. All personnel working in a healthcare setting should know the organization's policies regarding release of information and strictly adhere to them.

Faxed Information

Faxed information should be treated with extra care. Make certain you know the source of any faxed material that arrives in your office, and verify the source before putting the information in a patient's chart. If you have any questions about the source of faxed material, bring them to the attention of the physician immediately. Most fax machines print the source of incoming information on the faxed pages, but source information can be altered or obliterated. Faxed information should be treated like reports and be placed in a folder on the physician's desk for review before being added to the medical record. If the fax was printed on thermal paper, it should be photocopied before it is included in the chart, since information on this type of paper can fade over time.

> **Working Smart**
>
> If you make a copy of a thermal paper fax that contains confidential information, be sure to destroy the original.

Financial Records

Financial records, insurance billing and payment information, and data on collection procedures should never be included in a patient's medical record. That information could be interpreted as providing a basis for healthcare decisions and could lead to litigation. In addition, if financial records are part of a patient's medical record, and if the medical record is subpoenaed, the financial information is revealed to judges, attorneys, legal office assistants, and others who read the medical record. Financial information should be kept in a file separate from the medical record, and should be stored where it cannot be confused with the patient's chart.

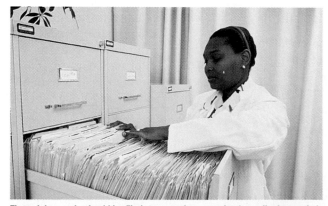

Financial records should be filed separate from a patient's medical records in order to ensure against a conflict of interest when providing medical care.

Closing a Medical Practice

A physician's practice may close for a number of reasons: retirement, death, disability, or a change of location or profession. Some reasons for closing a practice may be foreseeable and allow for planning, while others may arise suddenly, creating difficulty in deciding how to manage patients' medical records. Whenever a medical practice must be closed, it is wise to seek the counsel of an attorney experienced in legal issues related to medical practices. The local medical association may also be able to offer guidelines on closing the practice.

If there is an opportunity, patients should be notified in advance—by certified mail—and asked to arrange for transfer of their care to another physician before a given date. Doing this can help avoid any accusations of abandonment by the physician. The practice also should publish announcements in local newspapers and include any arrangements for medical records that it has established.

Once the patient has arranged for alternative care, the medical record can be transferred to the new physician after the patient signs a release. Medical records should be transferred by bonded courier or other secure method and clearly marked "Confidential" on the outside of the package.

> **Legal Issue**
>
> When transferring medical records, always mark the package as confidential.

If the practice must be closed suddenly, patients should be sent written notice as soon as possible and notices should be published in local newspapers and magazines. Letters and notices should include information about medical record transfers and ask patients to contact the office regarding their records. In some instances, the local medical association may be a contact point through which patients can arrange for transfer of their records. Whether the practice closes suddenly or with advance planning, there will usually be some medical records that are not transferred. These should be stored for a time period specified by the practice's attorney. Records containing immunization data may require special handling and long-term preservation.

Transcribing Medical Records

The ability to transcribe medical information—to type and format spoken material for addition to a medical record—is a valuable skill for medical assistants. Although some large medical practices have enough work to support a full-time transcriptionist, many

Procedure 9.2

Transcribing a Document

Purpose: To accurately transcribe a document.

Equipment/Supplies: Dictation machine and tape, computer, medical dictionary, drug reference, pen.

1 Make sure electronic equipment is turned on, clean, in good repair, and ready for use.
2 Assemble the dictation tapes, reference materials, supplies, patient charts, and any other necessary items before starting the transcription.
3 Review the information. Scan tapes by using the scan feature on the transcription machine and view reports of data to be transcribed from a digital system. Note the author, type of document to be produced, length, and any special instructions. Be alert for any corrections or other information on notes accompanying the work.
4 Based on your review of the transcription task, choose the format and the type of paper to be used. Set margins and spacing, and make other necessary adjustments.
5 Adjust the volume and speed of the dictation machine.
6 Use the foot pedals to start and stop recording. Use the reverse pedal to rewind the tape and the pause pedal if you need to catch up.

7 Transcribe the information as it was dictated. Supply punctuation and correct spelling where necessary, but do not alter the words or the word order, since this could change the meaning. If you have even a slight doubt about a word or phrase, make a note to mark the passage and request clarification from the speaker.
8 Proofread and edit your work on the computer screen. Look up the spelling of words you are unsure of, especially drug names. Check style and formatting points to be certain there are no errors.
9 Print the finished document and proofread it again. Make sure nothing went awry in the printing process. Look for pagination errors, printing that is crooked on the page, smearing, or other problems that could make documents difficult to read.
10 Flag any areas in question to alert the physician as she reads the transcribed material.
11 Place the document in a folder to maintain confidentiality, and put it on the physician's desk to be reviewed and initialed. If the transcribed material is a correspondence, the physician should sign below the closing and above the signature line.
12 Corrections must be made before a document is mailed or placed in a chart.

smaller offices expect medical assistants to include this in their duties. Procedure 9.2 outlines the steps of the transcription process.

Transcription Skills

Transcription is a skill that demands repeated, intensive practice to achieve the speed and accuracy today's medical offices require. You need to be able to type at least 60 words per minute accurately. Some offices require that medical transcriptionists be able to transcribe a minimum of 90 words per minute with 97% accuracy. A transcriptionist must also be able to use a computer or word processor; know grammar, punctuation, spelling, and word usage; and possess medical language skills. Attention to detail and the ability to maintain confidentiality are also important.

An important part of transcribing is understanding the various formats for different types of medical documents. While they can vary from one setting to another, most medical offices have selected formats for histories, physicals, progress notes, reports, and summaries. Formats specify such items as spacing, capitalization, punctuation, and use of abbreviations and numbers. A transcriptionist must be able to process spoken information in the correct format and according to accepted standards. Table 9.3 offers tips for transcription.

Transcription Equipment and Supplies

Dictation equipment is either analog or digital. Analog equipment uses cassette tapes to record the material to

Legal Issue

After a tape has been transcribed and the transcription checked by the physician, it should be erased. Most offices reuse dictation tapes several times before discarding them. Discarded tapes should be reviewed to make sure they have been completely erased before they are placed in the trash.

Table 9.3 Tips for Medical Transcription

- **Develop your listening skills.** When you transcribe, make certain that your mind is focused on what you are hearing. Avoid interruptions and distractions that could lead to errors. Think about what the speaker is saying, and be prepared to use your knowledge of medical terminology, including spelling and word usage. The inflection of the physician's voice can indicate where punctuation belongs or where a sentence or paragraph ends.

- **Check the context.** Pay close attention to the context of the dictation. Is the document an operative report or a progress note? Is the patient an elderly woman or a boy? Is the diagnosis congestive heart failure or dermatitis? Is the speaker a gastroenterologist or a pediatrician? Keeping the context in mind can help eliminate errors, minimize questions, and direct you to the proper spelling and punctuation.

- **Watch spelling as you type.** Spelling a word correctly the first time saves editing time. Keep your spelling skills sharp by noting spelling of new or unfamiliar words. List terms you are learning and review the list frequently until you can spell each word correctly on the first attempt.

- **Proofread, proofread, proofread.** You cannot be too careful in proofreading your transcribed documents, and you cannot proofread too much. Check and recheck your work. Research all questions until they are answered and you are certain the document is as free from error as you can make it.

- **Use resources.** A medical transcription workstation should have a minimum of one English language dictionary, two medical dictionaries, a volume of medical abbreviations and terms particular to your office's specialty, and a comprehensive drug reference book, such as the *Physicians' Desk Reference*. Finally, the *AAMT Book of Style*, published by the American Association of Medical Transcriptionists, can be used to answer questions of style and format.

- **Maintain confidentiality and ethical behavior.** Do not discuss the information being transcribed within hearing of patients, visitors, or others who should not have access to confidential information. Do not let coworkers listen to dictated tapes that have been assigned to you, and do not allow others in the office to see dictated material on your computer monitor or printed pages in your printer.

- **Refuse to compromise on accuracy.** Do not accept mistakes in the name of speed or timeliness. Never bluff, guess, or assume. If you question a word or passage, make certain it is brought to the attention of the speaker and reviewed thoroughly.

- **Double-check names.** Patient names can sound disturbingly similar, and it can be easy to mistake one patient's name for another. Make absolutely certain you are typing the correct patient name and identifying information on transcribed documents and that you file the documents in the proper chart.

be transcribed, while the newer digital models use computers and related accessories to capture voice data. Digital technology can also allow for dictation and transcription through telephone lines and can permit transcription that is almost simultaneous with the dictation. It can also provide for almost instantaneous sorting and selecting of various dictated files.

The dictation device may be similar to a tape recorder and can be anything from a small hand-held device about the size of a cellular phone to a larger desk model that also resembles a telephone. Almost any type of computer with good word processing capability and medical spellchecking software can be used for transcription. The computer system should be secure, and medical information should be protected by passwords and security software.

The transcription machine is usually controlled by foot pedals so the transcriptionist can have her hands free for keying the dictated information. Other features can include volume and speed controls, automatic backspace that rewinds the tape a few seconds each time it is stopped, a scanning control to let the user quickly review the entire contents of the tape, and an erase function. Most transcriptionists use headphones for comfort and convenience and to ensure privacy of the transcribed information.

Working Smart

If you have a question about the dictation you are transcribing, note the elapsed time on the machine's digital counter. Then, when you go over the question with the physician, you will know exactly where to find the area in question.

The future of transcription will include speech-recognition computer systems. In a speech-activated system, speech replaces keying or document scanning as the input medium. When using this type of system, your main role as a transcriptionist changes from keying dictated documents to reading and interpreting text, formatting documents, and editing voice-dictated drafts.

While there have been significant advances in voice and speech recognition, dialects and the inherent complexities of language continue to perplex inventors. Voice systems face three main challenges. First, the systems must be smart enough to understand words spoken by people with different accents. Second, conversational speech is, on average, at a rate of 120 words a minute, and many voice systems produce garbled or confused text at or close to that rate. Third, communication experts must design new systems for auditing, editing, and proofreading documents recorded via voice recognition. For example, such systems cannot accurately interpret proper names or homonyms.

Typical Medical Transcription Work

A wide variety of documents need to be transcribed in a medical office. Most of these are medical reports, but some are memos or letters. Any of the following may be dictated by physicians for transcription by a medical assistant.

HISTORY AND PHYSICAL History and physical (H&P) documents are required upon hospital admission and must be in the patient's chart before surgery. Some physicians require an H&P for every new patient seen in the office. H&P formats vary by physician, by office, and by hospital or institution, but many sections of the report are standard. In some offices, these standard sections are stored as computer files and retrieved by the transcriptionist as needed.

PROGRESS NOTES Some physicians prefer to write these notes directly in the chart while others like to dictate them for transcription. The physician should always sign dictated progress notes before they are added to the chart.

OPERATIVE REPORTS An **operative report** is an account of the events of surgery and the patient's response to the operation. It is written by the surgeon and placed in the patient's chart. An operative report notes any tissue samples that were sent to the pathology lab and includes any unexpected events during the operation.

CONSULTATION REPORTS **Consultation reports** are reports prepared by one physician for another (referring) physician. They contain a detailed account of the consulting physician's findings and recommendations concerning the patient who was referred. "Consult"

reports often use the same general format as the history and physical and may be included in a letter. The report requires the consulting physician's signature.

LABORATORY, PATHOLOGY, AND RADIOLOGY REPORTS Laboratory reports consist largely of numerical values and have a specific format using columns and rows to separate groups of items. They are generated by a laboratory technologist or pathologist who has performed blood, urine, or other testing ordered by the primary physician. Pathology reports give the findings of a pathologist who has examined samples submitted by another physician. These samples are often obtained during surgery, including surgery in the physician's office. Radiology reports are written by a radiologist after examining x-rays or other studies that the patient's primary physician has ordered.

DISCHARGE SUMMARIES A discharge summary is dictated by the patient's primary physician when the patient is released from a hospital or outpatient facility or by a registered nurse when the patient is released from home healthcare. It summarizes the events that occurred while the patient was in the facility or under the care of home health nurses.

LETTERS, MEMOS, AND OTHER CORRESPONDENCE Physicians often dictate correspondence that is not directly related to the medical field. This might be a letter confirming arrangements for a meeting or speaking engagement, a memo outlining an agreement for renovating the reception area, or an inquiry about investments. These nonmedical documents should be transcribed with the same care as entries in a patient's chart and should be treated with the same concern for confidentiality. The physician/author should specify the purpose of the dictation before beginning it so you can prepare the correct format. Follow the formats for business letters and memos outlined in Chapter 7, "Managing Communications: Telephones, Mail, and Correspondence."

Understanding the Vocabulary of Medical Records

Sound knowledge of medical terminology is essential to read and correctly interpret medical records as well as successfully transcribe documents. Understanding the construction of medical terms will help you deduce the word's meaning. It also helps to know general rules regarding the formation of plurals and to be familiar with the symbols and abbreviations used for medical terms.

The Construction of Medical Terms

Like the words you use in everyday conversation, most medical terms consist of word parts that are approximately equal to syllables. These word parts are defined in Figure 9.3.

These word parts can be mixed and matched to create thousands of medical terms. For example, the word *epigastric*, a term for above the stomach, can be broken down into *epi* (upon), *gastr* (stomach), and *ic* (pertaining to). Table 9.4 outlines steps that will help you understand an unfamiliar medical term.

It is important to recognize that some medical terms are not subject to the "word-part" approach, and their meanings must be memorized as whole terms. An example of this is Alzheimer's disease, characterized by degeneration of the brain cells, which is named after the physician who first described it. Appendix A, "Medical Language Handbook," lists common prefixes, roots (along with their combining forms), and suffixes.

Forming Plurals

In medical terminology, words based on Greek and Latin follow those languages' rules for forming plurals. The plural for other words is generally constructed by adding "s" or "es" to the singular form. For some words, the way the plural is formed does not follow any rules. Table 9.5 provides some examples of frequently used plural forms of medical terms. If you are uncertain of the correct plural of a term, check it in a medical dictionary.

Table 9.4 Steps for Deciphering a Medical Term

1 Scan the entire word.
2 Look at its context in the text for clues as to whether it is a surgical, pathological, or anatomical term. For example, in the sentence, "The patient was being treated for *mesophlebitis*," the words "treated for" would indicate that the word refers to a condition. It may be an anatomical condition or a pathological condition, but it is *not* a surgical procedure.
3 Look at the suffix, which usually indicates some form of action or state of being. For example, *itis* means inflammation.
4 Look at the root of the word, which usually indicates the body part or system being referred to. In this case, *phleb* refers to veins.
5 Look at the prefix. The prefix *meso* means middle.
6 Put the parts together to get a definition. *Mesophlebitis* means an inflammation of the middle layer of the wall of a vein. Check to see if that makes sense within the context of how the word was used.
7 If there is any doubt, look the term up in a medical dictionary.

Table 9.5 Frequently Used Plural Forms

Singular	Ending	Plural
vertebra	-a/-ae	vertebrae
diagnosis	-is/-es	diagnoses
phenomenon	-on/-a	phenomena
bacterium	-ium/-ia	bacteria
fungus	-us/-i	fungi
thorax	-ax/-aces	thoraces
apex	-ex/-ices	apices
appendix	-ix/-ices	appendices
cardiopathy	-y/-ies	cardiopathies
condyloma	-a/-mata	condylomata

Symbols and Abbreviations

Medical language uses a large number of abbreviations to save time. A few of them are standard, while a great many are recognized only in certain areas or by certain healthcare institutions. Any hospital, clinic, or

Figure 9.3 Word Parts

A prefix is a syllable attached to the front of a word, usually indicating an adjective that modifies the root. A root is the source of the word; in medical terminology, it usually refers to a body part. A suffix is a syllable attached to the end of a word, often indicating some kind of action.

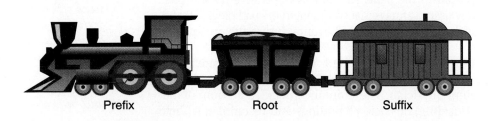

Prefix   Root   Suffix

other healthcare setting should have a printed list of the abbreviations it considers acceptable for charting. Ask for a list of accepted abbreviations where you work. If you are responsible for making decisions about charting in a medical office without an abbreviation list, you should establish one to avoid confusion and miscommunication.

Communication Challenge

If you are in doubt about an abbreviation, write the word out. Also, do not make up abbreviations; use the ones that are common in your medical office.

A comprehensive listing of commonly used symbols and abbreviations is lengthy and can be found in most medical dictionaries. In addition, entire books containing nothing but a lists of symbols and abbreviations used by healthcare professionals can be found in libraries and bookstores.

Challenging Situations

In today's world, many women keep their maiden name after marriage or continue to use their maiden name professionally after taking their husband's name. Some women use a hyphenated version of both last names. With divorce and remarriage so common, many children change last names or live with a parent whose last name differs from theirs. These things can cause confusion when filing medical records. It is important that the name of any patient in this situation be accurately cross-referenced so that a file can always be quickly accessed.

Many medical terms and medications sound alike. A small error or misspelling of a medical term could make a critical, even fatal, difference for a patient. It is important to become as well-versed in medical terminology as you can. Study new words when you come across them, and become familiar with the common prefixes, suffixes, and roots used in creating medical terms. Whenever you have a doubt, consult a medical dictionary. When transcribing, never assume or guess about a word. Also, reconfirm the word with the physician if you have a question. For the safety of the patient, a transcribed medical record must be 100% accurate.

Clinical Summary

- Medical records are used to communicate accurately, preserve data, and help provide quality patient care, and for billing and management purposes.
- Medical assistants are frequently responsible for initiating, maintaining, protecting, and storing medical records. In addition, many assistants are expected to transcribe the physician's dictation to be included in the medical record.
- Patient charts may be used for evaluating a patient's condition, monitoring care, educational purposes, increasing the quality of healthcare, research, and legal purposes.
- Medical records are kept confidential according to ethical standards and state and federal laws.
- Medical record formats may be organized chronologically (Source-Oriented Medical Record) or based on the patient's specific health problems (Problem-Oriented Medical Record).
- The POMR provides for coordination of a patient's healthcare, enhances communication among members of the healthcare team, and can encourage ongoing evaluation of a patient's condition.
- The POMR consists of four sections: the database, problem list, plan, and progress notes.
- Contents of a medical record may vary among institutions, or between an inpatient setting and an ambulatory care setting. The history and physical, patient data sheet, test results, reports, progress notes, and records of patient teaching are common to almost all medical records.
- Charting should be done according to accepted rules. Errors in a medical record should never be corrected by obliterating the original entry. Instead, a single line should be drawn through the error and the correction made above or beside it or in the margin. Corrections should be clearly noted, signed, and dated, and should be made only by the person who made the error.
- Medical records may be stored and managed in electronic files, manually on paper, or by a combination of electronic and paper-based methods.
- Managing medical records requires a plan for classifying and transferring files among classifications, retaining files, preserving and protecting records, and long-term storage of the records. Closing a medical practice presents special considerations in handling its records.
- Confidentiality is an important issue in medical records management. The medical office should have written policies regarding how the confidentiality of its records will be maintained.
- Labels, guides, and folders are all tools to make filing more efficient and accurate.
- Files may be organized alphabetically, numerically, or by subject. A chronological tickler file can help remind staff members of actions needed by a certain date.
- Medical transcription includes typing and formatting spoken material for addition to a medical record. Medical

assistants are often expected to perform transcription duties and need to be skilled in using computer hardware and software. They should be able to type rapidly and have excellent knowledge of medical language. Proofreading is essential in transcribing medical documents.

- Dictation/transcription equipment records and plays voice data, and is usually classified as analog (tape-based) or digital (computer-based). Digital dictation equipment is more expensive but offers several advantages over analog equipment.

- Steps in transcribing include readying equipment and supplies, reviewing information and planning the work, keying or processing the information, proofreading and editing, and printing.

- Medical transcription is easier if the transcriptionist has good listening skills, checks the context for clues to meaning, is careful of spelling and meticulous about proofreading, and uses resources when questions arise.

- The American Association of Medical Transcriptionists publishes the *AAMT Book of Style*, a manual that provides style points for uniformity and correctness in medical transcription.

- Medical transcription is very exacting, and medical assistants who function as transcriptionists must constantly be mindful of errors, confidentiality, and ethical behavior.

- Transcribed documents may include history and physical data, progress notes, operative reports, consultation reports, pathology reports, discharge summaries, radiology reports, and laboratory reports.

- Knowledge of medical terminology is essential to the medical assistant. Many medical terms are constructed from certain basic word parts and can be analyzed for meaning by defining the individual parts.

- Some medical terms are not subject to the "word-part" approach, and the term's meaning and spelling must be memorized.

- Plural forms of medical terms may be created according to English, Greek, or Latin rules.

- Medical language uses a huge number of abbreviations and symbols to save time. Most hospitals, clinics, and medical offices have a list of abbreviations that they consider standard.

The Language of Medicine

active files Files of patients currently receiving treatment.

consultation report Report prepared by a physician for a referring physician.

discharge summary A summary of the course of the patient's stay in the hospital, including condition and diagnoses at admission, tests, procedures, treatments, observations, progress, and condition upon discharge.

face sheet The first page of a patient's hospital chart, containing demographic data.

inactive files Files of patients who have not been a patient of a medical practice for a specified period (usually six months or more).

medical record The record of individual medical diagnoses and treatments; also called the patient chart.

operative report An accounting of a patient's surgery and response to the operation.

out guides Brightly colored cards used to mark where files have been removed.

patient data sheet A form containing demographic data about the patient; sometimes called the patient information sheet.

Problem-Oriented Medical Record (POMR) A record-keeping format centered on the patient's specific health problems.

progress notes Information provided by the patient and observations and examination results from healthcare personnel.

Source-Oriented Medical Record (SOMR) A record-keeping format in which data in the file are organized according to their source; also called narrative or diary format.

Signs/Symptoms of Progress

1 *Recall, Question, Connect*

Recall
Review the four major decisions that must be made when establishing a system for medical records.

Question
What questions do you have about establishing a medical records system?

Connect
Why does a medical assistant who is going to work in a long-established clinic need to know how the medical records system there was set up?

2 *Educating the Patient*

A patient has just been talking to the pediatrician about her four-year-old daughter. When you enter the room, she is sobbing. She tells you that the doctor has told her that her little girl has multiple sclerosis. She does not really know anything about the disease except that it is "terrible." You know that the doctor has diagnosed a mild form of scoliosis in the little girl.
1 What do you tell her mother?
2 Why is knowledge of medical terminology important when talking to patients?

3 *Exploring Perspectives in Teams*

Perspective involves the discipline of examining how ideas look from different points of view and recognizing that there are often multiple "answers" to complex questions. In small groups or on your own, reflect on possible alternative views or answers and summarize your findings.

1 You recently transcribed a progress report that included an unintelligible phrase. You think the tape says, "O_2 at two liters per nasal cannula," but a front office worker thinks it says, "owing to littering in the nasal canals. . . ." What do you do? What will you record in the patient's medical record?

2 Medical assistants use medical terms in transcribing, charting, and communicating with other staff members. For oral and written communication, think of three examples demonstrating how misuse of medical terms can harm patients.

3 Reread the case study presented in Exercise 2. What is the difference between multiple sclerosis and scoliosis? What skills, in addition to knowledge of medical terminology, would you use as you spoke with the confused and upset mother?

4 The medical team in your office is considering changing from dictation to voice technology. You have been asked to look into this area and list the major products. Research the products and write a memo summarizing their strengths and weaknesses.

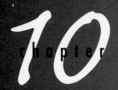
Learning Outcomes

- Use accounting terms correctly and explain the difference between accounting and bookkeeping.
- Identify manual and computer-based methods for recording financial transactions and charges and payments for medical services.
- Prepare checks for payments and bank deposits and reconcile a bank statement.
- List the employee forms and records that must be on file to maintain financial records.

Performance Objectives

- Use correct bookkeeping principles.
- Manage accounts receivable.
- Manage accounts payable.
- Process payroll.
- Document and maintain accounting and banking records.

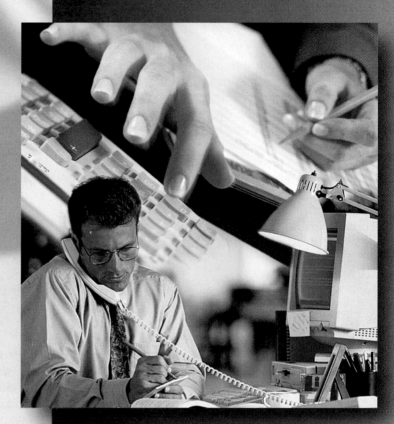

Handling Accounting Responsibilities

The purpose of accounting is to establish, maintain, and apply business data and to express this information in terms of money. A medical practice is a business and, like other businesses, detailed information must be kept concerning every aspect of its operation. All the money the physician earns, all payments for services, and all expenses involved in setting up and maintaining the practice must be entered into the accounting records.

A medical practice must keep complete and accurate records with supporting documents and summaries of business transactions. ***Bookkeeping*** *refers to keeping systematic records of financial transactions. The bookkeeping duties of the medical assistant will depend on the size of the practice. He is usually responsible for processing charges and payments for medical services provided to patients. In a small office, he may also be responsible for banking; paying bills for equipment, supplies, and office maintenance; and calculating the payroll and maintaining payroll records; as well as making appointments, filing insurance claims, and other administrative duties. In a large office,* *these duties are usually divided among several employees supervised by a medical assistant who acts as office manager.*

Patient Concerns

T he accounting responsibilities that directly affect the patient include accurate and efficient processing of charges and payments. When a patient has a question about a bill or a payment or feels that a mistake has been made, the medical assistant should be able to trace the transaction and provide answers. The assistant needs to be tactful and pleasant, and to display a caring attitude when trying to correct an error or clear up a misunderstanding about financial matters. Errors are less likely to occur when the medical assistant is knowledgeable about the procedures and bookkeeping involved.

Basic Accounting Principles

Accounting refers to a system of organizing, maintaining, and auditing business records; summarizing financial transactions; and interpreting the results. The larger the medical practice or organization, the more complicated the accounting process. In most medical practices, an outside specialist, such as a certified public accountant (CPA), develops financial plans, files tax forms, and oversees the accounting process, but it is typically the medical assistant's responsibility to record information and transactions on a daily basis. The assistant must be familiar with basic accounting principles to understand her role in the accounting process and to perform the bookkeeping duties that are essential to that process.

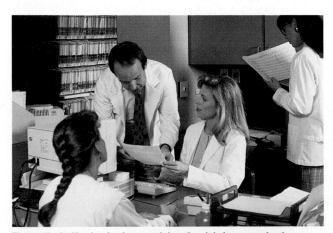

The medical office is a business and therefore it is important for the medical assistant to understand the accounting process and to accurately perform bookkeeping duties.

Record-Keeping

Good records are essential in monitoring the progress of the practice, preparing financial statements, keeping track of deductible expenses, and preparing tax returns. Charges, payments, purchases, payroll, and other transactions generate supporting documents such as invoices, receipts, credit card slips, canceled checks, deposit slips, account statements, and petty cash vouchers. These should be filed and kept in a safe place. Commonly, supporting documents are organized by year and by type of expense or type of income. The length of time that bookkeeping records are kept depends on the type of record and the reason it is kept. Even records that are no longer needed for tax purposes may be required by creditors or insurance companies. Accounting records are kept separate from medical records to preserve patient confidentiality. Additionally, the physician's business accounts are kept separate from his personal accounts for both legal and ethical reasons. Just as patient confidentiality is important, so is avoiding potential conflicts of interest for the physician.

Cash Versus Accrual Accounting

Accounting records may be based on cash or accrual methods. In the **cash method of accounting**, income and expenses are recorded only when they have been received or paid. Most businesses do not operate on a strictly cash basis. Most professional and service businesses, including the medical office, use a **modified cash method of accounting**. As in the traditional cash method of accounting, income is not recorded until cash is actually received and expenses are recorded only when paid. However, in the modified cash method of accounting, adjustments can be made for expenditures with an economic life of more than one year, such as the depreciation of equipment (because it wears out as it is used). The modified cash method also allows adjustments for prepayments of expenses such as insurance premiums and supplies. In the **accrual method of accounting**, income is recorded in the period it is earned, whether or not cash has been received, and expenses are recorded in the period they are incurred, regardless of whether they have been paid. It is mainly used in manufacturing and merchandising firms. The accounting method a medical practice uses will likely be developed by its CPA to clearly show income for the tax year and include a summary of business transactions.

The Accounting Equation

An **asset** refers to anything of value that is owned. Assets in a medical office include cash, money owed by patients (receivables), building and land, equipment, supplies, and office furniture. A **liability** is a debt owed. Liabilities in a medical office might include amounts owed for supplies, equipment and furniture purchased on credit, and a mortgage on equipment or the building. **Owner's equity** is the difference between assets and liabilities; it is the owner's share of the assets. These three terms are used in the **accounting equation**:

$$Assets = Liabilities + Owner's\ Equity$$

The accounting equation expresses the financial condition of a business. Both sides of the equation are always equal. Said another way, the accounting equation states that a business's assets will always equal the sum of its liabilities and owner's equity.

The parts of the accounting equation can be better understood by considering a few transactions. A **transaction** is a financial action or event that changes the amount of the assets, liabilities, or owner's equity. Imagine that you started a business by investing $25,000 of your personal funds. This transaction could be expressed in terms of the accounting equation as follows:

Asset	=	Liabilities	+	Owner's Equity
$25,000				$25,000
(cash)				(your share)

Assets (cash) increased because money came into the business. Owner's equity also increased because the money came from you, the owner. Liabilities did not increase because none of the money was borrowed.

Now, assume you made a $1,000 credit purchase of supplies for use in the office. This transaction affects the equation as follows:

Assets		= Liabilities	+	Owner's Equity
$25,000 +	$1,000 =	$1,000	+	$25,000
(cash)	(supplies)	(debt)		(your share)

Notice that the asset side of the equation is now $26,000, and the liabilities and owner's equity side is also $26,000. Also notice that this transaction did not affect owner's equity (because the business is not worth any more because of a credit purchase).

Now assume that you paid half your debt for supplies. The equation would then read:

Assets		= Liabilities	+	Owner's Equity
$25,000 +	$1,000 =	$1,000	+	$25,000
−500		−500		
$24,500 +	$1,000 =	$ 500	+	$25,000
(cash)	(supplies)	(debt)		(your share)

The left side of the equation now totals $25,500 (or $24,500 + $1,000), and the liabilities and owner's equity side also totals $25,500. The totals on both sides are always equal.

For one additional example, assume that you provided services to a patient and received $300 cash. The equation would read:

Assets		= Liabilities	+	Owner's Equity
$25,000 +	$1,000 =	$1,000	+	$25,000
−500		−500		
$24,500 +	$1,000 =	$ 500	+	$25,000
+300				+300
$24,800 +	$1,000 =	$ 500	+	$25,300
(cash)	(supplies)	(debt)		(your share)

In this transaction, cash (the asset side) increased by $300 while the owner's equity also increased by $300. Income increases the equity of the business.

A **balance sheet** is a statement of the financial condition of a business on a given date. Because assets, liabilities, and owner's equity are constantly changing, it "freezes" a moment in time and shows how the three elements of the accounting equation are balanced on a particular day. An example is shown in Figure 10.1.

Organizing the Transactions

An **account** is a record of financial transactions. Separate accounts are set up to record revenue (money coming in) and expenses (money going out), as well as transactions that are related to each asset or liability and each aspect of owner's equity. In the medical office, different accounts must be set up to handle patient charges and receipts (revenue) and employee salaries, payroll taxes, utilities, insurance, supplies and equipment, and office maintenance (expenses). Accounts may be added or deleted as needed. Each account is assigned a number, and all financial transactions are recorded in the appropriate account. Each category (revenue, expenses, etc.) is assigned a range of numbers, rather than a single number, so that new accounts can be added when needed.

A **chart of accounts** is a detailed listing of all of the business's accounts. These are usually listed in order of assets, liabilities, capital (owner's equity), revenue, and expenses. Organizing the financial recording by categories of accounts facilitates tracking of specific types of financial information. For instance, if you wanted to compare the cost of utilities this year with their cost last year, it would be a simple matter of looking at the utilities expense account. However, if utility expenses were mixed in with other expenses, such as supplies and equipment, it would take a considerable amount of time to go through the list and pick out the utility items. An example of a chart of accounts is shown in Table 10.1.

In accounting, **debit** refers to a transaction that increases assets and decreases liabilities, while **credit** refers to a transaction that decreases assets and

Figure 10.1
Balance Sheet

HEALTHY FAMILY PRACTICE
Balance Sheet

December 31, 20XX

Assets		Liabilities and Owner's Equity	
Cash	$47,000	Liabilities:	
Accounts Receivable	12,000	Accounts Payable	$82,050
Real Estate	215,000	Taxes Payable	18,100
Equipment & Supplies	250,000	Mortgage	107,000
Furnishings	21,050	Total Liabilities	$207,150
		Owner's Equity:	
		D. L. Jones	180,000
		J. A. Smith	157,900
		Total Owner's Equity	$337,900
	$545,050		$545,050

Table 10.1 Chart of Accounts

Assets (100–199)	Owner's Equity (300–399)
111 Cash	311 Dr. Smith, Capital
112 Accounts Receivable	312 Dr. Smith, Drawing
113 Office Supplies	
116 Office Equipment	Revenue (400–499)
117 Office Furniture	411 Service Revenue
Liabilities (200–299)	Expenses (500–599)
211 Accounts Payable	511 Rent
	512 Repairs

increases liabilities. The standard form of account is illustrated in Figure 10.2. A **T-account** is the skeleton version of the standard account form. Debits are entered on the left side, and credits are entered on the right. A helpful hint to remember when working with individual patient accounts in the medical office is that a debit is a charge and a credit is a payment. Debits

and credits are noted on the standard account form (Figure 10.2).

The **general ledger** is a collective record of all of the practice's accounts. It includes all the accounts in the chart of accounts, and contains the totals from all the journals. A **journal** is a sheet or book where all transactions are recorded in chronological order as they occur. Entries are then posted to the appropriate account in the general ledger. Journals used in a medical office include the **daily journal** (also called the **day sheet**, **daily log**, or **daily record**), which is a cumulative listing of all patient-related financial transactions recorded on a daily basis, and a check disbursement journal.

A **trial balance** is a listing of the balances of all accounts in the ledger, as of a specific date, to check the equality of debits and credits. A trial balance is usually prepared at the end of the month. It is also used in the medical office to total debits and credits on the day sheet to check for discrepancies.

Figure 10.2
Standard Account Form

(a) Account title and number. (b) Debits are listed on the left side. (c) Credits are listed on the right side.

Source: Adapted with permission from *Paradigm College Accounting, Fourth Edition*, by Dansby, Kaliski, and Lawrence. © Paradigm Publishing Inc.

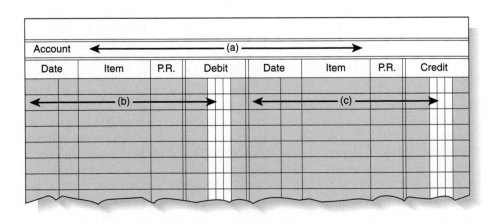

Step 1   Analyze transactions from source documents.

Source Documents

Any business paper that shows a business transaction has taken place. Examples include bills, receipts, and invoices.

Step 2   Record transactions in a journal.

Journal

A record in which both the debit and credit parts of an entry are recorded together in chronological order (data order).

Step 3   Post from the journal to the ledger.

Ledger

A record that summarizes data into individual accounts.

Step 4   Prepare a trial balance of the ledger.

Trial Balance

A report showing that debit balances in the ledger equal credit balances.

Figure 10.3
The First Four Steps in the Accounting Cycle

The medical assistant who handles accounting responsibilities will most likely handle the first two or three steps.

Source: Adapted with permission from *Paradigm College Accounting, Fourth Edition,* by Dansby, Kaliski, and Lawrence. © Paradigm Publishing Inc.

The Accounting Cycle

The **accounting cycle** refers to the steps involved in recording, processing, and summarizing financial transactions. Figure 10.3 shows the first four steps in the accounting cycle. The medical assistant would be responsible for the first two, and may be responsible for the third (**posting** transactions from the journal to the ledger). An accountant would most likely do the fourth step.

Analyzing Transactions from Source Documents

Every financial transaction entered into the system must originate with a document that contains the facts of the transaction. These are called **source documents**. For patient accounts, they might include charge slips, receipts for cash, credit card receipts, the doctor's record of her services to a patient in the hospital, personal checks received from patients, and payment checks from insurance companies.

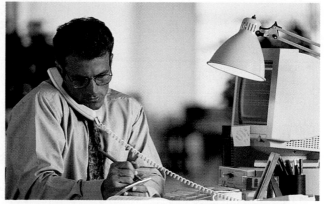

Many medical offices will hire a CPA to manage the accounting books, but the medical assistant will need to record the financial transactions on a daily basis.

When a patient comes in for an office visit, a charge slip (sometimes called a superbill or an encounter form) is attached to his chart. Most practices use forms printed specifically for the practice listing the services and procedures that are performed, along with procedure codes. (See Chapter 12, "Processing Insurance Claims," for detailed information on coding.) There may be space to record the next appointment date, balance remaining on the patient's account, and payments. These forms are designed to produce duplicate copies when filled out.

Before attaching the form to the chart, the medical assistant fills in the date, patient's name, and other information at the top of the form. When the doctor sees the patient, he checks the items on the form that apply to that patient, then gives the form to the patient to return to the reception desk. The medical assistant who handles the bookkeeping fills in the charges, accepts payment or processes the charge for billing to an insurance company and the patient, and gives the patient a copy. The form serves as a receipt as well as a bill. Figure 10.4 shows an example of a charge slip used by a family practice.

Recording Transactions in a Journal: Day Sheet

In most medical offices, all financial transactions involving patient accounts are listed in ink on the day sheet (daily journal) in the order in which they occur. A new day sheet is started each morning. The current date is written at the top of the sheet, along with the page number since there may be more transactions than can be recorded on one page. Each page should also have a space for the total number of pages used for the day. For example: Page _____ of _____. This prevents pages from being omitted.

The day sheet itself will vary from one office to another, depending on the bookkeeping system used, but all will provide space for recording the patient's

Healthy Family Practice
100 Oak Street, Shore City, VA 12312
(555) 123-1234

FAX (555) 456-7890   TAX ID # 00-0000000

PATIENT   ACCT. NUMBER   DATE OF SERVICE

GUARANTOR NAME AND ADDRESS

PRIMARY INSURANCE   CERTIFICATE NUMBER

SECONDARY INSURANCE   CERTIFICATE NUMBER

PHYSICIAN: [ ] D. I. Jones, MD   [ ] J. A. Smith, MD

✓	CPT	OFFICE VISIT	FEE
		OFFICE VISIT - NO CHARGE	
	99201	OV NEW - 1	
	99202	OV NEW - 2	
	99203	OV NEW - 3	
	99204	OV NEW - 4	
	99205	OV NEW - 5	
	99211	OV EST - 1	
	99212	OV EST - 2	
	99213	OV EST - 3	
	99214	OV EST - 4	
	99215	OV EST - 5	
		WELL VISIT	
	99381	OV WELL - NEW (AGE <1)	
	99382	OV WELL - NEW (AGE 1-4)	
	99383	OV WELL - NEW (AGE 5-11)	
	99384	OV WELL - NEW (AGE 12-17)	
	99385	OV WELL - NEW (AGE 18-39)	
	99386	OV WELL - NEW (AGE 40-64)	
	99387	OV WELL - NEW (AGE 65 AND OVER)	
	99391	OV WELL - EST (AGE <1)	
	99392	OV WELL - EST (AGE 1-4)	
	99393	OV WELL - EST (AGE 5-11)	
	99394	OV WELL - EST (AGE 12-17)	
	99395	OV WELL - EST (AGE 18-39)	
	99396	OV WELL - EST (AGE 40-64)	
	99397	OV WELL - EST (AGE 65 AND OVER)	
		ALLERGY	
	95115	ALLERGY Single	
	95117	ALLERGY Multiple	
		IMMUNIZATIONS	
	86580	PPD	
	86585	TINE	
	90701	DPT	
	90718	DT (AD)	
	90724	FLU	
	90731	HEP B	
	90737	HIB	
	90707	MMR	
	90712	OPV	
	90732	PNEUMVX	
		CHEMISTRY	
	84460	ALT (SGPT)	
	82040	Albumin	
	84450	AST (SGOT)	
	82250	Bili - Dir or Tot	
	82251	Bili - Dir & Tot	
	84520	BUN	
	82310	Calcium	
	82374	CO2	
	82435	Chloride	
	82465	Cholesterol	
	82550	CPK	
	82565	Creatinine	
	82977	GGT	
	82947	Glucose	
	83615	LDH	
	84075	Phos. Alk.	
	84100	Phos.	
	84132	Potassium	
	84155	Protein Total	
	84295	Sodium	
	84478	Triglycerides	
	84550	Uric Acid	
	80051	Electrolytes Panel	
	80061	Lipid Panel	

✓	CPT	CHEMISTRY	FEE
	80058	Hepatic Panel	
	80049	Metabolic Panel, Basic	
	80054	Metabolic Panel, Comp.	
		LABORATORY	
	84520	ANA	
	87070	Bacterial Culture	
	85025	CBC/Automated Diff	
	85024	CBC/partial auto Diff	
	83001	FSH	
	82948	Glucose, Reagent Strip	
	87205	Gram Stain	
	83718	HDL	
	82270	Hemocult	
	85018	HGB	
	85014	HCT	
	83036	Hgb A1C	
	86677	H. Pylori (Qual.)	
	87220	KOH	
	84447	Mono Strep ID	
	87177	OVA/ Parasites	
	88156	PAP	
	84703	Pregnancy, Serum	
	81025	Pregnancy, Urine	
	85610	Prothrombin time	
	84153	PSA	
	86430	RA	
	85651	Sed Rate	
	84436	T4	
	84443	TSH	
	81000	Urinalysis, Complete	
	81002	Urinalysis, Reagent Strip	
	87086	Urine Culture	
	36415	Venipuncture	
		DIGESTIVE	
	45330	Sigmoidoscopy, Flexible	
	45331	Sigmoidoscopy, Flexible w/Bx	
	46600	Anoscopy	
		EYES, EARS	
	65205	Foreign Body from Eye	
	69200	Foreign Body from Ear	
	65220	Foreign Body from Cornea	
	69210	Ear Wax Removal	
		GENITOURINARY	
	53670	Catheterization	
	57454	Culpo	
	57511	Cryocautery	
	57505	Endocervical Curett	
	58100	Endometrial Asp	
	56420	I & D Bartholin Abscess	
	53660	Urethral Dilatation	

✓	CPT	MUSCULOSKELETAL	FEE
	20550	Inj/Asp Trigger Point	
	20550	Inj/Asp Toes, Fingers, G-Cyst	
	20605	Inj/Asp Wrist, Elbow, Olecr, Ankle	
	20610	Inj/Asp Shoulder, Knee, Subacromial	
		FRACTURE SITE:	
		RADIOLOGY	
	73610	Ankle	
	71010	Chest PA	
	71020	Chest PA ? LAT	
	72040	C-Spine	
	72052	CS w/OBL	
	73080	Elbow/OBL	
	73140	Finger	
	73630	Foot 3 V	
	73130	Hand 3 V	
	73560	Knee	
	72100	L-Spine	
	72110	LS w/OBL	
	73030	Shoulder 3 V	
	70220	Sinus CMP	
	73660	Toes	
	73110	Wrist	
		SURGERY, BX, BURNS	
	11100	BX 1 Lesion	
	11101	BX Each Additional Lesion	
	16000	Burn, Initial 1st Degree	
		Excision: MAL. BENIGN SHAV	
	17000	Des Ben/Pre Malig Lesion 1st	
	17003	Des Ben/Pre Malig Lesion 2-14	
	17004	Des Ben/Pre Malig Lesions 15 or more	
	17110	Des Wart/Molluscum < 15	
	17111	Des Wart/Molluscum 15 or more	
	46320	Enucleation Thrombosed Hemorrhoid	
	10060	I & D Abscess	
	10061	I & D Abscess Compl	
	10080	I & D Pilonidal Cyst	
	10120	Incision, Removal Foreign Body	
	11200	Skin Tags < 15	
		PROCEDURES	
	93000	EKG & Report	
	94010	Spirometry	
	94060	Bronchospasm Eval	
	94664	Aerosol Treatment	
		MISCELLANEOUS	

DIAGNOSIS

1. _____
2. _____
3. _____
4. _____

ACCOUNT INFORMATION

Previous Balance: _____

Today's Charge: _____

Today's Payment: _____

NEW BALANCE: _____

NEXT APPOINTMENT: _____ Days _____ Weeks _____ Months DATE: _____

Figure 10.4
Patient Charge Slip

Source: Codes from CPT2000, courtesy of the American Medical Association.

name, the services provided, charges, and payments. Various source documents provide this information. Charges for service provided after the office closed the previous day (hospital visits, surgery, emergencies) should be listed along with each transaction that day. When the patient returns the charge slip to the reception desk at the end of the appointment, the bookkeeper transfers the information to the day sheet.

All checks or cash payments are recorded. Any adjustments made to a patient's account must be listed (discounts, write-offs, etc.). Even if there is no charge for the visit, the patient's name must still be listed on the sheet, along with the purpose of the visit, and "NC" (no charge) written in the charges column. When checks are received by mail, the amount and source is recorded on the day sheet and credited to the appropriate patient account. Often, checks from insurance companies include payment for more than one patient. When recording this transaction, each patient for whom payment was received, along with the amount the insurance company paid, should be listed separately.

At the end of the day, all charges and receipts are totaled and the sums recorded in the proof-of-posting box on the bottom of the sheet. By following the directions for calculating the amounts in the box, errors can be discovered and corrected. A current record of accounts receivable can be obtained by filling in the information in the accounts receivable box and calculating the total. Cash receipts can be controlled by keeping a daily record on the bottom of the sheet. The daily totals are recorded on a monthly summary sheet. In offices that use computerized systems, the day sheet is generated by computer at the end of the day. Figure 10.5 shows an example of a day sheet.

Post from the Journal to the Ledger: Patient Ledger Cards

A **ledger card** is a record of the amount each patient owes for services rendered. It provides a history of the

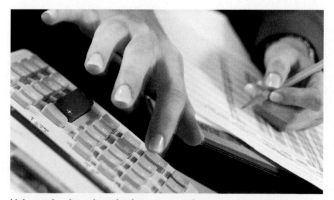

Make entries throughout the day as transactions occur to ensure accurate record keeping. At the end of the day, double-check your totals and reconcile any differences.

financial transactions for individual patient accounts. Ledger cards are kept in a separate file, not in the patient's medical record. Some offices use one card for a whole family rather than one for each member. The back of each patient ledger card lists the patient's or head-of-family's full name, address, telephone number, place of employment, and information about insurance coverage. Each charge, payment, and adjustment must be recorded on the front of the ledger card. This may be done when the transaction is recorded on the day sheet or as time permits during the day by referring to the day sheet listings. Ideally, the charge for each procedure should be shown, and the services and sources of payment should be described.

The current balance is always displayed at the bottom of the column on the right. Some offices send a photocopy of the ledger card as the monthly bill. This will be explained in more detail in Chapter 11, "Billing and Collecting Payments." In offices that use computerized systems, patient ledgers can be generated to meet selected criteria. For example, the medical assistant could print ledgers for all accounts that have a balance due.

Integrated Systems

Write-it-once (pegboard) bookkeeping is a system that is particularly well-suited to the medical office. Information is written only once to be recorded on several forms simultaneously, rather than being written in several separate records. It is used for accounts receivable and accounts payable. The method consists of a flexible writing surface with pegs along one side and forms with holes that will fit on the pegs to keep them properly aligned.

A day sheet is placed on the writing surface, and the patient's ledger, doctor's statement of services (superbill), and receipt forms are placed in the proper positions on top of it. As information is recorded on the top form, carbon copies appear on the forms underneath. One line on the day sheet is used for each transaction, with the day sheet providing columns for the date, patient's name, description of services rendered, charges, payments, adjustments, and current balance.

Other columns may be used to record data for use in business analysis summaries. The day sheet also includes a list of checks and cash to be deposited in the bank. Totals at the end of the day are recorded in the proof of posting, accounts receivable control, and accounts receivable proof boxes located at the bottom of the sheet. By following the directions for calculating the amounts in each box, errors can be discovered and corrected.

Summary Reports

As discussed previously, all transactions are recorded on a daily basis on the day sheet and patient ledger

Day Sheet Date _____ May 25, 20XX _____ Page ___1___ of ___1___

	Receipt No.	Name	Service	Charge	Payments Cash	Payments Checks	Adjust.	Current Balance.	Previous Balance.	Account No.
1	0110	Johnson, Sheneka	OV⁵⁵ Inj¹⁸	73.00	20.00			93.00	40.00	0245
2		Harmon, Jesse	CIGNA Ins.			123.00		27.00	150.00	1462
3		Smith, Howard	CIGNA Ins.			90.00		119.00	209.00	0947
4	0111	Yi, Choon	OV⁵⁵ Smear²⁵	80.00				80.00	—	0116
5	0112	Curtis, Phyllis	Post Op	NC	50.00			490.00	540.00	2345
6	0113	Clayton, Helen	Recheck Cast	25.00		48.00		25.00	48.00	1809
7		Sellars, Vivian	Medicare			110.00	20.00	—	130.00	1432
8	0114	Rodriguez, James	Biopsy	78.00				132.00	54.00	0765
9		Edwards, Janice	Hosp. Care	345.00				345.00	—	2081
10		Pitrer, Edna	Aetna Ins			260.00		430.00	690.00	7621
11		O'Malley, Peggy	ROA			120.00		85.00	205.00	0399
12	0115	Otero, Juan	Physical X	110.00		110.00		—	—	2418
13	0116	Dietrich, George	Flu inj	18.00				78.00	60.00	4111
14		Whitley, Charles	ROA			50.00		210.00	260.00	8041
15		Mackel, Jean	ROA			84.00		—	84.00	2121
16	0117	Goodman, Bryan	OV	55.00		20.00		35.00	—	0333
17	0118	Ashford, Brandon	OV⁵⁵ Lab³⁵	90.00				190.00	100.00	3000
18	0119	Duron, Stanley	OV⁵⁵ EKG⁵⁰	105.00		50.00		105.00	50.00	4186
19		Mitchell, Robert	Medicare			42.00	14.00	65.00	121.00	6514
20										
21										
22										
23										
24										
25										
26										
27										
28										
29										
30										
	Totals			Column A 979.00	Column B 70.00	Column C 1,107.00	Column D 34.00	Column E 2,509.00	Column F 2,741.00	

Proof of Posting

Column F Total	$ 2,741.00
Plus Column A Total	979.00
Minus Column B Total	70.00
Minus Column C Total	1,107.00
Minus Column D Total	34.00
Total	$ 2,509.00
	(Must equal Column E Total)

Accounts Receivable

Previous Balance	$ 2,080.00
Plus Column A Total	$ 979.00
Minus Column B Total	$ 70.00
Minus Column C Total	$ 1,107.00
Minus Column D Total	$ 34.00
Total Accounts Receivable	$ 1,848.00

Cash Control

Beginning Cash on Hand	$ 20.00
Plus Column B Total	$ 70.00
Minus Bank Deposit	$ 90.00
Closing Cash on Hand	$ —

Figure 10.5
Completed Day Sheet

cards, but the totals must be transferred to a monthly summary sheet. Information from the monthly sheets would be used to produce a yearly summary. A summary report is exactly what the name implies. It summarizes all the transactions during a specified period. Specific types of services may be targeted, so that total income and expenses associated with those services can be analyzed. If several physicians are associated in the practice, a summary report could provide a record of the revenue brought in by each one.

Bookkeeping Systems

There are several ways of recording the transactions that form the basis of the accounting process. These include manual procedures as well as computer programs that are designed for a specific type of business, such as a medical practice.

Double-Entry Bookkeeping

Double-entry bookkeeping is a system in which each transaction is recorded in at least two accounts. As we explained before, the accounting equation must remain in balance. To help with this task, accounts are grouped so that the total of all asset accounts can be confirmed to equal the combined total of the liability and owner's equity accounts. When you pay a debt, your liability decreases, but so does the cash account. For instance, if a check is written to pay a $360 utility bill, the cash account (asset) would decrease by $360. To balance this decrease, the accounts payable account (liability) would also decrease $360. One advantage of this type of bookkeeping is that errors are easily detected because a difference in the totals on the two sides of the equation indicates that a mistake was made. The disadvantage of double-entry bookkeeping is its complexity. This type of bookkeeping is not often done by the medical assistant, since it requires more accounting skills than he usually possesses.

Single-Entry Bookkeeping

Single-entry bookkeeping is a fairly simple method in which a transaction is recorded in only one account. In most healthcare offices, the medical assistant keeps records using a single-entry accounting system and the accountant transfers the information into a double-entry system. In a medical office where this type of bookkeeping is used, all transactions would be listed in a daily journal (day sheet) in the order in which they occur, and would then be copied onto ledger cards or other individual patient account records such as Figure 10.6.

Computerized Accounting Systems

Computerized accounting systems are widely used in medical offices to manage accounting and bookkeeping records as well as other administrative tasks such as recording patient information, scheduling appointments, and filing insurance claims. A number of computer programs are available written especially for use in the med-

Working Smart

No matter what system is used, any error must be found and corrected!

HEALTHY FAMILY PRACTICE
100 Oak Street
Shore City, VA 12312
(555) 123-1234

Name _____

Date	Family Member	Description of Services	Charge	Payment/ Adjustment	Current Balance

PLEASE PAY LAST BALANCE IN THIS COLUMN ▲

SERVICE CODES:		PAYMENT CODES:	
OV - Office Visit	ER - Emergency Room	C - Cash	CR - Credit
OS - Office Surgery	LAB - Laboratory	CK - Check	NC - No Charge
HC - Hospital Care	M - Medication	INS Insurance	ADJ - Adjustment
HV - Home Visit	BI - Biopsy	ROA - Received on Account	
INJ - Injection	TR - Treatment		
EKG - Electrocardiogram	X - X-Ray		

Figure 10.6
Patient Ledger Card

ical office setting. Although each one is different, all use a database consisting of information about patients, healthcare providers, insurance, diagnosis codes, procedure codes, and financial transactions. While the medical assistant is responsible for entering information in the databases, the computer software lets the assistant sort through the information in the database to generate the patients' billing statements, aging accounts reports (see Chapter 11, "Billing and Collecting Payments,"), and other business summary data electronically rather than manually. Computers save time and space, and reduce the chance of error, since information is entered only once. However, it is essential that the data be entered correctly and in the proper format. Follow the software manual's directions.

Accounts Receivable and Payable

Accounts receivable consist of money that has been earned but not yet received by the practice. Patient accounts are the primary example. These are recorded as assets as shown on the balance sheet. **Accounts payable** are debts owed to other businesses or individuals for goods and services. These are recorded as liabilities as shown on the balance sheet. Summary reports of accounts receivable and accounts payable are usually prepared monthly and at the end of each year.

Patient Accounts

Many medical offices require patients to pay their bills at the time of service. However, even though this may be office policy, there are always exceptions when payment cannot be collected immediately. Insurance companies must have time to process claims and pay their share of the bill. As discussed previously, the day sheet serves as a record of all transactions affecting patient accounts. To determine the amount of accounts receivable, add the unpaid balance on each patient ledger card (the last amount in the "Balance" column). The total represents the accounts receivable. Monthly statements (bills) are sent to all patients whose accounts show an unpaid balance.

Procedure 10.1 lists the steps to follow when managing charges and payments for medical services, or accounts receivable.

Practice Maintenance Accounts

Many expenses are involved in operating a medical practice, and these business expenses are usually kept

Technology Tip

Use the Internet to obtain information about medical practice management software. Many software companies offer free demonstrations which you can download to try in your office without financial obligation. The websites listed below offer product and cost information, updates, and free demonstrations. To locate others, do a web search for "medical billing software."

Medisoft:
www.medicalbillingsoftware.com/billing-software.html

CliniMed:
www.clinimed.com/body/intro.html

Medical Manager: www.medman.net/

MEDiCAT: www.nuesoft.com

Lytec Medical:
www.productsoftware.com

American Medical:
www.americanmedical.com/index.html

Procedure 10.1

Handling Accounts Receivable

Purpose: To set up and manage bookkeeping records for charges and payments for medical services.

Equipment/Supplies: Day sheet, patient ledger cards, source documents for payments and charges, pen.

1 Start a new day sheet at the beginning of the day by writing the date at the top of the sheet. Number the page and add pages when needed.

2 Place a charge slip on each patient's chart before he sees the physician.

3 Prepare a ledger card for each patient who does not already have one. Include the name, address, and telephone number of the responsible party, place of employment, and insurance information. *All information needed for billing should be handy without referring to the patient's medical record.*

4 After the patient sees the physician, record each charge and payment, along with the patient's name,

in the appropriate columns on the sheet in the order in which it occurs, using one line.

5 Give a copy of the charge slip or receipt to the patient, and retain a copy for your files. *These are source documents for the transactions, and a copy must be kept to support the entry in your books.*

6 Record each charge and payment on the patient's ledger card. Calculate the new balance.

7 At the end of the day, add the totals of all charges and all payments.

8 Enter the totals in the appropriate boxes at the bottom of the day sheet, and make the needed calculations.

9 Post the daily totals to the monthly summary sheet.

10 Deposit cash and checks in the bank daily or in accordance with office policy. *Money received that is kept in the office may be lost through fire or burglary.*

11 Record the amount of your bank deposit in the checkbook, and keep a copy of the deposit slip for the office files.

Procedure 10.2

Handling Accounts Payable

Purpose: To manage disbursement records.

Equipment/Supplies: Business checkbook, check register, source documents for disbursements, pen.

1 Inspect invoices and bills as they are received to make sure they are correct, and confirm that the product or service has actually been received. *Partial shipments of supplies may have been sent; some items may be on back order.*
2 Calculate any discounts.
3 Place the invoices temporarily in an accounts payable file.
4 Pay bills by the date indicated on the invoice. *Some suppliers may offer a discount for payment within 10 days;*

others may charge a penalty if the bill is not paid within 30 days.

5 List each check on a check register (also called a check disbursement journal or record of disbursements). In some offices, the checkbook stubs may serve as the record of disbursements. Include the check number, name of payee, amount of the check, date, and what item or service was purchased.
6 Subtract the amount of each check from the previous balance in the checkbook, and write down the new balance.
7 Keep a copy of each invoice or bill for your files, and write on it the date it was paid and the check number. *These are supporting documents, and a copy must be kept to support the entry made in your books.*

---

separate from the physician's personal finances. The medical assistant may be responsible for paying bills for supplies, utilities, and other expenses of running the office. Bills should be paid on a weekly basis, since some vendors offer discounts for prompt payment and others add charges when payment is overdue. An invoice that reads "2/10,n/30" means that a 2% discount can be subtracted from the price if payment is made within 10 days. Otherwise, the total invoice price must be paid within 30 days. All expenditures must be listed in chronological order in the record of disbursements. This record, also called the check register, should have space for recording the date, the name of the person or business to whom payment was made, the amount of the check, and the reason for the payment. Remember that you cannot sign checks unless you are authorized to do so and have a signature card on file with the bank for that account. Procedure 10.2 provides the steps to follow when paying bills.

Working Smart

Prompt payment can sometimes result in cost savings for the medical office. However, late payment will result in late payment fees. Always pay bills promptly.

Payroll

Preparing the payroll, keeping the necessary records, and distributing monies withheld for various government agencies can be a complicated process. For this reason, many physicians have it done by someone with an accounting background or experience. However, the medical assistant may be responsible for managing the payroll, which requires keeping time sheets on employees' hours worked, making out the payroll checks after withholding taxes and deductions, and submitting taxes to governmental units.

Employee Earnings

Employees may be paid **wages** or **salaries**. Salaried employees are paid a specific amount of money per pay period, regardless of the number of hours they work, while those who earn wages are paid on an hourly basis. An hourly minimum wage is set by the federal Fair Labor Standards Act and may change according to federal regulations. A record must be kept of the number of hours worked by each employee paid on an hourly basis and for some salaried employees. Compensation for working overtime (more than 40 hours per week) and on holidays is paid according to federal regulations. **Gross pay** is the amount earned before taxes, Social Security, and other deductions are made. **Net pay** is the amount of the paycheck. The **payroll** refers to the total paid to all employees for a pay period.

Consistent and accurate payroll data must be kept on every employee. Figure 10.7 shows an employee payroll sheet for recording the total wages and deductions withheld, including Social Security, Medicare, unemployment compensation, and federal and state

Name											Social Security Number					

Position _____ Address _____ Number of Exemptions _____ Year _____

HOURS							TOTAL HOURS		RATE		EARNINGS		TOTAL WAGES	Paid by Check No.	DEDUCTIONS				
SUN.	MON.	TUE.	WED.	THU.	FRI.	SAT.	Reg.	O.T.	Reg.	O.T.	Regular	Overtime			Social Security	Medicare	U.S. With. Tax	State With. Tax	Other
First QTR																			

Fourth QTR																			
TOTAL - YEAR																			

Figure 10.7
Employee Payroll Sheet

taxes. The net pay is paid to the employee by check or through an automatic deposit plan in which the money is sent directly to the employee's bank account. Payroll checks may be issued weekly, every two weeks, or monthly. Tables provided by the Internal Revenue Service (IRS) and state revenue departments show how much money must be withheld for federal and state taxes in various pay periods.

Taxes

Once an employee's gross pay for a period has been determined, deductions for federal, state, and sometimes local taxes must be withheld before a paycheck can be issued. This tax money must be remitted periodically to the appropriate government agency. Contributions to retirement plans and deductions for other reasons also may be withheld. A statement of all deductions must be given to the employee with the paycheck.

FEDERAL WITHHOLDING TAXES
The amount of money withheld from each paycheck is based on information the employee provides on Form W-4, shown in Figure 10.8. This form requires the employee's name and address, social security number, marital status, and number of dependents

Technology Tip
Visit www.taxsites.com/state.html for information on each state's tax laws and minimum wage, and links to each state's website.

(family members who depend on the employee for financial support).

Circular E, Employer's Tax Guide, has tables showing how much tax must be withheld from the employee's paycheck for federal income tax, based on the pay period and the employee's marital status. For example, a page from the Guide for 2000, shown in Figure 10.9, shows that $105 must be withheld from each check of a single employee who has one deduction and is paid $900 every two weeks.

SOCIAL SECURITY AND MEDICARE TAXES The employer also is required to withhold taxes for Social Security and Medicare. The Social Security tax is based on the **Federal Insurance Contributions Act (FICA)**. The base changes each January. For 2000, the rate was 6.2% on income up to $76,200. All wages also are subject to a 1.45% deduction for Medicare. This means that if your salary is $30,000 per year, you will have $1,860 withheld for Social Security and $435 for Medicare.

STATE WITHHOLDING TAXES
Employee wages are taxed in all states except Alaska, Florida, Nevada, New Hampshire, South Dakota, Tennessee, Texas, Washington, and Wyoming. The other forty-one states require

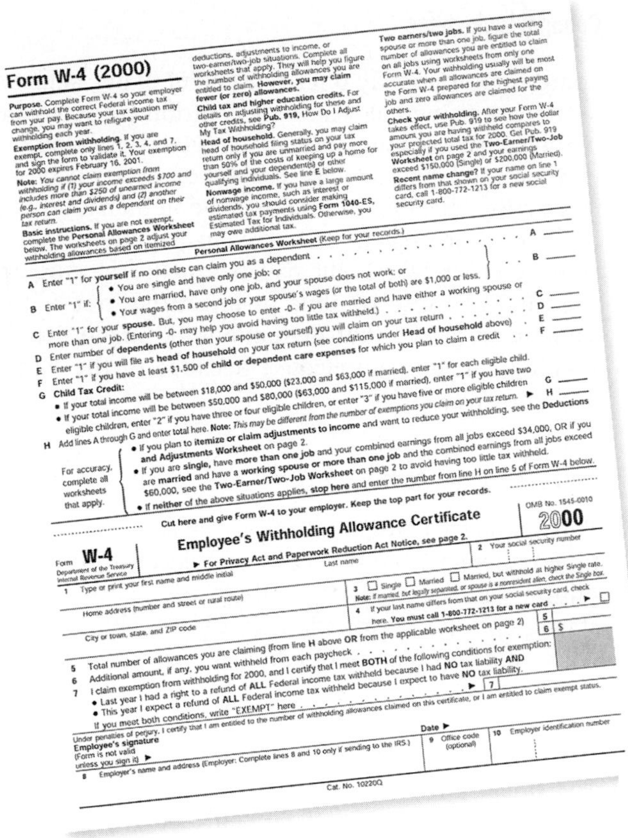

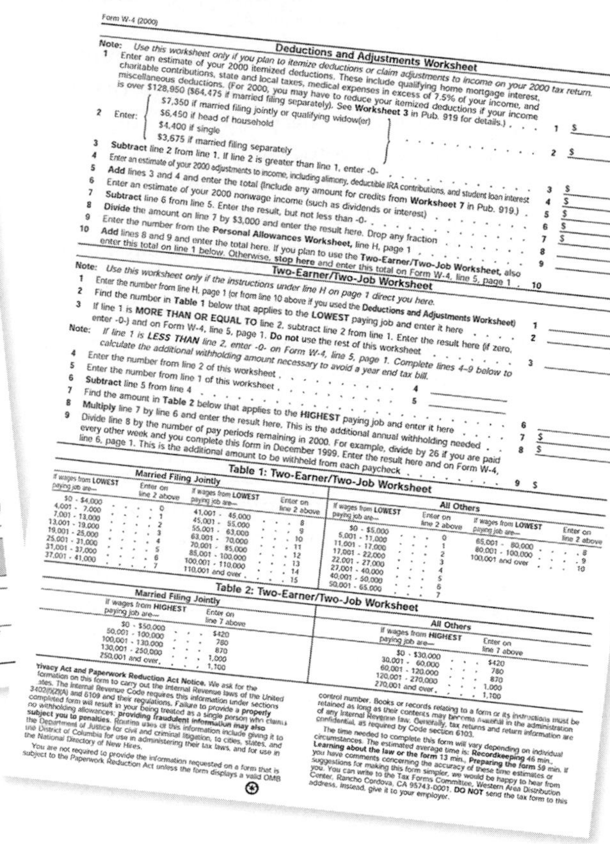

Figure 10.8
Withholding Form W-4

SINGLE Persons—BIWEEKLY Payroll Period
(For Wages Paid in 2000)

If the wages are—		And the number of withholding allowances claimed is—										
At least	But less than	0	1	2	3	4	5	6	7	8	9	10
		The amount of income tax to be withheld is—										
$800	$820	106	90	74	58	42	25	9	0	0	0	0
820	840	109	93	77	61	45	28	12	0	0	0	0
840	860	112	96	80	64	48	31	15	0	0	0	0
860	880	115	99	83	67	51	34	18	2	0	0	0
880	900	118	102	86	70	54	37	21	5	0	0	0
900	920	121	105	89	73	57	40	24	8	0	0	0
920	940	124	108	92	76	60	43	27	11	0	0	0
940	960	127	111	95	79	63	46	30	14	0	0	0
960	980	130	114	98	82	66	49	33	17	1	0	0
980	1,000	133	117	101	85	69	52	36	20	4	0	0
1,000	1,020	136	120	104	88	72	55	39	23	7	0	0
1,020	1,040	139	123	107	91	75	58	42	26	10	0	0
1,040	1,060	142	126	110	94	78	61	45	29	13	0	0
1,060	1,080	145	129	113	97	81	64	48	32	16	0	0
1,080	1,100	151	132	116	100	84	67	51	35	19	3	0
1,100	1,120	156	135	119	103	87	70	54	38	22	6	0
1,120	1,140	162	138	122	106	90	73	57	41	25	9	0
1,140	1,160	167	141	125	109	93	76	60	44	28	12	0
1,160	1,180	173	144	128	112	96	79	63	47	31	15	0
1,180	1,200	179	149	131	115	99	82	66	50	34	18	2

Figure 10.9
Withholding Table from Employer's Tax Guide

employers to withhold payments from their employees' paychecks. State departments of revenue issue booklets showing how to calculate the amounts to be withheld.

UNEMPLOYMENT TAXES Federal unemployment taxes, based on the **Federal Unemployment Tax Act (FUTA)**, are paid entirely by the employer. The FUTA tax, along with state unemployment taxes, provides unemployment payments to workers who lose their jobs. The FUTA tax for 2000 was 6.2% of the first $7,000 in wages. The FUTA tax is calculated each quarter and generally must be deposited on or before the last day of the first month after the quarter ends. An annual FUTA Form 940, shown in Figure 10.10, must be filed on or before January 31 of the year after the one for which the tax is due. If the employer is paying into a state unemployment fund, this amount may be subtracted from the federal FUTA tax.

Laws governing state unemployment tax vary among states. Some require that both employer and employee pay; however, in most states, the employer alone is responsible. Specific information should be obtained from the state employment commission, which has offices in many localities. Look in your local telephone directory for a number to call for details on unemployment tax.

Optional Deductions

Some employers may offer retirement plans, such as a 401K, to which employees may contribute a percentage of their salary before taxes are deducted. An employee may elect to have a certain amount of money deposited in a savings account or a savings bond plan after taxes have been deducted. Certain loan payments may be deducted from take-home pay. Normally, the employee can change these options at any time, but a court sometimes orders that deductions be made. Record-keeping can be complicated because of the various accounts involved.

Worker's Compensation

The employer is required to pay insurance premiums to compensate employees who suffer job-related injuries, illness, or death. Regulations vary among states. Specific information should be obtained from your state department of labor.

Depositing Withholding Taxes

The office practice will need two bank accounts for depositing the money withheld from employee paychecks.

Figure 10.10
FUTA Tax Form 940

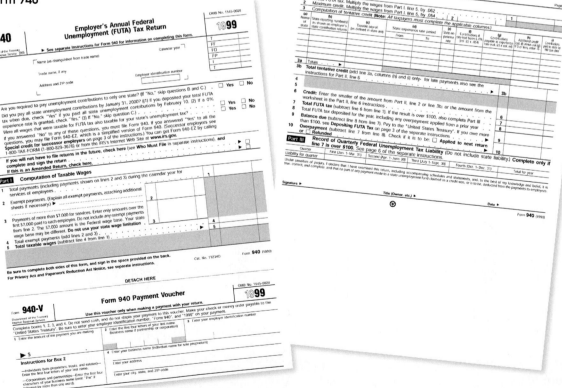

Technology Tip

Many tax forms can be downloaded and printed through the Internet. Forms I-9, W-4, SS-4, 940, and 941 are among hundreds that can be obtained this way. Other forms, such as the W-2 and W-3 that have multiple copies or are "machine readable," must be printed with special paper and inks and are not available from a website. However, these can be viewed for informational purposes, and the actual forms to file can be obtained from the IRS. Government publications can also be downloaded and printed. Circular E, Employer's Tax Guide (Publication 15) is one of these. The Internet address is: www.irs.gov/forms_pubs/. Check out the website and follow the information on your screen.

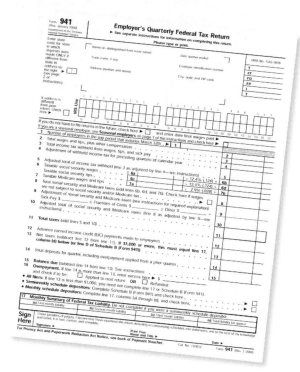

Figure 10.11
Employer's Quarterly Federal Tax Return

Federal, state, local taxes, and FICA taxes, which are paid by the employee, are deposited into one account. Employer payments, such as federal and state unemployment taxes, are deposited in the other account.

If your practice does not use the Electronic Funds Transfer program, you must submit employment taxes by deposit to a Federal Reserve Bank or an authorized financial institution. Cash, money orders, or checks are deposited using Federal Tax Deposit Coupons supplied by the IRS. Deposits are generally made every

WAGE AND TAX FORMS The amount of income tax and Social Security tax withheld from a paycheck must be recorded on a Wage and Tax Statement, IRS Form W-2. This form must be completed for each employee who had taxes withheld. These forms are filed with federal, state, and local agencies. Copies must be given to each employee by January 31 of the year following the taxable year. Figure 10.12 shows a 2000 Wage and Tax Statement Form, W-2.

Legal Issue

Employers are required to have an IRS tax identification number. This can be obtained by completing Form SS-4.

Figure 10.12
2000 Wage and Tax Statement Form W-2

month. However, every three months, an Employer's Quarterly Federal Tax Return (Form 941) must be filed listing the amounts withheld from employee paychecks. This quarterly tax return form (shown in Figure 10.11) is due on or before the last day of the first month after the end of the quarter.

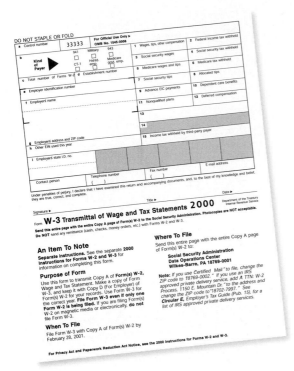

Figure 10.13
Transmittal of Wage and Tax Statements Form W-3

TRANSMITTAL OF WAGE AND TAX STATEMENTS The employer must submit a Wage and Tax Statements Form W-3, as shown in Figure 10.13, with the W-2 forms to the Social Security Administration. This form must be submitted on or before the last day in February.

Procedure 10.3 summarizes the steps to follow when processing a payroll in accordance with government regulations.

Banking

The responsibilities of the administrative medical assistant may include receiving payments in the form of cash or checks, preparing and making bank deposits, writing checks to pay for office supplies and maintenance, and reconciling bank statements.

Checks

Payment for medical services is usually made by check, either personal or from an insurance company. A **check** is a written order on a printed form directing a bank to pay money from a specific account to the party whom the check names. The person who writes the order is the **payer**, and the person or organization that is to receive the money is the **payee**. To write a check, the payer is required to have first deposited

sufficient money in a checking account with a financial institution.

Most checks received in a medical office will be personal checks (written by an individual) or insurance checks. However, patients may make payments in a variety of forms, including cash. A **cashier's check** is one that is purchased from a bank, and the money paid out when the check is cashed comes from the bank's account. A **money order** is similar to a cashier's check but can be purchased from the post office and some businesses as well as a bank. A **certified check** is an individual's personal check that has been guaranteed by the bank. The amount of money for which it is written is deducted from the depositor's account immediately, and the check is stamped "certified" or "accepted" and is signed by a bank employee.

Traveler's checks may also be purchased from a bank or other institution, such as the American Automobile Association, and used when personal checks are not acceptable. The signature of the purchaser is required when the checks are bought and again when they are used. A **voucher check** is one with a detachable portion that explains the purpose of the check. A good example is a payroll check.

RECEIVING CHECKS A check must be endorsed before it can be cashed or deposited. Figure 10.14 shows the different ways a check can be endorsed. A blank endorsement is simply the signature of the payee. Anyone could cash the check when it has been endorsed in this manner. A full endorsement is used to assign the check to another party. The words "Pay to the order of" followed by the name of the new payee and signed by the original payee allows the designated party to cash the check. A patient who signs over an insurance check to the physician might use this kind of endorsement. A restrictive endorsement indicates that the check is "For Deposit Only" followed by the name of the physician or organization. This type of endorsement prevents the check from being cashed if it is lost or stolen. This is the way that checks received in the medical office will be endorsed.

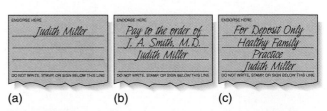

(a)   (b)   (c)

Figure 10.14
Check Endorsements

(a) A blank endorsement is the least restrictive and can be cashed by anyone. (b) A full endorsement can be cashed only by the person named on the back of the check. (c) A restrictive endorsement can only be deposited in the indicated account.

Procedure 10.3

Managing Payroll Responsibilities

Purpose: To process a payroll in accordance with government regulations.

Equipment/Supplies: *Circular E, Employer's Tax Guide,* Forms SS-4, W-4, 941, W-2, W-3, 940, 8109, and employee's compensation record, pen.

1 Complete Form SS-4 to obtain an Internal Revenue Service tax identification number if the practice does not already have one. *This number must be used on all reports and the deposit forms that accompany tax payments.*
2 Ask the employee to complete Form W-4 (Employee's Withholding Allowance Certificate). *Deductions are calculated based on the information on this form using withholding tables in* Circular E, Employer's Tax Guide.
3 Each payday:
  ■ Determine the number of hours worked and the hourly wage where applicable for each employee.
  ■ Calculate the employee's gross earnings.
  ■ Withhold federal income tax based on the employee's W-4 form and gross earnings.
  ■ Withhold the employee's share of Social Security (FICA) and Medicare taxes.
  ■ Withhold state and local income tax, based on the tax guides of your state and locality.
  ■ Withhold optional deductions.
4 Each month:
  ■ Deposit federal income tax and FICA tax withheld by submitting a check and Form 8109 (Federal Tax Deposit Coupon) to a Federal Reserve bank or

other authorized financial institution. **◉ NOTICE!** Some employers are on a semi-weekly deposit schedule. Consult *Circular E, Employer's Tax Guide* for more information.
  ■ Deposit state and local taxes according to local guidelines.
  ■ Deposit optional deductions to appropriate accounts.
5 Each quarter:
  ■ Deposit FUTA tax by submitting a check and Form 8109 (Federal Tax Deposit Coupon) to a Federal Reserve bank or other authorized financial institution.
  ■ File Form 941 (Employer's Quarterly Federal Tax Return).
6 Each year:
  ■ Give each employee a W-2 form (Wage and Tax Statement) on or before January 31.
  ■ Ask each employee to fill out an updated Form W-4 (Employee's Withholding Allowance Certificate) before the beginning of a new calendar year.
  ■ File copy A of all W-2 forms with the Social Security Administration, along with transmittal form W-3 (Figure 10.13).
  ■ File Form 940 (Employer's Annual Federal Unemployment [FUTA] Tax Return).
  ■ File state and local forms as required. Tax regulations vary from one locality to another. **◉ NOTICE!** Responsibilities for withholding, depositing, and reporting employment taxes can vary greatly depending on each employer's individual circumstances. See *Circular E, Employer's Tax Guide* for detailed information.

As a convenience, a stamp with the name of the physician or medical organization might be made available to patients who are paying in person for use in the "Pay to the Order of" space on the front of the check. This ensures that the check is made out to the proper payee, prevents misspellings, and is easier to read than handwriting.

Procedure 10.4 provides the steps to follow when receiving checks for payment in the medical office.

WRITING CHECKS The medical assistant may be responsible for writing checks to pay for supplies, utilities, or other expenses. Remember that you cannot sign checks unless the doctor has filled out the necessary forms at the bank authorizing you to do so. You must also have a signature card on file with the bank. If you are not authorized to sign checks, you should complete all other information on the check, attach it

to the appropriate invoice, and place it on the desk of the physician or other authorized person to be signed. Refund checks for patient care should be posted on the patient's ledger card and the current day sheet.

Some businesses use check-writing machines because the checks they write have small perforations across the amount and cannot be altered. Checks also can be printed electronically using computer software. Checkbooks should be kept in a locked drawer so that unauthorized persons do not have access to them. Computer software for check writing should be secured through the use of a password. When writing a check, follow the steps in Procedure 10.5.

Deposits

All cash, checks, and other funds received in the medical office should be deposited in the bank every day,

Procedure 10.4

Receiving Checks

Purpose: To process checks received as payment.

Equipment/Supplies: Checks, endorsement stamp, pen.

1 Inspect the check to make sure it is properly made out to the physician or medical organization, that the date is correct, and that there is no discrepancy between the amount written in numbers and the amount written in words on the face of the check. *Checks that are dated after the date of deposit may be returned. If the number amount and the written amount are different, the bank may not accept the check. If it is accepted, the bank will pay the amount written in words.*

2 Make sure that the check is signed. *The bank will not honor unsigned checks.*

3 Do not accept checks made out for more than the amount due. However, if a check received in the mail is made out for more than the amount due, credit the account with the amount of the check, leaving a negative balance due. *Accepting a check made out for more than the patient owes and giving the patient the difference as change might result in a loss, since the check might bounce.*

4 Do not accept checks marked "Paid in full" without

checking to make sure the check actually does cover the total debt. If a balance remains, write "Received as payment on account. Balance due: (indicate amount of balance remaining)" above the endorsement on the back of the check. Do not cross out "Paid in full." *Legal problems may result if you cross out "Paid in full." The note above the endorsement indicates that the amount owed is in dispute and that the balance may be collected.*

5 Do not accept third-party checks (ones made out to a payee other than the medical practice) unless specifically authorized to do so. Checks made out by an insurance company to the patient are usually accepted when endorsed by the patient.

6 Endorse the check immediately on the reverse side (within the 1½-inch area designated for endorsements) using a rubber stamp that includes the name of the physician or organization and the words "For Deposit Only." *This restrictive endorsement would keep an unauthorized person from cashing the check if it were lost or stolen.*

7 Place all checks in a secure place until they can be deposited.

---

or as soon as possible. A **deposit slip** (sometimes called a **deposit ticket**) is a form that must be completed and presented with the funds so they will be credited to the right bank account. Deposit slips are usually preprinted with the depositor's name, address, and account number. The slip provides a space for the date of deposit, the amount of currency (paper money) and coins, a listing of all checks, and the total amount of the deposit. Figure 10.15 is an example of a filled-out deposit slip.

To prepare the currency for deposit, arrange the bills with the faces up, all in the same orientation, grouped according to denomination (all $50s together, all $20s, all $10s, etc.) and placed in descending order with the largest denomination on top and the smallest on the bottom. Bills may be secured by wrapping them with a paper band provided by the bank. Coins should be counted, placed in an envelope, and sealed. Large numbers of coins are not usually handled in a medical office, but if needed, coin wrappers may be obtained from the bank. Coins are grouped according to denomination, and the appropriate amount is placed in each wrapper. The account number should be written on the wrapper. Checks should be arranged in alphabetical

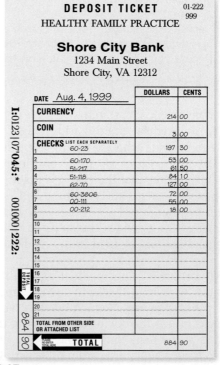

Figure 10.15
A Completed Deposit Slip

order according to the last name of the payer. List the checks in this order on the deposit slip and indicate the amount of each check and its **ABA number**, which was assigned by the American Bankers Association to identify the bank and its location. It appears on the face of every check as a fraction with two upper numbers joined by a hyphen.

The total amount of the checks is entered at the bottom of the column and also on the front of the slip. The total amount of the deposit is obtained by adding the amount of currency, coins, and checks. This should equal the total of all receipts on the day sheet since the last deposit. A copy of the deposit slip should be retained for the office's financial records.

When large numbers of checks are being deposited, most banks will accept an adding machine tape that has the amount of each check and the total printed on it, instead of listing the checks on the back of the deposit slip. The total on the tape would be entered on the front of the slip just as it would be if the checks were listed on the back. The checks should be kept in the same order that they were entered on the tape, and the tape should be secured to the checks with a rubber band or

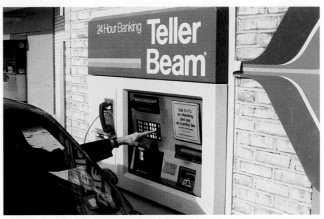

Many banks provide convenient 24-hour depositories for deposits. Here, deposits can be made after normal business hours.

paper clip. Some day sheets, such as the one used with the pegboard system, have a deposit slip attached that is filled out as the transactions are listed on the day sheet. If this is the case, add the cash amounts and the check amounts to get the total amount of the deposit.

Procedure 10.5

Writing a Check

Purpose: To fill out a check that is accurate, legible, not easily altered, and will be accepted by the bank.

Equipment/Supplies: Checkbook and non-erasable black or blue pen.

1 Write checks neatly and legibly in non-erasable black or blue ink. *Non-erasable ink makes it difficult for an unauthorized person to change the information on the check. Legible writing helps to prevent deciphering errors.*

2 Fill out the check stub completely before writing the check. Include the date, name of the payee, purpose of the check, and amount. ◎ **NOTICE!** Don't forget to subtract the amount of the check from the previous balance to obtain a new balance, and record it on the next stub.

3 Fill in the current date on the line at the upper right side of the check. *Post-dating or dating in advance may cause the check to bounce.*

4 Write the payee's name immediately following "Pay to the order of," leaving no space in front of the name. Do not use titles (Mr., Mrs., etc.). Draw a line to fill in any space left between the payee's name and the dollar sign at the end of the line. *Unused space on any line makes it easier for someone to alter the check.*

5 Immediately after the dollar sign, leaving no space, write the amount of the check in numbers.

6 On the next line, write the dollar amount in words and the cents as a fraction. "And" should be used only where the decimal occurs. Example: $127.50 would be written as "One hundred twenty-seven and 50/100." If there are no cents, write 00/100. Writing should begin at the extreme left of the line, and any space left after the amount should be filled in by drawing a line to the word "Dollars."

7 If a mistake is made while writing the check, write the word VOID in large letters across the face of the check and the stub. Do not destroy the check, but leave it attached to the stub to be filed with the canceled checks at a later date. *Checks are numbered in consecutive order, and all checks must be accounted for.*

8 State briefly what the check is for in the space provided.

9 Review the check to be sure it is completed correctly.

10 Obtain the physician's signature, or sign it yourself if authorized to do so. ◎ **NOTICE!** You cannot sign the check unless you have authorization from the physician and have a signature card on file with the bank.

11 Store the checkbook in a locked drawer. *Stolen checks can be forged.*

The money, checks, and deposit slip should be placed in a bag or envelope and taken to the bank. The total amount of the deposit should be recorded in the checkbook, and a copy of the deposit slip should be kept.

Reconciling Bank Statements

Each month, the bank will send a statement of all transactions that have occurred in the checking account, along with canceled checks that have been paid out of the account. Some banks will send photocopies instead of the original checks unless the originals are requested. The statement will show a beginning balance, a list of all deposits and all checks paid, withdrawals and any other transactions, service charges, interest earned, and ending balance. This statement must be **reconciled** (making the balances on the bank statement and in the checkbook agree) to assure that there are no discrepancies. The reconciliation must account for deposits made and checks written after the ending date of the statement as well as checks written earlier that have not been cashed. Figure 10.16 is a worksheet for reconciling your checkbook. Fill in the appropriate data on the blank lines to reconcile the bank's statement with your checkbook.

You may use this form or Procedure 10.6 to make sure the checkbook and bank statement agree. If you find a discrepancy, look for a mistake in the checkbook first. The automated equipment used by banks reduces the likelihood of errors on the statement; however, any error found on the statement should be reported to the bank immediately.

Procedure 10.6

Reconciling a Bank Statement

Purpose: To reconcile the bank's statement with the checkbook ledger.

Equipment/Supplies: Bank statement, checkbook ledger, canceled checks, black and red pens.

1 Check the beginning balance on the current statement and verify that it is the same as the ending balance on the previous statement. If these numbers are not the same, it may be because an error on the previous statement was corrected, changing the balance on the current statement. If you do not know the reason for the difference, contact the bank. *The reconciled balance on the checkbook and the bank statement will not be the same if the beginning balances are different.*

2 Compare the list of deposits on the statement with the deposits listed in the checkbook. Place a red check mark in the checkbook by each deposit listed on the statement. *A red mark by a deposit, withdrawal, canceled check, service charge, or interest recorded in the checkbook makes it easy to glance through the checkbook and determine which checks and deposits had not cleared the bank by the date of the statement. At the end of the reconciliation, all additions and subtractions shown on the bank statement should be marked in red in the checkbook.*

3 List all deposits in the checkbook that *do not* have a red check mark. Write down the total.

4 Arrange the canceled checks in numerical order and compare them with the check stubs in the checkbook. Place a red check mark in the checkbook on the stub of each check listed on the statement.

5 Go through the checkbook and list all checks that *do not* have a red check mark on the stub. Write down the total.

6 Compare the list of cash withdrawals on the statement with the withdrawals listed in the checkbook. Place a red check mark in the checkbook by each withdrawal listed on the statement.

7 List all withdrawals in the checkbook that *do not* have a red check mark. Write down the total.

8 Record in the checkbook any service charges or other fees listed on the bank statement. Subtract this from the last balance carried forward in the checkbook to obtain a new balance to be carried forward. Place a red check mark by the entry.

9 Record in the checkbook any interest credited to the account on the bank statement. Add this to the last balance in the checkbook to obtain a new balance to be carried forward. Place a red check by the entry.

10 On a separate sheet of paper, write down the new balance carried forward in the checkbook.

11 Subtract the total of the deposits not listed on the bank statement (Step 3) from the amount in Step 10. Write down the resulting amount.

12 To the amount calculated in Step 11, add the total of all withdrawals not listed on the bank statement (Step 7). Write down the resulting amount.

13 To the amount calculated in Step 12, add the total of the checks not listed on the bank statement (Step 5). Write down the resulting amount.

14 Compare the amount calculated in Step 13 with the ending balance on the bank statement. They should be the same. A difference indicates that an error has been made, and it must be found and corrected.

Checkbook balance:	$ _____
Bank charges:	– _____
Interest:	+ _____
Total of all outstanding checks not listed on bank statement:	+ _____
Total of deposits not listed on bank statement:	– _____
Total of withdrawals not listed on bank statement:	+ _____
Adjusted checkbook balance:	$ _____

Figure 10.16
Worksheet for Reconciling Checkbook and Bank Statement

The adjusted checkbook balance should match the ending balance on your bank statement.

If the adjusted checkbook balance does not agree with the ending balance on the bank statement, check the following:

- Have you entered the amount of each check in the checkbook correctly?
- Have all checks written been deducted from the checkbook?
- Are the deposit amounts entered in your checkbook the same as those shown on the statement?
- Did you deduct all charges from the checkbook?
- Did you recalculate the additions and subtractions in the checkbook?
- Did you check to make sure you brought forward the correct balance from one page to the next?
- Did you report errors to the bank promptly?

Petty Cash

Most offices find it convenient to have cash available when needed for minor expenses. But even though the amounts may be small, they must be accounted for. A petty cash fund is started by writing a check to "Cash" for a specific amount, cashing the check, and placing the money (in small bills and coins) in a box or envelope that is kept in a secure place in the office. One person is usually designated as responsible for the fund, but others may have access to it as well. Whenever money is paid out of the fund, a voucher must be completed and signed by the person receiving the money and the person making the disbursement.

The vouchers should be numbered consecutively and should show the date of the disbursement, the total spent, and the reason. If there is a receipt, it

should be attached to the voucher. The vouchers should be kept with the cash, and the total amount of all of the vouchers plus the amount of cash should always equal the amount placed in the fund. At the end of the month, or when the cash in the box seems no longer sufficient for future needs, the vouchers should be removed and the amounts totaled. The fund should be replenished to its original amount by writing and cashing a check equal to the total of the vouchers. Then the process starts again. The vouchers must be retained in an appropriate file, and each expenditure must be posted to its proper account. Do not use the petty cash fund to make change for patients who pay in cash.

Challenging Situations

*P*atients may become very upset when calling the office about a bill they have received that already has been paid or is in error. The medical assistant should always use a calm voice and treat the patient with respect.

Consider the call an opportunity to promote good customer relations. Before attempting to resolve anything, give the caller every opportunity to explain the whole problem. Take notes. Wait until the caller has told you everything before you respond with anything more than, "Please continue" or "Then what happened?" Have the caller clarify anything you do not understand. When you think you have all the details written down, ask if you can restate the problem to the caller to make sure you understand it. If the caller agrees with your statement, you may recognize where the problem lies based on your understanding of the office's procedures. If no obvious explanation comes to mind, you need to research the issue. At this point, it is appropriate to explain to the patient that some time will be needed to determine where the problem is. Before you hang up, make sure you have the caller's phone number.

Make every effort to solve the problem by referring to source documents, day sheets, the patient ledger, deposit records, and other records as necessary. Obviously, you will correct any error you find. Once you have determined the facts to the best of your ability, consider writing a letter explaining to the patient, in terms he can understand, what your understanding or resolution of the situation is. The advantage of a letter is that it documents both the fact that you responded and what your research found. You can also document your willingness to examine any evidence the patient can produce in support of his position. Finally, you can thank the person for *bringing this to the office's attention and for the patience that was needed to deal with the issue.*

When mistakes made in processing financial transactions are not discovered until later, it is not simply a matter of correcting the error on the patient's ledger or the day sheet. End-of-day totals must be recalculated and the correction carried forth on subsequent sheets. Summary reports may change as a result of the correction. The medical assistant must trace the error through all the records affected and make the necessary adjustments.

Clinical Summary

- The duties of the medical assistant may include book-keeping responsibilities, banking, handling the payroll, and maintaining a petty cash fund. To perform these duties efficiently, he must understand basic accounting principles and terminology.
- Double-entry bookkeeping is too complex for daily use in the medical office. Instead, single-entry bookkeeping, write-it-once systems, or computerized accounting systems are usually used.
- Business accounts are kept separate from the physician's personal accounts.
- Patient accounts are kept separate from practice maintenance accounts.
- Financial transactions originate with source documents and are listed in the appropriate account.
- Patient-related charges and payments are recorded on a day sheet in the order in which they occur and on the patient's ledger card.
- A restrictive endorsement is used for checks received as payment in the medical office.
- Bank statements must be reconciled with the checkbook to make sure there are no discrepancies.
- To sign checks, the medical assistant must have the physician's authorization and a signature card on file with the bank.
- Checks should be legible and properly written to be accepted by the bank and to minimize the likelihood of alterations.
- An employee earnings record must be kept that contains all information affecting the employee's pay, such as hours worked, pay rate, gross pay, deductions, net pay, earnings-to-date, Social Security number, and number of exemptions.
- A voucher should be filled out each time money from the petty cash box is used.
- Computer accounting software saves time and reduces the chance of errors.

The Language of Medicine

ABA number A number assigned to a bank by the American Bankers Association that identifies the bank and its location.

account A record of information and transactions related to each asset and liability, and each aspect of owner's equity.

accounting A system of organizing, maintaining, and auditing business records, summarizing financial transactions, and interpreting the results.

accounting cycle The steps involved in recording, processing, and summarizing financial transactions.

accounting equation The mathematical equation that expresses the financial condition of a business: Assets = Liabilities + Owner's Equity.

accounts payable Debts owed to other businesses or individuals for goods and services.

accounts receivable Money that has been earned, but not yet received.

accrual method of accounting The accounting method in which income is recorded in the period it is earned, whether or not cash has been received, and expenses are recorded in the period they are incurred, regardless of whether they have been paid.

asset Anything of value that is owned.

balance sheet A statement of the financial condition of a business on a given date based on the accounting equation.

bookkeeping The keeping of systematic records of financial transactions.

cash method of accounting The accounting method in which income and expenses are recorded only when they have been received or paid out.

cashier's check A check purchased from a bank.

certified check A personal check that has been guaranteed by a bank.

chart of accounts A detailed listing of all the accounts a business uses.

check A written order on a printed form directing a bank to pay money from a specific account to a designated recipient.

credit A transaction that decreases assets and increases liabilities.

day sheet (daily journal, daily log, daily record) A cumulative listing of all patient-related financial transactions recorded on a daily basis in chronological order.

debit A transaction that increases assets and decreases liabilities.

deposit slip (deposit ticket) A form that is completed and submitted with funds to ensure that they are credited to the right bank account.

double-entry bookkeeping A system in which each financial transaction must be recorded in at least two accounts.

Federal Insurance Contributions Act (FICA) The law establishing the Social Security tax and setting its rates.

Federal Unemployment Tax Act (FUTA) The law establishing federal unemployment taxes and setting the rate.

general ledger A record of all the accounts of a business.

gross pay The amount earned before deductions.

journal A sheet or book in which each business transaction is recorded from source documents.

ledger cards Individual patient account records.

liability Debt owed.

modified cash method of accounting The accounting method in which revenue is recorded only when money is received and expenses are recorded only when paid out, but adjustments are made for expenditures for items having an economic life of more than one year.

money order A form of check that may be purchased from post offices and certain businesses.

net pay The amount earned after deductions.

owner's equity The owner's share of the assets of a business.

payee The person or entity receiving money from a check.

payer The person or entity writing out a check.

payroll The total paid out to all employees for a pay period.

pegboard (See write-it-once.)

posting Transferring amounts from the journal to the ledger.

reconciled Made to agree, referring to the balances on a bank statement and in a checkbook.

salaries The pay for employees who earn the same amount per period regardless of the number of hours worked.

single-entry bookkeeping The bookkeeping method in which a transaction is recorded in only one account.

source documents Documents containing the information needed to record transactions.

T-account A skeleton version of the standard accounting form.

transaction A financial action or event that changes the amount of a business's assets, liabilities, or owner's equity.

traveler's checks Checks purchased from a bank or other institution to use when personal checks are not accepted.

trial balance A listing of the balances of all accounts in the ledger, as of a specific date, to check the equality of debits and credits.

voucher check A check with a detachable portion that explains the purpose of the check.

wages Pay earned on an hourly basis.

write-it-once (pegboard) A manual method of bookkeeping in which information is recorded on several forms simultaneously.

Signs/Symptoms of Progress

1 Recall, Question, Connect

Recall
List three bookkeeping or accounting systems that a medical assistant might use in a medical office.

Question
Think of questions you have regarding these systems for accounting in the medical office.

Connect
Why is it important for the medical assistant to be familiar with basic accounting principles?

2 Educating the Patient

During a physical exam, Dr. Jones discovers that Paula West, who has been his patient for several years, has an enlarged thyroid, and orders lab work to determine her thyroid function.

1 Where and how would the charges be recorded at the end of the visit?

2 When Ms. West calls a month later to find out if the insurance company has paid for her visit, where would you look to find the information?

3 Since the insurance company only covers those charges that relate to the thyroid problem, how should the charges have been recorded so that Ms. West can obtain a breakdown of them? How will you explain the information to her?

3 Exploring Perspectives in Teams

Perspective involves the discipline of examining how ideas look from different points of view and recognizing that there are often multiple "answers" to complex questions. In small groups or on your own, reflect on possible alternative views or answers and summarize your findings.

1 Dr. Jones's office manager has called a meeting of administrative personnel to discuss each person's duties and promote cooperation and efficiency among the staff. One member of your group should explain the bookkeeping system being used, how charges and payments are recorded, and what bookkeeping procedures are done at the end of the day. Another person should explain the guidelines for accepting checks and making bank deposits. A third person should explain how the petty cash fund operates. Each should challenge the others and ask questions about the standardization of procedures, accuracy, and problems that should be anticipated.

2 Go to two websites for companies that offer commercial medical billing software. Write a description of what the products do and compare their features. Which would you recommend to your supervisor?

3 The bank statement does not agree with your records. Write a memo to the office manager explaining how you will reconcile the two and avoid errors in the future.

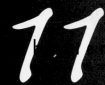

Learning Outcomes

- Describe how fees are set and the need for a fee schedule.
- Prepare billing statements, recognizing the importance of up-to-date information.
- Prepare an aging accounts report and explain why aging reports are important.
- Adhere to consumer protection laws that apply to collecting debts.
- Identify ways of making the patient aware of office policies regarding payment.

Performance Objectives

- Understand and adhere to managed care policies and procedures.
- Prepare billing statement and obtain reimbursement through accurate claims submission.
- Prepare aging reports and make collection phone calls.
- Follow federal, state, and local legal guidelines for billing and collections.

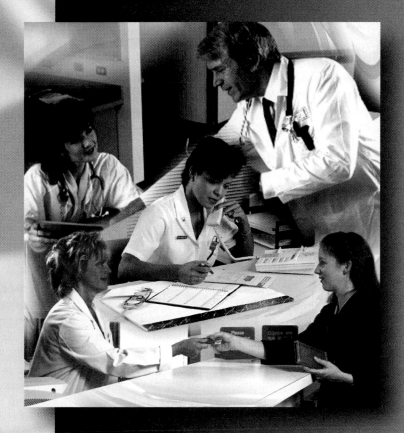

Billing and Collecting Payments

Any business must be paid for the goods and services it provides if it is to survive. Like other businesses, a medical practice must continue to pay salaries to its employees and pay for supplies, utilities, and other expenses, even though patients and insurance companies often do not pay until long after medical services are provided. If we as teachers, nurses, engineers, mechanics, secretaries, salespersons, and medical assistants had to wait several weeks or months to get paid for our work, we would be unhappy, and financial problems might result. Yet that is exactly what the physician must do. To prevent cash flow problems and compensate those who provide medical care, it is important to collect payment as soon as possible. Within the clinic, the medical assistant is usually responsible for collecting fees at the time of service, billing patients and insurance companies, handling overdue accounts, and discussing financial matters with patients.

Patient Concerns

Given the high cost of medical care today, it is reasonable for patients to be concerned about how much they are charged and how it is going to be paid. Some people may feel that charges are unreasonably high. Patients who know approximately what to expect before treatment and how fees are set are less likely to be upset when they get the bill and can consider various payment options. Listing the charge for each service provided helps to clarify the total bill.

Overdue accounts and the inability to pay may trouble some customers. The medical assistant should use a consistent and fair method of requesting payment for bills that are overdue. Some physicians may agree to provide care at no charge to a needy patient.

Payment Policies

As a business, a medical office must charge competitive and fair prices for services and must receive payment for those services in a timely fashion. Patients should be fully informed about the practice's fees and payment policies before they receive treatment. Even a patient with medical insurance is ultimately responsible for the bill if the insurance company refuses to pay or does not cover the full amount.

Charges

Physicians set their own fees for the services they provide based on experience, what competitors are charging, and the costs involved. Sometimes, the fee may be determined by "what the traffic will bear." A physician practicing in a wealthy community may charge more than one who practices in an economically depressed community. Insurance companies and government healthcare programs influence fees charged for specific services by establishing what they consider to be "usual, customary, and reasonable" fees. This means that the fee for a service is: 1) what the physician usually charges; 2) similar to what other physicians in the area charge; and 3) reasonable considering the difficulty involved. Many practices determine fees based on the **Resource-Based Relative Value Scale (RBRVS)**, which was devised by the federal government to control Medicare spending. Each procedure or service is assigned a unit value based on the time, skill, and expenses involved. The fee is calculated by multiplying this number by a dollar amount based on geographic location.

Ethical Issue

If fees are to be kept reasonable, costs must be monitored and controlled. Office employees should be aware of their role in controlling costs by using time on the job wisely, taking care not to waste supplies, and using and caring for equipment properly.

A **fee schedule** is a list of the services and procedures a physician usually performs, with the price of each. This list should be available for patients to review upon request. It can also be used as a source of information by the medical assistant. Figure 11.1 shows a partial fee schedule for a family practice. It is not unusual to hear patients complain about fees they consider to be excessive. However, one must keep in mind that the physician spent many years preparing for his profession, the investment in equipment is huge, and the overhead costs of operating an office are considerable.

Some physicians may charge for advice given by telephone, missed appointments, or appointments canceled at the last minute. These and all other payment policies should be made clear to both new patients and those seeking regular treatment. If payment in full is required at the time of service, this should be mentioned tactfully when a new patient calls for an appointment. A notice to this effect should be posted prominently in the office. Some physicians prefer payment at the time of service even if a patient's medical insurance will cover part or all of the bill. When this is the case, the patient is responsible for filing a claim for reimbursement with the insurance company.

One way to make patients aware of payment policies is to incorporate them into a brochure or **practice information sheet** such as the one shown in Figure 11.2. The sheet should list the physicians in the practice, their specialties, office hours, address, telephone number, how to reach the physician in an emergency, special services provided, payment policies and options, and other pertinent information. It would be distributed to new patients when they come into the office and to existing patients when there is a need. For example, when a new physician joins the practice or there is a change in office location, hours, or payment policy, the information could be mailed to all patients.

When a large fee is involved, the physician may give a written estimate of the charges for surgery or other procedures and for hospitalization, including her fee and the cost of anesthesiology, lab work, hospital room, operating room, and recovery room. The medical

HEALTHY FAMILY PRACTICE

100 Oak Street
Shore City, VA 12312
(555) 123-1234

FEE SCHEDULE   EFFECTIVE JANUARY 1, 20XX

CPT Code	Description	Fee
99211	Office visit, established patient, brief	$47.00
99212	Office visit, established patient, limited	$53.00
99213	Office visit, established patient, intermediate	$59.00
99214	Office visit, established patient, extended	$65.00
99215	Office visit, established patient, comprehensive	$75.00
99201	Office visit, new patient, brief	$59.00
99202	Office visit, new patient, limited	$65.00
99203	Office visit, new patient, intermediate	$71.00
99204	Office visit, new patient, extended	$76.00
99205	Office visit, new patient, comprehensive	$86.00
93000	ECG/interpretation	$65.00
90724	Flu immunization	$14.00
90732	Pneumonia immunization	$24.00
69210	Ear wax removal	$19.00
45330	Flexible sigmoidoscopy	$110.00
81002	Urinalysis, dip only	$13.00
81000	Urinalysis, complete	$22.00
82270	Hemocult	$18.00
36415	Venipuncture	$18.00
80061	Lipid panel	$54.00
82465	Cholesterol	$15.00
84153	PSA	$51.00
85018	Hemoglobin	$10.00
17000	Destruction of skin lesion, premalignant	$66.00
71020	Chest x-ray	$82.00

Figure 11.1
Partial Fee Schedule for a Family Practice

assistant should make sure the patient understands that the estimate is not a fixed price. A copy of the estimate should be filed in the patient's record.

Many patients are enrolled in managed care plans such as HMOs, which are discussed in Chapter 12, "Processing Insurance Claims." These plans vary in the way that they are administered and their impact on billing. Physicians who contract to treat these customers are paid according to the terms of their contract. Some plans pay a fixed amount per month for each patient, regardless of the services the patient receives. The medical assistant must collect the appropriate copayment, if any, each time the patient comes in for treatment. This amount is usually printed on the patient's insurance identification card. The medical assistant must also report the services the patient receives to the managed care plan's administrative office by sending in a copy of the encounter form, filling out an insurance claim, or some other reporting method.

Some physicians may treat other medical professionals or employees without charge or at a discount. Services extended as a **professional courtesy** still produce income since most of these customers have medical insurance and the "courtesy" is not extended to insurance companies. In such cases, the full amount is entered on the day sheet, charged to the patient's account, and billed to the insurance carrier. The ledger card should note that no bill will be sent to the patient. After the insurance company pays its portion of the charge, the remainder is adjusted or written off completely according to the physician's instructions. (A write-off is recorded as an adjustment.) If the patient is not covered by insurance, the charge after the discount is entered on the ledger card and the day sheet. If there is no charge, write "N/C" on the ledger card and the day sheet, and do not bill the patient.

The physician may provide free medical services to patients who are unable to pay, have no insurance, and

Figure 11.2
**Medical Practice
Information Sheet**

HEALTHY FAMILY PRACTICE
100 Oak Street
Shore City, VA 12312
(555) 123-1234

Dr. D. L. Jones   Dr. J. A. Smith
Board-Certified in Family Practice   Specializing in Women's Healthcare

Sharon Stillwater
Certified Family Nurse Practitioner

Office Hours by Appointment Only

9:00 A.M.–5:00 P.M. Monday, Tuesday, Thursday, and Friday
(Last appointment at 4:00 P.M.)
9:00 A.M.–1:00 P.M., 6:00–9:00 P.M. Wednesday
9:00 A.M.–12:00 P.M. Saturday

For appointments, call: (555) 123-1234
After hours, call: (555) 123-5678
Emergencies, call: 911

NEW PATIENTS WELCOME

- Specializing in Family Care
- CHAMPUS, Medicare, Medicaid Provider
- Complete Physical Exams
- Immunizations

*Payment is expected at the time of service.
For your convenience, we accept major credit cards.
There will be a $10 charge for appointments cancelled
less than 24 hours in advance.*

are not eligible for aid through social service agencies. N/C (no charge) is recorded on the charge slip, day sheet, and patient ledger. An alternative would be to record the routine charge for the service and then indicate that the charge was written off in full. In either case, no billing is involved and no income is realized.

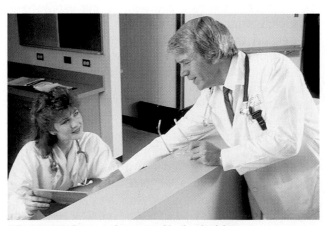

Adjustments to fees must be approved by the physician.

Payment Options

Prompt payment for services provided should be encouraged. After a patient sees the doctor and returns the charge slip to the business office, the amount owed usually must be filled in by the medical assistant based on the fee schedule. (See Figure 11.1.) The patient should then be told the amount owed for the visit and given an opportunity to pay immediately. The medical assistant might say, "Mrs. Edwards, the charge for today's visit is $55. Would you like to pay by cash or check?" Several methods of payment may be acceptable.

When payment is made in cash, the medical assistant should count the money carefully and give the patient a receipt, keeping a copy for office records.

The charge slip may serve as the receipt, since it usually has a space for payments to be recorded and the remaining balance entered. If there is no remaining balance, a zero should be entered. If there is no charge slip, a receipt book with the receipts numbered consecutively is used for cash payments. The receipt should state that the payment was in cash and include any remaining balance. The payment should be recorded on the day sheet and credited to the patient's ledger card, and the cash should be placed in an envelope or box and kept in a secure place until it can be deposited in the bank.

When a patient pays by check, the medical assistant must make sure the check is completed correctly, following the guidelines in Chapter 10, "Handling Accounting Responsibilities." As with cash, payments are recorded on the charge slip or a receipt, along with the remaining balance, and are also recorded on the day sheet and the patient's ledger card. The check should be stamped "For Deposit Only" and immediately placed in a secure place. It is not necessary to fill out a receipt for checks received by mail. If a check received in payment is returned by the bank because of insufficient funds, the patient should be notified by telephone and other arrangements should be made for payment. In the meantime, add the amount of the check (plus any penalty for returned checks) to the balance owed on the patient's ledger card and the current day sheet.

Most medical offices allow patients to use a major credit card to pay their bills. Physicians who do this must pay a fee to the company that issues the credit card. This reduces the amount the doctor actually receives for his service since, the fee cannot be added to the patient's bill. However, this method of payment may be cost effective in the long run because the physician is paid promptly, and the office staff does not have to expend time and effort collecting from the patient later. Special equipment and credit slips are needed to process credit card payments.

Credit and Collection Policies

For medical services that continue for a long time and as a result involve a large fee, the physician and patient

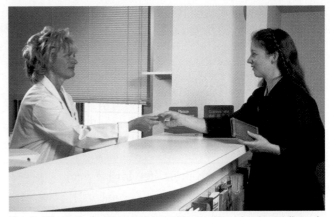

Many medical offices will accept payment in the form of major credit cards. However, the medical office will have to pay a fee to the company that issues the card, and this fee cannot be added to the patient's bill.

may agree to payment of the fee in several installments. When payment is to be made in more than four installments, federal regulations dictate that a **Truth in Lending Disclosure Statement** be completed and signed by the physician and the patient or responsible party. Figure 11.3 shows a form that meets the guidelines established by the **Truth in Lending Act**, Regulation Z of the Consumer Protection Act, which is administered by the Federal Trade Commission and protects consumers in their use of credit.

This law has two purposes. One is to ensure that the consumer is informed about all costs and conditions involved in using the credit. The other is to establish uniform terms that the consumer can use in comparing credit from different sources. The disclosure form must include:

1 The cash price of the service.
2 The amount of the down payment.
3 The total number of payments, the amount of each payment, and the date each payment is due.
4 The **annual percentage rate** of interest. This term must be included even when no interest is charged.
5 The total amount of all **finance charges**. This term must be used on the disclosure form.
6 The total cost including finance charges. The term **deferred payment price** must be used.
7 Any charges for late payments.

The Truth in Lending Act applies to a **bilateral agreement** between the physician and patient that includes more than four installments or a finance charge. It does not apply to an agreement in which the patient makes partial payments although the bill is for the full amount each month with no monthly payment indicated. The medical assistant is usually responsible

TRUTH IN LENDING DISCLOSURE STATEMENT

Patient: <u>Lena J. Coghill</u>   Physician: <u>D. L. Jones</u>
<u>2117 Union Station Ave</u>   <u>100 Oak Street</u>
<u>Shore City, VA 12313</u>   <u>Shore City, VA 12312</u>

Name and address of responsible party: <u>Same as patient.</u>

▪ Cash price (fee for service)	$2,100.00
▪ Cash down payment	$ 300.00
▪ Unpaid balance of cash price	$1,800.00
▪ Amount financed	$1,800.00
▪ FINANCE CHARGE	$ (none)
▪ ANNUAL PERCENTAGE RATE (yearly rate of the cost of credit)	$ (none)
▪ Total payments (amount financed plus finance charge)	$1,800.00
▪ DEFERRED PAYMENT PRICE (cash price plus finance charge)	$2,100.00

I agree to pay the total of payments shown above (<u>$1,800.00</u>) in <u>6</u> monthly installments of <u>$300.00</u> each to <u>D. L. Jones, M.D.</u> at his office at the above address. The first installment is due and payable on <u>July 1, 20XX</u> and each subsequent installment is due on the same day of each month thereafter until paid in full. The final payment is due on <u>December 1, 20XX</u>.

_____   _____
Date   Signature of Borrower (Patient or Responsible Party)

_____   _____
Date   Signature of Lender (Physician)

Figure 11.3
Truth in Lending Disclosure Statement

for discussing fees and payment policies with the customer, and must comply with government regulations covering the extension of credit. The assistant should make sure the patient understands the terms of the agreement before signing. After the document is signed, the medical assistant should give the original to the patient and keep a copy for the office records. It must be kept on file for at least two years after the final payment is made. The medical assistant will send the patient a monthly statement of account until the charge is paid in full.

The **Equal Credit Opportunity Act** protects consumers from discrimination in obtaining credit. A physician who extends credit to one patient must give all patients who request it the same opportunity. The only valid reason for denying credit is inability to pay. The doctor may ask you to do a credit check on a customer when a large fee is involved. Credit bureaus keep records on consumers who apply for credit. You can request a credit report that will show the patient's credit history and payment records for charge accounts, and may also include liens on property, bankruptcies, and other public information. When credit is refused, the consumer has the right to know why. You should send a letter stating the specific reason for denying credit. Include the name and address of the credit bureau that provided the report. The person can then check for inaccuracies and out-of-date or disputed information.

Billing

Two types of bills are used to collect payment for medical services—those sent to the insurer and those sent to the patient. The bill to the insurance carrier is submitted by filling out a claim form. The bill to the patient summarizes the charges and payments and lets her know how much is owed.

Even though patients are asked to pay for medical care when they receive it, extenuating circumstances often make paying the bill immediately unrealistic. Sometimes, it is a matter of not knowing how much of the charge, if any, the patient's insurance will pay. Established patients who are known and have a history of paying promptly when billed may expect (and be allowed by the physician) to continue paying as they have in the past. Sometimes, the patient may be temporarily unable to pay. In each of these situations, periodic billing by mail becomes necessary.

Billing Schedule

Statements (bills) are usually sent out on a monthly basis. Bills for all patients may be sent out at the end of the month, or **cycle billing** may be used to distribute the workload evenly throughout the month when there are a large number of statements to prepare. With cycle billing, bills are sent out periodically during the month based on the patients' last names. For example, bills might be sent out during the first week of the month to patients whose last names begin with A–F, during the second week to patients whose last names begin with G–L, during the third week for patients whose last names begin with M–R, and during the fourth week to patients whose last names begin with S–Z. Using this system helps to maintain an even cash flow, with income spread evenly throughout the month.

Format and Preparation

Patient ledger cards, as explained in Chapter 10, are used to prepare billing statements. In fact, a photocopy of the ledger card may be mailed out as a bill. Figure 11.4 is an example of both sides of a filled-out patient ledger card. Follow the steps in Procedure 11.1 to prepare a ledger card that can be photocopied and sent to the patient as a statement.

In the past, typewritten statements were prepared, but this time-consuming method has largely been replaced in the modern office by computer-generated statements. (See Figure 11.5.) Using computerized billing software has many advantages, including speed and accuracy in producing statements. The data the medical assistant enters from the charge slip can be used in different ways. Claims to insurance companies can be filed electronically, eliminating the need for paper forms. Some offices may use the software to print superbills that are tailored to meet their needs. In addition, receipts can be printed for patients who make a payment in the office. Patient billing statements can be created entirely by computer. Many offices insert preprinted statement forms into the printer, which then fills in data from individual accounts.

Whichever method is used, the statement should be itemized so the person responsible for payment knows exactly what charges are included in the bill. The bill should list the date of each visit during the billing period and the name of the person who was treated. Each procedure or service should be listed along with the fee. All payments or credits to the account should be listed, and the current balance shown. The patient is responsible for, and should be billed for, the entire balance, even though an insurance company is expected to pay part or all of the amount. When the insurance company pays, the transaction is recorded on the patient ledger card and the balance due is reduced accordingly. Including a return envelope along with the bill improves the payment rate. The statement may be printed on a form that can be folded and used as an envelope for payment by mail.

Some medical practices use an outside billing service to prepare and send out monthly statements. In these practices, the medical assistant will make sure that patient ledgers with outstanding balances due are

Working Smart

Start a **tickler file** to keep up with billing information. All you need is a small file box, dividers (guides) numbered 1–31 (one for each day of the month), and 3x5 cards. Make notes on the cards to "tickle your memory" about when a patient promised to make a payment on an overdue account, when you need to check on an insurance payment, or other tasks that need to be done at a later date. File the card under the appropriate day of the month. Then check the file each morning for items that should be taken care of that day.

(a)

Address in all caps using no punctuation

Name of family member if different from the patient

Service and payment codes used

Itemized list of services and charges

Last amount in column always shows what is due on the account

Codes explained on ledger

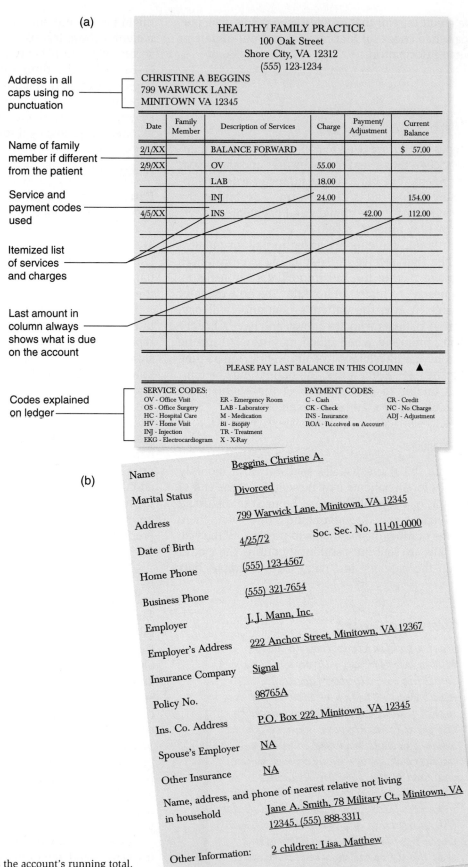

HEALTHY FAMILY PRACTICE
100 Oak Street
Shore City, VA 12312
(555) 123-1234

CHRISTINE A BEGGINS
799 WARWICK LANE
MINITOWN VA 12345

Date	Family Member	Description of Services	Charge	Payment/ Adjustment	Current Balance
2/1/XX		BALANCE FORWARD			$ 57.00
2/9/XX		OV	55.00		
		LAB	18.00		
		INJ	24.00		154.00
4/5/XX		INS		42.00	112.00

PLEASE PAY LAST BALANCE IN THIS COLUMN   ▲

SERVICE CODES:
OV - Office Visit   ER - Emergency Room
OS - Office Surgery   LAB - Laboratory
HC - Hospital Care   M - Medication
HV - Home Visit   BI - Biopsy
INJ - Injection   TR - Treatment
EKG - Electrocardiogram   X - X-Ray

PAYMENT CODES:
C - Cash   CR - Credit
CK - Check   NC - No Charge
INS - Insurance   ADJ - Adjustment
ROA - Received on Account

(b)

Name	Beggins, Christine A.
Marital Status	Divorced
Address	799 Warwick Lane, Minitown, VA 12345
Date of Birth	4/25/72 Soc. Sec. No. 111-01-0000
Home Phone	(555) 123-4567
Business Phone	(555) 321-7654
Employer	J. J. Mann, Inc.
Employer's Address	222 Anchor Street, Minitown, VA 12367
Insurance Company	Signal
Policy No.	98765A
Ins. Co. Address	P.O. Box 222, Minitown, VA 12345
Spouse's Employer	NA
Other Insurance	NA
Name, address, and phone of nearest relative not living in household	Jane A. Smith, 78 Military Ct., Minitown, VA 12345, (555) 888-3311
Other Information:	2 children: Lisa, Matthew

Figure 11.4
Patient Ledger Card

(a) The front of the card indicates the account's running total.
(b) The back of the card documents the insurance and contact information. This is for office use only.

Procedure 11.1

Preparing a Ledger Card/Billing Statement

Purpose: To prepare a patient ledger card that can be photocopied and sent to the patient as a bill.

Equipment/Supplies: Preprinted ledger form, completed patient information sheet, transaction source documents, typewriter.

1   Using the completed patient information sheet, fill in the items on the back side of the ledger pertaining to family, employment, insurance, and personal information. List names of family members whose charges may be billed to the account. *The information on the back of the ledger is for office use only and would not be photocopied for the billing statement.* ◉ **NOTICE!** Don't forget to write down both the home address and the mailing address if they differ.

2   On the front side of the ledger, type the name and mailing address of the patient or the person responsible for the bill in all capital letters, using no punctuation (except for the hyphen in the ZIP + 4 code), in the space indicated on the ledger form. *This is the format the U.S. Postal Service recommends to make mail technically compatible with the optical character readers it uses to sort mail.*

3   Type the amount of the balance brought forward under "Current Balance." If there is none, type -0-.

4   Using the charge slip, fill in the date and the name of the family member who was treated.

5   Under "Description of Services," type an itemized list of the services and record the charge for each in the "Charge" column. Use service codes printed on the front of the ledger to save space. *Breaking down the charges in this way lets the patient know exactly what she is paying for and may avoid time on the telephone answering questions about the bill. The service codes used must be easily understood by the patient.*

6   Add the charges to the balance brought forward and fill in the new current balance.

7   Record payments by filling in the date and describing the method of payment under "Description of Services." When checks are received from a third party, indicate the name of the payer. *A fee may be covered by more than one insurance company. Complete information makes it easier to trace transactions.*

8   Record the amount of each payment under "Payment/Adjustment."

9   Subtract the amount of the payment from the previous balance, and fill in the total under "Current Balance." If the total payments are for more than the amount owed, resulting in a credit balance, indicate this by placing a minus sign in front of the amount under "Current Balance." Overpayments may be refunded to the patient or used to reduce the amount owed by the patient on future visits.

---

provided to the service. The service will then prepare the invoices and mail them to the patients for payment.

Billing a Third Party

Most patients treated in the medical office today are covered by insurance. Even if the insurance company will not pay for service a patient receives, a claim must be filed because the charge may be part of a deductible amount on the patient's policy. Insurance billing is discussed in Chapter 12.

Occasionally, a company or an individual other than the patient may pay for medical services. In this case, the medical assistant should require a signed statement accepting responsibility for payment.

Collecting Delinquent Accounts

Many medical assistants consider bill collecting to be one of their least favorite duties. Most of us can identify with the patient who forgets to pay a bill or has

had a financial setback affecting his ability to pay. However, steps must be taken to collect sums owed to the physician that are not paid within the 30 days usually allowed. This is the responsibility of the medical assistant. Specifically, the assistant's duties regarding delinquent accounts include obtaining personal, employment, and insurance information that can be used in collecting debts; monitoring overdue accounts; sending collection notes and letters; making collection telephone calls; and attempting to trace patients who move without paying their bills.

Patient Information

The key to successful bill collection is good record-keeping. This begins when the patient first comes into the office for treatment. At that time, he should be asked to fill out an information sheet (registration form) that includes name, permanent address, telephone numbers at home and work, name and address of employer, insurance information, spouse's name and employer, family members, and name and address of the nearest relative not living in the same household.

MAKE CHECKS PAYABLE TO:

IF PAYING BY CREDIT CARD, FILL OUT BELOW.

CHECK CARD USING FOR PAYMENT

☐ VISA ☐ MASTERCARD

| CARD NUMBER | | EXP DATE |

| SIGNATURE | | |

HEALTHY FAMILY PRACTICE
100 OAK STREET
SHORE CITY VA 12312

STATEMENT DATE	PAY THIS AMOUNT	ACCT.#
04/13/XX	15.33	0000

Billing Questions: (555) 123-1234

PAGE # 1

SHOW AMOUNT
PAID HERE $

DELBERT JACKSON
889 KINGSTON AVENUE
MEADOWVILLE VA 33311

HEALTHY FAMILY PRACTICE
100 OAK STREET
SHORE CITY VA 12312

☐ **Please check box if above address is incorrect or insurance information has changed, and indicate change(s) on reverse side**

PLEASE DETACH AND RETURN TOP PORTION WITH YOUR PAYMENT

DIAG. CODE	DATE	PROCEDURE REFERENCE	PATIENT NAME	L O C	DESCRIPTION	PATIENT	INSURANCE
					BAL. FORWARD AS OF 03/12/99	.00	118.33
	03/16/XX	MY6939/030599			MEDICARE PYMT		-12.16
	03/16/XX	MY6939/030599			MEDICATE ADJ		-2.84
	03/16/XX	MY6939/030599			MEDICARE PYMT		-3.00
	03/16/XX	MY6939/030599			MEDICARE ADJ		-6.00
	03/16/XX	MY6939/030599			MEDICARE PYMT		-27.98
	03/16/XX	MY6939/030599			MEDICARE ADJ		-31.02
	03/16/XX				TRANSFER FROM MEDICARE		-7.00
	03/16/XX				TRANSFER TO CIGNA HC		7.00
	03/16/XX	MY6939/030599			MEDICARE PYMT		-3.65
	03/16/XX	MY6939/030599			MEDICARE ADJ		-9.35
	04/02/XX	CIGNA EOB			APPLY TO DEDUCTIBLE		.00
	04/02/XX				TRANSFER FROM CIGNA HCC		-15.33
	04/02/XX				TRANSFER TO PRIVATE	15.33	

**   YOUR INSURANCE HAS BEEN BILLED   **

CURRENT	OVER 30 DAYS	OVER 60 DAYS	OVER 90 DAYS	OVER 120 DAYS	PATIENT BALANCE DUE	INSURANCE
15.33	.00	.00	.00	.00	15.33	7.00

ACCOUNT NUMBER: 0000   PATIENT PAID YTD: .00
PLEASE REMIT TO: HEALTHY FAMILY PRACTICE   (555) 123-1234   10207

Figure 11.5
Computerized Billing Statement

The form usually includes questions regarding medical history and can be used to obtain the patient's signature for assignment of benefits and release of information to insurance carriers. A new form should be completed at least annually, and the information should be verified each time the patient comes in for an office visit. The medical assistant can use the data provided on the form to send monthly bills, collect from insurance companies, contact patients by telephone, and locate persons who move without paying their bills. Employer information is useful if legal steps are needed to obtain payment.

Aging Accounts

Accounts receivable should be continually monitored so that overdue accounts can be discovered and acted upon immediately. The chances of collecting an overdue bill diminish as time goes by. If computer software is used for accounting procedures, it is simple to print an **aging accounts report** when needed. (See Figure 11.6.) Data are analyzed and sorted by computer, and several types of aging reports can be obtained. Individual patient accounts may be displayed and printed with charges that are current, 30 days overdue, 60 days overdue, 90 days overdue, and over 90 days overdue, according to the date of the transaction. A computer-generated list of all overdue accounts, organized according to how long the money has been owed, can be printed. Insurance claims can be tracked in the same way, based on the date the claim was filed.

Aging reports can be done manually by going through the patient ledger cards and listing all overdue accounts.

Ledger cards that show overdue amounts should be flagged by applying color-coded, removable stickers, or in some other way, and actions such as phone calls or letters should be taken and noted on the card.

It is important to record exactly what services a payment covers. If the bill for a service remains unpaid while subsequent charges are reimbursed, the unpaid bill may not show up on an aging report. Procedure 11.2 provides the steps to be followed when preparing an aging account report.

Collection Plan

An agenda for actions to collect overdue accounts should be established so that all patients receive equal and consistent treatment. A firm, professional approach will usually bring results. The objective should be to collect the money without alienating the patient. Table 11.1 shows an example of a schedule for collecting overdue bills. The time frame for completing each step in the plan would depend on office policy. For example, the patient should be billed within 30 days of treatment. After 60 days, you might call the patient. After 90 days, 120 days, and 150 days, appropriate letters might be sent, and after 180 days, the account might be turned over to a collection agency.

CONSUMER PROTECTION LAWS The actions that can be taken to collect debts are subject to state and federal restrictions. The Fair Debt Collection Practices Act (FDCPA) and the Fair Credit Reporting Act (FCRA),

ACCOUNTS RECEIVABLE AGING REPORT

Date __February 1, 20XX__

Patient's name	Balance due	Date of charges	Current	Over 30 days	Over 60 days	Over 90 days	Over 120 days	Date of last payment	Notes
Conklin, Gayle	85.00	12/10/XX		85.00					
Gomez, Philip	146.00	10/18/XX				146.00		10/18/XX	Second Notice
Grafton, Maitland	55.00	11/15/XX	55.00						
Metz, Jason	72.00	11/7/XX		72.00					Called
Pittard, Diane	180.00	11/14/XX		180.00				12/4/XX	Called
Raymond, Dianne	69.00	12/19/XX		69.00					
Turner, Bradley	103.00	7/21/XX					103.00	7/21/XX	Collection agency
Williams, Letha	48.00	12/20/XX	48.00						

Figure 11.6
Aging Accounts Report

Procedure 11.2

Preparing an Aging Accounts Report

Purpose: To identify overdue accounts.

Equipment/Supplies: Patient ledger file, large sheet(s) of paper, pen.

1 Set up columns on the paper with the following headings: "Patient's name," "Balance due," "Date of charges," "Current," "Over 30 days," "Over 60 days," "Over 90 days," "Over 120 days," "Date of last payment." *This setup makes it easy to identify delinquent accounts at a glance.*
2 Start at the beginning of the ledger file and check each ledger card for outstanding balances.
3 For each account with a balance due, record:

- the patient's name in the appropriate column.
- the balance due.
- the amount owed in the appropriate column based on the date the services were provided.
- the date of the last payment. If no payment has been made, write NONE.

4 Add the amounts in each column and record the totals.
5 Add the amounts in the "Balance due" column and record the total.
6 Check the accuracy of your work by adding the total amounts in the "Current," "Over 30 days," "Over 60 days," "Over 90 days," and "Over 120 days" columns. This should equal the total in the "Balance due" column, and represents the total accounts receivable.

Table 11.1 Schedule for Collecting Payments after Treatment

within 30 days	bill patient
after 60 days	call patient requesting payment
after 90 days	first letter (polite request)
after 120 days	second letter (firmer but still polite)
after 150 days	third letter (final notice before action is taken)
after 180 days	account goes to collection agency or suit is filed

which are administered by the Federal Trade Commission, were initiated to protect consumers from harassment and misrepresentation. Under these laws, attempts to collect debts must not be made at times or places that are unusual or inconvenient. Repeated telephone calls and calls made during the night or very early in the morning are considered harassment. Abusive actions and threatening language must be avoided. For example, you could not say, "You'll be sorry if you don't pay this bill." Calls to the workplace cannot be made if the employer disapproves or if the patient tells you in writing not to call. When you call the workplace to locate the person who owes money, you must identify yourself, but not your employer. Do not reveal the purpose of your call until you reach the patient you are trying to contact.

You must not discuss financial obligations with anyone other than the patient. When you call the patient, you must identify yourself and cannot use any deception in trying to collect the debt. Any written message that is sent must be private and not easily accessible to other parties. For example, you cannot use postcards or com-

puterized billing statements whose contents can be seen on the envelope. If you threaten to take legal action or turn the account over to a collection agency, you must follow through. You may not try to collect the debt from the patient if you know she is being represented by an attorney regarding the debt. When you are given written notice that the debtor refuses to pay or wants you to stop trying to collect, you can no longer communicate with the debtor except to serve notice that you are turning the account over to a collection agency or taking legal action.

Legal steps to collect must be taken within the time each state sets in its statute of limitations. Each state determines its own limits depending on the type of account: an account with only one charge (single-entry), an account with multiple charges made from time to time (open-book), and accounts where there is a written agreement for payments over a period of time (written contract).

Table 11.2 Collection Guidelines

- Always be calm and professional when discussing overdue accounts with customers.
- Analyze the account history and select the best approach for the particular patient.
- Make phone calls between 8 a.m. and 9 p.m. Monday through Friday. Saturday and Sunday calls may be considered inconvenient. Avoid calling at meal times.
- Vary the style and content of the collection letters and phone calls to the same patient.
- Do not send the patient a bill after you have turned the account over to a collection agency.
- Do not try to collect from the patient if you know he is represented by an attorney regarding the debt.
- Try not to antagonize the patient; always treat the patient with respect.

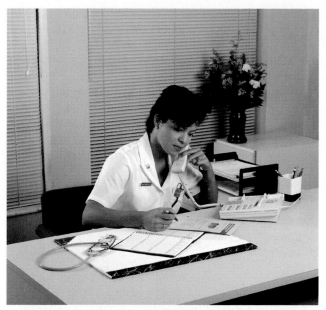

When making collection phone calls, make them in a private and quiet location, and review the history of the account before placing the call.

Table 11.2 provides some general guidelines for collecting debts.

COLLECTION PHONE CALLS When bills sent through the mail bring no response, sometimes a telephone call will work. This is the responsibility of the medical assistant. Before calling, you should take a few minutes to become familiar with the details of the account and decide on the best approach. Gather all necessary information. You will need pen and paper so that you can take notes. A tactful way to broach the subject is to say, "Hello, Mrs. Brown. I am (name) in Dr. Sutton's office. This is a courtesy call to remind you that we have not received payment for your last visit." Mrs. Brown may respond at this point by telling you why the bill has not been paid. If not, go on to explain that it is important to clear the account. Ask if she would like to charge it to her credit card or make other specific arrangements. (The conversation would continue, based on her response.) If you are unable to collect the total amount due, try to arrange for partial payment. Document the conversation. Procedure 11.3 outlines the steps you should follow when making a collection phone call.

Legal Issue

When you are trying to collect unpaid bills, be careful not to make an agreement with the patient that violates Truth in Lending Act regulations. As long as you bill the patient for the full amount each month and do not make explicit arrangements for payment in installments, you can accept partial payments.

Procedure 11.3

Making a Collection Phone Call

Purpose: To communicate effectively by telephone with a patient who has an overdue account.

Equipment/Supplies: Telephone, patient ledger card, paper, pen.

1 Inspect the patient's ledger card to familiarize yourself with the details of the account. *You will be better prepared to discuss the account with the customer if you know what the charges are for, what the insurance has paid, if anything, and how the patient has handled previous charges.*

2 Try to reach the patient at home first. ◉ NOTICE! If you call a patient at work, you must keep the reason for the call confidential.

3 Greet the patient and identify yourself.

4 State the reason for the call. Use a friendly but firm approach. ◉ NOTICE! The goal is to collect payment without antagonizing the patient.

5 Listen to what the patient has to say and try to find a mutually agreeable plan for payment. ◉ NOTICE! Avoid personal questions.

6 Take notes.

7 Be specific about the payment. Set a date when the payment is expected, and if the customer cannot pay the whole amount due, ask how much will be paid. ◉ NOTICE! Do not agree to an installment plan for payment without having the patient sign a Truth in Lending form. Instead, bill for the whole balance each month and ask the patient to pay as much as possible.

8 End the conversation by confirming the amount you will expect to be paid and the date by which you will expect it.

9 Document the conversation on the patient's ledger card.

10 Put a note in a tickler file to remind you when payment is expected. If it is not received, follow up with another call or letter.

COLLECTION LETTERS Letters are another means of communicating with the patient regarding unpaid bills. Form letters may be used that have spaces to fill in the amount owed and when it was due. A variety of letters may be stored on the computer and edited to include the customer's name and address, amount due, and length of time the bill is overdue. The medical assistant may be responsible for composing the letters, as well as sending them, but be sure the physician approves all letters before they are sent out. Each letter should be neatly printed on letterhead stationery and may be signed by the physician or the medical assistant, according to office policy. The tone of the letter and the message itself should be friendly and convey a desire for fairness. Use the best approach based on what you know about the individual and the way he has paid bills in the past. The letter should be brief and to the point. Never bully the patient; instead, try to gain her cooperation. Try to find out why she has not paid the bill. If the first letter goes unheeded, subsequent letters may be sent. The final letter should give a specific number of days before the account is turned over to a collection agency or suit is filed, as well as the date the action will be taken. If payment is not received, you *must* take the action described in your letter. Figure 11.7 shows examples of letters that are progressively firm in approach.

COLLECTION AGENCIES If the medical assistant is unable to collect a delinquent account, it may be turned over to a collection agency. The physician usually decides when a collection agency should be involved. Most agencies are paid on a **contingency fee basis**, receiving a percentage of the amount they recover. This can be quite expensive, so the medical assistant must make every effort to collect what is owed before this step is taken. The assistant must let the collection agency know what actions have been taken to collect the debt, including phone calls and letters. Once the account has been turned over to the collection agency, the physician's office must make no further attempts to collect. The patient must then deal with the collection agency, and it is illegal for the practice to send a bill to the patient at this point. In addition, the medical assistant must notify the collection agency when the physician's office receives a payment. Checks received from the agency should be posted to the patient's account.

SMALL CLAIMS COURT One option for collecting delinquent accounts is through small claims court. The cost is minor, and neither party is represented by an attorney. To file a suit in small claims court, the amount owed must not exceed the limit set by the state. The amount varies among states but is typically under $2,000. The medical assistant is responsible for obtaining a statement of claim form from the small claims court clerk, filling in the information, and returning it to the clerk. You and the patient will be notified when a court date is set. You may represent the physician in court and must be prepared to present evidence to the judge in the form of financial records, contracts, and copies of correspondence. One disadvantage of this method of recovering a bad debt is that even when the judge rules in the physician's favor, the problem of how to collect still remains. This may involve garnisheeing wages or putting a lien on the debtor's property. Specific information and instructions are available from the clerk of your local small claims court.

Special Collection Problems

Some collection problems will require special handling. These include the patient who cannot pay his bill, the patient who dies owing money to the practice, and the patient who moves leaving no forwarding address.

Bankruptcy

Occasionally, a patient who owes money to the physician will declare **bankruptcy** by filing a petition with the federal district court. Bankruptcy laws allow persons who cannot pay debts to resolve the debts through a supervised plan or to free themselves of financial obligations after their assets have been distributed. A person may petition for bankruptcy voluntarily, or creditors may force a debtor into involuntary bankruptcy. What happens next is determined by which section of the Bankruptcy Act applies. Assets may be liquidated and distributed among creditors, or the court may administer a plan to pay debts from future earnings over a period of time. Once the medical office is notified that a patient has filed for bankruptcy, it is illegal to send bills or try to collect from the patient. Instead, a claim must be made in the bankruptcy proceeding within the designated time limit.

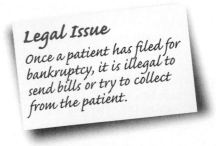

Legal Issue
Once a patient has filed for bankruptcy, it is illegal to send bills or try to collect from the patient.

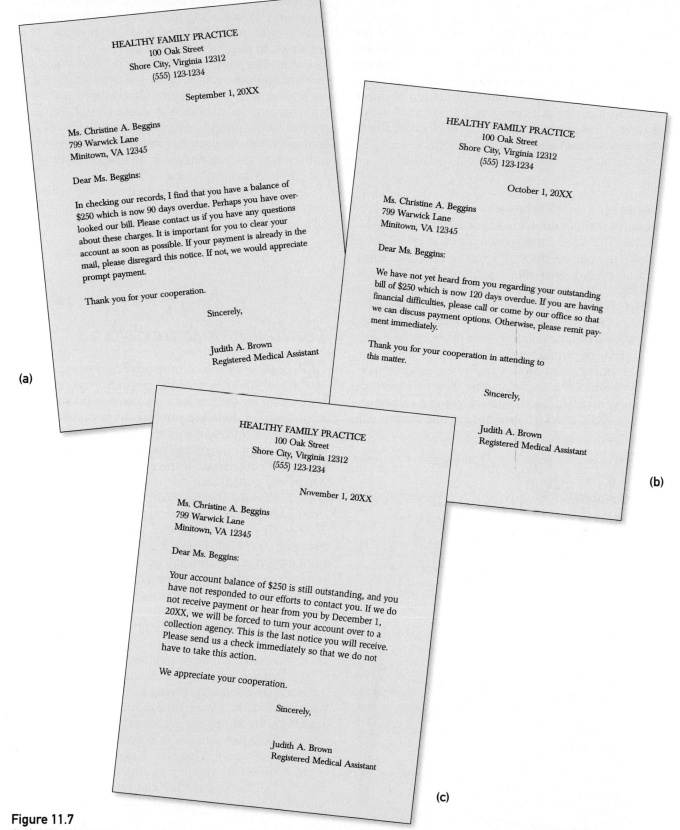

Figure 11.7
Collection Letters

(a) A courteous reminder that the bill is overdue. (b) A more urgent but still courteous demand for payment.
(c) Final notification indicating that action will be taken if the bill is not paid.

Deceased Patient

The debts of a person who dies are paid out of her estate by the executor (administrator) of the estate. The executor is named in the will, if the deceased has a will. If not, the probate court appoints an administrator. To collect unpaid medical bills, an itemized statement must be submitted to the executor within the time specified by state law. This limit varies among states but is typically three to four months.

Skips

Sometimes, a patient who owes money to the practice will move without notifying the office of the change of address. This may happen because of an oversight or because the patient is trying to avoid financial obligations. A person who moves without leaving a forwarding address to avoid paying a debt is referred to as a **skip**. When a bill is returned by the post office marked, "Return to Sender, Addressee Unknown," steps should be taken immediately to locate the patient and collect the money owed. First, call the home telephone number listed on the patient registration form. If it has been disconnected, a recording may refer you to a new number. Next, you might try calling the patient's work telephone number or the person who

was listed as the nearest relative not living in the same household. When trying to locate a person who owes money, you must identify yourself but not your employer, to anyone except the person you are trying to locate. You must not mention the debt—only the fact that you are trying to locate the person. Make only one call to each source. Other information on the registration form may be used in your investigation. Call the patient's insurance company to see if he is still covered and if the company has a new address. If you cannot contact the patient, it is advisable to turn the account over to a collection agency.

Occasionally, the physician may write off a bad debt instead of trying to collect in the interest of customer relations or when there are extenuating circumstances.

Challenging Situations

Because of their administrative and front office responsibilities, medical assistants may be responsible for talking with customers who are upset about charges. Whether you talk to the patient in person or on the telephone, you must respond to complaints in a calm, reasonable manner. Go over the charge for each service if there are any questions. Assure the patient that the fees are in line with what other physicians charge. You might explain that they must be high enough to cover overhead expenses, such as the cost of equipment, supplies, and personnel. You, as a medical assistant, do not have the authority to make any adjustments. If you cannot resolve the problem satisfactorily, refer the patient to the physician. Likewise, when a patient refuses to pay for medical services she has received, report the situation to the physician. Be sure to inform the physician of any patient complaints about the quality of the medical office's services.

If a patient refuses to pay because he feels that the service is or should be covered by insurance, the medical assistant should explain that it is the patient's responsibility to pay the doctor's office. The patient should direct concerns about coverage to the insurance company. However, if the patient says that a procedure wasn't performed and is being billed incorrectly, checking the file and resolving any discrepancies is your responsibility.

Technology Tip

Use the Internet to help find addresses and telephone numbers. Searches can be made at the following websites:

- www.aol.com — Click on "People," then on "AOL White Pages."
- www.excite.com — Click on "People Finder."
- www.hotbot.com — Click on "White Pages."
- www.yahoo.com — Click on "People Search."
- www2.switchboard.com — Click on "People Search."

Follow the directions for entering information. Searches can be made in cities, states, or nationwide.

Clinical Summary

- Physicians set their fees based on input from health insurance companies and government health programs.
- Office employees have an obligation to help control costs by using time wisely, not wasting supplies, and taking proper care of equipment.
- Fee schedules are sources of information for patients and medical assistants.
- Patients can be made aware of payment policies by incorporating them in an information sheet for new and existing customers.
- Payment for medical services before the patient leaves the office should be encouraged.
- Payment options include cash, checks, and credit cards in most offices.
- A disclosure form must be completed and signed when the physician and patient agree on an installment plan for payment.
- Information on the patient registration form is useful in collecting delinquent accounts.
- An established procedure should be followed when trying to collect delinquent accounts.
- The medical assistant's duties include making collection phone calls and sending collection letters for overdue bills.
- Once an account has been turned over to a collection agency, it is illegal for the medical office to bill the patient.
- When a person files for bankruptcy, assets may be liquidated and distributed among creditors, or the court may administer a plan to pay debts from future earnings over a period of time.
- If you cannot locate a "skip," it is advisable to turn the account over to a collection agency.
- Consumer protection laws must be observed when trying to collect debts.

The Language of Medicine

aging accounts report A list of overdue accounts showing the length of time each one is overdue based on the date of the transaction.

annual percentage rate The true interest rate of a debt based on the unpaid balance.

bankruptcy A legal proceeding that allows a debtor to free himself of financial obligations or resolve debts through a supervised plan.

bilateral agreement An agreement between two parties.

contingency fee basis A fee based on successful completion of a job.

cycle billing Distribution of billing throughout the month based on the patients' last names.

deferred payment price Total cost including finance charges.

Equal Credit Opportunity Act A federal law prohibiting discrimination against persons seeking credit.

fee schedule A list of services and procedures that a physician usually performs, with the amount charged for each.

finance charge The cost of credit.

patient ledger cards Individual patient account records.

practice information sheet Information for patients about office hours, payment policies, emergency procedures, and other aspects of the medical practice.

professional courtesy The practice of treating colleagues or employees at no charge or a reduced rate.

Resource-Based Relative Value Scale (RBRVS) A system of determining medical fees developed by the federal government in which each service is assigned a unit value based on time, skill, expenses involved, and geographic location.

skip A person who moves without leaving a forwarding address to avoid paying a debt.

tickler file A system the medical assistant can use as a reminder of time-sensitive activities such as sending or paying bills.

Truth in Lending Act Regulation Z of the federal Consumer Protection Act, protecting consumers who use credit.

Truth in Lending Disclosure Statement A written agreement between the physician and patient stating the terms under which a fee will be paid in more than four installments.

Signs/Symptoms of Progress

Recall, Question, Connect

Recall
How are fees for medical services and procedures determined?

Question
What questions do you have about fees for medical services and procedures?

Connect
What can you as a medical assistant do to keep medical costs down?

Educating the Patient

Dianne Davis is a new patient who came in for a physical examination. The charge for the visit is $170. Office policy states that patients must pay for the visit at the time of service. Ms. Davis states after being examined that she was unaware of the policy and considers the fee excessive.

1 What would you say to her about the amount of the fee?
2 What measures should have been taken to make sure she knew the fee was due at the time of the office visit?

3 What suggestions could you make regarding the method of payment?

Exploring Perspectives in Teams

Perspective involves the discipline of examining how ideas look from different points of view and recognizing that there are often multiple "answers" to complex questions. In small groups or on your own, reflect on possible alternative views or answers and summarize your findings.

1 Don Dinkin's account shows a balance of $125 that is 60 days overdue. When you call his home, there is no answer. When you try his office, someone there asks why you are calling. How should you answer this question? When you finally reach Mr. Dinkin, what is the best way to approach him and explain the purpose of your call?
2 Research the rules for filing bankruptcy. How does bankruptcy affect outstanding medical bills? Why should bankruptcy be considered a last resort?
3 Explain the purpose of the Fair Debt Collection Practices Act. From the patient's (consumer's) point of view, what situations might demonstrate a need for these laws? How do these laws affect the medical assistant who is trying to collect unpaid medical bills?

Learning Outcomes

- Describe different types of health insurance coverage.
- Use the terminology of insurance correctly.
- Differentiate between different kinds of insurance codes and their use.
- Prepare and file insurance claims using correct codes.
- Process insurance payments.
- Identify reasons why claims are rejected.
- Recognize ways to effectively monitor delinquent claims.

Performance Objectives

- Apply third-party guidelines.
- Obtain reimbursement through accurate claims submission.
- Monitor third-party reimbursement.
- Manage renewals of business and professional insurance policies.

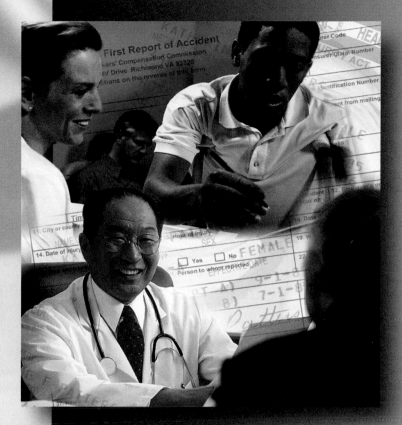

Health insurance coverage for every American has been a major political issue for many years, and Congress is constantly considering changes in the healthcare system. Federal programs have been established to help pay for healthcare for the elderly and the poor. Companies began offering healthcare coverage as a benefit for employees in the 1940s. With the high cost of medical care, it has become necessary to protect one's financial assets from the ruin that a significant health problem could cause. As a result, a large majority of the patients who seek medical services have some type of medical insurance coverage.

The medical assistant responsible for filing and maintaining insurance claims is expected to be the office expert when it comes to questions about insurance, how to file claims, and how much leading insurers can be expected to pay. The assistant's duties include obtaining information about coverage from the office's patients, obtaining the necessary claim forms, extracting pertinent information from the

12

Processing Insurance Claims

medical record, using insurance codes correctly, preparing and filing insurance claims, following up on unpaid claims, and processing payments. Proficiency in these skills enhances job opportunities for the medical assistant. A knowledge of medical terminology, anatomy and physiology, pathophysiology (the study of diseases), and diagnostic and treatment procedures is needed when processing insurance claims, along with excellent computer skills. Handling insurance in the medical office is a complicated process that requires the medical assistant to keep up with constantly changing insurance plans and filing rules, as well as the technology that makes it possible to file claims electronically.

Patient Concerns

*T*he patient is responsible for the payment of medical bills that are not covered by *insurance. Naturally, when insurance claims are rejected or payment is delayed because of processing errors, the patient feels some distress and anxiety and may suffer financially. The medical assistant can promote good customer relations by filing claims correctly and promptly. When claim forms are filled in completely and accurately, the physician will usually be compensated by the insurance company within a reasonable length of time. The medical assistant can investigate delayed settlements and rejected claims or assist the customer in appealing a denial of benefits.*

A History of Health Insurance and Key Terminology

Insurance is a contract through which one party agrees to compensate or reimburse another for any loss due to a specified cause. A person who buys automobile collision insurance, for example, has a contract with the insurer that covers reimbursement for damage to the vehicle if it is involved in an accident. For a patient protected by health insurance, the insurance company pays all or part of the cost of medical treatment. Health insurance in this country started in the mid-1800s and was intended as an income replacement for victims of accidents and certain diseases. Insurance coverage for hospital expenses began in 1929 when a group of schoolteachers in Texas contracted with a hospital to guarantee 21 days of hospital care for $6 a year. The idea proved to be popular,

and other groups of employees joined the plan, which later became known as the Blue Cross Plan. When wages were frozen during World War II, companies began to offer group health insurance to their workers as a fringe benefit. What began as a plan to protect patients from the major costs of hospitalization later expanded to include coverage for medical services in the physician's office and procedures to promote wellness. Government plans to cover the treatment of military dependents by civilian doctors, and to provide health insurance for the elderly, the indigent, and the disabled were established. Today, medical insurance is a large industry that serves as the major source of income for physicians, hospitals, and other healthcare providers.

As in any industry, there are special words that apply to insurance. The medical assistant must understand these common terms used in discussing insurance with customers and filing claims with insurance companies. Table 12.1 lists key insurance industry words and phrases.

Table 12.1 Insurance Terms

assignment of benefits	Agreement by the patient to the insurance company's payment of benefits directly to the physician.
beneficiary	A person designated by an insurance policy to receive benefits or funds.
benefits	Payments made by an insurance company.
carrier (insurer, underwriter)	The insurance company that contracts to pay benefits to the insured in the event of illness, injury, damage, or loss.
claim	A request for payment from an insurance carrier.
coding	Translating a diagnosis or procedure into numeric designations.
coinsurance	An arrangement whereby the patient pays a percentage of the cost of medical care and the insurer pays the rest.
coordination of benefits	The process of preventing duplication of payment when a patient is covered under more than one insurance plan so that the benefits received from the combined policies do not exceed 100% of the covered benefits.
copayment	An arrangement in which the patient pays a fixed fee when medical service is rendered and the insurer pays the remainder of the cost.
deductible	The amount the patient must pay before insurance begins paying for medical services.

(continues)

Table 12.1 Insurance Terms (continued)

elective procedures	Optional procedures that are not medically necessary.
exclusions	Conditions and circumstances for which the insurance company will not pay benefits.
explanation of benefits	A detailed explanation of the payments made for each charge submitted, which is sent to the patient and the provider. It indicates approved charges and amounts applied to the deductible, as well as any charge denied by the carrier.
fiscal agent	An organization with a contract to process claims for Medicaid, Medicare, or CHAMPUS; also call a fiscal intermediary.
indemnity	Compensation paid by an insurance carrier for damage, loss, or services rendered.
insured	Person or organization covered by an insurance policy.
insurer	Company or underwriter that provides insurance coverage.
preauthorization (precertification)	Approval or authorization obtained before a course of treatment.
pre-existing condition	A condition or disease that was present before an insurance policy was issued.
premium	Fee paid periodically to keep the insurance in force.
primary payer	The insurance company or health plan that assumes initial responsibility for paying benefits when the patient is covered by more than one plan.
provider	A person, organization, or institution that delivers healthcare services.
secondary payer	The insurance carrier that pays benefits after the primary payer pays the portion of the bill it is responsible for.
subscriber (policyholder)	The person who takes out an insurance policy or is covered through an employer.
waiting period	The time that must pass before a subscriber's pre-existing condition will be covered by an insurance policy.

Health Insurance Options

Health insurance can be obtained in three ways: participating in a group plan, buying a health insurance policy on an individual basis, or enrolling in a prepaid health plan.

When employers contract with an insurer to provide protection for workers and their dependents, a master policy covers all employees, and the coverage is the same for each participant. Some organizations also offer group plans to their members. Group insurance rates are usually lower than the rates an individual can obtain. Each person in the group is given an identification card (certificate of insurance) showing that he or she is covered and providing information such as the policy number, the names of the covered parties, and basic cost information. If circumstances change, an individual who is no longer eligible under the group contract may convert to an individual policy with the same insurer if the group contract has a conversion privilege clause. The federal COBRA act of 1986 requires that coverage be extended at group rates for up to 18 months to employees who are laid off or who terminate their employment. Extensions are also given to certain dependents in case of divorce or the death of the employee.

Many companies offer health insurance policies that individuals can buy to cover themselves and their families, though there may be some requirements or coverage limitations. A physical exam is usually necessary, and pre-existing conditions may be excluded from coverage or covered only after a specified period of time.

In prepaid health plans, subscribers pay a monthly or yearly fee in exchange for hospital, surgical, and medical benefits. Usually, the patient makes a small copayment at the time of service.

Types of Healthcare Plans

The first step in insurance billing is to obtain accurate and up-to-date information from the patient regarding coverage. Because so many plans and options are available, patients may not understand what their policy covers. The medical assistant should encourage patients to read the information booklet the insurer provides so that they are aware of benefits and can be sure the policy meets their needs. The medical assistant should help explain the policy information if necessary.

Blue Cross/Blue Shield

Blue Cross/Blue Shield is a nationwide association of independent insurers that operate primarily under state laws as non-profit organizations, although some have recently formed for-profit corporations and are traded on a stock exchange. Blue Cross was initially established to provide coverage for hospital expenses, while Blue Shield plans covered physicians' services. Now, however, both offer full healthcare coverage for their subscribers. In most states, they have become a single corporation, although in some they remain separate.

The Blue Shield concept began when employers in lumber and mining camps in the Pacific Northwest paid physicians a monthly fee to provide care for their workers. This evolved into "medical service bureaus" made up of groups of physicians. The Blue Cross Association and the National Association of Blue Shield Plans merged in 1982 to form the Blue Cross and Blue Shield Association.

A variety of plans are offered through Blue Cross/Blue Shield, including individual and family, group, preventive care, and managed care plans.

Health Maintenance Organization (HMO)

A **Health Maintenance Organization (HMO)** is a prepaid, **managed care** plan that covers hospital and physicians' services. Members must use participating providers and are enrolled for a specific period of time. Medical services are provided at an HMO-owned medical center or by a group of physicians who contract with the HMO to provide medical care. There are four basic types of HMOs.

- Staff: Medical services are delivered at HMO-owned centers by physicians who are salaried employees of the HMO or salaried employees of a specially formed group practice within the HMO.
- Group: Care is delivered in HMO-owned centers or clinics either by salaried physicians who belong to a legally separate medical group that serves only the HMO (closed panel) or where the HMO contracts for services with an existing independent group of physicians (open panel).
- Independent Practice Association: A group of physicians and other providers contract to provide services on a **fee-for-service** or **capitation** (uniform payment for each person) basis. The physicians practice in their own offices, are not employees of the HMO, and treat other patients as well as HMO members. Most HMO plans fall in this category.
- Network: An HMO contracts with a "network" of medical groups or medical clinics to provide services.

With many HMOs, the patient must choose a **primary care physician (PCP)** who is a part of the network. This physician is a **"gatekeeper"** who must arrange for specialists or hospitalization when needed. The PCP is usually a family practitioner, pediatrician, or obstetrician. HMO members are allowed unlimited visits to the primary care physician but are responsible for a copayment each time they receive service, which helps to control costs. When physicians are paid on a per-patient basis out of funds collected as premiums by

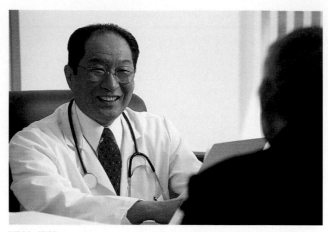

Within HMOs, a primary care physician provides care but also provides referrals for the patient to see a specialist or for hospitalization when necessary.

the organization that markets the health plan, a percentage of the fee may be withheld until the end of the year to cover operating costs. This serves as an incentive for the physicians to control costs, since they share any surplus funds.

HMOs are regulated by the Health Maintenance Organization Assistance Act of 1973 which provides financial support for the establishment of new HMOs that meet federal standards. To qualify, an HMO must provide certain basic benefits which include preventive healthcare, treatment for substance abuse, outpatient mental health services, and family planning services, as well as the usual hospital and physician services. The act requires businesses with 25 or more employees to make HMOs available to their employees as an alternative to other health insurance plans, and limits copayment amounts. Most HMO members are covered under a group plan through their employer.

Customer Service

Post a sign in the reception area urging patients to show their insurance cards to the receptionist when they check in for an appointment. When checking in a patient, the medical assistant should confirm that the patient's insurance will cover the appointment. If the patient is insured by a PPO, inform the patient if the physician is not a member of that network.

Preferred Provider Organization (PPO)

A **Preferred Provider Organization** is much like an HMO except that persons enrolled in a PPO plan can receive some benefits even if they seek medical care from physicians who are not part of the plan. HMO members are limited to health service providers who have agreements with the HMO, except in emergencies. PPOs contract with selected physicians, hospitals, and others to provide healthcare services at discounted rates in return for prompt payment. An insured who chooses a doctor not on the list of PPO member providers must usually pay a coinsurance of 20%–25%. This is intended to discourage patients from using providers outside the defined healthcare network.

Indemnity Health Insurance

Indemnity health insurance refers to the traditional health insurance plans that are designed to cover major medical expenses with coinsurance paid by the individual. It may be purchased on an individual basis from an insurance company or may be offered under a group policy through an employer or organization. This kind of insurance is more expensive for the patient than some other plans because a deductible amount must be met before the insurance begins paying for services. The deductible varies among insurance companies but often ranges from $200–$500. Claims are filed for services even when the insurance company is not expected to pay because they serve as a record of the patient's payments up to the deductible amount. Once the deductible has been met, the insurance pays the percentage of the cost stated in the policy, and the patient pays the rest. For example, if the charge for the service is $120, the insurance might pay $96 (80%) and the patient would pay $24 (20%).

To control costs, insurance companies establish **usual, customary, and reasonable rates (UCR)**. This is the maximum amount the company will pay for a service and is based on the prevailing fees in a geographic area. If a physician charges more than the "usual, customary, and reasonable" amount for a service, the patient is responsible for the difference.

Most indemnity policies set a maximum out-of-pocket amount that the insured pays each year. After that figure is reached, the insurer pays 100% of the covered expenses incurred.

Medicare

Medicare is a national health insurance program for persons who are 65 or older, disabled, on kidney dialysis, or have kidney transplants. It was introduced in 1966 and is administered by the Health Care Financing Administration (HCFA), a federal agency in the Department of Health and Human Services. Coverage under Medicare is divided into two categories: Part A and Part B.

Medicare Part A covers inpatient hospital treatment and also helps pay for care in a skilled nursing facility, skilled healthcare at home, hospice care for the terminally ill, and blood after the first three pints. There is no premium for those who are receiving retirement benefits from Social Security or the Railroad Retirement Board or who are eligible to receive these benefits. The patient is responsible for paying the coinsurance, which varies according to the length of stay.

Medicare Part B is medical insurance that helps pay for services in a doctor's office, hospital, or nursing home; outpatient hospital care; x-rays and laboratory tests; various other medical services; and certain medical equipment prescribed by a doctor for use at home. Part B picks up where Part A leaves off. It is optional, and participants must pay a monthly fee for this coverage which is deducted from their Social Security or Railroad Retirement check.

Enrollment in both Medicare parts is automatic for those who are receiving Social Security or Railroad Retirement benefits when they become 65 years old. Part B must be canceled if it is not wanted. Others must apply for this coverage. Participants are given an identification card showing what coverage they have, a Medicare claim number, and the date coverage began.

In some areas, persons covered by Medicare can choose a fee-for-service plan or a managed care plan. Those who choose fee-for-service can seek care from almost any healthcare provider, and Medicare will pay its share of the bill. Under a managed care plan, the patient must use healthcare providers that are a part of the plan, except in emergencies. Plans vary from one

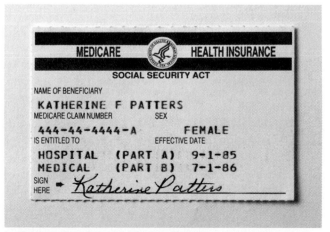

The Medicare ID card provides important information such as the patient's name, the claim number, the type of coverage (Part A and/or Part B), and the effective dates for the coverage.

area to another but usually involve a monthly premium and a copayment whenever service is provided.

Medicare claims must be filed with **Medicare intermediaries** or carriers. These are private insurance companies that have a contract with the federal government to handle Medicare claims. Carriers vary from one state to another, and sometimes, there are different carriers in different parts of the state. Some major carriers that operate in several states are Blue Cross/Blue Shield, MetraHealth, Aetna Life Insurance, CIGNA, and Xact Medicare Services.

When a physician "accepts assignment" for Medicare, the practice agrees to accept the amount approved for a particular service and will not charge the patient more than the 20% coinsurance. Physicians who do not accept assignment must, by law, limit their fees to no more than 15% above the amount approved by Medicare. Non-participating physicians must notify patients in writing of the estimated charge, estimated Medicare allowable charge, and the difference between the two in advance of elective surgery. An example of a blank form for informing a patient of

an estimated surgical charge is provided in Figure 12.1. Under the direction of the physician, the medical assistant will need to fill out this form and obtain the necessary signatures. Similarly, any doctor who provides services that Medicare may determine to be unnecessary should notify the patient in writing before performing the service.

Medicare may be the primary or secondary payer. If an eligible patient is covered under an employer's group health insurance or a liability plan, Medicare becomes the secondary payer. For example, if a 68-year-old man covered by Medicare slipped and fell in a puddle of spilled liquid while shopping in a grocery store, the store's liability policy would be the primary payer and Medicare would be the secondary payer. In such cases, you would file a claim with the primary payer. A patient questionnaire such as the one shown in Figure 12.2 can help you determine which insurer to bill first. After payment is received, you would file a Medicare claim and attach a copy of the payment report or check. Mark or stamp in red "Medicare Secondary Payer" on the front of the form. Do not bill

Figure 12.1
Medicare Estimate of Surgical Charges Form

This form is used to inform a Medicare patient of the estimated cost of a surgical procedure and the portion of that cost that Medicare is expected to pay.

In accordance with Medicare regulations, the following estimate of surgical charges is hereby submitted:

Patient _____

Address _____

City _____ State _____ ZIP _____

Proposed surgical procedure(s) _____

    Estimated charge $_____

    Estimated Medicare payment $_____

    Estimated payment by patient $_____

This estimate is based on the planned surgical procedure(s) listed above, and does not include any modifications that might be necessary at the time of the actual surgery.

Signature of provider _____ Date _____

I have received the information concerning the surgery specified above and understand my financial obligations with respect to the estimated charges. I understand that changes in the surgical procedure(s) may need to be made at the time of surgery and additional charges may be necessary.

Signature of patient _____ Date _____

Please answer the following questions to help us in determining who is responsible for coverage of your medical expenses.

1. Is your injury or illness due to any of the following? Please check the items that apply.
   _____ a work-related accident or condition
   _____ a condition covered under the Federal Black Lung Program
   _____ an automobile accident
   _____ an accident other than an automobile accident
   _____ the fault of another party
   If you have checked any of the above, please explain briefly.

   _____

   _____

2. Are you eligible for coverage under the Veteran's Administration?　　　　　　　Yes _____ No _____

3. Are you eligible for coverage under the United Mine Workers of America?　　　　　Yes _____ No _____

4. Are you employed?　　　　　　　　　　　Yes _____ No _____
   Do you have coverage under an employer group health insurance plan?　　　　　　Yes _____ No _____

5. Is your spouse employed?　　　　　　　　Yes _____ No _____
   Do you have coverage under your spouse's employer group health insurance plan?　　Yes _____ No _____

6. Are you a dependent covered under a parent or guardian's employer group health insurance plan?　Yes _____ No _____

Figure 12.2
Insurance Eligibility Questionnaire

This form will help you determine who is the primary payer and who is the secondary payer for a patient's medical claim.

Medicare and another insurer for the same service at the same time.

The time limit for filing Medicare claims is the last day of the year following the year of service. The physician may be penalized by a fine, reduction in payment, or loss of compensation for sending in claims after the deadline. Medicare claims are submitted on form HCFA-1500.

Working Smart
Medicare claims are due by the last day of the year following the year of service. File all claims promptly.

Medicaid

Medicaid is a program that provides medical assistance for the needy and disabled persons in long-term care nursing facilities. The program became law in 1965 under Title XIX of the Social Security Act. It is jointly funded by state and federal governments. Each state administers its own program and establishes its own eligibility standards. The services covered and the payment rates vary from one state to another. Some states use a managed care plan. The physician, if he decides to treat Medicaid patients, cannot be selective

in treating them on a case-by-case basis. Also, this physician must accept the Medicaid compensation as payment in full.

Potential participants in the program must apply at their local welfare office. If accepted, they are given a form or card verifying the dates of eligibility. Identification cards are issued periodically, sometimes as often as twice a month in some states, so it is important for you to check the expiration date of the card each time the patient visits the office. Prior authorization is needed for some services.

Working Smart
Check the expiration date on all patients' insurance cards, especially Medicaid cards. Since Medicaid identification cards are issued very frequently by some states, it is important to check the expiration date on the card each time a Medicaid patient visits the office.

Claims for Medicaid reimbursement are submitted to the fiscal agent in your area or, in some cases, to the local department of social services. When a patient who is covered under Medicaid is also covered under another health insurance plan, the other plan is designated as the primary carrier and must be billed first. Medicaid becomes the secondary carrier and is billed next. Claims for a patient covered by both Medicare and Medicaid are sent to Medicare as the primary carrier. After Medicare has processed the claim, it will be transferred automatically for processing by Medicaid.

Medigap

Medigap is a health insurance plan offered by private entities that is designed specifically to supplement Medicare benefits by filling in gaps not paid by Medicare. It may pay for deductibles or coinsurance as well as some services. Companies that offer Medigap insurance must be approved by Medicare and are regulated by Medicare laws. When the medical assistant files Medicare claims for patients who are covered by Medigap insurance, an authorization signed by the patient should be sent in with the claim instructing Medicare to forward bills for services that it does not cover to the Medigap insurer. This is known as a **crossover claim** and eliminates the need for the provider to submit a separate claim for Medigap. Your local Medicare contractor keeps a list of companies authorized to offer Medigap policies.

CHAMPUS/TRICARE/CHAMPVA

CHAMPUS (Civilian Health and Medical Program of the Uniformed Services) is a government program that covers dependents of active duty and retired military personnel, military retirees, and dependents of members of the military who died while on active duty. Administered by the Office for the Civilian Health and Medical Program of the Uniformed Services (OCHAMPUS), it provides for treatment in civilian healthcare facilities or by private physicians, and is designed to supplement the healthcare services available at military-owned hospitals. Service members on active duty are not covered.

Patients living within 40 miles of a military treatment facility must obtain authorization from the military hospital stating that it cannot provide the services needed (Nonavailability Statement, Form 1251) before they can seek treatment from civilian providers. The forms are entered into the Defense Enrollment Eligibility Reporting System (DEERS), a computerized database, for claims processing. The patient is usually responsible for a copayment or deductible amount.

Dependents who are age 10 or older must have a CHAMPUS identification and privilege card; others can use a parent's card. Both sides of the card should be photocopied for office records.

TRICARE is a managed care program that is being phased in to help control costs and standardize benefits for CHAMPUS members. There are three options: TRICARE Standard, TRICARE Prime, and TRICARE Extra. The TRICARE Standard plan is the same as CHAMPUS. The patient is responsible for the deductible and a percentage of the cost of care. TRICARE Prime is an HMO-style plan that offers standard services plus preventive care such as periodic physicals and immunizations. Participants must enroll and pay an annual fee (except for families of active duty personnel). A physician chosen or assigned as a primary care manager provides care and makes referrals when necessary. TRICARE Extra is a PPO with reduced rates offered for services from providers who are part of its network. Service is on a visit-by-visit basis, and there is no annual fee.

CHAMPVA (Civilian Health and Medical Program of the Veterans Administration) is much like the CHAMPUS program except that it covers dependents of veterans with total, permanent, service-related disabilities (or survivors of veterans who died as a result of such disabilities) who are not eligible for CHAMPUS. Claims are filed on the same form as Medicare. Contact the nearest military hospital or medical clinic if you have questions or need more information.

Worker's Compensation Insurance

Worker's compensation insurance provides benefits for employees suffering from job-related accident or illness, and their dependents. Benefits include providing an income when the employee is unable to work as a result of the accident or illness, as well as compensation for medical care. Federal laws cover coal miners, longshoremen, workers employed by the federal government, and workers in the District of Columbia. All other workers are covered under state laws, which vary.

Some states require employers to insure workers through a state fund, while others let employers buy insurance from private companies. Premiums are paid by the employer. Some employers may qualify as self-insurers.

There are three kinds of worker's compensation claims: non-disability, temporary disability, and permanent disability. Non-disability claims are made when the employee sees a doctor but the injury or illness is

Legal Issue

If a medical clinic agrees to treat Medicaid patients, Medicaid reimbursement must be accepted as payment in full.

not serious enough to prevent her from working. Temporary disability claims pertain to conditions that prevent the employee from working for a period of time, while permanent disability claims involve impairment that prevents the worker from returning to work.

When a physician treats a patient who is already a customer of the practice for an injury or illness covered by worker's compensation, a separate medical record and ledger should be set up. Only the information and charges regarding the current condition should be recorded in the new record. This protects patient confidentiality, since claims adjusters and employers are allowed access to records pertaining to a covered injury.

The patient covered by worker's compensation should bring authorization for treatment under the plan from his employer to the physician's office. The employer must complete a First Report of Accident form (Figure 12.3), and the physician must complete the first medical treatment report within the time limit the state requires. Figure 12.4 shows an example of the physician's report. Some states require that the form be sent in immediately, while others allow a few days. Contact your state worker's compensation commission to determine the state regulations and for instructions on obtaining forms. If treatment is prolonged, a monthly progress report and bill should be sent to the state fund or private insurance company. The physician may be required to sign a release form similar to the one shown in Figure 12.5 before the patient can return to work.

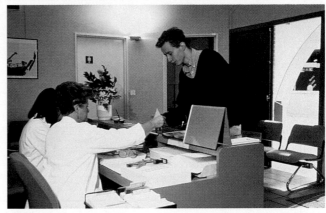

Insurance information must be checked with the patient to make sure the office records are up-to-date. A patient's claim cannot be processed efficiently without having current information.

Billing Requirements

Insurance plans provide a significant portion of the income for most medical practices. For this reason, most physicians encourage the office staff to assist patients by processing insurance claims for them to make the process of reimbursement easier for the patient. Even offices with a policy of collecting the full fee from patients should still give them the information needed to file claims themselves.

When filing claims for reimbursement from insurance companies, you must be sure to have all the information necessary to expedite the process. Claims that are returned because of inaccurate or incomplete information cause extra work for you and delay the payment of benefits.

Patient Information

The claim process begins when the patient comes into the office. Each new patient should complete a registration form, which should be updated annually and verified at each office visit. The form should contain employment and insurance information as well as demographic data. Ask for an insurance identification card, check its expiration date, and photocopy both sides. When you greet the patient on subsequent visits, ask if the insurance coverage has changed. If so, update your records by photocopying the new card and noting the change.

Insurance Provider Information

The identification card issued to patients by their insurance provider will tell you the policy number, type of coverage, address for mailing in claims, and telephone number for verifying eligibility, obtaining precertification (prior approval that a service will be covered), and asking questions about claims. Do not hesitate to call the insurance company if you are in doubt about benefits or coverage. A medical assistant cannot be expected to know everything about insurance, but she should know where to find answers and information.

Some patients may be covered by more than one insurance plan. Be sure to obtain information about all insurance coverage. Most policies include a coordination of benefits statement that prevents duplication of payments by different insurers for the same service. The primary insurance is billed first, and charges it does not pay are billed to the secondary carrier. When children are covered under

Working Smart

Be sure to document in the patient's medical record when prior approval (precertification) is obtained from the insurer.

Employer's First Report of Accident

Virginia Workers' Compensation Commission
1000 DMV Drive Richmond VA 23320
See instructions on the reverse of this form.

The boxes to the right are for the use of the insurer	VWC File Number	Reason for filing
	Insurer Code	Insurer location
	Insurer Claim Number	

Employer

1. Name of employer	2. Federal Tax Identification Number 3. Employer's Case No. (if applicable)
4. Mailing address	5. Location (if different from mailing address)
6. Parent Corporation (if applicable)	7. Nature of business
8. Insurer (name and location)	9. Policy number 10. Effective date

Time and Place of Accident

11. City or county where accident occurred	Did accident occur on	12. Employer's premises? ☐ Yes ☐ No	13. State property? ☐ Yes ☐ No
14. Date of injury 15. Hour of injury	16. Date of incapacity	17. Hour of incapacity	
18. Was employee paid in full for day of injury? ☐ Yes ☐ No	19. Was employee paid in full for day incapactiy began? ☐ Yes ☐ No		
20. Date injury or illness reported 21. Person to whom reported	22. Name of other witness	23. If fatal, give date of death	

Employee

24. Name of employee (Last, First, Middle)	25. Phone number	26. Sex ☐ Male ☐ Female
27. Address	28. Date of birth	29. Marital status ☐ Single ☐ Divorced
	30. Social security number	☐ Married ☐ Widowed
31. Occupation at time of injury or illness	32. Department	33. Number of dependent children
34. How long in current job? 35. How long with current employer?	36. Was employee paid on a piecework or hourly basis? ☐ Piece work ☐ Hourly	
37. Hours worked per day 38. Days worked per week	39. Value of perquisites per week	
40. Wages per hour $ 41. Earnings per week (inc. overtime) $	Food/meal $ Lodging $ Tips $ Other $	

Nature and Cause of Accident

42. Machine, tool, or object causing injury or illness	43. Specify part of machine, etc.	Were safeguards or safety equipment	44. Provided? ☐ Yes ☐ No
46. Describe fully how injury or illness occurred			45. Utilized? ☐ Yes ☐ No

47. Describe nature of injury or illness, including parts of body affected

48. Physician (name and address)	49. Hospital (name and address)		
50. Probable length of disability	51. Has employee returned to work? ☐ Yes ☐ No	If yes 52. At what wage? $	53. On what date?
54. EMPLOYER: prepared by (name, signature, title)	55. Date	56. Phone number	
57. INSURER: processed by	58. Date	59. Phone number	

This report is required by the Virginia Workers' Compensation Act

First Report of Accident
VWC Form No. 3 (rev. 10/1/91)

Figure 12.3
Employer's First Report of Accident

This form is from the Virginia Workers' Compensation Commission. Each state has its own form.

Attending Physician's Report

Virginia Workers' Compensation Commission
1000 DMV Drive Richmond VA 23220
See instructions on the reverse of this form.

The boxes to the right are for the use of the insurer	Reserved	VWC file number
	Insurer code	Insurer location
	Insurer claim number	

Employee

1. Patient's name BARNABY HILTON

2. Phone number (757) 555-1111

3. Address 228 PINE STREET HANLEY VA 20000

4. Date of birth

5. Sex [X] Male [ ] Female

6. Social security number

Background Information

7. Name of employer HOME CONSTRUCTION INC

8. Address of employer 1100 INDUSTRIAL ROAD HANLEY VA 11122

9. Date of injury or illness 09/08/XX

10. Patient's account of how injury or exposure to occupational disease occurred

Patient states, "I was closing a big warehouse door and lost my balance.
I fell and caught myself with my left hand."

11. Date of first visit 09/08/XX

12. Date of discharge

13. Person authorizing treatment

Findings and Diagnosis

14. Findings upon examination, including results of x-rays, laboratory studies, etc. Please note any prior injuries and pre-existing conditions. Provide additional comments on the reverse side of this form.

Pain, swelling, and contusion of left forearm. X-ray showed a simple fracture of the distal end of the left radius.

15. Diagnosis

Simple fracture left radius, distal end.

16. Is diagnosed condition due to the occurrence described by the patient? [X] Yes [ ] No [ ] Unknown

17. Nature of treatment

Closed reduction of fracture and cast application.

18. Dates of your treatment 09/08/XX

19. Provide names and addresses of other health care providers to whom patient was referred

20. Was there any fracture or amputation? [X] Yes [ ] No [ ] Unknown

21. Please describe (If yes) Simple fracture distal end of left radius.

22. Was there disability for work? [X] Yes [ ] No [ ] Unknown

23. Date disability began (If yes) 09/08/XX

24. Date able to return to light work

25. Date able to return to regular work

26. Will there be any permanent defect or disfigurement? [ ] Yes [X] No [ ] Unknown

27. Please describe (If yes)

28. Has patient reached maximum medical improvement? [ ] Yes [X] No

Attending Physician

29. Name of attending physician JOHN DOE MD

30. Address 333 MEDICAL WAY HANLEY VA 01234

31. Date of this report 09/09/XX

I certify that I personally examined and treated this patient

Signature *John Doe* M.D.

This report is required by the Virginia Workers' Compensation Act

Attending Physician's Report
VWC Form No. 6 (rev. 10/1/91)

Figure 12.4
Attending Physician's Report

This form is from the Virginia Workers' Compensation Commission. Each state has its own form.

Figure 12.5
Physician's Release to Return to Work Form

I have examined _____ and do hereby certify that, as
(Name of Patient)

of _____ , he or she is medically able to return to work subject to the
(Date)

following restrictions, if any:

_____ NO RESTRICTIONS on usual and customary work
activities due to the injury or its residual effects.

_____ Work activities to be RESTRICTED as follows:

_____

_____

_____   _____
(Physician's Signature)   (Date)

Physician's Name _____

Address _____

_____

Phone No. _____

both parents' insurance plans, the birthday rule has been adopted in most states. Under this rule, the insurance plan of the parent whose birthday falls earliest in the year would be the primary carrier, while that of the other parent would be the secondary carrier.

Permission to Release Information

The information in a patient's medical record that relates to treatment and conditions is considered "privileged" and must be kept confidential. It cannot be released, even to the insurance company, without the patient's permission. The patient must give the medical office written permission to release the information for filing a claim. This signed release of information form should be kept on file so that the patient does not have to sign each claim form. Instead, in the space for the patient's signature, note "SIGNATURE ON FILE." The insured also must sign an agreement for the insurer to pay the physician directly. An assignment-of-benefits statement and release of information statement may be included on the registration form (Figure 12.6.). Authorization is not needed for the release of non-privileged information unrelated to the patient's treatment, such as demographic data.

Legal Issue

Authorization is not needed for the release of non-privileged information such as demographic data. However, facts related to a patient's treatment or health status cannot be made available without the patient's consent.

Coding

Coding is the process of converting words that describe diseases, conditions, and procedures to numbers when filing insurance claims. Using codes describes medical services more uniformly and accurately, and allows for more systematic processing of claims. Coding is a complicated process, and the medical assistant must understand medical terminology, anatomy, physiology, and pathophysiology to apply codes correctly.

The assistant must extract the pertinent information from the patient's chart to complete the claim form,

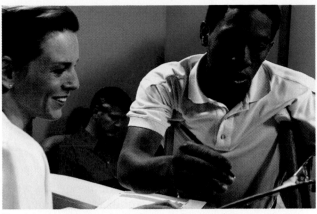

The patient must give the medical office written permission to release information for filing a medical claim.

and then must use the correct codes to denote the physician's diagnosis, services rendered, and procedures performed.

Incorrect coding can result in billing the insurance company for an amount less than the physician is entitled to, or it can result in overbilling, which is considered fraud.

Always refer to up-to-date code books. The intro-

Legal Issue
Coding must be done correctly. Mistakes can be considered fraudulent.

ductory material at the front of the coding books will help you understand how to use them properly. Take advantage of workshops and coding classes offered in your vicinity. When in doubt about which code to use, always check with the physician. Two major coding systems are used: procedure codes and diagnosis codes.

Procedure Codes

The CPT coding system was developed by the American Medical Association and is published in a text called *Current Procedural Terminology*. This listing of descriptive terms and the codes assigned to them is revised annually to include new procedures and modifications of existing techniques. CPT codes are made up of five-digit numbers that have been assigned to each diagnostic and therapeutic procedure used by physicians. The codes are highly refined to precisely describe medical services. When complications or special circumstances make a procedure more difficult or time-consuming, a two-digit modifier is added to the five-digit code number.

CPT divides the codes into six sections:

- evaluation and management
- anesthesia
- surgery
- radiology
- pathology and laboratory
- medicine

Guidelines at the beginning of each section and explanatory notes in the sections help the coder select the correct codes and modifiers. An index in the back of the *Current Procedural Terminology* text lists procedures alphabetically. Table 12.2 lists some codes from the CPT code book. You can obtain a copy of the book for your office by contacting the American Medical Association at 515 North State Street, Chicago, Illinois 60610 or calling 800-621-8335. Other code books can also be ordered from the AMA.

HCPCS (Health Care Financing Administration Common Procedure Coding System) was developed for the Medicare program. It is an alphanumeric coding system based on the CPT system and consisting of three levels of coding:

Level I: CPT codes and modifiers.
Level II: Alphanumeric codes assigned by the HCFA and used nationwide for equipment, supplies, and services not included in the CPT system.
Level III: Codes assigned and used by local intermediaries for services not included in the CPT system or HCFA codes.

I, the undersigned, do hereby request that authorized insurance benefits be paid directly to _____ for services furnished by this provider. I authorize the provider to release all information necessary to secure the payment of said benefits. I understand that I am financially responsible for all charges for the services provided, whether or not paid by the insurer.

_____
Signature of Patient or Responsible Party

_____
Date

Figure 12.6
Release of Information and Assignment of Benefits Statement

Table 12.2 A Partial List of CPT Codes for External Ear Procedures

69000	Drainage external ear, abscess, or hematoma; simple
69005	Drainage external ear, abscess, or hematoma; complicated
69020	Drainage external auditory canal, abscess
69090	Ear piercing
69100	Biopsy external ear
69105	Biopsy external auditory canal
69110	Excision external ear; partial, simple repair
69120	Excision external ear; complete amputation (for reconstruction of ear, see 15120 et seq)
69200	Removal of foreign body from external auditory canal; without general anesthesia
69205	Removal of foreign body from external auditory canal; with general anesthesia
69210	Removal of impacted cerumen (separate procedure), one or both ears

Source: Excerpted from *Current Procedural Terminology*, CPT, 2000. Chicago: American Medical Association, 1999. Used with permission.

You can order the *HCFA Common Procedure Coding System, Non-CPT-4 Portion* from the U.S. Government Printing Office.

In this system, each procedure code indicates a charge, and sometimes more than one code is needed to obtain reimbursement for a service. For example, when a patient receives an immunization for pneumonia, both the immunization code (90732) and the administration code (G0009) are used in billing. You must list each service separately on the claim form. If all relevant service codes are not listed, the physician will not receive the financial compensation she is entitled to.

As with any coding system, you must be very careful to use the correct codes. You would *never* use a code for a higher level of service than the patient received. For example, if an established patient came into the office to have you check her blood pressure and did not see the doctor, you would use code 99211 in charging the patient, *not* code 99213 which indicates the doctor spent about 15 minutes with the patient. Miscoding could result in severe penalties.

Diagnosis Codes

ICD-9-CM *(International Classification of Diseases, Ninth Revision, Clinical Modification)* is used for coding diagnoses on insurance claims. It is published in three volumes, two of which are used in the physician's office. Volume 1 lists diseases and conditions in numerical order, while Volume 2 lists the same diseases and conditions in alphabetical order. Volume 3 lists procedures and is primarily used in hospitals.

ICD-9 codes consist of a three-digit number often followed by a decimal point and one or two additional digits which further specify the disease. Always use the highest possible level of specificity. Remember that you are using numbers instead of words to describe a diagnosis, and you must find the code that exactly represents the patient's condition. Table 12.3 lists examples of ICD-9 codes.

To find the correct code in the ICD-9 system, you would first look up the key word in the diagnosis in Volume 2, the Alphabetic Index. For example, if the diagnosis is "acute otitis media," look up the word "otitis." Search through the subheadings under the main term until you find a match for the diagnosis in the patient's record. Then verify the code number by looking it up in Volume 1, the Tabular Index.

Unicor Medical, Inc. publishes the *ICD-9-CM Easy Coder*, which is an abbreviated version that is completely alphabetical and simpler to use than the original ICD-9 volumes. Diagnoses are listed alphabetically by the key word, anatomic site, or the first word of the diagnosis as it is written in the patient's chart. An excerpt is shown in Table 12.4.

A patient may be treated for more than one problem during an office visit. The code for each must be used on the claim form, and the sequence in which they are listed is very important. Remember that the problem that brought the patient to the office is listed first, unless the physician discovers a more serious problem. In that case, you would list the diagnosis that demanded more of the physician's attention and effort first.

The diagnosis code(s) used on the insurance claim form should reflect the services rendered. For example, if a patient with hypertension comes into the office for treatment of dermatitis, the code for dermatitis, not hypertension, would be used on the

Technology Tip

Keep up-to-date on the latest coding guidelines at www.hcfa.gov/medicare/icd9cm.htm

Table 12.3 ICD-9 Coding Examples

Diagnosis in Patient's Record	ICD-9 Code Options	Correct Code
Viral pneumonia	pneumonia: 486 viral pneumonia: 480.9	480.9
Essential hypertension, benign	essential hypertension: 401 essential hypertension, benign: 401.1	401.1
Sickle-cell anemia trait	sickle-cell anemia: 282.6 sickle-cell anemia trait: 282.5	282.5
Chronic thyroiditis	subacute thyroiditis: 245.1 chronic thyroiditis: 245.8	245.8

Table 12.4 ICD-9-CM Easy Coder Examples

41.4	E COLI INFECTION OR ORGANISM
771.8	E COLI INFECTION INTRA-AMNIOTIC (FETUS OR
756.71	NEWBORN)
362.18	EAGLE-BARRETT SYNDROME
	EALES' DISEASE OR SYNDROME
388.8	EAR
0	ABSENCE
388.7	ABSENCE CONGENITAL, SEE 'EAR ANOMALY'
0	ACHE
388.9	ANOMALY, SEE 'EAR ANOMALY'
380.50	ATROPHY
388.60	CANAL OBSTRUCTION
388.69	DISCHARGE
388.61	DISCHARGE BLOOD
384.20	DISCHARGE CEREBROSPINAL FLUID
	DRUM PERFORATION (SEE ALSO 'TYMPANIC
	MEMBRANE PERFORATION')

Source: Excerpted from *ICD-9-CM Easy Coder* (p. 165), published by Unicor Medical, Inc. Used with permission.

Technology Tip

Use the Internet to order CPT, ICD-9-CM, and HCPCS code books and HCFA-1500 forms. Instructional material and coding software are also available at these websites:

Medbooks:
www.medbooks.com/book_prices.html
(You can also order by calling 1-800-443-7397.)
Medical Book Store:
www.medicalbookstore.com
A-Z Technical Books:
www.technical-books.com/icd9cm.html

insurance form. Chronic conditions are not listed on the claim form unless medical service relating to the condition was given.

ICD-9 codes are used as a basis for the **diagnosis-related group (DRG)** system of patient classification in hospitals. A computer program assigns DRGs based on the principal diagnosis that led to hospitalization. Under this system, the hospital is paid a fixed fee instead being reimbursed for the time the patient spends in the hospital or the services rendered. The medical assistant plays an important role in the DRG assignment when calling the hospital to arrange admission of a patient. You must be sure to give the correct admitting diagnosis. If there is more than one, be sure to inform the hospital of all of them. Follow the coding guidelines presented in Table 12.5.

Table 12.5 Coding Guidelines

- Use the most current code books available. Keep your library up-to-date.
- Read the directions at the beginning of the code books so you will know how to use them properly and know what the symbols mean.
- Make sure you understand the medical terminology the physician uses in the patient's chart.
- Code only the condition(s) the patient is being treated for in a specific visit.
- Do not code suspected diagnoses. Use only the diagnosis, symptom, complaint, or problem reported.
- Always use both Volume 1 and Volume 2 of the ICD-9-CM code books.
- Code to the greatest degree of specificity possible.
- If you are unsure of the code to use, check with the physician.

Claims Processing and Understanding Claims for Review

Insurance claims may be sent to the carrier by mailing a paper claim form or may be submitted electronically directly to the carrier or via a clearinghouse. A **clearinghouse** is a third-party administrator that reformats claims according to the requirements of the various insurance carriers and distributes them to the carriers electronically. Paper forms should be filled out using a typewriter or computer printer. Claims must be submitted within the time limits the insurer specifies.

Universal Claim Form

A basic health insurance claim form, HCFA-1500, was developed by the Health Care Financing Administration for the filing of Medicare claims. This form has been adopted by OCHAMPUS, approved by the American Medical Association Council on Medical Services, and accepted for use by most private insurance carriers, eliminating the need for each insurer to have its own form. If a patient is insured by a company that does not accept the universal claim form, you should ask him to obtain a form from the insurer for you to complete and submit.

The HCFA-1500 form was revised in 1990 and printed in red ink for optimal scanning. Some Medicare carriers will accept a black-and-white copy of the form, but confirm this before submitting it. The upper portion of the form is used for information about the patient and her insurance carrier(s), and the lower portion is for information about the services provided and the physician or other supplier. Figure 12.7 is an

PLEASE
DO NOT
STAPLE
IN THIS
AREA

CARRIER

| | PICA | | **HEALTH INSURANCE CLAIM FORM** | PICA | |

| 1. MEDICARE MEDICAID CHAMPUS CHAMPVA GROUP HEALTH PLAN FECA BLK LUNG OTHER | 1a. INSURED'S I.D. NUMBER (FOR PROGRAM IN ITEM 1) |

(Medicare #) (Medicaid #) (Sponsor's SSN) (VA File #) (SSN or ID) (SSN) (ID)

| 2. PATIENT'S NAME (Last Name, First Name, Middle Initial) | 3. PATIENT'S BIRTH DATE MM DD YY SEX M   F | 4. INSURED'S NAME (Last Name, First Name, Middle Initial) |

| 5. PATIENT'S ADDRESS (No., Street) | 6. PATIENT RELATIONSHIP TO INSURED Self Spouse Child Other | 7. INSURED'S ADDRESS (No., Street) |

| CITY | STATE | 8. PATIENT STATUS Single Married Other | CITY | STATE |

| ZIP CODE | TELEPHONE (Include Area Code) (   ) | Employed Full-Time Student Part-Time Student | ZIP CODE | TELEPHONE (INCLUDE AREA CODE) (   ) |

| 9. OTHER INSURED'S NAME (Last Name, First Name, Middle Initial) | 10. IS PATIENT'S CONDITION RELATED TO: | 11. INSURED'S POLICY GROUP OR FECA NUMBER |

| a. OTHER INSURED'S POLICY OR GROUP NUMBER | a. EMPLOYMENT? (CURRENT OR PREVIOUS) YES NO | a. INSURED'S DATE OF BIRTH MM DD YY SEX M   F |

| b. OTHER INSURED'S DATE OF BIRTH MM DD YY SEX M   F | b. AUTO ACCIDENT? PLACE (State) YES NO | b. EMPLOYER'S NAME OR SCHOOL NAME |

| c. EMPLOYER'S NAME OR SCHOOL NAME | c. OTHER ACCIDENT? YES NO | c. INSURANCE PLAN NAME OR PROGRAM NAME |

| d. INSURANCE PLAN NAME OR PROGRAM NAME | 10d. RESERVED FOR LOCAL USE | d. IS THERE ANOTHER HEALTH BENEFIT PLAN? YES NO *If yes*, return to and complete item 9 a-d. |

READ BACK OF FORM BEFORE COMPLETING & SIGNING THIS FORM.

| 12. PATIENT'S OR AUTHORIZED PERSON'S SIGNATURE I authorize the release of any medical or other information necessary to process this claim. I also request payment of government benefits either to myself or to the party who accepts assignment below. SIGNED _____ DATE _____ | 13. INSURED'S OR AUTHORIZED PERSON'S SIGNATURE I authorize payment of medical benefits to the undersigned physician or supplier for services described below. SIGNED _____ |

PATIENT AND INSURED INFORMATION

| 14. DATE OF CURRENT: MM DD YY ◄ ILLNESS (First symptom) OR INJURY (Accident) OR PREGNANCY(LMP) | 15. IF PATIENT HAS HAD SAME OR SIMILAR ILLNESS. GIVE FIRST DATE MM DD YY | 16. DATES PATIENT UNABLE TO WORK IN CURRENT OCCUPATION MM DD YY MM DD YY FROM TO |

| 17. NAME OF REFERRING PHYSICIAN OR OTHER SOURCE | 17a. I.D. NUMBER OF REFERRING PHYSICIAN | 18. HOSPITALIZATION DATES RELATED TO CURRENT SERVICES MM DD YY MM DD YY FROM TO |

| 19. RESERVED FOR LOCAL USE | | 20. OUTSIDE LAB? YES NO $ CHARGES |

| 21. DIAGNOSIS OR NATURE OF ILLNESS OR INJURY. (RELATE ITEMS 1,2,3 OR 4 TO ITEM 24E BY LINE) 1. ⌐____.____ 3. ⌐____.____ 2. ⌐____.____ 4. ⌐____.____ | 22. MEDICAID RESUBMISSION CODE ORIGINAL REF. NO. 23. PRIOR AUTHORIZATION NUMBER |

24. A DATE(S) OF SERVICE From To MM DD YY MM DD YY	B Place of Service	C Type of Service	D PROCEDURES, SERVICES, OR SUPPLIES (Explain Unusual Circumstances) CPT/HCPCS MODIFIER	E DIAGNOSIS CODE	F $ CHARGES	G DAYS OR UNITS	H EPSDT Family Plan	I EMG	J COB	K RESERVED FOR LOCAL USE
1										
2										
3										
4										
5										
6										

| 25. FEDERAL TAX I.D. NUMBER SSN EIN | 26. PATIENT'S ACCOUNT NO. | 27. ACCEPT ASSIGNMENT? (For govt. claims, see back) YES NO | 28. TOTAL CHARGE $ | 29. AMOUNT PAID $ | 30. BALANCE DUE $ |

| 31. SIGNATURE OF PHYSICIAN OR SUPPLIER INCLUDING DEGREES OR CREDENTIALS (I certify that the statements on the reverse apply to this bill and are made a part thereof.) SIGNED _____ DATE _____ | 32. NAME AND ADDRESS OF FACILITY WHERE SERVICES WERE RENDERED (If other than home or office) | 33. PHYSICIAN'S, SUPPLIER'S BILLING NAME, ADDRESS, ZIP CODE & PHONE # PIN# GRP# |

PHYSICIAN OR SUPPLIER INFORMATION

(APPROVED BY AMA COUNCIL ON MEDICAL SERVICE 8/88)   **PLEASE PRINT OR TYPE**   FORM HCFA-1500 (12-90), FORM RRB-1500, FORM OWCP-1500

Figure 12.7
HCFA-1500 Form

example of this HCFA-1500 form. Forms may be purchased from the Government Printing Office or through medical forms suppliers. Procedure 12.1 lists step-by-step instructions for completing Form HCFA-1500.

You must be very meticulous in filling out the forms accurately. When a form has incomplete or inaccurate information, Medicare will reject the claim. You will then have to make corrections and resubmit it. Claims can be filed electronically using the NSF (National Standard Format) or the ANSI (American National Standards Institute) format. Electronic filing saves time, cuts down on errors, and provides immediate confirmation that the claim has been received. Reimbursement is made in about half the time it takes when a paper claim is filed. Medicare is encouraging a complete conversion to automated filing. Contact your local carrier for specific information and instructions.

Technology Tip

The HCFA-1500 form can be printed off the website www.hcfa.gov/medicare/edi/1500info.htm. The site also lists the states that accept black-and-white copies of the form.

Procedure 12.1

Completing Form HCFA-1500

Purpose: To complete the universal health insurance claim form accurately and completely for filing with an insurer.

Equipment/Supplies: Patient's health record, ledger card, and insurance information; Form HCFA-1500; typewriter or computer.

Fill in the information indicated below for each block on the form. Type in all caps using no punctuation except for hyphens in names and numbers.

Block 1 — Type of insurance: Check patient's insurance card and place an X in the box that applies to the claim.

Block 1a — Insured's ID number: Enter the number on the patient's identification card that corresponds to the type of insurance checked in Block 1. Some insurers, such as CHAMPUS, use the patient's social security number.

Block 2 — Patient's name: Copy *exactly* as it appears on the insurance card, last name first.

Block 3 — Date of birth: Use six or eight digits (Example: 02/07/56 or 02/07/1956). Type an X in the box for male or female.

Block 4 — Insured's name: Leave this blank if Medicare is the primary insurance. Otherwise, if the patient is the insured person, enter the word SAME. If the claim is for Worker's Compensation, enter the employer's name.

Block 5 — Patient's mailing address and telephone number: Enter the street address on the first line, the city and state on the second line, and the ZIP code and phone number on the third line.

Block 6 — Patient's relationship to insured: Check the appropriate box when Block 4 is completed. For Worker's Compensation, check "Other."

Block 7 — Insured's full address and telephone number: Write SAME if the address is the same as the patient's. Leave it blank if Medicare is the primary insurance.

Block 8 — Patient status: Check appropriate box for marital status. Check appropriate box for employment status. Leave blank for Medicaid and Worker's Compensation.

Block 9 — Other insured's name: For Medicare claims, this item and its subdivisions must be completed by participating physicians and suppliers only when the patient wants to assign Medigap benefits to the physician. Enter MEDIGAP followed by the policy number. Other supplemental coverage should not be listed on a Medicare claim. For other third-party payers, enter the name of the other person whose insurance covers the patient.

Block 9a — Other insured's policy or group number: Enter the policy number for other coverage. For Medigap, if the patient is the insured, type SAME.

Block 9b — Other insured's birth date and sex: Enter the birth date using six or eight digits, and check the box for "Male" or "Female."

Block 9c — Other insured's employer's name or school name: For Medicare, leave blank if the Medigap Payer ID is entered in Block 9d. Otherwise, enter the claims processing address of the Medigap insurer. Enter the information indicated for other third-party payers. Leave blank for Worker's Compensation.

Block 9d — Other insured's insurance plan name or program name: Enter the name of the Medigap insurer or its nine-digit payer ID number. For other third-party payers, enter the name of the other insurance plan. Leave blank for

Procedure 12.1 Completing Form HCFA-1500 (continued)

Worker's Compensation. Caution: Medicare participating providers must complete Blocks 9, 9a, 9b, and 9d for the Medicare carrier to forward the claim to the Medigap insurer.

Block 10   Status of patient's condition: Check the appropriate box for items a–c regarding employment and accident. If an accident, use the two-letter postal code to indicate the state. A "Yes" answer on a Medicare claim indicates that other insurance may be primary. Leave blank for Worker's Compensation.

Block 10d   Reserved for local use: Used for Medicaid. Enter the patient's Medicaid number preceded by MCD. Leave blank for other claims unless you need to include information about another insurance carrier. In this case, type the word ATTACHMENT and attach a sheet with the name and address of the other carrier.

Block 11   Insured's policy group or FICA number: This item must be completed on Medicare claims. If no insurance is primary to Medicare, enter NONE and go to Block 12. Otherwise, enter the insured's policy or group number.

Block 11a   Insured's birth date and sex: Enter the birth date and check the appropriate box for "Male" or "Female."

Block 11b   Insured's employer's name or school name: Enter the information indicated. If there has been a change in status because of retirement, type RETIRED and the date of retirement.

Block 11c   Insurance plan name or program name: Enter the nine-digit payer ID number or the plan name of the primary insurer. Leave blank for Medicaid and Worker's Compensation.

Block 11d   Is there another health benefit plan?: Leave blank for Medicare, Medicaid, and Worker's Compensation. If the answer is "Yes" for other third-party payers, the information in Block 9, a–d, must be completed.

Block 12   Patient or authorized person's signature for the release of medical information: The patient or authorized representative must sign and date this release of medical information for the claim to be processed. An alternative is to have the patient sign a statement authorizing the release of medical information and payment of benefits to the service provider. The statement must be retained by the physician or the insurer. If this is the case, type SIGNATURE ON FILE.

Block 13   Insured or authorized person's signature authorizing payment of benefits: This item must be signed for the insurer to pay the physician. Enter SIGNATURE ON FILE if it is. For Medigap, a separate authorization must be on file.

Block 14   Date of current illness: Enter date of current illness, injury, or pregnancy. Use date of last menstrual period for pregnancy. Leave blank for Medicaid. Enter the date using six or eight digits as you did in Block 3.

Block 15   Date of same or similar illness: Leave blank for Medicare and Medicaid. For others, complete if appropriate.

Block 16   Dates patient unable to work in current occupation: Leave blank for Medicaid, and complete for others, if appropriate and the patient is employed.

Block 17   Name of referring physician: Enter the name of the referring or ordering physician. All Medicare claims for items and services that result from a physician's order or referral, like lab tests or consultations, must include that physician's name and National Provider Identifier (NPI). This item must be completed when the provider filing the claim is not the one who requested the service. When the performing physician is also the ordering physician, as with in-office lab tests, the performing physician's name and NPI go in Blocks 17 and 17a. File separate claims when there are multiple ordering/referring physicians.

Block 17a   ID number of referring physician: Fill in the referring/ordering physician's NPI number assigned by the HCFA. Use the following surrogate NPIs for physicians or other professionals who have not been assigned an NPI:

RES00000   interns and residents
RET00000   retired physicians
VAD00000   physicians in the military or Department of Veterans Affairs
PHS00000   physicians in the Public Health or Indian Health Services
NPP00000   nurse practitioners and others

Block 18   Hospitalization date related to current services: Enter if appropriate.

Procedure 12.1 Completing Form HCFA-1500 (continued)

Block 19   Reserved for local use: May be used when special circumstances or special services apply and for additional narrative information.

Block 20   Outside lab work: Place an X in the "Yes" block if some entity other than the physician performed the service and it is included on the claim. "No" indicates that no purchased tests are included on the claim. If yes, enter the purchase price and complete Block 32.

Block 21   Diagnosis or nature of illness or injury: Use ICD-9 codes and list in priority order. More than one code can be used if the patient received services for each diagnosis. The problem that brought the patient to the office should be listed first, unless the physician discovers a more serious problem. Do not list chronic conditions unless treated at the time of the visit.

Block 22   Medicaid resubmission code: Complete if applicable.

Block 23   Prior authorization number: Complete if applicable.

Block 24a   Date of service: Enter six-digit dates for each procedure or service.

Block 24b   Place of service: Indicate the place of service by using the appropriate code. A partial list follows:
- 11   Office
- 12   Home
- 21   Inpatient Hospital
- 22   Outpatient Hospital
- 23   Emergency Hospital
- 25   Birthing Center
- 32   Nursing Facility
- 71   State or Local Public Health Clinic

Block 24c   Type of service: Leave blank for Medicare and third-party payers. This is used for the Medicare Remittance Advice document codes.

Block 24d   Procedures, services, or supplies: List service using the appropriate CPT or HCPCS code with modifiers when necessary. Leave the "Modifier" column blank if not needed. Use Block 19 to explain unusual circumstances, or include an attachment.

Block 24e   Diagnosis code: For each service, enter the line item reference of the diagnosis it relates to in Block 21. Only one diagnosis code can be used for each service.

Block 24f   Charges: Enter the charge for each service. Do not use dollar signs or decimal points.

Block 24g   Days or units: Used for multiple visits or supplies. Enter 1 if only one such service is performed on the visit(s) being billed. If more than one, enter the appropriate number. Example: If 5 hospital visits were made on consecutive days, enter 5.

Block 24h   EPSDT: This stands for "Early, periodic, screening, diagnosis, and treatment" and is used for Medicaid. Enter E for these services and F for family planning. Leave blank for other third-party payers.

Block 24i   EMG: Applies to Medicaid. Enter X if emergency services were given in a hospital emergency room. Leave blank for other third-party payers.

Block 24j   COB: Coordination of benefits. Check if applicable.

Block 24k   Reserved for local use: Use to list the NPI(s) of the performing providers if they are members of a group practice. When several providers in a group are billed on the same form, enter the individual NPI for each item. Type the first two digits of the NPI in Block 24j and the other six digits in Block 24k.

Block 25   Federal tax ID number: Enter the physician's social security number or tax ID number (Employer Identification Number), and mark the appropriate box.

Block 26   Patient's account number: Optional. You may enter the account number assigned by the service provider.

Block 27   Accept assignment: Check "Yes" or "No."

Block 28   Total charges: Add all charges and enter the total.

Block 29   Amount paid: Enter any amount paid by the patient or another insurer for the charges listed on the claim.

Block 30   Balance due: Enter the balance due. Leave blank for Medicare.

Block 31   Signature of physician or supplier: Should be signed by the physician and dated.

Block 32   Name and address of facility where services were rendered: Complete this item for service rendered anyplace other than in the physician's office or the patient's home.

Block 33   Physician's name, address, and telephone number: Enter the appropriate information. Enter the NPI for a performing provider who is not a member of a group practice. When the provider is part of a group practice, enter the group NPI.

A number of practice management software programs can file insurance claims electronically to Medicare, Medicaid, Blue Cross/Blue Shield, and commercial carriers. Claims may be filed individually or in batches. Insurers may give preferential treatment on turnaround time to claims that are submitted electronically. Some software programs will automatically check the claim for omissions and typical data-entry errors. Features such as electronic eligibility verification and referral authorization/status may also be included. Some programs let you receive the Explanation of Benefits (EOB) electronically and automatically post payments to a patient's account. Medical Manager, MediSoft, Lytec Medical, Merlin, and AccuMed are medical office programs that allow for the submission of "paperless claims," more efficient insurance bookkeeping, and improved productivity and cash flow.

Payment Processing

When a claim is processed by an insurance company and the amount eligible for reimbursement is determined, a check is sent to the physician with an Explanation of Benefits (EOB) statement. Sometimes the check covers more than one patient. The EOB lists each patient covered, the date(s) of service, the total charges, any amount not covered, the covered amount, the amount applied to the deductible, the amount due from the patient, and the payment amount. The amount paid must be entered on each patient's ledger card and on the day sheet. The insurer also sends an EOB to the patient.

Technology Tip

Use the Internet to learn more about filing Medicare claims. You can download free interactive Medicare training software from the website www.medicaretraining.com/cbt.htm Course topics include:

- HCFA-1500 (Part B)
- HCFA-1450 (Part A)
- fraud and abuse
- ICD-9-CM diagnosis codes
- world of medicare
- front office
- medicare secondary payer
- home health benefits

Once the courses are installed on your computer, a number of users can take—and retake—them. You may use this for in-service training of both beginners and more experienced staff members.

Date filed	Patient's name	Insurer	Amt. billed	Payment Date	Amt.	Difference	Follow-up date	Settled ✓

Figure 12.8
Insurance Claims Log

Use a registration log like this to keep track of insurance claims.

Procedure 12.2

Processing Insurance Claims

Purpose: To follow an established method for filing claims and monitoring the status of insurance billing.

Equipment/Supplies: Claims registration log, alphabetic "claims pending" file, source documents, pen.

1 Complete the insurance claim form.
2 List the information in the claims registration log. *This provides a method of keeping up with outstanding claims.*
3 Make a copy of the claim and place it in the alphabetic "Claims pending" file according to the patient's last name. *If the claim is lost or there is a question about items submitted, you need a copy for reference.*
4 Note on the patient's ledger card that the insurance was billed. Include the date.
5 Submit the claim to the insurer.
6 When payment is received, list the amount and date in the log. Determine the difference, if any, between the amount billed and the amount received. If they are the same, place a check mark in the "Settled" column. When all claims on a page have been settled, draw a diagonal line across the page. *This helps you quickly spot claims that have not been paid.*
7 Post the payment on the day sheet and the patient's ledger card, and make necessary adjustments. *Medicare-approved amounts may differ from those submitted on the claim, and the physician's charges may have to be adjusted accordingly.*
8 Process the check for deposit.
9 Remove the claim form from the "Pending" file, attach a copy of the explanation of benefits, and place it in the inactive insurance file.
10 Check the log daily for delinquent claims and take the appropriate action.

Delinquent Claims

The medical assistant is responsible for processing insurance claims from the time charges are incurred through settlement. Careful records must be kept, and follow-up action must be taken when an insurance claim is not paid within a reasonable time. There are several ways to establish an audit trail to keep up with the status of claims. One method is to set up a claims registration log and filing system for pending claims. (See Figure 12.8.)

Delinquent claims can be monitored easily by checking the register, and copies of the claim forms are easy to locate in the alphabetic file. List each claim in chronological order in the log, based on the filing date. Keep log sheets in a loose-leaf binder so that new sheets can be added. When payment is received, record the amount and date in the log. You can tell at a glance which claims are outstanding by looking at this column and can follow up as necessary. Make a copy of each claim. Set up an alphabetic file for pending claims, with copies filed according to the patient's last name. When a claim is settled, pull the form from the pending file and place it in an inactive file. Procedure 12.2 explains the steps involved in processing insurance claims.

When payment is overdue, the medical assistant should contact the carrier to determine the reason. Insurance payments may be delayed or denied for a number of reasons. Table 12.6 lists common reasons for rejection of claims and delays in payment.

Claims with incorrect or missing information and claims that have been lost must be resubmitted. Claims may be denied, among other reasons, because:

- The service is not covered by the policy.
- Treatment was for a pre-existing condition not covered by the policy.
- The patient was not insured at the time of service.
- The service needed prior authorization.

You should notify the patient immediately when a claim is denied. Keep all correspondence. A denied claim can be appealed by the medical office on behalf of the patient for reasons that include:

- a payment amount reduced from what is usually allowed
- unusual circumstances involving the treatment or procedure that were not reflected in the amount of reimbursement
- special circumstances regarding precertification
- no reason was given for denial

Appeals must be made in writing within each plan's time limit, which is usually indicated on the EOB. Send a letter explaining the reason for the appeal and attach copies of pertinent information or documents that

Table 12.6 Common Reasons for Rejection of Claims and Payment Delays

- Incorrect ID numbers or policy numbers. Double-check all numbers to make sure they have been entered on the form correctly.
- Inaccurate or incomplete patient information. Review and update patient information periodically to be sure it is correct. Identify all insurance that a patient has.
- Diagnosis code that is missing, inaccurate, or not appropriate for the treatment given. Use the most recent edition of the code books, and make sure that the reported diagnosis is relevant to the service provided. Inconsistency may indicate a coding error.
- Neglecting to indicate whether the patient's condition is related to employment or an accident. This information is used by the primary insurer to determine whether the service should be covered by worker's compensation or liability insurance.
- Total charges not equal to the amounts itemized. Always check to make sure calculations are correct.
- Invalid or incorrect procedure codes. Use the most recent edition of code books to make sure you do not use codes that have been deleted or changed.
- Missing signatures. Make sure the patient signs either the claim form or an authorization to release information and assignment of benefits form to be kept on file. Make sure the physician signs the claim.
- Inconsistent data, e.g., an inappropriate diagnosis for the patient's gender. Review each claim for accuracy before submitting it to the insurer.
- Missing supporting or explanatory attachments. Make sure the patient's name and identification number are on each attachment. Type "ATTACHMENT" in Block 10d of HCFA-1500.
- Billing of the secondary, instead of the primary, insurer. Determine the primary payer from the patient information sheet or from details given at the time of the visit. For example, if the patient was injured on the job, worker's compensation would be primary instead of the patient's insurance plan.

support your argument. An example might be an operative report detailing complications of a usually straightforward surgical procedure. When a claim is lost, send a copy of the original claim marked "copy of original submitted on (date)."

Working Smart

Avoid confusion when ascertaining the status of Medicare claims by using proper terminology. **Claim status** indicates that you are inquiring about a claim for which you have received no response. **Review status** means you are appealing or requesting a review of a claim that has already been processed.

Business and Professional Insurance

In addition to understanding insurance that covers patient services, the medical assistant needs to be knowledgeable about other kinds of insurance related to the practice of medicine. The physician needs insurance that protects against property loss and malpractice. In addition, he needs personal health insurance, and may offer health insurance as a benefit to employees under a group plan. The medical assistant may be responsible for paying premiums, keeping up with renewal dates, and maintaining insurance files. Use a separate filing system for business insurance. Keep a calendar or set up a tickler file to remind you when premium payments and renewals are due.

Professional liability insurance protects the physician from damages resulting from a malpractice suit. High malpractice insurance premiums reflect the increase in such suits filed by patients in recent years and the tendency of courts and juries to make generous awards when they rule in favor of the suing patient. Other medical professionals, including medical assistants, should also purchase malpractice insurance.

Personal liability insurance covers damages that result from accidents unrelated to the practice of medicine that happen in the physician's office or on her property. This may be packaged with a property loss policy. In addition, a supplemental "umbrella" policy covering these losses may be purchased which offers protection of $1 million or more.

Fire and smoke damage, theft, vandalism, and other causes of loss are covered by property loss insurance. Office furniture, equipment, and supplies should be inventoried and appraised so that if property loss occurs, there is a record of the items lost or damaged and their value.

Automobile insurance covers the physician's personal automobile and also may be purchased to cover an employee who uses her own car for job-related errands. You may be covered under this policy if you drive your car to pick up office supplies, make bank deposits, or perform other medical assisting duties for the practice.

As discussed previously, worker's compensation insurance covers employees who suffer from job-related illness or are injured while carrying out their work responsibilities. As an employer, the physician is required by law to provide worker's compensation insurance for you and other employees.

A fidelity bond offers insurance against embezzlement by employees. Bonding may cover a specific job, an individual, or all employees. In these instances, a background investigation may be required.

Challenging Situations

*S*ometimes, an insurance company may repeatedly delay payments without a valid reason. In such cases, a formal complaint should be sent in writing to the state insurance commission. This body monitors the activities of insurance companies to make sure they comply with insurance laws. The number of complaints against an insurance company may affect its rating, and consumers in some states have access to this information. The state insurance commissioner cannot force companies to make payments, but they are more likely to pay promptly if future business could be affected. Even the threat of filing a complaint can motivate an insurance company to pay what it owes.

The practice may occasionally see a patient who has no medical insurance coverage. Patients who are 65 or older are automatically covered with Medicare Part A. Medicare Part B coverage requires an additional monthly fee. The medical assistant should urge the patient to contact the local Social Security Administration office for information.

Trying to collect a fee when an insurance policy has lapsed can be a problem for the medical assistant. This situation could be prevented by contacting the insurance carrier in advance of costly treatment. The patient's insurance identification card usually lists a telephone number that can be called to check on eligibility or verify benefits.

Medical insurance plans and claims processing are constantly being revised and modified. Keep up with changes by attending workshops in your area sponsored by the American Association of Medical Assistants and by reading bulletins and information booklets sent out by Medicare, Medicaid, and other insurers.

Clinical Summary

- Handling insurance in the medical office is a complicated process that requires the medical assistant to keep up with constantly changing insurance plans and claims processing procedures, as well as the technology for filing claims electronically.
- Patients may be covered under group plans, individual plans, or prepaid health plans.
- HMOs and PPOs are managed care plans in which patients make a copayment each time they visit the office.
- Medicare is a national health insurance program that covers persons at least 65 years old, disabled persons, and kidney dialysis or kidney transplant patients.
- Medicare Part A is hospital insurance, and Medicare Part B covers physicians' services.

- When a patient is covered by Medicare and Medicaid, Medicare is the primary payer.
- Dependents of military personnel are covered by CHAMPUS.
- A separate medical record should be set up for worker's compensation patients.
- New patients should fill out a registration form that should be updated annually and verified at each office visit.
- Both sides of the patient's insurance identification card should be photocopied for office records.
- Medical information cannot be released to an insurance company on a claim form unless the patient signs a release of information statement.
- Accurate coding of procedures and diagnoses is essential in collecting the amount due the physician, while avoiding overbilling.
- Claims must be filed within the time limits various insurance plans set.
- The medical assistant must make sure that insurance information for each patient is current, and must be able to extract the information needed to file a claim from the patient's record.
- Paper claims for Medicare, Medicaid, CHAMPUS, and most private insurance companies are submitted using form HCFA-1500, the universal claim form.
- Filing claims electronically improves accuracy and leads to quicker payment than submission of paper claims.
- The medical assistant must be able to communicate with patients and insurers concerning the processing of claims.
- Accuracy and good record-keeping are essential when handling insurance claims.
- The medical assistant should establish an audit trail, monitor delinquent claims, and follow up on claims not paid within a reasonable time.
- The medical assistant may be responsible for handling business and professional insurance as well as processing health insurance claims for patients.

The Language of Medicine

assignment of benefits Agreement by the patient to the insurance company's payment of benefits directly to the physician.

beneficiary A person designated by an insurance policy to receive benefits or funds.

benefits Payments made by an insurance company.

Blue Cross/Blue Shield A nationwide association of independent healthcare insurers; many are non-profit organizations.

capitation The type of plan in which healthcare providers contract to provide care for a group at a fixed amount per person per month.

carrier An insurance company that underwrites healthcare policies.

CHAMPUS/TRICARE/CHAMPVA CHAMPUS is a government health insurance program covering mainly dependents of military personnel; TRICARE is a managed care program to control costs and standardize benefits for

CHAMPUS members; CHAMPVA is a program similar to CHAMPUS covering dependents of veterans with total, permanent, service-related disabilities.

claim A request for payment from an insurance carrier.

claim status The status of a claim that has been filed to which there has been no response.

clearinghouse A third-party administrator who reformats medical claims according to the requirements of various insurance carriers and distributes them to the carriers electronically.

coding Translating words that describe a diagnosis or procedure into numeric designations.

coinsurance An arrangement in which the insured must pay a percentage of the cost of medical services covered by the insurer.

coordination of benefits A process to prevent duplication of payment when a patient is covered under more than one insurance plan.

copayment An arrangement in which the patient pays a fixed fee when medical service is rendered and the insurer pays the rest of the cost.

crossover claim Automatic forwarding of a bill by Medicare after it has paid its portion of the costs to a Medigap insurer that will pay the remainder.

deductible The amount of a bill that the patient must pay before insurance begins payment for medical services.

diagnosis-related group (DRG) A system of patient classification used in hospitals for reimbursement based on a fixed fee instead of fee-for-service.

elective procedures Optional procedures that are not medically necessary.

exclusions Conditions and circumstances for which the insurance company will not pay benefits.

explanation of benefits (EOB) An explanation of the payments made for services which the insurer sends to the patient and the provider.

fee-for-service A payment method in which the patient is charged a specific fee each time a specific service is provided.

fiscal agent (fiscal intermediary) An organization that has a contract to process claims for Medicaid, Medicare, or CHAMPUS.

gatekeeper A primary care provider who controls patients' access to specialists.

Health Maintenance Organization (HMO) A prepaid managed care plan in which members must use participating providers and are enrolled for a specific period of time.

HCPCS The Health Care Financing Administration Common Procedure Coding System, an alphanumeric coding system developed for Medicare.

ICD-9-CM The International Classification of Diseases, Ninth Revision, Clinical Modification, which is used for coding diagnoses on insurance claims.

Indemnity Compensation paid by an insurance carrier for damage, loss, or services rendered.

indemnity health insurance Traditional health insurance plans for major medical expenses that include coinsurance paid by the individual.

insurance A contract whereby one party agrees to compensate or reimburse another for any loss due to a specified cause.

insured A person or organization covered by insurance.

insurer A company or underwriter that provides insurance coverage.

managed care A healthcare plan that promotes cost-effectiveness by establishing selective relationships with providers.

Medicaid A nationwide program of medical assistance for the needy.

Medicare intermediary A private insurance company that has a contract with the federal government to handle Medicare claims.

Medicare Part A A national health insurance program that covers hospitalization of the elderly and other qualified persons.

Medicare Part B A national health insurance program that covers physicians' services and other medical services for the elderly and other qualified persons.

Medigap A health insurance plan offered by private entities to supplement Medicare benefits by filling in gaps not covered by Medicare.

preauthorization (precertification) Submission of a treatment plan to an insurance carrier for approval before proceeding with the plan.

pre-existing condition A condition or disease that was present before an insurance policy was issued.

Preferred Provider Organization (PPO) A managed care plan in which enrolled persons may receive benefits, though at a lower rate, even if they choose a physician who is not part of the plan.

premiums The fees paid periodically to keep insurance in force.

primary care physician A physician who manages the healthcare of patients in an HMO or PPO plan, and serves as a gatekeeper.

primary payer The insurance company or health plan that assumes initial responsibility for paying benefits when the patient is covered under more than one plan.

professional liability insurance Insurance that physicians buy to protect themselves against damages resulting from a malpractice suit.

provider A person, organization, or institution that delivers healthcare services.

reimbursement Repayment for expenses or losses incurred.

review status The status of a claim on which the insurer's action is being appealed or for which a review is requested.

secondary payer The insurance carrier that pays benefits after the primary payer has paid the portion of the bill for which it is responsible.

subscriber (policyholder) A person who takes out an insurance policy or is covered through an employer or other group plan.

usual, customary, and reasonable rates (UCR) Maximum amounts that insurance companies will pay based on prevailing fees in a geographic area.

waiting period The time that must pass before a subscriber's pre-existing condition will be covered by an insurance policy.

worker's compensation insurance A government program providing benefits for employees suffering from job-related accident or illness, and their dependents.

Signs/Symptoms of Progress

Recall, Question, Connect

Recall

What is the difference between Medicare Part A coverage and Medicare Part B coverage?

Question

What questions do you have about these coverages?

Connect

Which part of Medicare would cover flu shots given in the office?

Educating the Patient

Catherine Jenkins, whose husband is on active duty in the military, brings her seven-year-old son to Dr. Jones's office because he hurt his wrist playing basketball. She says she did not take him to the medical facility on the nearby base because there would have been a long wait before he could see a doctor. When you check DEERS, neither Ms. Jenkins nor her son is listed.

1 What insurance program covers the dependents of active duty military personnel?

2 How do you explain to Ms. Jenkins why the program will not cover her son's treatment today?

3 What managed care options are available through this program?

Exploring Perspectives in Teams

Perspective involves the discipline of examining how ideas look from different points of view and recognizing that there are often multiple "answers" to complex questions. In small groups or on your own, reflect on possible alternative views or answers and summarize your findings.

1 An administrative staff meeting has been called to discuss what can be done to reduce errors and the time it is taking for insurance claims to be paid. Attending are the physician, office manager, insurance clerk, and bookkeeper. Confer on the problem of errors and delays. Answers these questions: What kinds of problems can cause late payments? Specifically, how do errors or omissions on the claim form affect payment? What procedures could reduce errors? Which of the responsibilities discussed affect the role of the medical assistant?

2 Create a chart detailing the advantages and disadvantages of HMOs and PPOs. Illustrate your conclusions with specific family profiles and hypothetical disease conditions.

3 What is an audit trail, and why is it important?

4 If you were the insurance commissioner for the country, what changes would you recommend to make the system less confusing for patients?

Learning Outcomes

- Understand how to manage and supervise the office staff.
- Explain the importance of team building.
- Demonstrate motivational and leadership qualities.
- Understand how payroll records are managed.
- Recognize the importance of interpersonal and problem-solving skills.
- Manage the recruiting and hiring of new employees.
- Train, monitor, and evaluate employees.
- Understand the function of public relations and marketing.

Performance Objectives

- Manage and facilitate staff meetings.
- Supervise and assess employees.
- Hire and train employees.
- Write and review job descriptions.
- Develop public relations materials.

The office manager is responsible for running the office efficiently and for maintaining an environment that enables all employees to operate at their highest levels. This may involve managing one other person or several other people, depending on the size of the clinic. In a small office, the manager works under the supervision of the physician, while in a large office, the office manager may report to a human relations manager. The office manager directs the work of the other office employees and interacts daily with physicians, patients, and other service providers. Responsibilities may include payroll activities as well as personnel management.

Promotion to the position of office manager—usually involving increased pay and responsibilities—may be offered to a medical assistant who demonstrates management potential and key skills important to the organization. If you are highly organized, enjoy working with people, demonstrate flexibility, and are respected by

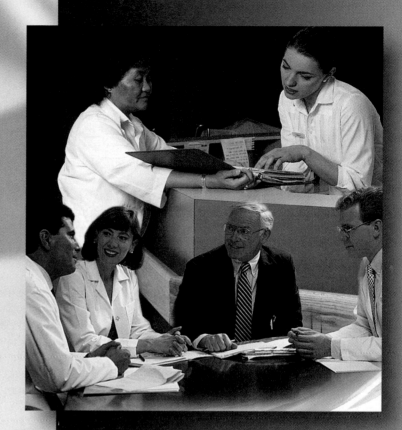

Chapter 13

Supervising the Front Office

your colleagues, you may be offered this position when a vacancy occurs. All medical assistants do not wish to assume managerial tasks, but if you are a self-starter and like new challenges, you may aspire to this job either in your office or in another medical setting.

Patient Concerns

*M*aria Slater was waiting to be called in for her appointment to see the doctor. She sat in the office for over thirty minutes. That did not bother her so much, but what happened during that time did. First, she—and everyone else in the waiting room—heard an argument between the receptionist and a nurse. A few minutes later, a doctor rushed through the front office area berating the receptionist because of a scheduling problem. Then, Maria heard a receptionist barking orders to one of the medical assistants in a very unpleasant tone of voice. Although Maria waited to see the doctor, she made a mental note to change to another medical practice

where the atmosphere in the waiting area would be less unpleasant. Because Maria liked her physician, she wrote a letter telling her why she was thinking about changing to another clinic.

Usually, when patients come to the medical office they are already concerned about their health. They do not need additional reasons to be anxious. The clinic staff must convey the message that the office is well-organized and that the staff members genuinely care about each other and the patients they serve. The office manager is ultimately responsible for developing this atmosphere in the medical office.

Modeling the Qualities of an Efficient Office Manager

It is essential that the office manager be flexible and ready to meet daily challenges. This includes the ability to smooth over differences among staff members and to instruct them about the importance of keeping disputes from public view. The office manager is responsible for creating a warm and friendly environment for patients who are waiting to see the medical practitioner. In this role, she can set the tone for the entire office by being warm, friendly, and patient. These interpersonal skills, along with excellent organizational and leadership abilities, are essential for the office manager.

Organizational Skills

The organizational skills the office manager must possess include the ability to set priorities, be detailed and careful in both written and oral communication, and work in a systematic way. You need to be confident in delegating tasks to subordinates. This requires that you clarify employees' assignments, specify the area and limits of their responsibilities, and establish controls for monitoring performance.

The office manager will be responsible for setting and maintaining all office schedules, including those of

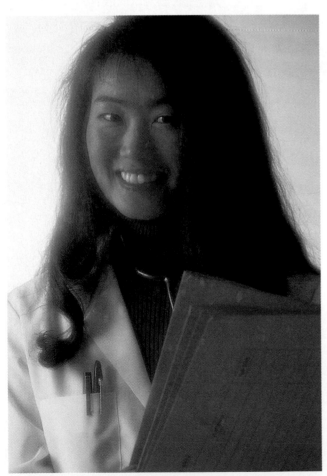

A medical assistant must be highly organized and have excellent interpersonal skills in order to be an effective office manager.

Working Smart

When your supervisor gives you an assignment, be sure to get answers to these questions:

- What is the timeline?
- What is the budget?
- What outcome is expected?
- How should I report my progress?

the physician, staff, and patient visits. While input on scheduling should come from all office personnel, the office manager ultimately is responsible for establishing and implementing the schedule. Problems with schedules will have to be resolved by you. As discussed in Chapter 8, "Scheduling Appointments and Managing Time," this may be done by performing a time study. Major difficulties may require that you deal with the problems during a staff meeting and possibly assign a team to propose solutions.

File management will be under the supervision of the office manager. While other staff members may keep the files, the office manager is responsible for establishing a coherent and organized filing system. Files should be orderly and periodically updated as explained in Chapter 9, "Managing Medical Records." Sloppy file management cannot be tolerated in a medical office, as files contain critical and confidential information on patient treatment and care.

Leadership Skills

The office manager who understands how to lead will do more than just manage the daily tasks involved in running the office. He serves as a role model by inspiring and motivating others to reach their highest potential. An office manager with leadership skills has a vision for the office, constantly striving to improve efficiency while maintaining an atmosphere of warmth and caring.

Interpersonal Skills

It is essential to possess good interpersonal skills such as:

- communicating honestly
- showing empathy
- being patient
- being trustworthy

Accurately assessing your own strengths and weaknesses can help in your relationships with others. The self-assessment survey in Figure 13.1 can help you look at some of your behavioral characteristics. If you score low on characteristics such as decision-making, problem-solving ability, flexibility, and assertiveness, you can improve these areas through goal-setting,

---

Circle the number that best represents your response to each statement.

		Never						Always
1.	I work well in teams.	Never	1	2	3	4	5	Always
2.	I complete job assignments on time.	Never	1	2	3	4	5	Always
3.	I see myself as competent in a variety of tasks.	Never	1	2	3	4	5	Always
4.	I usually react slowly and deliberately.	Never	1	2	3	4	5	Always
5.	I am a good decision-maker.	Never	1	2	3	4	5	Always
6.	I like to see others do well on the job.	Never	1	2	3	4	5	Always
7.	I contribute frequently to discussions.	Never	1	2	3	4	5	Always
8.	I can accept other people's ideas.	Never	1	2	3	4	5	Always
9.	I like to seek out new experiences and challenges.	Never	1	2	3	4	5	Always
10.	I look people in the eye when speaking.	Never	1	2	3	4	5	Always
11.	I consider myself an organized person.	Never	1	2	3	4	5	Always
12.	I manage time efficiently.	Never	1	2	3	4	5	Always
13.	I share my personal feelings when it is appropriate.	Never	1	2	3	4	5	Always
14.	I introduce myself in social gatherings.	Never	1	2	3	4	5	Always
15.	I can produce quality work on my own.	Never	1	2	3	4	5	Always
16.	I know my own strengths and weaknesses.	Never	1	2	3	4	5	Always
17.	I am aware of what I do not know.	Never	1	2	3	4	5	Always
18.	I know how to achieve group consensus.	Never	1	2	3	4	5	Always

Scoring: The items in this survey are desirable qualities for a leader. Look at any items on which you scored 1 or 2. Consider how you could strengthen yourself in these areas.

Figure 13.1
Self-Assessment Survey

attending development seminars for medical assistants, and reading appropriate educational materials. Becoming aware of problems may be enough to start you working conscientiously to change these behaviors. For example, if you tend to be a procrastinator, someone who puts off making decisions (as well as taking action), try writing down the decision that needs to be made and setting a deadline for making it.

Communicating honestly with patients and other staff members is essential. Most patients respond favorably to open and honest discussion, while deception or avoidance of issues is usually met with suspicion and distrust. While honest communication may be painful, it is absolutely necessary. Often, a patient or member of the patient's family will ask you for a medical opinion. While you cannot give this, you can respond honestly by saying, "I'm sorry, but I'm not authorized to discuss such information; perhaps you should speak with the physician to clarify your treatment options," rather than, "I don't know."

Similarly, your communication with staff members must be honest. If an employee asks for your opinion of her work, your responsibility is to give her an honest answer. If you feel that some areas need improvement, you must discuss them in an open and frank manner. Even though you may feel uncomfortable discussing negative aspects of the employee's performance, you will be providing an opportunity for her to improve and grow. If you can make your suggestions in a warm, friendly, and supportive manner, most employees will be appreciative and strive for improvement.

Showing **empathy** to both employees and patients indicates that you care about them and their concerns. This does not mean that you become overly involved

with other people's problems but that you display concern about their particular situation.

Showing concern often is difficult, particularly when an employee or patient is rude or argumentative. It is difficult to do when you are tired and have had a day full of problems. However, expressing concern always brings the best result. It is hard for a person to keep up a barrage of insults if you are responding patiently to the outburst. Most unpleasant situations can be moderated by your quiet and calm manner. Of course, if a bad situation goes on too long, or if violent behavior starts, you need to have the physician intervene.

Building trust with both patients and employees is absolutely essential. This means that you do not repeat gossip or talk about people behind their backs. Similarly, you do not pass on information that has been given to you in confidence. You must always remember that patient and employee records are confidential, and you have no right to share that information with other patients or employees. Nor should you share personal information patients have disclosed to you with anyone other than the physician (in cases where the information is medically relevant).

Understanding Management Duties and Responsibilities

The office manager sees that the physician's office runs smoothly. This involves overseeing all the day-to-day organizational tasks and managing the office staff. Duties will vary depending on the size of the office and the employees' specialized skills. For example, if the office employs an accountant or bookkeeper, the office manager may not have hands-on responsibilities for financial matters. However, it is still important that the office manager understand the business side of office management. The manager's administrative duties fall into three major categories: financial responsibilities, public relations, and personnel management.

Financial Responsibilities

The office manager's financial duties will vary with the size of the office. In a large office, an accountant may oversee many of the financial and record-keeping duties. In a small office, the office manager may be responsible for some or all of the following tasks:

- maintaining employee time sheets
- preparing payroll records
- withholding taxes
- making bank deposits of withheld funds
- preparing W-2 forms and filing federal and state government reports

As was discussed in Chapter 10, "Handling Accounting Responsibilities," a number of government publications and numerous books on tax reporting can help you with these tasks. However, if you are totally unfamiliar with basic financial and tax reporting, you may need to work with a tax adviser or other professional to acquire these skills. If that is not possible, you may be able to take a home study or web-based course on payroll management and tax reporting, or a continuing education seminar provided by the American Association of Medical Assistants (AAMA). Colleges and universities also offer courses on these subjects. Before you take on this responsibility, talk with your employer to see what level of expertise is expected of you and how willing he is to provide you with outside professional support while you are learning these tasks. If you are replacing a person who knows these functions, it may be possible to have her train you before she leaves.

You may also be expected to prepare the office's annual budget. A **budget** is a financial document that shows the estimated revenues and expenditures for a given period of time, usually a year. Budgeted expenses will include such items as salaries, rent, and supplies. Projected income will be based on estimated fees paid through patient billings and insurance payments for the same period. In a large clinic, the expense budget

Expense Budget for the Park Medical Clinic

ITEMS	MARCH	APRIL	MAY
Payroll	$54,000	$54,000	$70,000
Medical Supplies	2,000	2,000	2,000
Equipment Rental	1,200	1,200	1,200
Maintenance Contract	500	0	0
Office Rental	3,600	3,600	3,600
Office Supplies	350	350	350
Telephone	350	350	350
Insurance	1,000	1,000	1,000
Postage and Mailing	350	400	400
Training Costs	225	225	225
Quarterly Tax Payment	30,260	0	0
Total Monthly Expenses	**$93,835**	**$63,125**	**$79,125**

Figure 13.2
Sample Medical Office Budget

may be allocated by department. Figure 13.2 shows a three-month expense budget for a medical practice.

A computerized **spreadsheet** program is useful for developing budgets and is much faster than preparing a budget with paper and pencil. A spreadsheet consists of columns and rows of cells in which budget figures are inserted. Once all the numerical data are inserted, the computer calculates how items interrelate. For example, you can automatically adjust for variations in income or a seasonal increase in expenditures.

Some integrated software programs let you create budgets and track expenses against the budget as they are incurred. There are many programs designed for use in the medical office. Monthly or quarterly budget reviews enable you to spot trouble areas and make adjustments to avoid financial problems. For example, if a quarterly review shows that billings were under the projected figure, you may have to reduce expenditures in the next quarter by delaying purchases or reducing staff hours. Conversely, if revenues were much higher than expected, you may decide to buy a needed item that had not been included in the budget. You also can calculate the salary and tax impact on the budget of adding a new employee.

Public Relations and Marketing

A medical office uses **public relations** and **marketing** activities to convince the public that the practice provides excellent medical services, respects and values each patient, and operates efficiently. While public

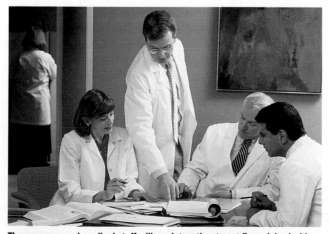

The manager and medical staff will work together to set financial priorities and goals that will be reflected in the annual budget.

relations and marketing are interrelated, good public relations may be less formal than some other marketing activities. For example, public relations starts with courtesy on the telephone, which is often a patient's first contact with the office. How the call was answered can determine whether the patient's first opinion of the office is positive or negative. Good public relations are fostered by such factors as a friendly and caring staff, efficient and polite service, clear and timely written communication, cleanliness of the facility, and accurate record-keeping.

Customer Service

It takes a number of positive incidents to make up for a single negative one. Up to 95% of dissatisfied customers will give you another chance if you move quickly to resolve their complaint.

How patients feel about the office often depends on how they are treated by not only the physician but by the office staff as well. The office manager is responsible for seeing that the atmosphere in the office is pleasant. Some ways to ensure that the office has a warm and friendly feeling are:

- establishing and maintaining a pleasing and orderly environment
- providing brochures, newsletters, and other information relating to the practice for patients in the waiting room
- encouraging professional office staff interaction with patients
- maintaining a competent staff by encouraging staff members to participate in continuing education
- informing the public about the medical office by preparing press releases
- offering seminars for patients and staff
- promoting staff recognition events

MARKETING PLANS AND DOCUMENTS Marketing activities are specific actions that promote and inform the public about services your practice provides. As office manager, you may be expected to provide a marketing plan, and possibly to prepare marketing materials supporting the plan, for any one or a number of these services. The plan should include a mission statement and goals, strategies to accomplish the goals, specific activities, completion dates, and a budget for marketing activities.

SEMINARS AND PRESENTATIONS Some offices may offer seminars on specific health subjects such as surgical aftercare, caregiver survival skills, managing high blood pressure, dealing with arthritis, and healthy eating plans. Seminars should be tailored to fit the audience. For example, one designed for young patients would differ considerably from a program for seniors.

INFORMATION SHEETS AND BROCHURES Many offices provide a variety of information sheets and brochures. These may be set out on a table or bookcase, but a special rack for the materials works best. Simple one-page information sheets can be reproduced on the office copier, and they and brochures can be created on an office computer. However, if the budget allows the expenditure, work with a printer who can help with layout and design. Prepare the text carefully, and check it for accuracy, clarity, and readability level. Be sure it is edited for spelling and grammatical errors. Avoid fancy, distracting design features. Whenever possible, use high-quality paper and an easy-to-read type font.

PRESS RELEASES AND NEWSLETTERS A **press release** is information for an article that is submitted to a newspaper for publication. Press releases may be used to announce news such as staff additions or promotions, added services, seminars, employee recognition,

---

PRESS RELEASE

From Sandy Holgren
Park Medical Clinic
19 Third Avenue
Bloomville, MN 55000
612-555-9589

Date: November 6, 20XX

PARK MEDICAL CLINIC ANNOUNCES NEW LOCATION

Bloomville, November 6, 20XX

The Park Medical Clinic announced today that it is moving into a new, larger facility on December 1, 20XX. The practice will occupy the first floor of the newly remodeled Norwest Office Complex at the northwest corner of Highways 62 and 494.

The 4,000-square-foot space will have five office suites, two conference rooms, and a state-of-the-art laboratory. The new office will include a large play area for young children, a patient education center, and a large aquarium.

The Park Medical Clinic, established in 1985, employs three general practitioners, two pediatricians, and a dermatologist.

An Open House will be held on Saturday, December 13, from 2 to 5 P.M. All current and prospective patients are invited to attend. Refreshments and gifts for the children will be provided. For further information, please call Sandy at 612-555-9589.

Figure 13.3
Sample Press Release

and extended hours. They should follow the format shown in Figure 13.3. A press release includes a headline, the date of release, and a contact person's name and phone number.

Newsletters keep patients in contact with the office. They may include articles on a variety of topics such as new staff members, new facilities, staff promotions, staff recognition, health tips, reviews of books on health-related topics, recipes, and exercise routines. The physicians and office staff should be encouraged to suggest topics for the newsletter. A newsletter can be produced in the office or by a printing house. As with brochures, you must check and recheck the text for accuracy and readability.

SPECIAL EVENTS Inviting the public to special events helps promote the services the office provides. Some events that could be well attended are blood pressure screenings, blood drives, and lectures by specialized healthcare providers. Invite members of your office team to suggest topics for special events and to help plan them. These may be organized in conjunction with other community activities such as health fairs and allied health education programs and promotional activities.

Personnel Management

Personnel responsibilities will not be the same in every office. However, the office manager should be prepared to assume any or all of these staff-related tasks:

- hiring
- orientation and training
- supervision
- performance evaluation
- disciplining
- developing and communicating office policies and procedures
- keeping office records

It may even be necessary for you to dismiss an employee. The office's procedure manual should list the steps you should carefully follow for dismissal. If such a list has not been developed, consult an attorney before acting.

Managerial Tasks

Establishing a work schedule for staff members, managing inventory and ordering supplies, maintaining files, budgeting, communicating with the staff, overseeing and evaluating staff members, and keeping personnel records are tasks that most office managers perform. Today, computers in most offices have soft-ware programs that can help you perform these tasks quickly and efficiently.

ESTABLISHING A WORK SCHEDULE The office manager usually establishes the work schedule for the staff. This includes monitoring and approving vacation schedules so that a full staff is working on all business days. The office manager may set cutoff dates for non-emergency requests for time off. Coordinating staff time with the patient appointment scheduling is crucial. Usually, a physician's schedule is posted before patient appointments for that physician are scheduled. The office's appointment book, either manual or computerized, must accurately reflect the physician availability for a given day. Overseeing the scheduling of work hours and out-of-the-office time is the office manager's responsibility. Hours and days worked by each staff member should be documented in the office's permanent record.

COMMUNICATING WITH THE STAFF Harmony and efficiency in the medical office often depends on the clarity of communication. While much of the office manager's communication will be oral, there will be times when a written document is useful. The memorandum, usually called a memo, is an effective way to

---

MEMORANDUM

TO: Medical Office Staff
FROM: Janna Black
Office Manager

DATE: NOVEMBER 16, 20XX

SUBJECT: COMPENSATORY TIME

It has come to my attention that there is some misunderstanding about the accumulation and use of compensatory time. I hope that the following paragraph from the Clinic Policy Manual will clarify this.

> Par.V. 1a: Compensatory time is accumulated only when the employee is requested by the office manager to work more than 7.5 hours per day or 37.5 hours in a given week. Compensatory time is calculated in .5 hours and may be taken upon prior approval from the office manager.

If you have any questions regarding this policy, please call me.

Figure 13.4
Memo to Staff

communicate information to employees. A major advantage over oral communication is that employees can keep the document for reference. For example, Figure 13.4 contains information on a compensatory time policy. Memos should be limited to one page. They are usually printed on plain paper and follow a standard format. Refer to Chapter 7, "Managing Communications: Telephones, Mail, and Correspondence," for more information on written communication.

If all members of the staff have access to e-mail as part of their job responsibilities, it may be appropriate to e-mail messages about office policies. It is not appropriate to rely on e-mail for office communication if everyone does not have access to it. In a busy office, the most appropriate way to make important announcements might be in a formal memorandum or orally at a staff meeting.

Oral communication with staff members and patients should be direct and clear. Always establish eye contact with your listener and speak in a well-modulated voice. Use brief sentences so there is no doubt as to what you say or mean. Avoid medical jargon when talking with patients. Sometimes, you may need to repeat what you have just said, but be careful not to insult your listeners by excessive repetition. Be sure to offer your listeners a chance to respond to you and ask questions. Being a good listener is as important as being a good speaker. Be careful how you use your facial expressions. Communication experts say that as much as 55% to 75% of the impact of a message results from non-verbal factors such as body language, facial expressions, and tone.

KEEPING PERSONNEL RECORDS A personnel file must be maintained for each employee. Data in it should include date of employment, official transcript of education, position description, dates and details of employee reviews, records of any disciplinary action, compensation history, educational training and continuing education, commendations, and other relevant information pertaining to job performance.

Building a Team

When you assume the role of office manager, you may find a team in place. If that is the case, you should be sensitive to how the team functions and cautious about suggesting changes in team behavior. If the employees are used to operating independently without any team structure, the office manager will need to explain the benefits of teamwork. This can be accomplished by describing how teams work and how they benefit the staff and patients. It is absolutely essential to give the

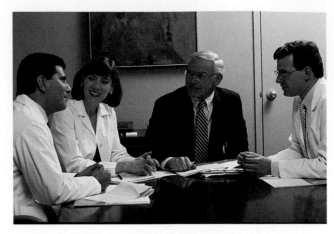

The office staff will be more successful if they work together as a team.

staff time to understand and "buy into" the concept of a team operation. Without staff consent and support, efforts at team building can be disappointing and may even fail. Successful teamwork in the office can result in higher employee morale, less staff turnover, higher efficiency, and improved patient service.

Successful team building requires a common goal or vision. The office may already have a goal statement prominently displayed. If so, the office manager can begin with this statement. For example, a first step in team building could be to ask for each employee's response to the current goal statement. Ideally, this would be done at a meeting for this purpose.

Working Smart

A team will operate more effectively if:
- goals are clearly stated and are achievable
- everyone participates
- openness and honesty are encouraged
- members listen respectfully to each other
- members speak respectfully to each other
- the team leader encourages members but does not dominate them
- members feel free to critique or give feedback about the process
- members are willing to accept task assignments

Encouraging all employees to react to a goal statement without fear of being criticized is very important. If there is considerable disagreement or confusion about the statement, ask employees to rewrite the statement and bring their new versions to the next meeting for discussion. Even if there is agreement on a goal statement, it is likely that problems in implementing it will be mentioned. This is the opportunity for the office manager to suggest that a team approach be designed to correct these problems.

For example, a goal statement in a physician's office could be, "A patient will wait no more than fifteen minutes after a scheduled appointment to see the physician." If this goal is frequently not being met, the office manager has an excellent opportunity to seek a team solution to the problem. At a meeting to discuss this goal, physicians and staff members can state their views on why it is not met. The resulting discussion could generate several possible solutions, such as rewriting the goal statement to permit exceptions, changing the schedule to prevent such occurrences, or dropping the goal statement altogether.

> **Working Smart**
>
> Effective teams can boost productivity and job satisfaction. Accept—even encourage—differing views. The results will generate fresh opinions and allow new perspectives.

Teamwork should not be reserved just for dealing with problems. Routine office practices can benefit from team input. For example, scheduling, policies and procedures, benefits, patient management, record-keeping, continuing education, and public relations may all benefit from team involvement. Research has shown that employees who feel they have some control over their work are more dedicated to their jobs. Being a member of a team gives an employee that sense of control. Naturally, everything cannot be decided by employees, but an amazing amount of daily activity can be positively affected by employee team decisions.

Empowering the Team to Find Solutions

Teams can be very effective in solving office problems if they believe that their recommendations will be valued. This requires trust between management and staff. The office manager plays a key role in creating this trust. A team should not be given a problem to solve before that trust is established. Never ask a team to solve a problem if there is little chance that the team's recommendations will be taken seriously. If management is well represented on the team, this should not be a problem.

The first step in resolving a problem is to clearly identify it. Every team member should agree on what is at stake. This can be done several ways in a group setting. Generally, at a team meeting, the group leader (usually, but not always, the office manager) asks team members to describe the problem. Responses are written on a chalkboard or flip chart. Then they are discussed and evaluated until consensus is reached on the exact description of the problem. It may be stated in a brief sentence.

The following example shows how an inner city medical clinic handled a problem:

> The physicians wanted to extend office hours to evenings and Saturdays. They wanted to use the current staff for this as much as possible without incurring overtime costs. The employee team was asked to suggest scheduling options that might encourage the present staff to consider working evenings and Saturdays.

First, the problem was reduced to one question: "What incentives would encourage present staff members to work evenings and Saturdays?"

Then the team held a **brainstorming** session. This requires that team members be encouraged to throw out the first idea that comes to mind. All ideas are accepted at this point, and no idea is criticized. The group leader writes down all the ideas on a flip chart or blackboard.

Then, the members are invited to respond seriously to each idea. Gradually, impractical suggestions are eliminated, leaving a manageable list for discussion and evaluation. The final list might include the following options:

- alternate evening and Saturday hours among staff members
- offer full-time positions to part-time employees
- full-time, senior employees would not work as many evening and weekend hours
- hire part-time staff to cover the additional hours

> **Working Smart**
>
> When brainstorming, every idea is a good idea. Being critical will squelch the creative process.

The next step is to rank these options. The team might decide to rank them according to what the members think is most acceptable or by cost.

A technique similar to brainstorming is **concept mapping**. The team leader draws a big circle that represents the problem. Team members are asked to offer one-word solutions. Each word is attached with a line to the center of the circle. A concept map for the problem in the medical practice previously discussed might look like Figure 13.5. The results of this activity could lead to a different list of activities such as:

Procedure 13.1

Conducting a Team Brainstorming Session

Purpose: Use brainstorming techniques to solve a defined office problem.

Equipment/Supplies: Flip chart with erasable magic markers, conference room with chairs and table.

1 Appoint someone to be the note-taker. Explain that this person will provide a written summary of the group's work at the end of the discussion.

2 Set a time limit for the session.

3 Ask each staff member to identify and describe the problem in one or two sentences. Write down exactly what each person says. Number each description. Encourage everyone to contribute, but do not force anyone to do so.

4 Discuss each person's description of the problem and gradually rewrite or rework the problem so that everyone clearly understands it. The brainstorming session should not proceed until all agree on the statement of the problem.

5 Tell members that brainstorming begins with all ideas being offered, and that no criticism is allowed. Encourage everyone to contribute any idea, no matter how wild or unrealistic. At this point, it is important to make everyone feel relaxed. Be sure that you, as the leader, respect each individual's contribution.

6 Write each idea on the flip chart and number it. You will have enough ideas to consider when you have one or two sheets filled. However, don't stop taking ideas before the group has agreed that there are enough possible solutions to discuss.

7 Give the group fifteen minutes to discuss the solutions and begin a process of elimination. One way to eliminate ideas is by asking the group to list pros and cons for each idea. Try to reduce the list to no more than three possible solutions.

8 On a new sheet of paper, summarize the group's top suggestions.

9 Explain how the group's recommendations will be used. Never ask a group to work on a problem unless you will seriously consider its suggestions.

10 Set a date for a follow-up meeting to discuss how the group's recommendations are being used to correct the problem. Also set a date for when the summary of the meeting (assigned in Step 2) will be delivered to management.

- Look into how competitors deal with extended hours.
- Research and resolve safety concerns for night workers.
- Consider continuing education opportunities for extended-hour workers.
- Provide childcare for extended-hour workers.
- Establish a bonus pay schedule for evening and Saturday workers.

Both brainstorming and concept mapping can help the team to come up with solutions for evaluation and discussion. The office manager may use both methods or can develop another system for arriving at group solutions. The nature of the problem and time constraints may determine the best method.

It is important to follow up on the suggestions and to provide a written summary of the team's findings. Sometimes, it will be necessary to assign team members to provide information on the feasibility of the suggestions. The office manager should assemble team member findings and present this information to the group. A complex problem may take many meetings to resolve. While every team member may not agree with the group's recommendations, it is important that each member feel involved in the process.

Conducting Staff Meetings

Regular staff meetings provide an opportunity for management and staff to communicate their concerns to one another. In most offices, the office manager sets the date and conducts the meetings. An **agenda** is prepared and distributed before each meeting. Employees should be encouraged to suggest topics for discussion. Open and free discussion should be encouraged. Contentious or complex items can be assigned for further study. In fact, meetings are more productive if follow-up assignments are given and employees are expected to do follow-up work. A sample agenda might look like the one shown in Figure 13.6.

The meetings should be held regularly. In some offices, they are weekly; in others, monthly. Many offices have Monday morning staff meetings where the entire week is mapped out and assignments clarified. The timing will depend on the

Working Smart

Start and end meetings on time. This will communicate that you value the time of the participants.

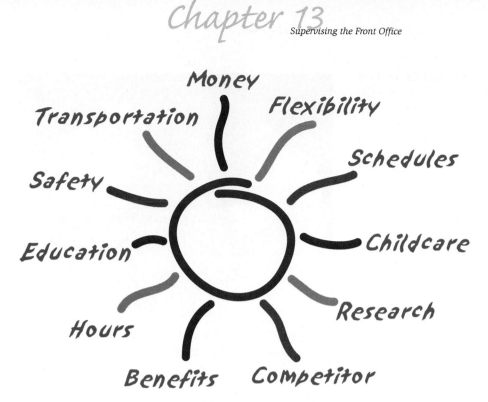

**Figure 13.5
Example of a Concept
Map Developed During a
Brainstorming Session**

office schedule, but the meeting should be held either before patients arrive or after office hours later in the day. A definite adjournment time must be set.

PARKVIEW COMMUNITY CLINIC
December 11, 20XX
7:30 A.M.–8:30 A.M. in Conference Room A

AGENDA

1. Call to order.
2. Approval of minutes from November 13 meeting.
3. Introduction of new employee.
4. Discussion of telephone policy.
5. Report on staff Christmas party plans.
6. Report on winter semester continuing education offerings at Metropolitan State College.
7. Office hours and schedule for staff during the holidays.
8. Other business.
9. Adjournment, 8:30 A.M.

**Figure 13.6
Sample Agenda**

Employees should be encouraged to contribute in the meetings. As issues arise, assign employees to bring information to the next meeting. Meetings will be more effective when everyone participates through discussion and assigned responsibilities. Some offices will have the office manager act as the meeting facilitator, while others may rotate this responsibility. By sharing this role, staff members learn to take the meetings more seriously, to recognize the work that goes into effective meeting planning, and to understand the importance of participation.

The office manager (or someone appointed) is responsible for providing notes on the meeting to any employee who is absent. Failure to do this can result in misunderstandings, particularly when important issues are decided at the meeting. Periodically, employees should be asked to evaluate the effectiveness of the staff meetings. Suggestions for improving them should be taken seriously. In some cases, a small team might be assigned to suggest ways to increase meeting productivity and effectiveness.

Providing Motivation and Recognition

Staff morale can be built through periodic recognition of employee contributions to the smooth running of the office. One or more employees might be singled out for outstanding performance under unusual circumstances. More often, a team may be rewarded for the time and effort its members contributed to solving a problem. This reward could be in the form of a recognition lunch or dinner, or might consist of tickets to a special event. Sometimes, an individual might receive a plaque or a pin. The type of reward will depend on the office culture and the budget allocated for awards. Remember that praise and affirmation for good work should be offered frequently. Do not fail to praise individuals by name in a meeting. Some offices like to post pictures of employees and their titles in the office area. This helps make employees feel important and also helps patients recognize them.

Developing Policies and Procedures

A policy refers to a plan or course of action. A procedure describes how a policy will be implemented step by step. Some offices put policies and procedures in one document. This is acceptable, but you should remember that they are not the same thing. When policies and procedures are included in one document, the policy is usually stated at the top of the page, followed by a list of the procedures to carry out the policy.

Policy Manual

The **policy manual** describes the office philosophy and goals. It also contains an organizational chart showing the lines of authority. Biographies of each physician may be included, listing educational background, medical training and specialties, board certifications, state license number, and professional memberships. The manual provides a guide for employees regarding professional dress and conduct. It describes working conditions such as office hours and policies concerning scheduling, breaks, holidays, sick days, overtime, pay periods, vacations, benefit packages, payment for continuing education, salary and performance evaluation, use of equipment, public relations, bookkeeping, billing, criteria for promotion and bonuses, grievances, termination, and severance pay. Policy manuals tend to expand over time. They must be reviewed periodically. Outdated policies must be deleted and new policies added.

Procedure Manual

Every medical office needs a **procedure manual** to describe the services the office provides and how they are delivered. The manual lists every task and its rationale, who performs it, when and where, and how the task is recorded and billed.

The procedure manual usually is kept in a loose-leaf three-ring binder so that insertions and deletions are easy to make. Each task should be numbered, dated, and reviewed annually. Listing procedures in a standardized format enables the information to be presented

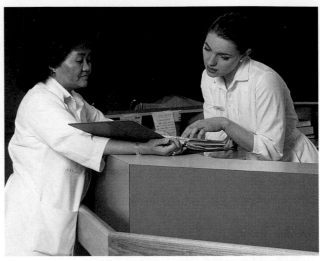

Keeping the office procedure manual complete and up-to-date will help ensure an organized work environment and will reduce stress and confusion.

clearly and consistently. All the office forms and document templates for standard letters belong in this manual. Maintaining the manual is an important responsibility of the office manager.

If you are working in an office that does not have a procedure manual, you should discuss its importance with your employer. It may be that procedures are written but not well organized. Sometimes, you will find that they are tacked up on bulletin boards, in file cabinets or desk drawers, or attached to other office documents. Offer to locate all these pieces of information and organize them by topic in a three-ring binder. Once the binder has been completed, review the contents with the staff. Some procedures may be outdated. Others may need to be written down for inclusion in the binder. Every employee should have access to this resource. It is particularly important that new employees be familiar with the manual.

Hiring and Reviewing Employees

The office manager may be authorized to hire new employees. Or, in some offices, the physician or a team of employees may want to meet with prospective candidates. In either case, your responsibility will be to prepare the job description, advertise the position, evaluate the applications, resumes, and interview impressions, and either recommend one individual for the job or submit more than one name for the physician or team to consider. If all the applicants appear to be acceptable, you may rank them and offer the position to the highest-ranked candidate. If that person turns down your offer, you still have other viable choices. Once the job is filled, write thank-you notes to the applicants who interviewed for the position. New employees usually go through a trial period specified in the policy manual, often 90 days. During this time, the employee may be terminated without showing cause.

Preparing Job Descriptions

A job description is a written document listing the responsibilities of the position and the qualifications needed to fill it. Job descriptions for every position in the office should be filed in the procedures manual, dated, and revised annually.

A job description has at least three parts: description of the position; educational and experience qualifications; and job tasks. It may also list the person to whom the employee reports and a salary range for the position. If you are expected to write job descriptions when you are new to the job, discuss the position requirements with the physician and other staff members. The job description also is useful when placing an ad for the position or listing it with an employment agency. A sample job description is shown in Figure 13.7.

JOB TITLE:	Medical Assistant
QUALIFICATIONS:	High school diploma, degree from a 2-year medical assistant program, and CMA or RMA certification
JOB RESPONSIBILITIES:	Prepare treatment room Measure vital signs Clean and sterilize instruments Contact specialists or other medical facilities for tests Give injections and other treatments Keep treatment records Prepare insurance forms Other responsibilities as assigned
SALARY RANGE:	$22,000 to $25,000 depending on experience
SUPERVISOR:	Head clinic physician or nurse practitioner

Figure 13.7
Job Description for the Position of Medical Assistant

MEDICAL ASSISTANT/CERTIFIED MEDICAL ASST. Seeking FT CMA or RMA for busy 24-physician cardiology clinic in Minneapolis. Clinical experience in phlebotomy required, and ECGs preferred. Hours are 8:30–5:00 Monday thru Friday. Candidates should mail or fax resume to Office Manager, Minneapolis Heart Clinic, 2025 Centre Pointe Blvd., Ste. #200, Minneapolis, MN 55407. Fax (651) 555-7570, E-mail to Heartclinic@emcp.com. Equal Opportunity/Affirmative Action Employer.

MEDICAL ASSISTANT Ancillary Coordinator, 32 hours/week/days. OB/GYN clinic is seeking an individual to coordinate communications & documentation about clinic patients' care. Computer skills, working knowledge of med terms and medical transcription required. Send resume to Office Manager, Human Resources, 625 Smith Street, St. Paul, MN, 55100, Fax: 651-555-1249 EOE.

Figure 13.8
Classified Ads for Medical Assistant Positions

Recruiting

There are several ways to fill staff vacancies. In a practice with several levels of job opportunities, a current staff member may wish to apply for an open position. Even if all staff members know about the vacancy, the job description for the opening should be posted on the office bulletin board. If none of the current staff is interested, you may do one, some, or all of the following: advertise the position in local newspapers or trade journals, contact employment agencies, or call local colleges and technical schools that provide medical assistant training. Figure 13.8 provides a sample of two medical assisting positions that were advertised in a classified section. Procedure 13.2 suggests steps to follow when recruiting new employees for the medical office staff.

Screening and Interviewing Applicants

Applicants may be asked to fill out an application form and/or send a resume. These documents provide background information to help you assess the applicant's qualifications. After screening all the applications, arrange personal interviews with the best of the candidates who fit your job needs. Try to keep your interview list short, as the interview process is time-consuming. If your first interviews do not provide you with a viable employee, review the applications and schedule more interviews if you can identify other suitable candidates.

Prepare for the interview carefully. Be aware that certain questions of a personal nature may not be asked. For instance, you cannot ask if the person is married, has children, or has debt. Federal law also prohibits discriminating against job applicants because

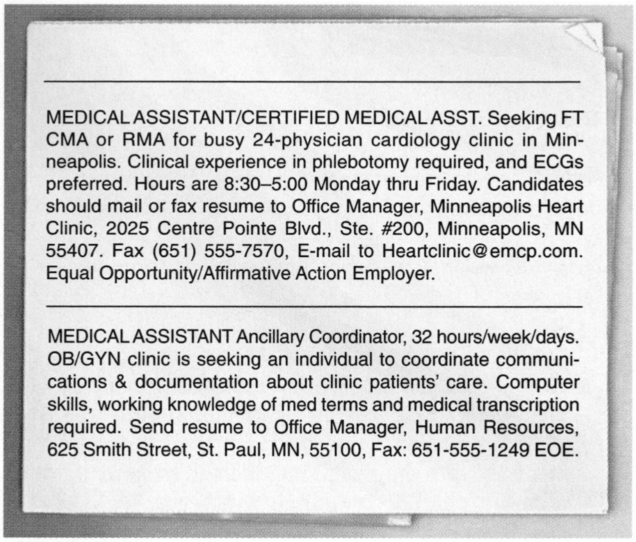

Procedure 13.2

Recruiting an Employee

Purpose: To fill a newly created position or replace a departing employee.

Equipment/Supplies: Pen, paper, typewriter or computer, telephone.

1 Confer with the physician and the team to identify the required skills if the position is new. If you are replacing an employee, an existing job description will list the skills needed. Even so, review the job description carefully with other staff members to be sure that it is accurate and reflects your current needs.
2 Post the job description in your office and on public bulletin boards in your building or neighborhood.
3 Write an advertisement describing the position and submit it to the major newspapers in your area. Be sure it is listed in the classified section's Health Careers category.
4 Call the placement offices of local colleges and technical schools. Ask them to post your opening on bulletin boards and in their newsletters or other informational publications.
5 Attend job fairs for health professionals whenever possible. Students and counselors attend these and may provide a link to potential employees.
6 Submit your advertisement to appropriate medical trade journals.
7 Call several employment agencies. Be sure to clarify who pays the fee if you hire an applicant an agency sends you—the employee or the employer.
8 Ask colleagues if they know of anyone who might be qualified and interested in the position.

---

of their country of origin, age, race, sex, sexual preference, or religion. A standardized interview form will ensure that you ask the same questions of each interviewee. This does not mean that you do not deviate occasionally from your script so that the interview does not seem stiff. However, it is important that each candidate have an opportunity to cover the same subject matter in the interview.

Open-ended questions will elicit the most information from the candidate. Avoid questions that can be answered with a simple "yes" or "no." Be sure to allow the candidate ample opportunity to ask you questions about the job as well. These questions often indicate the level of interest and desire that the person has in the job. Also, the candidate's communication style can be noted. A person with poor speech or a hesitant speaking style may not be right for a position that requires frequent patient interaction. Table 13.1 provides questions you may want to ask during an interview. You will want to adapt some of them to your own office and the specific job opening.

Legal Issue

Federal law prohibits discrimination based on country of origin, age, race, sex, religion, marital status, and sexual preference. Do not ask questions about these aspects of a prospective employee's life during an interview.

Table 13.1 Suggested Questions for Interviewing an Applicant

- Why are you interested in this position?
- What jobs have you held? How were they obtained? Why did you leave?
- Why did you become a medical assistant?
- In what kind of a setting do you want to work?
- What do you know about our office?
- What qualifications do you have that you think suit you for this position?
- Why do you think you would like this job?
- Do you enjoy working with others or mostly by yourself?
- How did you get along with other employees at your previous jobs?
- What are your long-term goals?
- How does this position fit with those goals?
- Are you planning to seek further education?
- What do you consider your strengths?
- What do you consider your weaknesses?
- If offered this position, when could you start?
- What are your outside interests?

You also will need a checklist for observing such traits as grooming, eye contact, interest in and enthusiasm for the position, distracting mannerisms, and openness. Allow time in the interview to explain carefully the tasks that the job entails, and the office's policies on subjects such as working hours, dress code, salary, benefits, vacation, time off, continuing education, and promotional opportunities.

Ask the interview candidates to give you the names of references you may contact by phone. These phone interviews should be brief but to the point. Have a list of

Table 13.2 Questions You May Ask a Reference

- What were Jane's responsibilities in your office?
- How long did she work there?
- How well did she work with other employees?
- Why did she leave?
- What are her strengths? Her weaknesses?
- Was she a dependable and hardworking employee?
- Is she eligible for rehire?

questions prepared before you call. Table 13.2 lists questions you may wish to ask a reference. Keep in mind that if someone calls you as a reference for an employee, these are the only questions you should answer.

Since people are very reluctant, because of legal considerations, to say anything negative about a person, you will have to listen carefully to how the reference answers the questions. Sometimes, the tone of voice or a hesitation will give you a clue. Phone references, while not totally reliable, are still useful in choosing a future employee.

Each prospective employee must have a Social Security identification number or a work permit/visa. Application forms may be obtained at a local Social Security office or post office. Assuming the applicant has a Social Security number, several forms must be filled out before the person can be hired. He must complete and sign form I-9 (Employment Eligibility Verification) showing that he is a U.S. citizen or is legally authorized to work in this country. A

Technology Tip

You can obtain a copy of the I-9 form and instructions at the Immigration and Naturalization Service's website at www.ins.usdoj.gov.

Table 13.3 Proof of Employment Eligibility

An individual with one of these documents is eligible for employment.

- U.S. Passport (unexpired or expired)
- Certificate of U.S. Citizenship
- Certificate of Naturalization
- unexpired foreign passport with I-551 stamp or attached INS Form I-94 indicating unexpired employment authorization
- Alien Registration Receipt Card with photograph
- unexpired Temporary Resident Card
- unexpired Employment Authorization Card
- unexpired Reentry Permit
- unexpired Refugee Travel Document
- unexpired Employment Authorization Document issued by the INS with photograph

An individual with one document from the first column and one from the second column is eligible for employment.

Documents That Establish Identity	*Documents That Establish Employment Eligibility*
<ul><li>driver's license or ID card issued by a state or outlying possession of the U.S. if it contains a photograph or information on name, date of birth, sex, height, eye color, and address</li><li>ID card issued by federal, state, or local government agencies or entities if it contains a photograph or information on name, date of birth, sex, height, eye color, and address</li><li>school ID card with photograph</li><li>voter registration card</li><li>U.S. military card or draft record</li><li>military dependent's ID card</li><li>U.S. Coast Guard Merchant Mariner Card</li><li>Native American tribal document</li><li>driver's license issued by a Canadian government authority</li><li>If under age 18, and not able to present the above, the following items are acceptable:<ul><li>school record or report card</li><li>clinic, doctor, or hospital record</li><li>day-care or nursery school record</li></ul></li></ul>	<ul><li>U.S. Social Security card issued by the Social Security Administration</li><li>certification of Birth Abroad issued by the Department of State</li><li>original or certified copy of a birth certificate issued by a state, county, municipal authority, or outlying possession of the U.S. bearing an official seal</li><li>Native American tribal document</li><li>U.S. Citizen ID Card</li><li>ID card for use of resident citizen in the United States</li><li>unexpired employment authorization document issued by the INS</li></ul>

Source: Form I-9, 1991.

job applicant must present proof of eligibility for work in the form of a birth certificate, an original Social Security card, a current or expired U.S. passport, or other acceptable document. Table 13.3 lists acceptable documents, according to the I-9 form.

Orienting and Training New Employees

New employees who go through a systematized and thorough orientation process are much more likely to perform well and stay with the office. Nothing is so frustrating for a new employee as being thrown into a situation without a clue as to how things work. Even though the new employee may have worked in other offices, your office and some of its rules and customs will be different. No matter how intelligent or skilled the new employee is, she still needs assistance to become an effective team member in a new setting.

Orientation Process

Basic **orientation** procedures should be listed in the office procedure manual. The orientation process includes introducing the new employee to everyone in the office, providing the employee with a copy of the procedure manual, meeting with the employee's director, supervisor, or mentor, and walking the employee through the daily routine. A carefully followed orientation process will assure that the new employee feels comfortable and is able to work effectively from the very beginning.

Ongoing Supervision

Some employees require close supervision for weeks or months. Others, based on previous experience and skills, may need little oversight. However, it is important that the office manager carefully observe each new employee's work. You will want to note general characteristics such as punctuality, neatness, ability to listen and follow instructions, attitude, and oral and written skills. Specifically, note the employee's ability to fulfill the assigned responsibilities. Is she careful, accurate, and knowledgeable? Does she know when to ask questions to avoid error? How well does she interact with other staff members and patients? What are her strengths? Keep all these observations in a file so that you can discuss them with the employee. Remember to stress your positive observations as well as noting areas needing improvement.

Mentoring

Assigning a **mentor** to a new employee is an effective way to orient him. An experienced colleague who

---

Procedure 13.3

Orienting a New Employee

Purpose: To guide a new employee through job orientation.

Equipment/Supplies: Pen, paper, policy manual, procedure manual, timesheets.

1 On the first day of employment, meet with the employee and provide background information about the office and the staff members the employee will be working with. Encourage him to ask you questions at this time, and to feel free to ask questions of you and other staff members during the orientation period.
2 Show the employee where he will be working. Tour the facilities, pointing out coat closets, supply cupboards, conference rooms, labs, staff offices, restrooms, and the lunchroom. If you are in a large building with other facilities such as a coffee shop or workout room, be sure to visit those areas.
3 Introduce the new employee to the rest of the staff.
4 Review with the employee the tasks he is expected to perform.

5 Give the new employee a copy of the office policy and procedure manuals and arrange a time to go over these documents later after the employee has studied them.
6 Give the employee a timesheet and explain how hours are recorded.
7 Introduce the employee to his immediate supervisor or mentor.
8 Check with the new employee frequently during the first few days of work to be sure things are going well.
9 Arrange to meet weekly for the first few months to review any concerns or problems, and to offer praise and encouragement when warranted.
10 Check with physicians and staff members for their impressions of how the new employee is fitting in and performing the required tasks.
11 Keep notes on your meetings with the new employee and comments from coworkers. *These will help you talk meaningfully with him during your meetings and provide a basis for the employee's performance evaluation.*

understands how the office is run can be extraordinarily helpful to the new employee. Mentors use different styles. Some assign a certain time each day for the new employee to ask questions or discuss concerns. Others keep the meetings more informal but work by building trust with the new employee. When the new employee and the mentor are comfortable with each other, they usually interact informally, sometimes over coffee, during breaks, at lunch, or while sharing duties.

Working Smart

Taking time to express appreciation for those you work with pays off. Most employees report that lack of recognition creates stress for them. Consider jotting a note on your calendar to remind you to recognize your staff for work well done.

Figure 13.9
Performance Review Form

PERFORMANCE REVIEW
Treatment Assistant

Name: _____

Date: _____

Reviewed by: _____

RATING

	Needs Improvement								Excellent	

Communication Skills

	1	2	3	4	5	6	7	8	9	10
1. tactfulness	1	2	3	4	5	6	7	8	9	10
2. effective oral communication	1	2	3	4	5	6	7	8	9	10
3. effective written communication	1	2	3	4	5	6	7	8	9	10
4. directness and candor	1	2	3	4	5	6	7	8	9	10

Staff Relations

	1	2	3	4	5	6	7	8	9	10
1. attitude toward staff	1	2	3	4	5	6	7	8	9	10
2. teamwork	1	2	3	4	5	6	7	8	9	10
4. decision-making	1	2	3	4	5	6	7	8	9	10
5. work without supervision	1	2	3	4	5	6	7	8	9	10
6. use of time	1	2	3	4	5	6	7	8	9	10

Maturity

	1	2	3	4	5	6	7	8	9	10
1. ability to empathize	1	2	3	4	5	6	7	8	9	10
2. objectivity	1	2	3	4	5	6	7	8	9	10
3. dependability	1	2	3	4	5	6	7	8	9	10
4. honesty	1	2	3	4	5	6	7	8	9	10
5. self-confidence	1	2	3	4	5	6	7	8	9	10
6. patience	1	2	3	4	5	6	7	8	9	10

Personal Characteristics

	1	2	3	4	5	6	7	8	9	10
1. punctuality	1	2	3	4	5	6	7	8	9	10
2. appearance	1	2	3	4	5	6	7	8	9	10
3. personal hygiene	1	2	3	4	5	6	7	8	9	10
4. diplomacy	1	2	3	4	5	6	7	8	9	10
5. adherence to "uniform and personal appearance policy" as defined in the office policy manual	1	2	3	4	5	6	7	8	9	10

Technical Skills

	1	2	3	4	5	6	7	8	9	10
1. prompt and adequate preparation of treatment room and/or conference room for each patient	1	2	3	4	5	6	7	8	9	10
2. sterilize instruments according to recommended procedures promptly and effectively	1	2	3	4	5	6	7	8	9	10
3. anticipate the doctor's needs when assisting	1	2	3	4	5	6	7	8	9	10
4. implement technical procedures correctly	1	2	3	4	5	6	7	8	9	10
5. prompt and effective seating and dismissing of patients	1	2	3	4	5	6	7	8	9	10
6. maintain medical equipment as indicated in employee responsibilities for treatment assistant	1	2	3	4	5	6	7	8	9	10
7. maintain adequate room inventory	1	2	3	4	5	6	7	8	9	10

Record-keeping Skills

	1	2	3	4	5	6	7	8	9	10
1. legibly records patient treatment information	1	2	3	4	5	6	7	8	9	10
2. accurately records dates of visit and treatment involved on patient's record if asked to do so by doctor	1	2	3	4	5	6	7	8	9	10
3. completes all information in all designated areas on the patient's records	1	2	3	4	5	6	7	8	9	10

Evaluating Employees

The effective office manager helps and encourages employees to reach their highest potential. The manager looks for ways to praise employee performance when it is deserved, and also looks for constructive ways to help employees with performance problems.

Methods of Assessing Performance

A periodic **performance assessment** serves several functions. It offers the opportunity to praise and motivate employees who are performing very well. It also is the time to discuss any work-related problem the employee may have. If an employee has been underperforming, it may be appropriate to offer counseling.

A standard form should be used when you conduct a performance review. The performance review form in Figure 13.9 provides an example of the types of items usually discussed during the review. This kind of form lets you and the employee review the characteristics and skills required for the job. Items that receive a low rating should be discussed and plans made for improving performance in these areas. Dates for improvement should be noted.

Annual performance reviews may be used as the basis for salary adjustments. Though increases usually are based on the office salary schedule, they may also be related to the cost of living index. Salary increases presume that the employee is performing well. If an employee needs to correct certain deficiencies, the increase may be delayed. Setting performance goals, along with a higher salary goal, may help improve the employee's performance.

A carefully drafted job description may be used to evaluate a new employee's job performance. Use the tasks on the job description as a checklist to determine how well the employee is performing them. If she appears to be working well but attending to different tasks, something may be wrong with the job description, or the employee simply may prefer to do other tasks. Use the task list as a baseline for discussing and

reviewing the job assignment with the new employee. You may find that she has been doing tasks that needed to be performed but were not on the list, or that the tasks on the list were being done by someone else. By discussing the job description with your employee, you can clarify what she should be doing. This may require that you revise one or more job descriptions.

Managing Performance Problems

Serious performance problems must be addressed immediately. The policy manual should list the disciplinary measures applied for employee misconduct. For example, most offices call for the immediate suspension of an employee found sleeping on the job, stealing, using drugs, or breaching confidentiality. Any employee suspected of these or other serious acts of misconduct is suspended with pay until a thorough investigation is made. If the charges are unfounded, the employee should be reinstated, but if the charges are true, the employee is fired.

Minor problems often are dealt with less harshly. For example, an employee who is often absent or late may be put on probation. He should be given a written notice that includes the specifics of the problem, suggestions for correcting it, timeline for compliance, and consequences of failing to comply.

Suspension and firing are serious events. When they become necessary, you must make an incident report describing the reason for the disciplinary action. Be sure to include: 1) the employee's name; 2) date of the incident; 3) description of the incident; 4) date of employee notification; and 5) content of the oral and written notification given the employee. Figure 13.10 is an example of an incident report form documenting an employee's attendance problem. The form may be modified to document tardiness, excessive personal phone calls, or other inappropriate behavior.

Assessing Job Performance and Promotional Opportunities

Personal observation of the employee's performance during the first weeks of employment helps determine how well she fits the job. In addition, other employees' remarks provide information on the employee's skill level and ability to work with the staff and patients.

When considering promotion of an employee to another level of responsibility, you should evaluate how well she accepts change, takes responsibility, and works with people. For example, if the promotion involves a large amount of patient contact, you need to be confident that the employee enjoys working with patients, has a friendly attitude, and remains calm under all circumstances.

Working Smart

Beware of upward delegation. When staff members come to you with a problem, be careful not to make their assignment your own. Discuss possible solutions that the employee can implement and offer to review the finished work.

INCIDENT REPORT

TO:

FROM:

SUBJECT: **Probation Status—Attendance**

DATE:

On _____ you received a written warning advising you that further discipline would result if your attendance did not improve. Since then, you have been absent _____ days. As a result of your failure to improve your attendance record, you are hereby being placed on a 90-day probationary period from this date. Absences will continue to be unpaid and will require a physician's verification of illness.

Any further absences during this probationary period may result in your termination before the end of the probationary period.

If your attendance improves and you are retained, your attendance record must be maintained at a satisfactory level. Failure to maintain a satisfactory attendance record could result in your termination without further warning.

I have read and received a copy of this notification.

_____   _____
Employee Name   Date

_____   _____
Supervisor Name   Date

Figure 13.10
Incident Report Form

Promoting Educational Opportunities

Physicians expect staff members to stay current in their medical specialties. Since new therapies and techniques are being developed rapidly, medical personnel must continually read and study about their fields. The office manager can see that a variety of educational opportunities are available for the staff.

MEDICAL OFFICE EMPLOYEE EDUCATION PLANS Most offices will encourage their employees to seek additional educational opportunities. Office policy will vary, but some offices pay for attendance at seminars or for short courses in subjects related to the medical practice. The office manager can help employees become aware of advanced educational opportunities and the degree of available support if they wish to take advantage of the opportunities.

The manager can also provide in-house educational opportunities for staff members. When new medical therapies are introduced, the office manager, in consultation with the physician, may arrange for a specialist in the new therapy to hold a seminar for the staff. If that is not possible, written materials on the therapy may be prepared and discussed in a group session with employees. Videos and professional publications relating to the office practice should be available for group or individual use.

CONTINUING EDUCATION OPPORTUNITIES AND BENEFITS Continuing education for medical assistants is offered in a variety of settings. Courses are offered on college campuses, at seminars and workshops, through professional medical organizations, through home study, and on the World Wide Web. Participating in continuing education assures that you will be current in your field. Some offices require medical staff members to earn a certain number of continuing education credits to advance on the pay schedule.

The office manager should establish a system for recording staff participation in educational opportunities. Attendance at seminars and completion of relevant

Technology Tip

Because of the changing nature of medical technologies, continuing your education is necessary to staying current in the medical field. A growing number of training and certification courses are available on the Internet, and many will let you proceed at your own pace.

courses should be noted in the record of each employee who presents evidence of having fulfilled the seminar or course requirements.

PROFESSIONAL MEDICAL ASSOCIATIONS There are many benefits to belonging to a professional medical organization. Foremost is the opportunity to take part in seminars and courses that award Continuing Education Units (CEUs) which can be applied toward the requirements for recertification.

Two professional health organizations that are particularly well suited for medical assistants are the American Association of Medical Assistants (AAMA) and American Medical Technologists (AMT). These organizations have chapters in most states. Through participation in one or both of them, you can attend workshops and conferences, meet other health professionals, receive journals and newsletters, and earn continuing education credits. Membership in professional organizations assures that you will grow professionally and stay current in your field.

Challenging Situations

*T*he office manager's responsibility is to see that the office runs smoothly. You will often have to deal with patient complaints. For example, you will have to calm the occasional patient who gets angry when he has been kept waiting or has been treated rudely by a staff member. No matter how angry a patient may be, your function is to calm her. Keep your voice low and soothing, explain the cause of the delay, and express your empathy for the inconvenience. It is never appropriate for you to react with anger to a patient's rudeness or outbursts.

If the patient is complaining because of perceived rudeness by a staff member, pay careful attention to what is said and assure the patient that you will take note of the complaint. However, never criticize a staff member in front of a patient. Should a patient become abusive or threatening, notify a physician or supervisor in the office immediately. If no physician or supervisor is on the premises, ask the person to leave. If she refuses, notify building security or call 911.

Sometimes your toughest challenge is dealing with a staff member who is extremely competent but whose personal habits annoy coworkers. Staff complaints about a colleague should be taken seriously, but you should be sure they are valid. If you believe the complaints are valid, discuss them with the employee.

A complaint that involves personal use of the telephone during office hours can be dealt with as a policy issue. Most practices strictly forbid personal telephone calls during office hours unless the situation is an emergency. Usually, a discussion with the employee about office policy regarding use of the phone during office hours will take care of this problem.

Complaints of a more personal nature, such as talking too loudly, telling offensive jokes, or wearing too much perfume, must be handled directly and diplomatically. Explain carefully why a particular behavior is distracting or annoying to other employees. Most staff members will try to accommodate their colleagues. If the employee becomes defensive or angry about the criticism, you may have to consider probation or even dismissal.

Clinical Summary

- The office manager sets the tone for the office. She creates an environment where physicians and staff members can work efficiently without distractions.
- Public relations and marketing activities help create awareness about the medical practice and its services.
- The office manager knows how to build a team and be its leader.
- The team can be used to effectively solve office problems.
- The office manager recruits, hires, supervises, and evaluates employees.
- Before a person can be hired for a job, he must complete an Employment Eligibility Verification form and must have a Social Security identification number.
- Policies and procedures should be documented in office manuals, which should be updated and reviewed annually.
- Staff orientation and periodic job assessments are critical components of the office manager's duties.
- The office manager promotes educational opportunities for staff members to grow in their chosen fields through continuing education courses, home study, membership in professional organizations, or in-house educational seminars.

The Language of Medicine

agenda A list of items for discussion at a meeting.

brainstorming A process in which all ideas for solving a problem are initially considered and no criticism of them is allowed.

budget A financial document showing estimated revenues and expenditures for a given period of time, usually a year.

concept mapping A process in which circles and lines are used to represent problems and solutions.

empathy An attitude marked by conscious awareness of and insight into another person's actions and behavior. Understanding and being sensitive to another person's feelings.

marketing Activities designed to promote the medical practice and inform the public about its services.

mentor A knowledgeable person who counsels and guides less-experienced employees.

orientation The process by which new employees are introduced to the work environment.

performance assessment/evaluation/review A formal process in which a supervisor examines the quality of an employee's work and informs the employee of the conclusion.

policy manual A document listing the organization's guiding principles.

press release Information for an article about the medical practice that is submitted to a newspaper for publication.

procedure manual A document listing the steps for performing specific tasks.

public relations Activities designed to create a favorable public view of the medical practice.

spreadsheet A software program for inputting and manipulating numerical data to facilitate a wide variety of financial activities.

Signs/Symptoms of Progress

Recall, Question, Connect

Recall
Think of the organizational skills that an office manager needs. List ways you are organized in your own life that you might apply to an office setting.

Question
What could you do to improve your own organizational skills?

Connect
What specific tasks is an office manager responsible for that require good organizational skills?

Educating the Patient

Many patients in your clinic are elderly. Most of them do not drive cars but are not comfortable taking public transportation. Often they are late for their appointments because of transportation difficulties. Many of them depend on family members or friends for a ride. Even though they are apologetic about being late, they seem reluctant to discuss this problem with the people who provide their transportation.

1 What can the office manager do to help these people get to the office on time?

2 What kind of information might help the office manager deal with this problem?

3 Identify types of written material that might be used in this situation.

Exploring Perspectives in Teams

Perspective involves the discipline of examining how ideas look from different points of view and recognizing that there are often multiple "answers" to complex questions. In small groups or on your own, reflect on possible alternative views or answers and summarize your findings.

1 Management experts say that leaders need to be respected but not to be liked. Do you agree or disagree? Why? Is a person who is liked a stronger leader?

2 The office is serving 30% more patients than last year. You need to hire an office assistant. Discuss what the responsibilities will be and draft a job description. Be sure to include the required technical and interpersonal skills.

3 Review the traits of leaders. Are you a natural leader? Is anyone in your group a natural leader? Why or why not?

4 Discuss the concepts of motivation and recognition. What motivates you? How do you want to be recognized on the job? As office supervisor, what techniques would you use to motivate others? Use the brainstorming techniques discussed in the chapter to arrive at your answer.

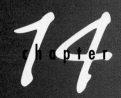

Learning Outcomes

- Describe the examination area of the medical office and specify the activities that occur in each part of the area.
- Identify the responsibilities of the medical assistant for medical asepsis and the order and safety of the examination suite.
- State the need for appropriate handwashing technique and detail the steps involved.
- List the steps for surface disinfection and indicate how and when this should be done.
- Contrast and compare the responsibilities of the medical assistant in maintaining the examination room at the end of the day with those responsibilities during the day between patients.
- Manage the inventory of supplies and equipment and understand the requirements for storage procedures.

Performance Objectives

- Prepare and maintain examination and treatment areas.
- Demonstrate the best practices in aseptic technique and infection control.
- Demonstrate correct handwashing technique.
- Comply with established risk management and safety procedures.
- Maintain supply inventory and recommend equipment and supplies.

As Pasteur and Koch established in the late 1800s, preventing germs that cause disease from entering the body will help prevent disease. Since then, much of the work of modern medicine has focused on infection control and asepsis. Their pioneering work in the area of infection control is so significant that they likely deserve most of the credit for the decline in death rates in the twentieth century. Life expectancies in much of the world have roughly doubled; in effect, modern medicine has given us virtually a second lifetime.

The problem is that disease agents, from microscopic organisms to larger parasites, live

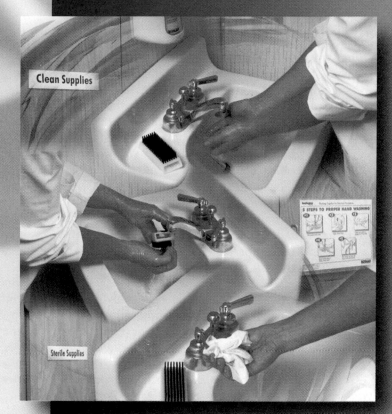

Managing the Clinical Environment

everywhere. These types of organisms, primarily bacteria, viruses, fungi, protozoa, and helminths, can be found in the air, in beverages, on dust particles, food, and plants; on and in animals and humans; in soil and water; and on nearly every surface. If you encounter an organism when your immune system is weak or you have not built up a resistance to it, illness results.

One of the most important responsibilities of the medical assistant is to provide an environment free of exposure to infectious agents. This requires that you know disinfection practices and follow them diligently. You are responsible for the general maintenance, orderliness, and efficient use of the examination suite. The cleanliness of the equipment, supplies, and examining room itself is of utmost importance. For example, the examination table, scale, blood pressure machine, and counter tops all require frequent disinfection. Furthermore, handwashing, a procedure critical to the goal of medical asepsis, must be done thoroughly and frequently.

The medical assistant is also responsible for maintaining the functioning of all examination equipment and ensuring that items are repaired or replaced as necessary. Supplies are inventoried each day and restocked on a scheduled basis.

Finally, the medical assistant must be acutely aware of the patient's physical and emotional comfort. The waiting area should be clean, comfortable, and orderly. Once the patient is brought into the examination room, privacy should be assured. The patient has a right to know the medical procedures and activities being planned, and the medical assistant should help answer any questions or direct the questions to the provider. A patient-centered, hospitable, and functional examination suite will communicate to the patient that the medical office provides high quality medical care.

Patient Concerns

*A*lthough some patients come to the medical office for routine checkups, most have one or more medical problems. These may include contagious conditions such as the common cold, flu (influenza), or pneumonia. Since these conditions can be easily spread from one person to another, patients who do not cover their mouth and nose when they cough or sneeze or do not dispose of used tissues in waste containers put other patients, as well as the healthcare team, at risk of infection. In addition, patients can be exposed to germs in the healthcare environment, resulting in infections. The *medical assistant is responsible for decreasing the potential for these infections by disinfecting and sanitizing equipment and surfaces properly.*

Examination Suite: Managing the Back Office

The **examination suite,** sometimes called the "back office," is the section of the medical office where the patient is interviewed to determine the reason for the visit, the examination takes place, and appropriate care is planned. This is the area where the medical assistant does clinical procedures including taking blood pressure readings, performing electrocardiograms (tracing the electrical impulses responsible for the heart's pumping cycle), and obtaining and processing blood and urine specimens for diagnostic purposes.

Some medical offices are solo practices. However, in recent years, two or more physicians have tended to join together to form a partnership. The examination suite will therefore vary in size and contents depending on the number of physicians in the practice. The suite usually has one or more examination rooms, a consultation room, a laboratory area, various diagnostic areas depending on the physicians' practice and/or specialty, and one or more bathrooms.

Examination Rooms

Most of the patient's care is provided in the examination rooms. It is in these private spaces that the patients meet with members of the healthcare team. The medical assistant plays an important role in managing these rooms by cleaning up between patients and stocking the supplies needed in the rooms. By performing these tasks efficiently, the assistant ensures that the rooms are ready as soon as possible for the next patient. The larger the medical practice, the more patients who will be seen daily and the more rooms that will be used for exams. We will discuss the importance of these rooms and the medical assistant's role in maintaining them later in this chapter.

Consultation Area

Many medical offices have an area available where the physician can meet with the patient and family members to discuss the patient's condition and treatment plan. All physicians in the practice might share this area or each physician might have his or her own consultation room. In this location, the physician needs adequate writing space, most likely

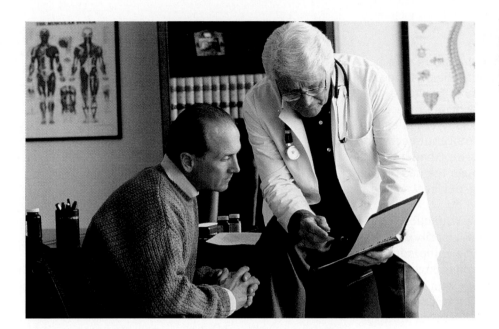

The consultation area, like all areas that patients visit in the medical office, should be designed and decorated in a way that accommodates both the physician and the patient.

provided by a desk, and comfortable chairs for the patient and family members. The area usually has a phone and an intercom to the reception area as well as medical reference materials. Physicians tend to "personalize" this area, making it as appealing as possible for their patients.

Laboratory Area

Within the examination suite is a designated laboratory area that includes the laboratory supplies and equipment the medical practice uses. Some relatively simple, portable devices might be kept there if testing is done on-site: for example, checking blood specimens for glucose levels to identify the presence of diabetes or hemoglobin levels to assist in diagnosing anemia. Other tests may be performed on urine to determine urinary tract infections or on feces to identify abnormal bleeding that might be due to ulcers or colon cancer. The supplies and equipment will vary depending on which procedures are performed in the office and which are done by outside laboratories. Your professional responsibilities may also include assisting with maintenance of the laboratory equipment, processing specimens, and ordering and replacing supplies for laboratory testing.

Some form of refrigeration will be available for storing specimens obtained during a physical examination. *Only* specimens should be kept in this designated refrigerator. It should not be used for storing medications or food since food sources can contain bacteria and medications can become contaminated by the specimens or food.

Biohazard labels, which indicate that the labeled item might contain microorganisms that can spread

> *Dangerous Situation*
>
> To protect medical personnel from acquiring infections from contaminated specimens, all personnel in areas where potentially infectious materials are present are not allowed to eat, drink, smoke, chew, apply cosmetics, or touch the mouth or eyes.

disease, must be placed on the outside of the refrigerator containing specimens obtained during physical examinations as well as on the door to the lab. The medical assistant is responsible for maintaining the cleanliness and orderliness of the office's laboratory area.

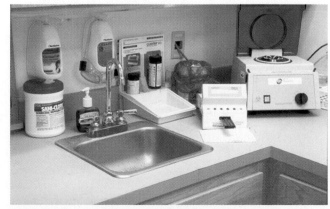

A medical office may need only a small area for lab procedures.

Diagnostic Areas

Depending, again, on the needs of the specific practice, a variety of diagnostic procedures may be performed in the medical office. Radiologic procedures, such as taking x-rays, are performed in some general practice and specialty medical offices while others refer patients to radiologic centers. In the medical office, unnecessary or inappropriate radiation exposure of patients and personnel must be eliminated through the use of lead shields and exposure monitoring devices worn by office personnel.

Electrocardiograms and pulmonary function testing (done to evaluate lung volume and capacity) are performed in some medical offices. The equipment may be stored in the examination suite and brought into the exam room when needed, or it may be kept in a specific room where these procedures are performed. The medical assistant is responsible for ensuring that the

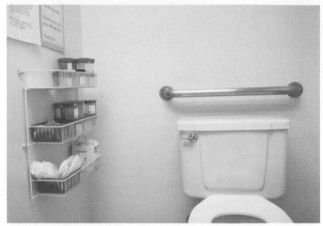

Restocking bathroom supplies when needed is part of the medical assistant's responsibilities.

equipment is functioning properly and that adequate supplies are available. Because electric currents from other machines sometimes obscure electrocardiogram readings, the medical assistant should make sure all other electrical devices in the exam room are turned off when the electrocardiograph is in use.

Bathrooms

Bathrooms should be exceptionally clean and neat to protect the people who use them from infection. Trash cans for waste disposal should have disposable liners and foot-operated lids to reduce exposure to disease-producing microorganisms. The medical assistant should empty these at least daily, or more often if they become full. Adequate toilet paper, filled soap dispensers, and paper towels for hand-drying should be available. The medical assistant needs to monitor these supplies and restock them throughout the day, even if a maintenance service is responsible for cleaning and restocking them between examination days. Containers for routine urine collection may be provided in the bathroom for patients' convenience. Handrails should be installed for those who need them.

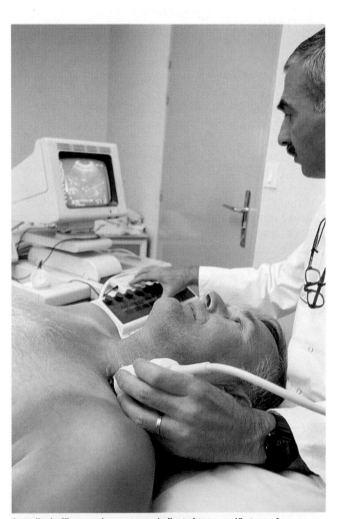

A medical office may have a room dedicated to a specific type of diagnostic test.

Safety and Assurance Responsibilities for the Medical Assistant

The medical assistant is responsible for maintaining the overall cleanliness, order, and safety of the examination suite. This will ensure that patients are served efficiently and effectively. Keeping the examination area clean (including properly disinfecting all work surfaces) is essential in preventing the spread of infection. The single most important action the medical assistant must take to ensure cleanliness is appropriate handwashing. Hands that are not properly cleaned can spread infectious microorganisms simply because the medical assistant constantly uses his hands when working with patients. In addition, the assistant must work to keep the medical office environment safe for both staff and patients by eliminating hazards.

The Importance of Handwashing

In 1847, Ignaz Semmelweiss was the first person to determine the benefits of handwashing. He noted that the patients of physicians who performed autopsies had a higher frequency of infection than those of midwives who did not perform autopsies. We now know that when your hands touch areas where microorganisms are present, the chances that you will pick up and transmit germs increase. Additionally, Semmelweiss found that the use of chlorine in handwashing before contact with patients reduced the mortality rate from 18% to 1.2%. Therefore, his policy of requiring everybody to wash their hands in a chlorine solution significantly cut the infection rate at the Vienna hospital's obstetrics unit where he practiced. As a medical assistant, your hands come into contact with a large number of items and people, many of whom are sick with contagious or infectious diseases. Each time this happens, you are at risk of picking up germs and transmitting them to someone or something else. When you do not wash your hands properly, you may be exposing patients, your coworkers, or yourself to infection and disease. It is, therefore, imperative that you wash your hands properly.

Acquiring appropriate handwashing technique is essential for everyone who works in the medical office. Handwashing is a form of **medical asepsis** by which disease-producing **microorganisms** (germs) are eliminated or controlled. Germs survive best in warm, moist, dark environments. Soap, water, and friction are the essential elements in handwashing to reduce the number of microorganisms.

> **Working Smart**
> Liquid soap should be used whenever possible. If only bar soap is available, it should be placed on a rack or holder where water can drain from the soap. Liquid soap dispensers should be cleaned each time they are refilled. If you use a hot air blower to dry your hands, turn it on with an elbow so you don't touch the knob with your clean hand.

Handwashing technique depends on the purpose of the handwashing. Procedure 14.1 identifies the appropriate handwashing technique for maximum medical asepsis. In practice, you may find that time does not always permit the thorough cleaning described. However, always follow this method before assisting with invasive procedures, before and after coming in contact with wounds or changing dressing, after taking care of an infected patient, and after handling contaminated equipment, supplies, or organic material. For routine handwashing, a vigorous rubbing together of all surfaces of lathered hands for at least 10 seconds, followed by thorough rinsing under a stream of water is recommended by the Centers for Disease Control. Hands should be washed:

- before you start and after you finish your work day
- before and after each patient contact
- after using the restroom
- before and after eating or handling food
- after handling any contaminant
- before putting on gloves and after removing them
- before and after handling specimens
- any time you feel it is needed

Surface Disinfecting

Medical asepsis is carried out within the examination area to reduce the number of disease-producing microorganisms. All surface areas in the examination suite need to be disinfected at the end of the day and whenever the surface has been contaminated with any body fluid. Surfaces include counter tops, floor coverings without carpeting, examination tables, and all equipment and/or its plastic or vinyl coverings exposed to air.

> **Working Smart**
> To prevent the spread of infection, fingernails should be kept short and clean. Avoid fingernail polish since it can crack and harbor germs. It is also best not to wear jewelry when working directly with patients. Jewelry harbors microorganisms, may cause tears in gloves, and may be damaged by frequent handwashing.

Procedure 14.1

Washing Hands (Medical Asepsis)

Purpose: To reduce the number of microorganisms on your hands that cause infection and disease, thus reducing the incidence of transmission.

Equipment/Supplies: Sink with hot and cold running water (preferably with foot- or knee-operated control), antimicrobial soap (preferably liquid), paper towels, nail stick or brush, waste basket with foot-operated lid and plastic disposable liner.

1 Remove watch and other jewelry and put in a safe place. *Jewelry provides a place for microorganisms to hide during handwashing.*
2 Turn on the water and adjust flow and temperature to be lukewarm.
3 Wet forearms and hands, keeping fingers pointing downward. Figure 1. *Water helps soap to lather and free contaminants and germs. It should flow from least contaminated to most contaminated areas; arms are considered less contaminated than the hands.*

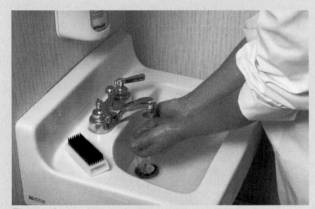

Figure 1

4 Apply enough soap to lather your hands well. **CAUTION!** If using bar soap, rinse it off as you replace it in the holder. Work soap into a good lather.
5 Using a brush or your fingertips, scrub the palms and backs of your hands, wrists, and fingers. Be sure to clean the front, back, sides, and between all fingers. Scrub for one full minute. Figure 2.
6 Using a brush or nail stick, clean under your fingernails and around your cuticles.
  Rinse from the forearm to the fingertips with your hands pointed downward for one full minute. *By rinsing from the forearm to the fingertips, germs will be rinsed downward and away.* **WARNING!** Do not touch the inside of the sink.
7 Obtain paper towels without touching the towel dispenser or any other surface. **CAUTION!** If paper

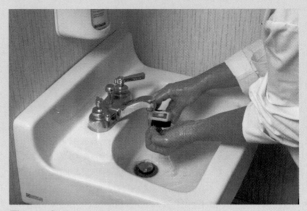

Figure 2

towels are in a rolled dispenser, use your elbow to activate the dispenser.
8 Use a clean paper towel to dry each hand and then discard it. Start at the forearm and dry downward.
9 Turn off the water. Figure 3. **WARNING!** If faucets are manually operated, turn the handles with a dry, clean paper towel. *All areas of the sink, including the faucets, are considered contaminated since many people have touched them.*

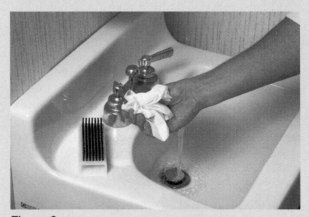

Figure 3

10 Discard paper towels in waste container. **WARNING!** Do not touch the lid of the waste container since it is considered contaminated. Use the foot control.
11 Replace watch and other jewelry. **CAUTION!** Contaminated jewelry must be washed before replacing it on your hand. Contamination is not always visible.
12 Apply lotion to prevent drying or cracking of skin on hands.

Procedure 14.2

Disinfecting Surfaces

Purpose: To reduce the number of microorganisms in the examination area by disinfecting surfaces.

Equipment/Supplies: Gloves, protective eyewear, disinfectant solution (10% bleach solution or EPA-approved disinfectant), paper towels, tongs, dust pan and brush, disposable cloth, pail, biohazard waste receptacle, sharps container (if cleaning up broken glass or other sharp objects).

1 Put on protective eyewear. Wash hands and put on gloves. *Observe Standard Precautions.*
2 Pick up any broken glass or sharp item with tongs or sweep it into a dustpan. With a brush or tongs, direct the sharp objects into a sharps container without touching them. *Using tongs or a brush and dustpan will reduce the possibility of puncturing your gloves.*
3 Absorb any visible spills with paper toweling and discard into a biohazard waste receptacle. Use a disposable cloth to wipe the surface with disinfectant solution and allow the area to air dry.
4 Pour the disinfectant solution down a drain or toilet (or as directed by your state's guidelines) and rinse the pail thoroughly in running water. *The disinfectant solution is considered contaminated after use and should not be used again.* ✹ WARNING! Pails used for disinfectant solution should be labeled to prevent their use for other purposes.
5 Discard the disposable cloth and then the gloves in the biohazard waste receptacle. *They are considered contaminated and should not be reused.*
6 Wash your hands and remove goggles.

A 10% solution of household bleach in water is the most convenient approved disinfecting solution. It needs to be mixed just before use since it loses its potency when stored. Other chemical disinfectants, such as glutaraldehyde (Cidex®), also have been approved for this use by the Environmental Protection Agency (EPA).

See Procedure 14.2 for the required steps in surface disinfecting and cleanup tasks. Although this procedure is standard, the medical assistant should follow the facility-specific procedure approved within a particular medical office, which should be included in its procedure manual. In most medical offices, each area will have a cleaning/disinfection log for tracking these activities. The log (Figure 14.1) will contain columns for noting the date and type of cleaning, the type of disinfection solution used, and the name of the person performing the cleanup.

Technology Tip
Consult the EPA's website at www.epa.gov for more information.

Legal Issue
It is against the law not to follow appropriate cleanup protocol. According to the Bloodborne Pathogen Standards of the U.S. Occupational Safety and Health Administration (OSHA), "contaminated work surfaces shall be decontaminated with an appropriate disinfectant after completion of procedures; immediately or as soon as feasible when surfaces are overtly contaminated or after any spill of blood or other potentially infectious materials; at the end of the work shift if the surface may have become contaminated since the last cleaning."

Examination Room 5

Date	Time	Cleaning Solution	Comments	Name

Figure 14.1
Sample Log for Recording Surface Disinfecting Procedures

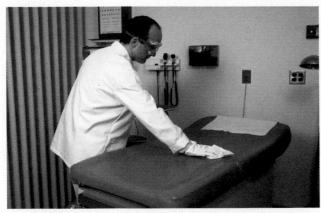

Gloves and protective eyewear should always be worn when disinfecting surfaces in the medical office.

These logs provide a quick reference as to when the area was last cleaned. However, if there is any doubt as to the cleanliness of an area, the medical assistant should assume it is not clean and should perform the appropriate disinfection procedure.

Ideally, floor surfaces in the examination area should be linoleum or another surface that can be easily disinfected with a 10% household bleach solution, a commercially prepared disinfectant, or a cleanup kit. This will permit the medical assistant to immediately disinfect any area that is contaminated with a spill or splatter. The examination rooms and the laboratory are areas that can become contaminated most easily and should, therefore, have floors that can be easily disinfected. In some instances, the physician might prefer that the hall and the consultation areas be carpeted. If this is the case, daily vacuuming and a schedule for carpet shampooing and disinfection need to be established. A spill or splatter in a carpeted area should be cleaned up as well as possible using Procedure 14.2. The area should then be covered with a non-absorbing material and marked with a brightly colored floor sign so that patients and staff will not walk on it. At the end of the examination day, the area will need to be treated with an EPA-approved solution.

The medical assistant is also responsible for **disinfecting** (reducing or eliminating infectious organisms) and/or cleansing all diagnostic equipment between patients. This includes instruments such as otoscopes, nasal speculums, vaginal speculums, proctoscopes, percussion hammers, and stethoscopes. The medical assistant should clean electrocardiograph electrodes after each use to prevent residual buildup of electrolyte product. Use a mild detergent (such as dishwashing liquid) to clean the electrode surfaces and rubber straps.

It is a common oversight to assume something has been cleaned when it has not. When cleaning a room,

assume that all the equipment and surfaces will need to be disinfected and do not allow a new patient into a room until it has been thoroughly cleaned. In addition, make sure that the 10% bleach solution is mixed properly daily. It loses its effectiveness if it sits overnight or is diluted to less than 10%.

Waste Disposal

The medical assistant may be responsible for arranging for disposal of the waste generated by the medical office. Ordinary office waste (paper and plastics) does not require any special handling, but medical (infectious) waste, including sharps, must be handled properly. (See Table 14.1.)

Generally, sharps must be disposed of and transported in locked, puncture-proof containers. Other medical waste must be double-bagged, in sturdy red plastic bags preprinted with the biohazard symbol. Be careful choosing a company to haul and dispose of the waste your office generates. Consider checking with the Better Business Bureau or local Chamber of Commerce to see if any unresolved complaints have been filed.

The handling and management of hazardous items or substances are closely regulated by OSHA and the EPA. State and local governments may also have laws that apply to hazardous waste. Information is available from federal, state, and local agencies and your office's waste disposal contractor.

Physical Hazards

One does not think of an office as a dangerous workplace, but the physical hazards of a medical office can injure medical and administrative staff and patients alike. Tripping and falling are real possibilities. Strategies to prevent this type of injury include closing file drawers when they are not being used; keeping walkways, aisles, and stairs free of obstructions; and posting cautionary signs to warn of wet floors.

Compressed air tanks are another physical hazard. Tanks of oxygen and other compressed gases must be

Table 14.1 Medical Waste

- soiled or bloodied bandages
- culture dishes or other glassware
- discarded surgical or exam gloves
- discarded surgical or exam instruments
- needles used to give shots or draw blood
- cultures and swabs used to inoculate cultures
- removed body tissue
- lancets

chained to a wall to prevent them from falling. If the regulator apparatus were damaged in a fall, the escaping compressed gas could propel the tank around the office like a jet engine. Oxygen from leaking cylinders can result in fires or explosions if exposed to flames or sparks.

The Examination Room

The examination room is at the heart of the medical office. This is where the physician will evaluate the patient and establish a plan of care. As a medical assistant, it will be your responsibility to maintain this room so that it meets the needs of its occupants. It should provide a private environment in which the patient will feel safe and confident that the care he receives will be of the highest quality. For the physician to be able to work effectively, the space must be well organized and have all the necessary equipment to diagnose and possibly treat the patient's condition.

Understanding the Patient's Needs

As the primary customer of the medical office, it is important that the patient feels comfortable in the examination room. Although the medical assistant may not have much influence on the layout of the office environment, the assistant can help make the patient's visit more pleasant by attending to details such as privacy, décor, educational materials, temperature, and accommodations for patients with disabilities. The medical assistant should assure the patient that she is in a private and safe environment.

PRIVACY It is very important that the medical office respond to the patient's need for privacy. Often, it is the medical assistant who will escort the patient to the examination room. Unoccupied rooms that are ready for a patient should have the doors open. After entering a room with a patient, close the door.

Confirm that the record you have is for the right patient, and ask why the patient is there. If a urine sample has been ordered, have the patient provide it before putting on the examination gown, unless the exam room has an attached, private bathroom. Once you have settled the patient into the examination room, ask him to undress and put on the gown if needed. The medical assistant should allow the patient to change into the examination gown in privacy. Before leaving the room, show him where he can hang his clothes, and whenever possible, provide hooks, a clothes tree, or a hanger to keep the patient's clothes neat. The medical assistant should leave the room and

close the door at this point. After an adequate amount of time, the assistant should knock on the door and ask permission to enter. This will communicate to the patient that you value his privacy. After confirming that the patient has changed, you can tell the physician the patient is ready for the examination. Make sure you give the patient an opportunity to ask questions before you leave the room.

Do not leave the chart in the examination room with the patient. Although the chart is about the patient, the documentation belongs to the medical office and should not be given to the patient for review. If the patient has questions about his or her medical record, the medical assistant can review it and answer specific questions. However, the assistant needs to remember to be sensitive to the timing of sharing information with a patient who is upset. Also, it is not appropriate to discuss prognosis information with the patient.

In some offices, the medical assistant will place the patient's chart in a chart rack outside the exam room. This, along with a light in the hallway or some other notification system, will indicate to the physician that the patient is ready for the examination.

> ## Working Smart
>
> A chart rack outside the examination room will provide a convenient and accessible spot for the patient's medical record. Place the chart in the rack so the patient's information is not visible.

DÉCOR The examination room itself should offer a friendly, comfortable environment for the patient and family as well as the office personnel. Although there are a variety of décor options, the colors and decorative features, including window treatments and wall hangings, should be comforting in nature. Colors ranging from red to yellow to yellow-green communicate

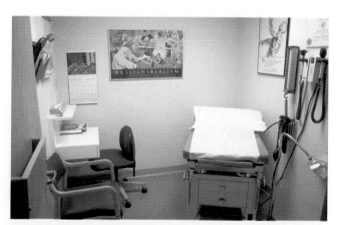

The examination room should offer the patient privacy and a safe, comfortable environment.

warmth and relaxation. Cool colors, from green-blue to blue to violet, tend to evoke tranquility and are excellent for waiting rooms and examination rooms.

Rarely will the medical assistant have influence over the décor of an examination suite, but the assistant should make sure the room is clean and orderly to ensure safety. Lighting should be bright but not harsh. The room should not be cluttered, and the medical assistant should make sure that stools, chairs, and electrical cords are not in places where they can be easily tripped over.

EDUCATIONAL MATERIALS Since patients may have to wait in the examination room while the physician is attending to other patients, the medical assistant should make sure that patient education materials are prominently displayed and available. Information about the need for appropriate and frequent handwashing may be posted in the bathroom. Recommendations for influenza and pneumonia vaccinations could be displayed on a bulletin board. Pictures of low-cholesterol foods might hang on the walls. A wall rack may include informational pamphlets on subjects such as warning signs of cancer or breast self-exam technique. The Patient's Bill of Rights should also be posted for patients' reference.

Educational materials provided in the examination room can be geared to the physician's specialty. In a pediatric practice, educational toys should be available. In an obstetric practice, instructional pamphlets about breast feeding and warning signs during pregnancy can be prominently displayed. In a gerontology practice, information regarding osteoporosis and heart risk factors may be available. The medical assistant should consider the particular interests and educational needs of the office's patients when planning these materials for the office and examination suite.

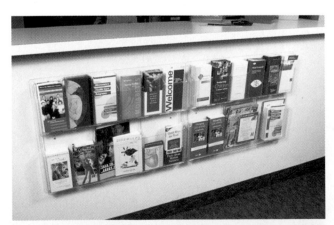

The medical assistant should make sure healthcare information is available for the patient on the way to the exam room or when leaving the office so that the patient can read the information in private.

TEMPERATURE Since the patient will, in most instances, change into a cotton or disposable gown for the examination, the medical assistant should ensure that the room temperature is appropriate. Anxiety, apprehension, and fear can cause the patient to feel chilled. Altering the environmental temperature to meet individual needs based on a patient's age and condition is an excellent way of ensuring patient comfort. The medical assistant should also evaluate the examination room for exposure to drafts from windows and doors and should correct these situations whenever possible. If the temperature in a cold room cannot be adjusted, give the patient an additional sheet or blanket if possible. The room's temperature should be set so that the patients and staff members who use it are comfortable.

> ### Customer Service
>
> The elderly population is more sensitive to lower temperatures because of loss of insulating fat and reduced circulation. The medical assistant should check with elderly patients regarding their comfort and should provide a blanket and modify the examination room temperature if necessary.

ACCOMMODATING DISABILITIES A patient with a disability would expect the medical office to be equipped or constructed in such a way as to handle the handicap. The office staff should also know how to deal effectively with handicapped individuals.

According to the U. S. Census Bureau, 20.6% of non-institutionalized Americans have a disability that limits their functioning, and the disabilities of 9.9% are severe. Functional limitations include the inability to:

- go up a flight of stairs
- lift a bag of groceries
- hear what is said in normal conversation
- see words or letters in ordinary newsprint, even with glasses
- have one's speech understood
- walk a quarter of a mile

The Americans with Disability Act of 1990 is a wide-ranging civil rights law that prohibits discrimination against people with disabilities. It covers people with physical and mental impairments that substantially limit activities such as walking, talking, seeing, hearing, or caring for themselves. The act requires that reasonable accommodation be made for individuals with disabilities. This includes making existing facilities accessible or usable and making tasks achievable. The U.S. Equal Employment Opportunity Commission and the Department of Justice have issued guidelines to help define "reasonable." In a medical office, this would include:

- a minimum doorway width of thirty-two inches
- slip-resistant flooring
- door hardware that can be grasped with one hand and does not require twisting
- door closures that allow sufficient time for wheelchairs to enter and exit
- grab bars in bathrooms

Individuals who have AIDS or are HIV-positive are protected under the Americans with Disabilities Act. Reasonable accommodations must be provided for them, and they cannot be denied reasonable care because of their diagnosis.

Assisting the Physician

The medical assistant will also be responsible for assisting the physician during the patient examination. In some examinations, the assistant will adjust equipment or help position the patient.

Equipment in the examination room must be positioned for the physician and staff to perform their functions. For effective management, arrange the instruments and supplies where the doctor has safe and easy access. Every physician has individual preferences as to how the instruments should be arranged. Make certain you are familiar with these preferences. Arrange the instruments in the same place for every exam. Table 14.2 lists routine equipment that is generally in the examination room and its use.

In all instances, a flat surface will be required in the examination room for use by both the physician and the medical assistant when writing entries in the medical record. The area should be clutter-free and large enough for the patient's medical record, prescription pads, and writing implements.

The examination table is the major piece of equipment in the exam room. The table can be adjusted to various positions to help keep the patient comfortable and facilitate the examination. Most tables also have a pullout step to help patients get onto it more easily. The upper portion of the table usually can be elevated so the patient can sit up while speaking with the physician and the medical assistant. The table might contain drawers for storage of supplies. There is usually also a section that will hold table coverings. The table usually should be placed in the center of the room with the foot away from the door so that the physician can examine the patient from all sides while maintaining the patient's privacy.

In addition to the equipment in the examination room, there are a variety of items that the medical assistant may be required to store and have available upon request. Newly purchased supplies such as sterile dressings and syringes will require special precautions by the medical assistant. Since these items

> ### Technology Tip
> More information on accessibility and accommodation is available at the ADA home page, www.usdoj.gov/crt/ada/adahom1.htm

> ### Legal Issue
> Providing access to quality medical care for patients with disabilities is a legal and ethical responsibility of healthcare professionals.

Table 14.2 Routine Equipment in the Examination Room

Equipment	Use
biohazardous waste containers	proper disposal of biohazardous waste (should have a foot-operated cover)
chairs	seating for patient and family members
examination table	positioning the patient for comfort and facilitating examination by physician
light source	illumination of areas of the patient's body for examination
metal garbage container	disposal of waste materials (use replacement liners for appropriate disposal and infection control)
ophthalmoscope	inspection of eye grounds and internal structure of the eye; checking pupil reaction (dilation and constriction)
otoscope	inspecting the inner ear; has varying sizes of disposable specula
percussion hammer	testing of reflexes
rolling stool	facilitating movement by physician during the exam
sharps containers	proper disposal of needles and other sharps (must be puncture-proof)
sphygmomanometer	measurement of blood pressure (either attached to wall or freely movable)
stethoscope	listening to heart, lung, and bowel sounds
tuning fork	determining nerve conduction hearing loss
vaginal speculum	visual examination of the vagina and cervix

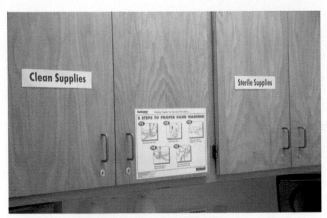

Labeling of storage areas speeds access to supplies.

are sterile, they must not be exposed to wet or damp storage conditions. They should be placed in an area in the examination room or storage area that needs to be clearly labeled "sterile supplies." Syringes and needles need to be kept in a locked area. Supplies that are not sterile may be placed in the examination room or storage area, and, again, this area should be labeled as clean storage.

In addition to instruments, other supplies are needed:

- Disposable items that are discarded after one use. For the physical examination, these include: cervical scraper, cotton balls, applicators, disposable needles and syringes, gauze dressings and bandages, glass slides, gloves (sterile and unsterile), tissues, specimen containers, and tongue depressors.
- Consumable supplies that are used repeatedly if not emptied such as fixative (cervical) spray to preserve specimens for further study; isopropyl alcohol (70%) for skin cleansing; and K-Y Jelly, a lubricant for vaginal or rectal examinations.

These supplies as well as prescription pads and medications are generally kept locked out of the patient's sight. The particular disposable and consumable needs will vary depending on the individual medical office.

Preparing the Examination Room

The medical assistant should never escort a patient into a room that has not been adequately cleaned and prepared. After the patient has been examined and the physician has determined a treatment plan, the patient will change back into his street clothing and leave the room. The medical assistant will then prepare the room for the next patient.

The assistant will need to sanitize the examination table and routine instruments used by the physician. If

any spills occurred, the medical assistant will sanitize the area as described in Procedure 14.2. The assistant will place specimens in the laboratory area for processing and refrigeration as necessary. The medical assistant also will put any small items that require sterilization in the area designated for that purpose.

The assistant will return items such as the rolling stool, gooseneck lamp, and sphygmomanometer to their original places in the examination room and will replace any needed supplies.

EQUIPMENT The medical assistant needs to check daily to be sure all equipment and instruments are in working order. Since there is a wide variety of medical instruments, the assistant must be aware of the use, replacement requirements, and appropriate handling of each item. All equipment used daily should be checked daily. All other equipment should be checked at least weekly. This includes ECG machines, audiometers, and ultrasound equipment. Information about these instruments should be obtained from the manufacturer or marketing representative and kept in a file established and maintained by the medical assistant. For each piece of equipment, this should include the date of purchase; manufacturer's address and phone number; disinfecting, sanitizing, and sterilizing recommendations; supplies needed; and any other pertinent information.

VENTILATION Gases, toxic fumes, and even trapped dust can pollute indoor air. Table 14.3 lists common causes of poor quality indoor air and preventive actions the medical assistant can take to reduce them. Over extended periods, an individual exposed to these pollutants can experience irritated eyes, a runny nose, scratchy throat, coughing, headaches, and fatigue.

Poor indoor air quality has been a growing problem since the energy crisis of the 1970s. In response to the need for energy efficiency, buildings have been built "tighter," with less air exchange between the outside and inside. As a result, moisture, carbon dioxide, and other compounds are trapped inside the buildings.

Improving ventilation and airflow is basic to improving air quality. If the medical office has windows that open, the medical assistant should ventilate the examination room to outside air each day. Ideally, this should occur at the end of the day, with doors and windows opened for ten to fifteen minutes to allow the room air to mix with environmental air and reduce contaminants. Another way to improve air quality is by using an air filtration system that increases ventilation while recapturing heat and saving energy. These devices can be installed in window units or as part of a central air system. Air purifiers may also be purchased and are especially recommended for medical practices that treat patients with respiratory conditions.

Table 14.3 **Common Causes of Poor Quality Indoor Air**

Element	Cause	Preventive Action by Medical Assistant
gases from burning fuels	Burning fuel, such as natural gas, may release pollutants, the most dangerous of which is carbon monoxide.	Have central heating system inspected annually. Be sure equipment is working properly and is vented to outdoors. Install carbon monoxide detectors and check functioning frequently.
chemicals	Cleaning solutions can release toxic fumes.	Never mix chemical products. Chlorine bleach should not be mixed with ammonia cleaners. Follow instructions for use of all chemicals. Use chemicals only in well-ventilated areas.
dust and moisture	Dust mites (microscopic insects found in dust) can cause severe allergy although they are not technically considered pollutants. Damp conditions increase the level of dust mites.	Vacuum and dust often. Have heating and cooling ductwork cleaned frequently. Clean drain pans under refrigerator and air conditioners. Use vented fans in bathrooms and dehumidifiers in high humidity areas.

Working Smart

Newly laid carpet and freshly painted surfaces can give off irritating fumes. When areas have been newly carpeted or freshly painted, open them to outside air and run fans during the first few days. Before having carpet laid, ask the installer to unroll the carpet and air it in a well-ventilated area.

LAUNDRY AND DISPOSABLE MATERIAL All laundry items, including cloth gowns, patient drapes, and blankets that have been exposed to bodily fluids, need to be considered infectious and handled with gloves and placed in a covered hamper containing a biohazardous plastic bag. In most medical offices, the laundry is cleaned by a professional cleaning service.

Any paper gowns and/or examination table coverings should be placed in a lined trashcan with a lid operated by a foot pedal.

The disposable paper covering the examination table is a barrier to infection and contamination during the physical exam. It should be changed after each patient. This paper generally comes on a roll that fits under the head of the examination table. If a pillow is used, a clean cover is put on it after each patient. In removing the paper, roll it tightly for disposal. If the paper is contaminated with visible blood or body fluid, dispose of it in a biohazard container. If it is not visibly soiled, dispose of it in the trash. The medical assistant should then wash his or her hands before re-covering the examination table.

Challenging Situations

*I*f a patient states a false assumption that he must have a contagious disease because he sees the medical assistant wash her hands both before and after she has performed a procedure, it is important for the assistant to explain why she is performing the handwashing procedure. This might be an opportunity for the medical assistant to instruct the patient about proper handwashing.

Although it is unlikely that the patient will see the medical assistant performing routine surface disinfection or instrument sterilization, the patient might see instruments removed for sterilization or, if an accidental spill occurs, might see surface disinfection performed. Once again, the patient may become concerned about possible exposure to infection. The medical assistant will need to explain why the procedures are being performed.

If a disabled person enters the examination suite, try to see the environment from her perspective. Are there clutter or other obstacles to safe travel? Is there a place to wait before being seen that is not "in the way"? Is there a way for the patient to talk to the person behind the desk without having to shout or look up at someone looming over her? Remember, persons with disabilities only want to go where others can go. Try to make the medical office environment accessible and welcoming to all patients.

Clinical Summary

- The examination area of the medical office is where the patient is interviewed, examined, and appropriate care is planned.

- In the consultation area, the patient's condition and treatment plan are discussed.
- Specimens of blood, urine, and feces are processed in the laboratory area.
- Radiologic procedures, electrocardiograms, and pulmonary function testing may be performed in the diagnostic area.
- The medical assistant is responsible for maintaining overall cleanliness, order, and safety in the examination area.
- The medical assistant recognizes that appropriate handwashing is essential to reduce the spread of infection and follows the correct procedures.
- The medical assistant is responsible for disposing of infectious materials safely.
- Equipment needs to be checked for proper functioning and, if necessary, repaired.
- Supplies should be monitored, ordered, and restocked as necessary.
- The examination room should be private, adequate in size, comfortable, well-lighted, and adequately ventilated.

- The examination suite should be designed to accommodate the disabled population.

The Language of Medicine

biohazard (**bi**-O-haz-rd) A substance or object that may contain microorganisms that can spread disease.

disinfecting Reducing or eliminating infectious organisms.

examination suite The "back office" area of a medical facility where the patient is interviewed to determine the reason for the visit, is then examined, and appropriate care is planned.

medical asepsis The technique used to clean the medical office to eliminate pathogenic organisms.

microorganism (mI-krO-**org**-ah-niz-um) A germ, a minute living body invisible to the naked eye.

Signs/Symptoms of Progress

Recall, Question, Connect

Recall
Review the ways a medical assistant can assure that the office is a safe environment for patients and staff.

Question
What questions do you have about safety concerns for specific types of patients?

Connect
What specific steps would you take to assist a patient who uses a walker?

Educating the Patient

Mrs. Pozanski, thirty-five years old, enters the medical office with complaints of watery eyes, muscle aches, and a cough. She says the symptoms are getting worse and that she's concerned her children will also become ill. Mary Ann Flood, CMA, finds Mrs. Pozanski's temperature elevated and notes that she has a runny nose and productive cough. Mrs. Pozanski asks if she will be okay and wonders if she has pneumonia.
1 What should Mary Ann say to Mrs. Pozanski?
2 The physician asks Mary Ann to explain to Mrs. Pozanski how she can limit exposure of her children to her microorganisms. What explanation should Mary Ann offer?

3 What suggestions might Mary Ann give Mrs. Pozanski about reducing the number of microorganisms in the home environment?

Exploring Perspectives in Teams

Perspective involves the discipline of examining how ideas look from different points of view and recognizing that there are often multiple "answers" to complex questions. In small groups or on your own, reflect on possible alternative views or answers and summarize your findings.
1 The author credits Pasteur's and Koch's medical advances with helping to double our life spans. Can you think of other pioneers who deserve credit too? What other factors may have contributed to an increased life span? What issues do people who live longer have to deal with?
2 Why does infection control continue to be such a major problem? Will disease-producing microorganisms ever be eliminated? Why or why not?
3 We know that standards of cleanliness vary from culture to culture, but minimum health standards should be universal. How would you communicate those standards to your coworkers? How would you communicate them to a patient who does not understand the standards?
4 Does the Patient's Right to Know include receiving complete copies of her or his files and doctor's charts and notes? Why is it not a good idea to let the patient leave the medical office with the medical record? When would it be appropriate to give a patient or a patient's family member access to the documents on file?

Appendix A
Medical Language Handbook

Table A.1 Common Prefixes

Prefix	Meaning	Example	Prefix	Meaning	Example
a- an-	without, not	apnea—without breathing anhydrous—without water	hemi-	half	hemicardia—half of the heart (right or left)
ab-	away from	abnormality—away from normal	semi-		semilunar—half moon
ad-	toward, to, near	adduction—toward the center	hyper-	above or excessive; extreme	hyperkalemia—excess potassium (in the blood)
ambi-	both	ambidextrous—use of both hands	hypo-	deficient; below	hypoglycemia—low blood sugar
ante-	before	antepartum—before labor or childbirth	infra-	under; below	inframammary—below the breast
pre- pro-		prenatal—before birth procephalic—anterior part (before) of the head	sub-		subdural—below the dura mater
anti- contra-	against; opposed to	antibiotic—against bacteria contraindication—opposed to a certain treatment	inter- mal-	between bad	intercellular—between cells malaise—bad comfort; discomfort
auto-	self	autoimmune—immunity to self	meso-	middle	mesophlebitis—inflammation of the middle layer of the wall of a vein
bi- di-	two; both	bilateral—both sides didactylism—condition of two digits on a hand or foot	meta-	beyond; after; change	metastasis—extension of disease from one part of the body to another
bio-	life	biology—study of life	micro-	small	microcardia—small heart
brady-	slow	bradycardia—slow heart rate	mono-	one	mononuclear—one nucleus
circum-	around; circular movement	circumorbital—around the orbit (eye)	uni- neo-	one new	unilateral—one side neonatal—new birth
peri-		pericardium—around the heart	pachy- pan-	thick all	pachyderma—thick skin panimmunity—immune to all diseases
con-	with or together	consanguineous—with blood (common ancestry)	para-	abnormal; alongside; beside	paracystic—alongside the bladder
sym- syn-		symbiotic—with life synergy—with energy	per-	through	percutaneous—through the skin
de-	not; from; down	decalcify—removal of calcium	poly-	many	polycythemia—many (red) blood cells
dia- trans-	across or through	diathermy—through heat transurethral—across the urethra	multi-		multidisciplinary—many areas of study
dis-	apart; separate	disease—separate from ease	post- quadri-	after four	postmortem—after death quadriplegic—paralysis of all four limbs
dys- e-	faulty; painful; difficult out; away	dysuria—painful urination efferent—conduction away from	tetra-		tetradactylism—condition of only four digits on a hand or foot
ec-		ectomorphic—away from form	re- retro-	again or back backward or behind	resorb—absorb again retroflexion—backward bending
ex- ecto- exo- extra-	outside	excrete—separate, cast out ectoderm—outer layer of skin exothermic—release of heat extracellular—outside the cell	sub-	under, below	subvaginal—below the vagina
en- endo-	inside; within	enclosed—contained within endocardium—innermost layer (lining) of the heart	super- supra-	above or excessive outside or beyond	superficial—near the surface suprascleral—outside the sclera
intra-		intra-abdominal—within the abdomen	tachy- tri-	fast three	tachycardia—rapid heart rate trigeminy—three abnormal heart beats
epi-	upon	epigastric—upon (above) the stomach	ultra-	beyond, excessive	ultrasonic—excessive sound
eu-	normal or good	eupnea—normal breathing			

Table A.2 Common Root Words and Combining Forms

Root Word	Combining Form	Meaning
abdomin-	abdomin/o	abdomen
angi-	angi/o	vessel
bacteri-	bacteri/o	bacteria
bio-	bio	life
carcin-	carcin/o	cancer; cancerous
cardi-	cardi/o	heart
cephal-	cephal/o	head
cyst-	cyst/o	sac or cyst containing fluid; urinary bladder
cyt-	cyt/o	cell
electr-	electr/o	electricity
enter-	enter/o	intestines
fibrin-	fibrin/o	fiber
gnath-	gnath/o	jaw
gynec-	gynec/o	woman, female
hem-	hem/o	blood
hemat-	hemat/o	blood
hepat-	hepat/o	liver
irid-	irid/o	iris
kerat-	kerat/o	keratin (a protein)
lip-	lip/o	fat
mast-	mast/o	breast
necr-	necr/o	death
nephr-	nephr/o	kidney
onc-	onc/o	tumor
path-	path/o	disease
pelv-	pelv/o	pelvic
radi-	radi/o	x-rays
ren-	ren/o	renal, the kidney
sarc-	sarc/o	flesh
sial-	sial/o	saliva, salivary glands
thromb-	thromb/o	clot
trache-	trache/o	trachea
uter-	uter/o	uterus

Table A.3 General Suffixes

Suffix	Meaning	Example
-ac	pertaining to	hemophiliac—pertaining to an individual with hemophilia
-al		temporal—pertaining to the temporal lobe of the brain
-ar		clavicular—pertaining to the clavicle
-ry		sensory—pertaining to the senses
-eal		esophageal—pertaining to the esophagus
-ic		gastric—pertaining to the stomach (gastrum)
-ose		adipose—relating to fat
-ous		cutaneous—pertaining to the skin
-tic		spermatic—pertaining to sperm
-blast	immature	osteoblast—immature bone cell
-cyte	cell	osteocyte—bone cell
-e	noun marker (indicates this form of the word is a noun)	melanocyte—pigment-producing skin cell
-gram	record	electroencephalogram—record of brain activity
-graph	instrument for recording	electroencephalograph—instrument for recording brain activity
-graphy	process of recording	electrocardiography—process of recording the electrical activity of the heart
-meter	instrument for measuring	arthrometer—instrument for measuring motion in a joint
-metry	process of measuring	arthrometry—process of measuring joint motion
-iatric	treatment	psychiatric—treatment of the psyche

(continues)

Table A.3 General Suffixes (continued)

Suffix	Meaning	Example
-iatry	study of	psychiatry—study of the psyche
-logy		urology—study of urine
-logist	one who specialized in the treatment or study of	cardiologist—one who specializes in the treatment or study of the heart
-icle	small	ventricle—small pouch or cavity, particularly within the heart or brain
-ole		arteriole—small artery
-ula		macula—small spot
-ule		pustule—small lesion (pimple) with pus
-ium/-eum	tissue or structure	periosteum—structure surrounding bone
-ize	make; use; subject to	anesthetize—subject to anesthesia
-ate		impregnate—make pregnant
-or	one who	medicator—one who gives medicine
-poiesis	formation	erythropoiesis—formation of red blood cells
-scope	instrument for examining	cystoscope—instrument for examining the bladder
-scopy	examination	cystoscopy—examination of the bladder
-stasis	stop or stand	hemostasis—stop bleeding

Table A.4 Suffixes Related to Conditions, Symptoms, or Diagnoses

Suffix	Meaning	Example
-algia	pain	myalgia—muscle pain
-dynia		arthrodynia—pain in a joint
-cele	pouch, sac, or hernia	cystocele—hernia of the bladder
-emesis	vomit	hematemesis—vomiting blood
-emia	condition of blood	anemia—condition of insufficient iron in the blood
-form	like or resembling	vermiform—resembling vermin
-oid		osteoid—resembling bone
-genic	beginning, origin, or	pyogenic—production of pus
-genesis	production	pathogenesis—origin of disease
-ia	condition of	dysuria—condition of painful urination
-ism		hirsutism—condition of excessive hair
-iasis	formation of; presence of	lithiasis—formation of stone
-itis	inflammation	tendinitis—inflammation of a tendon
-lysis	breaking down	hemolysis—breaking down of blood
-malacia	softening	osteomalacia—softening of bone
-megaly	enlargement	cardiomegaly—enlargment of the heart
-oma	tumor	osteoma—tumor of bone
-osis	condition	psychosis—condition of the psyche
-penia	abnormal reduction; lack of	leukocytopenia—abnormal reduction of white blood cells
-phage	eat; devour	macrophage—large cell that devours
-phagia		geophagia—eating dirt
-phagy		aerophagy—swallowing air
-phile	attraction for; love for	pedophile—abnormal adult attraction to children
-philia		hemophilia—attraction for blood
-phobia	fear of	photophobia—fear of light
-plasia	formation	dysplasia—faulty formation
-pnea	breathing	apnea—without breathing
-ptosis	drooping; falling or downward displacement	mastoptosis—drooping breast
-rrhage	to burst forth	hemorrhage—bursting forth of blood
-rrhagia		hemorrhagia—condition of bleeding
-rrhagic		hemorrhagic—relating to condition of bleeding
-rrhea	discharge or flow	amenorrhea—absence of menstrual flow
-rrhexis	rupture or breaking	trichorrhexis—breaking of hair
-spasm	involuntary contraction	laryngospasm—involuntary contraction of the larynx
-trophy	development	hypertrophy—excess development (enlargement)
-y	condition or process of	ambulatory—process of ambulation (walking)

Table A.5 Suffixes Related to Procedures

Suffix	Meaning	Example
-centesis	puncture to remove fluid	amniocentesis—puncture of the amniotic membrane to remove fluid
-desis	binding	arthrodesis—binding of a joint
-ectomy	excision; surgical removal	splenectomy—removal of the spleen
-pexy	surgical suspension or fixation	uteropexy—surgical fixation of the uterus
-plasty	surgical repair or reconstruction	hernioplasty—surgical repair of a hernia
-rrhaphy	suture	myorrhaphy—suture of muscle
-stomy	surgical creation of an artificial opening	colostomy—creation of an artificial opening in the colon
-tomy	incision	tracheotomy—incision into the trachea
-tripsy	crushing	lithotripsy—crushing of stones

Table A.6 Word Parts

a- . . . . without, not
ab- . . . . away from
abdomin/o . . . . abdomen
-ac . . . . pertaining to
acous/o . . . . hearing
ad- . . . . toward, to, near
aden/o . . . . gland
adip/o . . . . fat
adren/o . . . . adrenals
aer/o . . . . air
-al . . . . pertaining to
-algia . . . . condition of pain
algia/i . . . . pain
alveol/o . . . . hollow sac
ambi- . . . . both
ambly/o . . . . dull
amni/o . . . . . amnion (sac around fetus)
an- . . . . without, not
andr/o . . . . male, masculine
angi/o . . . . (blood) vessel
anis/o . . . . unequal
ankyl/o . . . . . . crooked, fusion, stiffness
ante- . . . . before
anti- . . . . against; opposed to
aort/o . . . . aorta
aque/o . . . . water
-ar . . . . pertaining to
-arche . . . . first
arteri/o . . . . artery
arteriol/o . . . . arteriole
arthr/o . . . . joint
articul/o . . . . joint
-ase . . . . enzyme
asthen/o . . . . loss of strength
-ate . . . . make; use; subject to
ather/o . . . . . . deposit of pasty material
atri/o . . . . atrium
audi/o . . . . hearing, sound
aur/o . . . . ear
auricul/o . . . . ear
auto- . . . . self
bacteri/o . . . . bacteria
balan/o . . . . glans penis
bas/o . . . . Greek for base, basis
bi- . . . . two; both
bi/o . . . . life

-blast . . . . immature cell, germ, bud
blast/o . . . . immature cell, germ, bud
blephar/o . . . . eyelid
brady- . . . . slow
bronch/o . . . . airway
bronchiol/o . . . . bronchiole
carbo- . . . . carbon atom
carcin/o . . . . cancer; cancerous
cardi/o . . . . heart
-cele . . . . pouch, sac, or hernia
celi/o . . . . abdomen
-centesis . . . . . puncture to remove fluid
cephal/o . . . . head, brain
cerebell/o . . . . cerebellum
cerebr/o . . . . cerebrum
cervic/o . . . . neck
cheil/o (chil/o) . . . . lips
chol/o (chol/e) . . . . bile
choledoch/o . . . . common bile duct
chondr/o . . . . cartilage
chrom/o . . . . Greek for color
circum- . . . . . around; circular movement
col/o . . . . colon
colp/o . . . . vagina
con- . . . . with or together
conjunctiv/o . . . . conjunctiva
contra- . . . . against; opposed to
corne/o . . . . cornea
coron/o . . . . crown or circle
crani/o . . . . head, cranium
cutane/o . . . . skin
cyan/o . . . . blue
cyst/o . . . . sac or cyst containing
                      fluid; bladder
cyt/o . . . . cell
-cyte . . . . cell
dacry/o . . . . tear
dactyl/o . . . . fingers or toes
de- . . . . not; from; down
dent/o . . . . teeth
dermat/o . . . . skin
-desis . . . . binding
di- . . . . two; both
dia- . . . . across or through
dipl/o . . . . double
dis- . . . . apart; separate

duoden/o . . . . duodenum
-dynia . . . . pain
dys- . . . . faulty; painful; difficult
e- . . . . out; away
-e . . . . noun marker
-eal . . . . pertaining to
ec- . . . . out; away
echin/o . . . . prickly
ecto- . . . . outside
-ectomy . . . . . excision; surgical removal
electr/o . . . . electricity
embry/o . . . . embryo
-emesis . . . . vomit
-emia . . . . condition of blood
emmetr/o . . . . correct measure
en- . . . . inside; within
encephal/o . . . . related to the brain
endo- . . . . inside; within
enter/o . . . . intestines
epi- . . . . upon
erythr/o . . . . red
estr/o . . . . female
eu- . . . . normal or good
-eum . . . . tissue or structure
ex- . . . . out; away
exo- . . . . outside
extra- . . . . outside
fibrin/o . . . . fiber
-form . . . . like or resembling
gamet/o . . . . gamete
gangli/o . . . . swelling, connection
gastr/o . . . . stomach
-genesis . . . . beginning, origin,
                      or production
-genic . . . beginning, origin, or production
gingiv/o . . . . gums
glauc/o . . . . gray
gli/o . . . . gluey substance
gloss/o . . . . tongue
gluc/o . . . . glucose (sugar)
glyc/o . . . . sugar
gnath/o . . . . jaw
gonad/o . . . . sex organs, seed
-gram . . . . record
granul/o . . . . granular, granules
-graph . . . . instrument for recording

(continues)

Table A.6 Word Parts (continued)

-graphy	process of recording
gyn/o	female
gynec/o	woman, female
hem/o	blood
hemat/o	blood
hemi-	half
hepat/o	liver
hepatic/o	liver
herni/o	rupture, hernia
hidr/o	sweat glands
hydr/o	water
hyper-	above or excessive; extreme
hypo-	deficient; below
hyster/o	uterus
-ia	condition of
-iasis	formation of; presence of
-iatric	treatment
-iatry	study of
-ic	pertaining to
ichthy/o	fish (scales)
-icle	small
ile/o	ileum
ili/o	ilium; hip
immun/o	immune, protected
infra-	under; below
inter-	between
intra-	inside; within
irid/o	iris
-ism	condition of
-itis	inflammation
-ium	tissue or structure
-ize	make; use; subject to
jejun/o	jejunum
kary/o	nucleus
kerat/o	keratin (protein), horny tissue; also cornea of eye
kinesi/o	movement
labi/o	lips
lacrim/o	tears
lact/o	milk
lapar/o	abdomen
laryng/o	larynx
leuk/o	white
lip/o	fat, lipid
-lith	stone (calcification)
lith/o	stone, calcification
-logist	one who specializes in the treatment or study of
-logy	study of
lumb/o	lower back
lymph/o	lymph
-lysis	breaking down
macro-	large
mal-	evil; disease
-malacia	softening
mamm/o	breast
mandibul/o	lower jaw
mast/o	breast
meat/o	passageway
-megaly	enlargement
melan/o	black, pigment-producing
men/o	menses, menstruation

mening/o	membrane covering brain and spinal column
meso-	middle
meta-	beyond; after; change
-meter	instrument for measuring
metr/a, o	uterus
-metry	process of measuring
mi/o	less
micro-	small
mono-	one
morph/o	shape
multi-	many
muscul/o	muscle
my/o	muscle
mydr/o	widen
myel/o	bone marrow or spinal cord
myring/o	tympanic membrane
nas/o	nose
necr/o	death
neo-	new
nephr/o	kidney
neur/o	nerve
neutr/o	neutral
nucle/o	nucleus
o/o	egg
occipit/o	occiput (back of the head)
ocul/o	eye
odont/o	tooth
-oid	like or resembling
-ole	small
-oma	tumor
onc/o	tumor
onych/o	nail
oophor/o	ovary
ophthalm/o	eye
opt/o	eye/vision
-or	one who
orchi/o	testis (testicle)
orchid/o	testis (testicle)
organ/o	organ
orth/o	straight
-ose	pertaining to
-osis	condition
osse/o	bony
oste/o	bone
ot/o	ear
-ous	pertaining to
ov/o	egg
ox/o	oxygen molecule
pachy-	thick
palpebr/o	eyelid
pan-	all
pancreat/o	pancreas
para-	abnormal; alongside; beside
pariet/o	relationship to a wall
path/o	disease
pelv/o	pelvis, basin
-penia	abnormal reduction; lack of
per-	through
peri-	around; circular movement
-pexy	surgical suspension or fixation
phac/o	lens of the eye

phag/o	eating
-phage	eat; devour
-phagia	eat; devour
-phagy	eat; devour
pharyng/o	pharynx (throat)
phas/o	speech
-phile	attraction for; love for
-philia	attraction for; love for
phleb/o	vein
-phobia	fear of
phon/o	sound
phot/o	light
phren/o	diaphragm
pil/o	hair
-plasia	formation
plasm/o	formed; plasma
-plasty	surgical repair or reconstruction
pleur/o	rib area
pne/o	breath
-pnea	breathing
pneum/o	lung, air
-poiesis	formation, production
poikil/o	irregular
poly-	many
post-	after
pre-	before
presby/o	old age
pro-	before
proct/o	rectum, anus
prostat/o	prostate
-ptosis	drooping; falling or downward displacement
pulmon/o	lung
pupill/o	pupil
purpur/o	purple
pyel/o	renal pelvis
pylor/o	pylorus (gatekeeper)
quadri-	four
rachi/o	spine
radi/o	x-rays
re-	again or back
rect/o	rectum
ren/i (o)	renal, the kidney
reticul/o	reticulum (a fine network of cells)
retin/o	retina
retro-	backward or behind
rhin/o	nose
-rrhage	to burst forth
-rrhagia	condition of bursting forth
-rrhagic	relating to bursting forth
-rrhaphy	suture
-rrhea	discharge or flow
-rrhexis	rupture or breaking
-ry	pertaining to
sacr/o	sacrum
salping/o	tube
sarc/o	flesh
scapul/o	scapula
schist/o	split
scler/o	sclera (outer membrane), hardening

(continues)

Table A.6 Word Parts (continued)

-scope . . . . instrument for examining	artificial opening	tympan/o . . drum (pertaining to hearing)
-scopy . . . . examination	sub- . . . . under; below	typhl/o . . . . cecum
scot/o . . . . dark	super- . . . . above or excessive	-ula . . . . small
seb/o . . . . sebum (secretion from	supra- . . . . outside or beyond	-ule . . . . small
sebaceous glands)	sym- . . . . with or together	ultra- . . . . beyond, excessive
semi- . . . . half	syn- . . . . with or together	uni- . . . . one
sept/o . . . . partition	tachy- . . . . fast	ur/e (a), (o), (i) . . . . urea or urine
ser/o . . . . serum (fluid part of blood)	tars/o . . . . tarsal bones in the ankle	ureter/o . . . . ureter
sial/o . . . . saliva, salivary glands	tempor/o . . . . temporal (skull bone)	urethr/o . . . . urethra
sider/o . . . . iron	tend/o; tendin/o . . . . tendon	urin/o . . . . urine
sigmoid/o . . . . sigmoid colon	tetra- . . . . four	uter/o . . . . uterus
somat/o . . . . body	thel/o . . . . nipple	uve/o . . . . uvea
-spasm . . . . involuntary contraction	thorac/o . . . . chest	vagin/o . . . . vagina (sheath)
sperm/o . . . . semen, spermatozoa	thromb/o . . . . blood clot	varic/o . . . . twisted, swollen vein
spermat/o . . . . semen, spermatozoa	thym/o . . . . thymus	vas/o . . . . vessel
spher/o . . . . sphere shaped	thyr/o . . . . thyroid	vascul/o . . . . vessel
sphygm/o . . . . relating to the pulse	-tic . . . . pertaining to	ven/o . . . . vein
splen/o . . . . spleen	-tomy . . . . incision	ventricul/o . . . . ventricle
spondyl/o . . . . vertebrae	tox/o . . . . poison	vertebr/o . . . . vertebra
squam/o . . . . pertaining to scales	trache/o . . . . trachea, windpipe	viscer/o . . . . internal organs
-stasis . . . . stop or stand	trans- . . . . across or through	vitre/o . . . . glassy
sten/o . . . . narrowing, constriction	-tripsy . . . . crushing	vulv/o . . . . vulva (covering)
stern/o . . . . chest	tri- . . . . three	xanth/o . . . . yellow
steth/o . . . . relating to the chest	troph/o . . . . .nutrition	-y . . . . condition or process of
stom/a . . . . mouth	-trophy . . . . development	zyg/o . . . . yoke; a type of joining;
stomat/o . . . . mouth	-tropic (tropin) . . . turning toward, changing	the cheek bone
-stomy . . . . surgical creation of an	tub/o . . . . tube (little tube)	

Anatomy Handbook

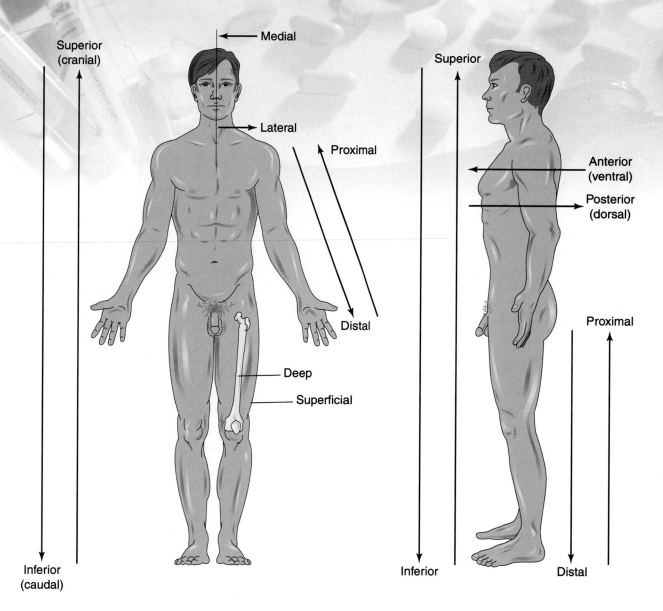

Figure B.1
Anatomical Position

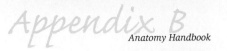

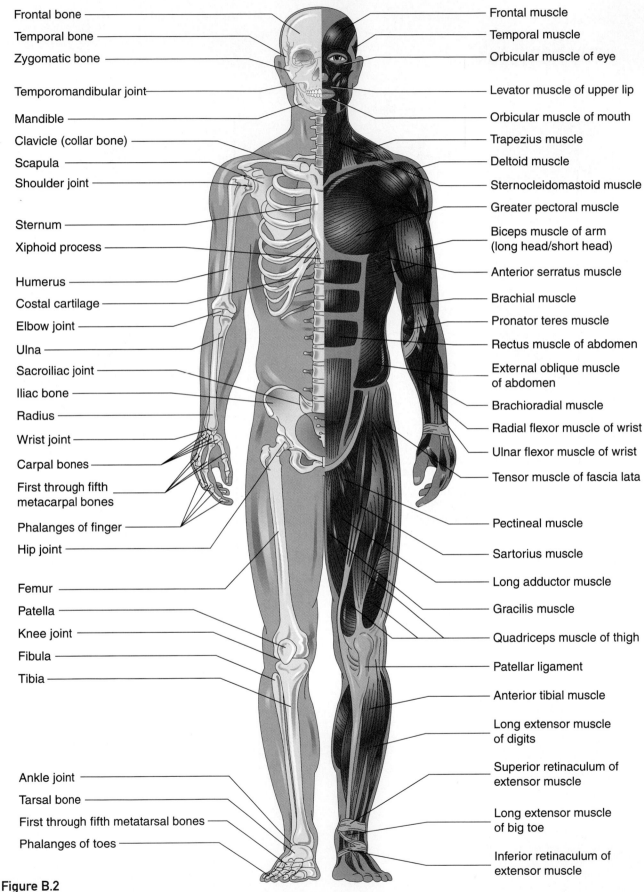

Frontal bone

Temporal bone

Zygomatic bone

Temporomandibular joint

Mandible

Clavicle (collar bone)

Scapula

Shoulder joint

Sternum

Xiphoid process

Humerus

Costal cartilage

Elbow joint

Ulna

Sacroiliac joint

Iliac bone

Radius

Wrist joint

Carpal bones

First through fifth
metacarpal bones

Phalanges of finger

Hip joint

Femur

Patella

Knee joint

Fibula

Tibia

Ankle joint

Tarsal bone

First through fifth metatarsal bones

Phalanges of toes

Frontal muscle

Temporal muscle

Orbicular muscle of eye

Levator muscle of upper lip

Orbicular muscle of mouth

Trapezius muscle

Deltoid muscle

Sternocleidomastoid muscle

Greater pectoral muscle

Biceps muscle of arm
(long head/short head)

Anterior serratus muscle

Brachial muscle

Pronator teres muscle

Rectus muscle of abdomen

External oblique muscle
of abdomen

Brachioradial muscle

Radial flexor muscle of wrist

Ulnar flexor muscle of wrist

Tensor muscle of fascia lata

Pectineal muscle

Sartorius muscle

Long adductor muscle

Gracilis muscle

Quadriceps muscle of thigh

Patellar ligament

Anterior tibial muscle

Long extensor muscle
of digits

Superior retinaculum of
extensor muscle

Long extensor muscle
of big toe

Inferior retinaculum of
extensor muscle

Figure B.2
Musculoskeletal System

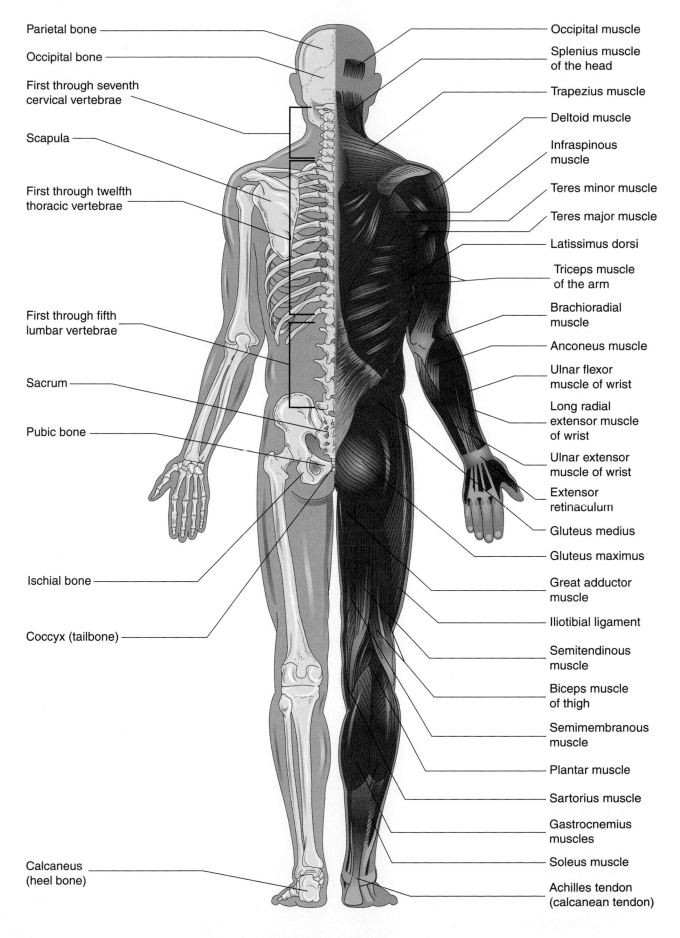

Parietal bone

Occipital bone

First through seventh
cervical vertebrae

Scapula

First through twelfth
thoracic vertebrae

First through fifth
lumbar vertebrae

Sacrum

Pubic bone

Ischial bone

Coccyx (tailbone)

Calcaneus
(heel bone)

Occipital muscle

Splenius muscle
of the head

Trapezius muscle

Deltoid muscle

Infraspinous
muscle

Teres minor muscle

Teres major muscle

Latissimus dorsi

Triceps muscle
of the arm

Brachioradial
muscle

Anconeus muscle

Ulnar flexor
muscle of wrist

Long radial
extensor muscle
of wrist

Ulnar extensor
muscle of wrist

Extensor
retinaculum

Gluteus medius

Gluteus maximus

Great adductor
muscle

Iliotibial ligament

Semitendinous
muscle

Biceps muscle
of thigh

Semimembranous
muscle

Plantar muscle

Sartorius muscle

Gastrocnemius
muscles

Soleus muscle

Achilles tendon
(calcanean tendon)

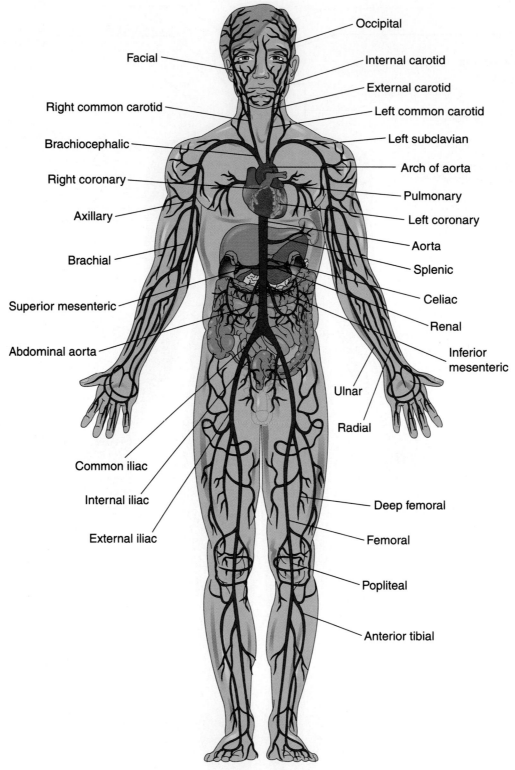

Figure B.3
Major Arteries of the Body

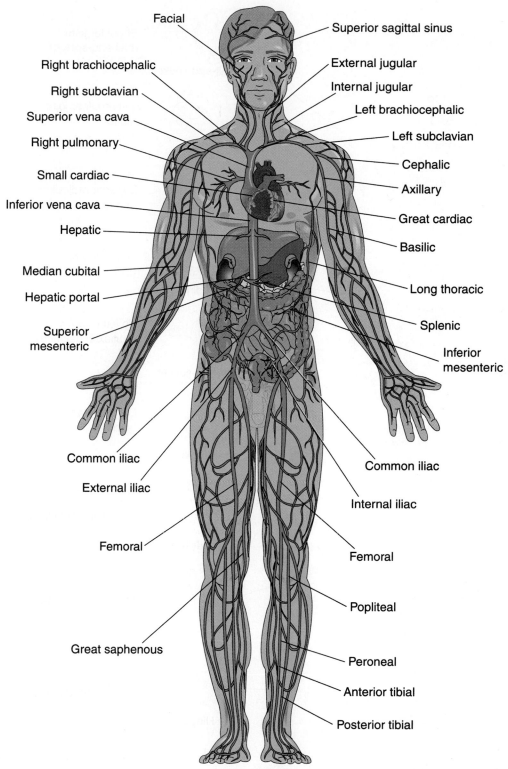

Facial

Superior sagittal sinus

Right brachiocephalic

External jugular

Right subclavian

Internal jugular

Superior vena cava

Left brachiocephalic

Right pulmonary

Left subclavian

Small cardiac

Cephalic

Inferior vena cava

Axillary

Hepatic

Great cardiac

Median cubital

Basilic

Hepatic portal

Long thoracic

Superior mesenteric

Splenic

Inferior mesenteric

Common iliac

Common iliac

External iliac

Internal iliac

Femoral

Femoral

Popliteal

Great saphenous

Peroneal

Anterior tibial

Posterior tibial

Figure B.4
Major Veins of the Body

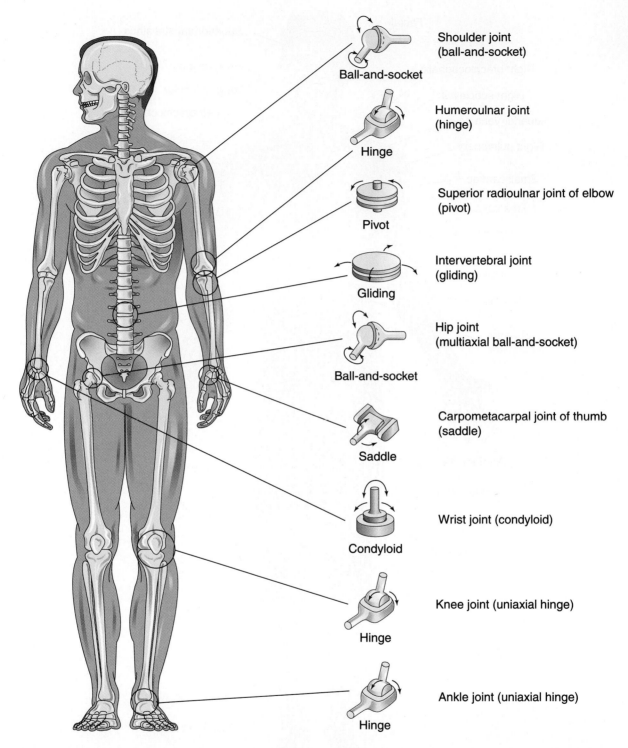

Shoulder joint
(ball-and-socket)

Ball-and-socket

Humeroulnar joint
(hinge)

Hinge

Superior radioulnar joint of elbow
(pivot)

Pivot

Intervertebral joint
(gliding)

Gliding

Hip joint
(multiaxial ball-and-socket)

Ball-and-socket

Carpometacarpal joint of thumb
(saddle)

Saddle

Wrist joint (condyloid)

Condyloid

Knee joint (uniaxial hinge)

Hinge

Ankle joint (uniaxial hinge)

Hinge

Figure B.5
Types of Diathroses and Their Functions

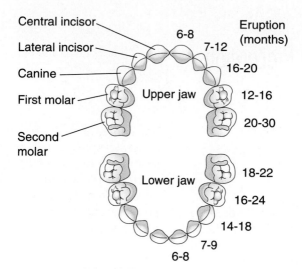

Central incisor — 6-8

Lateral incisor — 7-12

Canine — 16-20

First molar — 12-16 — Upper jaw

Second molar — 20-30

Lower jaw — 18-22

16-24

14-18

7-9

6-8

Eruption (months)

Figure B.6
Deciduous (Baby) Teeth

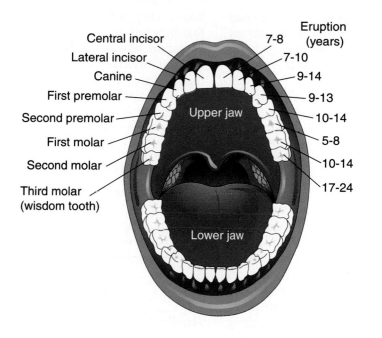

Central incisor — 7-8

Lateral incisor — 7-10

Canine — 9-14

First premolar — 9-13

Second premolar — Upper jaw — 10-14

First molar — 5-8

Second molar — 10-14

Third molar (wisdom tooth) — 17-24

Lower jaw

Eruption (years)

Figure B.7
Adult Teeth

Standard and Universal Precautions

Standard Precautions

1 Handwashing

a. Wash hands after touching blood, body fluids, secretions, excretions, and contaminated items, whether or not gloves are worn. Wash hands immediately after gloves are removed, between patient contacts, and when otherwise indicated to avoid transfer of microorganisms to other patients or environments. It may be necessary to wash hands between tasks and procedures on the same patient to prevent cross-contamination of different body sites.

b. Use a plain (nonantimicrobial) soap for routine handwashing.

c. Use an antimicrobial agent or a waterless antiseptic agent for specific circumstances (e.g., control of outbreaks or hyperendemic infections), as defined by the infection control program.

2 Gloves

Wear gloves (clean, nonsterile gloves are adequate) when touching blood, body fluids, secretions, excretions, and contaminated items. Put on clean gloves just before touching mucous membranes and nonintact skin. Change gloves between tasks and procedures on the same patient after contact with material that may contain a high concentration of microorganisms. Remove gloves promptly after use, before touching noncontaminated items and environmental surfaces, and before going to another patient, and wash hands immediately to avoid transfer of microorganisms to other patients or environments.

3 Mask, Eye Protection, Face Shield

Wear a mask and eye protection or a face shield to protect mucous membranes of the eyes, nose, and mouth during procedures and patient-care activities that are likely to generate splashes or sprays of blood, body fluids, secretions, and excretions.

4 Gown

Wear a gown (a clean, nonsterile gown is adequate) to protect skin and to prevent soiling of clothing during procedures and patient-care activities that are likely to generate splashes or sprays of blood, body fluids, secretions, or excretions. Select a gown that is appropriate for the activity and amount of fluid likely to be encountered. Remove a soiled gown as promptly as possible, and wash hands to avoid transfer of microorganisms to other patients or environments.

5 Patient–Care Equipment

Handle used patient-care equipment soiled with blood, body fluids, secretions, and excretions in a manner that prevents skin and mucous membrane exposures, contamination of clothing, and transfer of microorganisms to other patients and environments. Ensure that reusable equipment is not used for the care of another patient until it has been cleaned and reprocessed appropriately. Ensure that single-use items are discarded properly.

6 Environmental Control

Ensure that the hospital has adequate procedures for the routine care, cleaning, and disinfection of environmental surfaces, beds, bed rails, bedside equipment, and other frequently touched surfaces and ensure that these procedures are being followed.

7 Linen

Handle, transport, and process used linen soiled with blood, body fluids, secretions, and excretions in a manner that prevents skin and mucous membrane exposures and contamination of clothing, and that avoids transfer of microorganisms to other patients and environments.

8 Occupational Health and Bloodborne Pathogens

a. Take care to prevent injuries when using needles, scalpels, and other sharp instruments or devices; when handling sharp instruments after procedures; when cleaning used instruments; and when disposing of used needles. Never recap used needles, or otherwise manipulate them using both hands, or use any other technique that involves directing the point of a needle toward any part of the body; rather, use either a one-handed "scoop" technique or a mechanical device designed for holding the needle sheath. Do not remove used needles from disposable syringes by hand, and do not bend, break, or otherwise manipulate used needles by hand. Place used disposable syringes and needles, scalpel blades, and other sharp items in appropriate puncture-resistant containers, which are located as close as practical to the area in which the items were used, and place reusable syringes and needles in a puncture-resistant container for transport to the reprocessing area.

b. Use mouthpieces, resuscitation bags, or other ventilation devices as an alternative to mouth-to-mouth resuscitation methods in areas where the need for resuscitation is predictable.

9 Patient Placement

Place a patient who contaminates the environment or who does not (or cannot be expected to) assist in maintaining appropriate hygiene or environmental control in a private room. If a private room is not available, consult with infection control professionals regarding patient placement or other alternatives.

Source: Garner, Julia S., Guidelines for Isolation Precautions in Hospitals, 1 January 1996, < http://aepo-xdv-www.epo.cdc.gov/wonder/prevguid/p0000419/entire.htm > (4 October 2000).

Universal Precautions

1 **Barrier protection** should be used at all times to prevent skin and mucous membrane contamination with blood, body fluids containing visible blood, or other body fluids (cerebrospinal, synovial, pleural, peritoneal, pericardial, and amniotic fluids, semen and vaginal secretions).

Barrier protection should be used with <u>ALL</u> tissues.

The type of barrier protection used should be appropriate for the type of procedures being performed and the type of exposure anticipated. Examples of barrier protection include disposable lab coats, gloves, and eye and face protection.

2 **Gloves** are to be worn when there is potential for hand or skin contact with blood, other potentially infectious material, or items and surfaces contaminated with these materials.

3 Wear **face protection** (face shield) during procedures that are likely to generate droplets of blood or body fluid to prevent exposure to mucous membranes of the mouth, nose, and eyes.

4 Wear **protective body clothing** (disposable laboratory coats, Tyvek) when there is a potential for splashing of blood or body fluids.

5 **Wash hands or other skin surfaces** thoroughly and immediately if contaminated with blood, body fluids containing visible blood, or other body fluids to which universal precautions apply.

6 **Wash hands immediately** after gloves are removed.

7 **Avoid accidental injuries** that can be caused by needles, scalpel blades, laboratory instruments, etc., when performing procedures, cleaning instruments, handling sharp instruments, and disposing of used needles, pipettes, etc.

8 Used needles, disposable syringes, scalpel blades, pipettes, and other **sharp items are to be placed in puncture-resistant containers** marked with a biohazard symbol for disposal.

Source: National Institute of Environmental Health Sciences, Universal Precautions, 22 December 1998, < www.niehs.nih.gov/odhsb/biosafe/univers.htm > (5 October 2000).

Self-Check

The following are the answers to the "Signs/Symptoms of Progress" feature at the end of each chapter. Answers for the "Exercise 3: Exploring Perspectives in Teams" section are not provided due to the nature of the questions. For many of the questions in this exercise type, there is no one right answer and open-ended discussions are encouraged. However, as you assess your individual or group responses to these questions, consider the following criteria.

- Did your response suggest a reasonable level of mastery of the subject?
- Did your response reveal a personalized, thoughtful, and coherent grasp of the question?
- Did your response show insightful consideration?
- Did your response reveal an appreciation for another's views?
- Did your response address the major points discussed or considered in the question?

CHAPTER 1

Exercise 1: Recall, Question, Connect

Recall: Responses will vary. The attributes listed may include: professionalism; a strong sense of ethics; initiative; a sense of responsibility; the ability to work as a team player; good time management skills; the ability to prioritize and to perform multiple tasks; adaptability; the willingness to work towards professional certification; and an on-going interest in education.

Question: Again the responses will vary, but will include one or more of the above.

Connect: You should explain how you will develop the particular professional attributes mentioned in the Question part of the exercise. Answers might include actions such as education, practice, and accepting constructive criticism.

Exercise 2: Educating the Patient

1. Caution Ms. Babcock that "chat" room discussions are truly that, just discussions. The people who participate are not necessarily experts in the information they are discussing. While acknowledging that chat rooms can be very helpful to those seeking support and understanding from others sharing their medical concern, the medical information found in a chat room may be unproven or untrue. Suggest that Ms. Babcock cautiously evaluate the chat room information and discuss any issues it raises with her physician.
2. Provide a listing of reliable websites for medical information. Start with those provided in Table 1.8.

Also, tell Ms. Babcock that ".edu" and ".gov" sites are generally reliable and that ones ending in ".com" may be less reliable because they are commercial or run by special interest groups.

CHAPTER 2

Exercise 1: Recall, Question, Connect

Recall: Elderly patients requiring long-term care have a variety of settings in which this care might be provided. A nursing home is one option. Other options include home care with or without the assistance of a home health agency, assisted living facilities, adult day care centers, and hospices.

Question: Responses will vary. Questions may include: What support services can the family provide? What gaps in the availability of time or resources of the family might be filled by a home healthcare agency? What will happen if a home caregiver needs to take a break, go back to work, or can no longer care for the patient? Does the patient have emotional or social needs that might be best met in an adult day care setting? If a nursing home is the best choice, how desirable is 24-hour nursing care? Is the long-term care patient dying? If so, is home hospice care or a separate hospice facility the better choice for the patient in his last days?

Connect: As a medical assistant, you need to be familiar with the various placements and/or agencies that can provide support for long-term patients because you may be charged with helping patients sort out and understand their options. You might also choose to work in one of these settings. In order to educate yourself about which long-term facilities and services exist in your community, you should make a plan to visit a number of them. Arrange an appointment with a staff worker at the facility who can tell you about the facility and the kinds of services it offers. You can collect a number of brochures or handouts to give to your patients or to keep for your own reference. You will act as a link in helping patients choose between options by understanding the needs of the patients and their families, the options available for long-term care in your community, insurance coverage of these options, and community agencies that might provide additional resources to help patients with these decisions.

Exercise 2: Educating the Patient

1. A PPO (preferred provider organization) is a loose form of managed care that arranges with a limited number of healthcare providers to provide services to a defined group of individuals. Enrollees who use the

preferred providers pay a small co-payment. Enrollees may seek care from healthcare providers not in the plan and are then susceptible to a deductible and a co-payment.

In an HMO (health maintenance organization) the enrollee must use the plan's physicians and generally needs a primary care physician's referral or plan approval before visits to a specialist, tests, surgery, or hospitalization. The enrollee also makes a co-payment.
2. As a medical assistant, you have responsibilities for both the health of the patient and the success of the practice. However, your concern in maintaining Ms. Radice as a patient should be secondary to making sure that she has access to the medical care that best meets her needs. Provide Ms. Radice with all the information you have about the two plans, and have her review the materials that were provided by her employer. Emphasize that there are benefits and shortcomings to all plans and that she should carefully consider both options before making a decision. Questions to ask her may include: Are there any doctors in the HMO with whom you would feel comfortable? Would it bother you to have to get a referral every time you need a test, surgery, or visit to a specialist? What is the cost difference between the two plans?

CHAPTER 3
Exercise 1: Recall, Question, Connect

Recall: A Living Will, a Durable Power of Attorney for Healthcare, and a Healthcare Proxy are three ways an individual can make her wishes regarding medical treatment and end-of-life issues known.
Question: Responses will vary. They may include questions such as: Can a patient change a Durable Power of Attorney? What is the difference between a Durable Power of Attorney and a Healthcare Proxy? Do you always need a lawyer to draw up one of these documents? How can a healthcare professional find out what advance directive a patient has? What do these documents look like? Where are they filed? A student can find the answers to these questions by researching at the library or on the Internet. The American Bar Association will also provide information. The law firm that works with the medical practice in which a medical assistant works can also clarify issues about advance directives.
Connect: A thorough understanding of advance directives is necessary to ensure that state laws are understood and complied with. It is important that the patient's preferences regarding their care are known and respected. Also, the physician will need to know exactly who should be included in discussions of medical care and who can make the final decisions for a patient.

Exercise 2: Educating the Patient
1. Gently ask Mrs. Jacobson if she has given any thought to issues that will be coming up concerning her care. Ask her if she has made her preferences known and if they are documented anywhere. If she hasn't made these decisions yet, ask her if she would like information about advance directives, or if she would like help in getting her wishes documented.
2. Mrs. Jacobson's family should be informed as to what her wishes are regarding her end-of-life care so that they are clearly understood by all parties. If Mrs. Jacobson has her preferences in writing, her family needs to know where the document is.

CHAPTER 4
Exercise 1: Recall, Question, Connect
Recall: Factors such as stress, age, gender, economic status, disability, ability to speak English, culture, and emotions such as anger, or personality traits such as shyness, can all affect communication in the medical office.
Question: Responses will vary. Questions may include: How can I identify what the barrier to communication is? How can I find out more about the different cultures of the patients coming into the office? What ways can I help a child or teenager feel comfortable talking to me? Are there any factors about me that affect how I communicate?
Connect: The medical assistant is the communication link between the patient and the physician, and the information she relays is critical in promoting wellness or diagnosing and treating disease. Since the medical assistant is often the first provider that the patient sees during the office visit, the patient is often more comfortable speaking to her than any other staff member. The medical assistant must know how to communicate with the patient and the physician so that the essentials of the patient's visit are conveyed.

Exercise 2: Educating the Patient
1. Express empathy in a nonverbal attitude of active listening, eye contact, a gentle tone of voice, and an unhurried atmosphere. Let her know that many people feel the same way as she does about needles, yet they learn how to give themselves shots successfully and without much pain. Explain how important it is for her to be able to control her condition without depending on others. Also, provide pamphlets or other written or visual resources to Ms. Freeman for her to review once she gets home.
2. The best way to know whether Ms. Freeman understands your instruction is feedback. Ask her to repeat the instructions; have her demonstrate to you that she knows how to give herself the injection.

CHAPTER 5

Exercise 1: Recall, Question, Connect

Recall: Although some traditional medical practitioners in the United States might not approve of any of the holistic and alternative approaches to healthcare presented in this chapter, osteopathy and chiropractic therapy have been approved by the American Medical Association.

Question: Student responses will vary. Questions may include: What exact criteria should a therapy meet before it is considered acceptable? What scientific information is there to back up each alternative therapy? How were these alternative therapies developed? Should the West be more open to alternative ideas? What obligations does a physician have to learn about alternative medicine? What cultural factors are there to consider when dealing with a patient who uses an alternative therapy?

Connect: A medical assistant needs to be knowledgeable about alternative therapies for several reasons. Some are becoming an accepted part of Western medicine, and may be used in the office in which the medical assistant is working. Also, the medical assistant will need to be aware of aspects of alternative therapy that a patient is using so that she can let the physician know of things that may interfere or affect the care that he recommends to the patient.

Exercise 2: Educating the Patient

1. State that you have some understanding of traditional Chinese medicine, but ask her to elaborate on why she believes this is so.

2. You should ask her to tell you about any alternative therapies she may be using and the rationale for their use. Medical assistants should always ask patients about other therapies they may be using, as such methods may interfere with medical treatments or prescriptions.

3. Discuss with Ms. Si the importance of informing the physician about all treatments that the traditional Chinese doctor is using because of the danger of interference between the therapies. Inform the physician about what Ms. Si has told you so that he can take the traditional Chinese treatment into consideration as he plans her care. Since it is important to acknowledge and respect diversity in patient care, be open, respectful, and positive as Ms. Si describes the alternative therapy. But remember that the AMA has not approved many such alternative treatments, so be careful not to either encourage or recommend them.

CHAPTER 6

Exercise 1: Recall, Question, Connect

Recall: Medical offices use computer software for word processing; desktop publishing; spreadsheet, database, and presentation creation; and virus protection and security.

Question: Student responses will vary. They may include questions such as: Are all medical offices using computers? What computer skills does a medical assistant need? How does computer use impact patients? How safe is medical information on a computer? How are files maintained and updated? Who has access to the computerized information?

Connect: A physician could use a computer to check her schedule, to look up a patient file, to research information, to compose a letter or report, to collect and respond to e-mail, and to communicate with the office. Information can be transferred over the Internet or by saving it on a diskette.

Exercise 2: Educating the Patient

1. You will need to find a way to transfer inactive files to the new computer, perhaps by downloading the patient files from the old computer onto diskettes to be loaded into the new system. You may need to retrieve hard copies of patient files that are in storage. Until the problem is resolved, the office will need to have one computer connected to the old system so that inactive files can be retrieved when necessary.

2. Thank the staff member for bringing the matter to your attention, and ask everyone to be on the lookout for any other problems that may arise with the transition to the new system.

CHAPTER 7

Exercise 1: Recall, Question, Connect

Recall: Correspondence can be transmitted via letter, e-mail, and fax.

Question: Student responses will vary. Questions may include: When is it necessary to send a fax instead of a letter? Are there times when a letter is the only acceptable means of communication? What are the costs associated with each method? Is it necessary to keep a copy of every e-mail? Is there a style for e-mail?

Connect: A letter is the appropriate method of communication when you need formality, a good hard copy, and need to ensure confidentiality. The advantage of a fax is speed. E-mail is informal, quick, and is included in the cost of the Internet service. Faxes and e-mail must be used with caution when sending confidential information.

Exercise 2: Educating the Patient

1. You cannot give out any medical information about Ms. Martin without her consent.

2. Tell Ms. Jones that you cannot discuss her medical condition, but that you will mention to Ms. Martin that she was concerned.

3. These symptoms could indicate a serious problem such as a stroke. Thank Ms. Jones for the information and inform the physician. Contact the patient.

CHAPTER 8

Exercise 1: Recall, Question, Connect

Recall: A time study is made by tracking each patient's arrival time, the type of appointments, wait for the physician, and length of visit with the physician, as well as noting the appointment type over a period of several weeks.

Question: Answers will vary. Questions may include: Who does the timing? How are the times recorded? Does the physician know he is being timed? How often should a time study be conducted?

Connect: A time study will reveal whether you are allocating the correct amount of time for each appointment slot. It can also indicate whether the office is opening too early or closing too soon, or if there is a need to adjust for the number of cancellations and no-shows. There will be fewer scheduling conflicts if problems indicated by a time study are addressed.

Exercise 2: Educating the Patient

1. The woman would be considered a new patient. You may want to tell the woman to arrive early for her appointment to fill out the necessary paperwork. If the physician requires that every new patient receive a complete physical, you would need to take that into account when making the appointment.

2. You would want to offer the woman directions to the office and any special information about the practice that a new patient would need to know.

CHAPTER 9

Exercise 1: Recall, Question, Connect

Recall: When a medical records system is established, decisions must be made concerning how files will be classified and transferred between classifications; how long records will be retained; how active records will be protected and preserved; and how records will be stored long-term.

Question: Responses will vary. Questions may include: Who is responsible for setting up the medical records management system? What are the laws in the state where I work concerning medical records? How far away should inactive files be stored, in case one needs to access them? How have computers impacted decisions regarding medical records?

Connect: The medical assistant will be using the medical records on a daily basis, and will be responsible for initiating, maintaining, protecting, and storing the records. He will work more efficiently and accurately if he knows exactly how and why the medical records management system was set up in the office. On occasion, the system will need to be revised or updated, the laws concerning medical records may change, or the medical assistant could move to a new office where a medical records management system will need to be started from scratch. A thorough knowledge and understanding of the decisions that need to be made will assist him in those situations.

Exercise 2: Educating the Patient

1. Tell the woman what the correct diagnosis is. Explain to her that although they sound alike, scoliosis and sclerosis are two completely different conditions. Define scoliosis for her. Let her know that her daughter has a mildly crooked spine. Assure her that what her daughter has is treatable and is in no way life-threatening.

2. Many medical terms sound alike, and a patient could easily misinterpret a term that they hear. (In this case, both words have the suffix *-osis*, meaning condition. Scoliosis is derived from a Greek word meaning crooked, whereas sclerosis refers to a hardening of body tissue.) It is important to make certain that the patient understands all medical terminology being discussed. A medical assistant will want to be familiar with terminology used in the office so that she will be able to clearly explain what the medical terms mean.

CHAPTER 10

Exercise 1: Recall, Question, Connect

Recall: Three bookkeeping or accounting systems used in a medical office are single-entry, write-it-once (pegboard), and computerized.

Question: Responses will vary. Questions may include: Which system takes the most time? Which system is the easiest to learn? Does an office ever use more than one system? What are the advantages and disadvantages of each system?

Connect: The medical assistant must be familiar with accounting principles in order to understand his or her role in the accounting process and to perform bookkeeping duties.

Exercise 2: Educating the Patient

1. Charges would be recorded on the day sheet and the patient's ledger card according to the bookkeeping system being used in the office.

2. Information regarding an insurance payment would be in the patient's ledger card.

3. Medical services should be itemized on the ledger card.

CHAPTER 11

Exercise 1: Recall, Question, Connect

Recall: Physicians set their own fees, which are usually based on fees established by government health-care programs and insurance companies.

Question: Responses will vary. Questions may include: How often are fees raised? Are fees higher in some areas of the country than in others? What other factors impact the amount that a physician charges? Are all office costs passed on to the patient?

Connect: The medical assistant can help keep medical costs down by using his time on the job wisely, being careful not to waste supplies, and using and caring for equipment properly.

Exercise 2: Educating the Patient

1. Answers will vary. Possible responses by the medical assistant include telling Ms. Davis that the fee is similar to what other physicians charge for the same service and that the fee is based on the physician's skill and knowledge. Also, fees must cover overhead costs.

2. She should have been informed at the time she made the appointment. A sign to this effect should be displayed in the office. Payment policies should be incorporated in an information sheet or brochure to be given to new patients when they fill out a registration form.

3. The medical assistant might suggest payment by credit card or check, whichever Ms. Davis prefers.

CHAPTER 12

Exercise 1: Recall, Question, Connect

Recall: Medicare Part A covers inpatient hospital care, care in a skilled nursing facility, skilled care in the home, and hospice care for the terminally ill, while Medicare Part B covers physicians' services, outpatient hospital care, x-rays, and lab tests.

Question: Responses will vary. Why would a patient not carry Part B? Does Part B cost the same all over the country? Can a physician agree to provide services for one part but not another? How can a medical assistant find out the details of these two types of coverage? Are there some medical settings where Medicare would never be used?

Connect: Medicare Part B.

Exercise 2: Educating the Patient

1. CHAMPUS covers dependents of active-duty military personnel.

2. The treatment will not be covered because advance authorization is needed.

3. TRICARE Prime (HMO), TRICARE Extra (PPO), and TRICARE Standard are available through this program.

CHAPTER 13

Exercise 1: Recall, Question, Connect

Recall: The organizational skills needed by an office manager include the ability to set priorities, to be detailed and careful in both written and oral communication, and to work in a systematic way. Examples of ways in which you are organized in your life will vary. They may include things such as responsibilities you have had in previous jobs; your ability to prioritize and complete homework in school; your experience balancing your checking account and handling your personal budget; being treasurer for a school club or record-keeper for the softball league; or assigning chores and planning menus for a household.

Question: Answers may vary. Volunteering to run a Boy Scout troop, taking a computer class, or setting a budget for yourself are all ways that you can learn and practice organizational skills.

Connect: Planning and keeping to a budget; setting a schedule and delegating job responsibilities; monitoring performance; keeping personnel records up-to-date; planning and carrying out public relations activities.

Exercise 2: Educating the Patient

1. Answers may vary. The office manager could help the patient find appointment times that are more convenient for the driver, or offer to call the patient's residence and remind the driver of the appointment. If the budget permits it, perhaps the office could pay cab fare for elderly who meet a needs test.

2. The office manager should find out what type of transportation the patient will be using and what alternatives are available. Social Services or the AARP may have information that would help the office manager better understand how to communicate with the elderly and understand their concerns, as well as ideas on transportation options for those who don't drive.

3. Bus schedules, the name of cab companies, AARP information.

CHAPTER 14

Exercise 1: Recall, Question, Connect

Recall: The office should be clear of any hazards that may cause anyone to trip or fall, such as toys on the floor or a file drawer left open. Stairs and aisles should be clear. Any wet floor must be marked with a cautionary sign. All bathrooms should have grab bars. Doorways should be wide enough to accommodate a wheelchair.

Question: Responses may vary. Questions may include: What safety hazards are particular to children? To the elderly? To patients with vision problems? To patients in a wheelchair? To patients who cannot read English? To mentally disabled patients? How can I make the office safer for them? *Connect:* Check that the hall to the room and the room itself are clutter-free and there is sufficient space to accommodate the width of the walker. If at all possible use the examination room closest to the reception area. Walk behind the patient if a family member is not with the patient. Ask the patient if she would like assistance with changing into the examination gown. Assist the patient into a chair until the physician is ready to examine the patient. When the physician is ready for the exam, assist the patient onto the examination table and stay with the patient during the exam. If a urine specimen is needed, accompany the patient to the bathroom. Instruct the patient about the use of handrails.

Exercise 2: Educating the Patient

1. Explain that her temperature is elevated and that the physician will need to examine her and provide the appropriate treatment for her condition.

2. Mary Ann should explain the necessity of hand-washing whenever Mrs. Pozanski coughs, sneezes, or blows her nose. She should also wash her hands before she prepares food for the children. She should dispose of tissues into a waste receptacle immediately after use.

3. Mary Ann might suggest the use of 10% bleach solution for cleaning areas such as counter tops, sinks, and linoleum or tile floors; opening windows and doors to outside air; installation of air filtration or air purification system; vacuuming and damp-dusting often; cleaning drain pans under refrigerator and air conditioners; and the use of vented fans in bathrooms and kitchen.

Glossary

A

abandonment A physician's halting of treatment without proper notification to the patient.

ABA number A number assigned to a bank by the American Bankers Association that identifies the bank and its location.

ABC Initials for the first things an emergency responder should check: airway, breathing, and circulation.

abduction Movement of a limb away from the body.

abortion Termination of pregnancy.

abscess A deep, infected cavity that usually results from bacteria entering the skin through a puncture, laceration, or surgical incision.

absorption The process through which drugs enter the bloodstream.

account A record of information and transactions related to each asset and liability, and each aspect of owner's equity.

accounting A system of organizing, maintaining, and auditing business records, summarizing financial transactions, and interpreting the results.

accounting cycle The steps involved in recording, processing, and summarizing financial transactions.

accounting equation The mathematical equation that expresses the financial condition of a business: Assets = Liabilities + Owner's Equity.

accounts payable Debts owed to other businesses or individuals for goods and services.

accounts receivable Money that has been earned, but not yet received.

accreditation A process by which an outside agency evaluates a program and certifies that it meets a set of standard requirements.

Accrediting Bureau of Health Education Schools (ABHES) An agency that accredits educational programs in either a hospital, private vocational institution, or public postsecondary institution.

accrual method of accounting The accounting method in which income is recorded in the period it is earned, whether or not cash has been received, and expenses are recorded in the period they are incurred, regardless of whether they have been paid.

accuracy The proximity of a value to the true or known value.

acne vulgaris (**ak**-nee vul-**gah**-ris) A common skin disease resulting from obstruction of sebaceous glands and increased production of sebum and bacteria.

Acquired Immune Deficiency Syndrome (AIDS) The final stage of the bloodborne pathogen disease caused by the human immunodeficiency virus (HIV).

acromegaly (ak-rO-**meg**-ah-lee) A chronic condition of the anterior pituitary lobe in which excess growth hormone is secreted.

active-assistive ROM Range of motion exercises in which both the patient and the practitioner participate.

active files Files of patients currently receiving treatment.

active immunity Immunity developed through exposure to a disease: antibodies are produced that protect the body upon subsequent exposure.

active listening A form of listening in which a person listens closely to what another says with few interruptions, seeking to understand what is being communicated.

active ROM Range of motion exercises in which the patient performs the movements as instructed by the practitioner.

activities of daily living (ADL) Activities human beings perform to remain independent as they function in society.

acuity (ah-**kyoo**-ih-tee) Clearness of vision and focusing ability.

acupressure (**ak**-yoo-presh-er) A method of relieving pain or altering the function of a system of the body by applying gentle, firm pressure with the fingers and hands.

acupuncture (**ak**-yoo-pungk-cher) A method of relieving pain or altering the function of a system of the body by inserting fine, wire-thin needles into the skin at specific sites on the body along a series of lines, or channels, called meridians.

acute care Healthcare in which a patient is treated for an abrupt episode of illness, for the complications of an accident or other trauma, or during recovery from surgery, usually given in a hospital.

acute phase The period of an infection during which symptoms are at their peak.

addiction Psychological and/or physical dependence on a drug.

Addison's disease A condition in which there is partial or complete failure of adrenocortical function.

adduction Movement of a limb toward the body.

adipose Fat tissue.

administrative competencies Skills that the medical assistant usually uses in the "front office." These may include clerical functions, handling insurance claims, accounting, bookkeeping, greeting patients, answering the telephone, and general office management tasks.

adrenal glands (ah-**dree**-nal glandz) The triangular endocrine glands on top of the kidneys.

adrenalin (a-**dren**-a-lin) See epinephrine.

adrenal medulla The portion of the adrenal gland that releases epinephrine and norepinephrine to help the body respond to stress.

adrenergic (ad-ren-**er**-jik) A substance that constricts blood vessels.

advance directive A living will, durable power of attorney for healthcare, or healthcare proxy specifying what treatment the patient wants or does not want if the patient cannot voice those decisions, and/or designating a person to make those decisions at that time.

adverse reaction A harmful, unintended reaction to a drug administered at normal dosage.

aerobic bacteria (ayr-**O**-bik bak-**tee**-ree-ah) Bacteria that require oxygen to grow.

afferent nerves Sensory nerves, those that receive information from the environment.

agar (**ag**-ahr) A gelatinous substance to which other nutrients may be added to support the growth of bacteria.

agenda A list of items for discussion at a meeting.

agglutination (ah-gloo-tih-**nay**-shun) Visible clumping of red blood cells caused by antibodies attaching to them. The process by which an antibody molecule binds to more than one antigen.

aging accounts report A list of overdue accounts showing the length of time each one is overdue based on the date of the transaction.

air conduction Transmission of sound through the ear canal, tympanic membrane, and ossicular chain.

albumin (al-**byoo**-min) A common protein found in blood. When present in the urine, it indicates an abnormality of the kidneys.

aldosterone (al-**dos**-ter-On) A mineralocorticoid hormone that regulates the resorption of sodium and the excretion of potassium by the kidneys.

allergic rhinitis (ah-**ler**-jik rI-**nI**-tis) Hay fever, a common Type I hypersensitivity disorder.

allergist The medical specialist who diagnoses and treats allergic disorders.

allergy A hypersensitive reaction to intrinsically harmless antigens, most of which are environmental.

alligator forceps Forceps whose jaw closure is similar to that of an alligator.

alopecia (al-O-**pee**-shee-ah) Complete or partial loss of hair.

Alzheimer's disease (**alts**-hI-merz) A chronic, progressive, neurodegenerative disorder characterized by cerebral atrophy, particularly of the frontal lobes.

ambulatory care (**am**-byoo-la-tor-ee kayr) A wide range of services provided to non-institutionalized patients which generally include primary care treatments such as checkups, immunizations, tests, x-rays, and therapies. Ambulatory care settings include physician's offices, outpatient surgery centers, and freestanding emergency centers.

ambulatory electrocardiography (Holter monitoring) Recording the heart's electrical activity for 24 or 48 hours while the patient is walking or moving about.

American Association of Medical Assistants (AAMA) A national professional organization that represents medical assistants and their profession.

American Medical Technologists (AMT) A national professional organization that represents medical assistants and their profession.

Americans with Disabilities Act A federal law prohibiting discrimination against the disabled in the workplace and mandating full accessibility for them in all public places.

amniocentesis (am-nee-O-sen-**tee**-sis) A diagnostic procedure performed by inserting a hollow needle through the patient's abdominal wall into the uterus to withdraw a small amount of fluid from the sac surrounding the fetus. The fluid is then analyzed for information about the status of the fetus.

ampules (**am**-pyoolz) Small, sealed glass containers that hold a single dose of parenteral medication.

anabolism (ah-**nab**-O-liz-em) The process through which the body uses food molecules as building blocks, and in which simple substances are converted into more complex substances.

anaerobic bacteria (an-er-**O**-bik bak-**tee**-ree-ah) Bacteria that do not require oxygen to grow.

analgesic (an-al-**jee**-zik) A medication that reduces or relieves pain without loss of consciousness.

anaphylactic shock A hypersensitivity reaction in which the airways swell so that breathing is impossible and the blood vessels expand so that the heart has no blood to pump.

anaphylaxis (an-ah-fih-**lak**-sis) A systemic form of immediate hypersensitivity that causes dramatic vascular and bronchial changes leading to profound hypovolemia and severe respiratory distress. A sudden onset of a severe allergic response.

anemia A clinical condition in which there is a decrease in red blood cells or hemoglobin.

anencephaly (an-en-**sef**-al-ee) A condition in which the brain is incomplete or missing.

anesthesia (an-es-**thee**-zhah) Medication that reduces or eliminates pain. Local anesthesia covers a relatively small area, regional anesthesia a larger area (the legs and pelvis, for example), and general anesthesia, the entire body, generally accompanied by unconsciousness.

anesthetic (an-es-**thet**-ik) A substance that produces a lack of feeling.

angiography (an-jee-**og**-rah-fee) An imaging technique in which a contrast agent is injected into the bloodstream to illustrate the vascular anatomy of a region.

annual percentage rate The true interest rate of a debt based on the unpaid balance.

anorexia nervosa (an-O-**rek**-see-ah ner-**vO**-sah) A psychological disorder of primarily young women characterized by a refusal to eat for fear of becoming obese; emaciation may result.

antacid A substance that decreases acid.

antecubital (an-tih-**kyoo**-bih-tl) The region between the forearm and upper arm commonly used for venipuncture.

antiarrhythmic (an-tee-ah-**rith**-mik) A substance that controls cardiac arrhythmia.

antibiotic (an-tI-bI-**ot**-ik) A substance that kills microorganisms.

antibody (**an**-tih-bod-ee) A protein-containing structure made in response to a specific antigen to destroy the cell or microorganism. An immunoglobulin that reacts to a specific antigen and protects a person from the effects of a disease.

anticipatory guidance Information given to caretakers during a well-child visit to help them anticipate changes in their growing child.

anticoagulant (an-tI-kO-**ag**-yoo-lant) A substance that prevents or delays blood clotting.

anticonvulsant (an-tI-kon-**vul**-sant) A substance that reduces the likelihood of convulsions.

antidepressant (an-tI-dee-**pres**-ant) A substance that prevents or relieves symptoms of depression.

antidiarrheal (an-tI-dI-ah-**ree**-al) A substance that prevents or relieves diarrhea.

antidiuretic hormone (ADH) The hormone produced by the hypothalamus that regulates the excretion of water by the kidneys; also called vasopressin.

antidote A substance that counteracts poisons and their effects.

antiemetic (an-tee-ee-**met**-ik) A substance that prevents or relieves nausea and vomiting.

antifungal (an-tI-**fung**-gal) A substance that fights against fungus.

antigen (**an**-tih-jen) A protein or glycoprotein of a cell or microorganism. It has a specific structure and can stimulate the production of antibodies. A foreign invader of the body.

antihistamine (an-tI-**his**-tah-meen) A substance used to treat allergies by opposing the action of histamine.

antihypertensive (an-tI-hI-per-**ten**-siv) A substance that lowers or prevents high blood pressure.

anti-inflammatory (an-tee-in-**flam**-ah-tor-ee) A substance that prevents inflammation.

antineoplastic (an-tih-nee-O-**plas**-tik) A substance that prevents the replication of cancer cells.

antipyretic (an-tI-pI-**ret**-ik) A substance that reduces fever.

antiseptic (an-tih-**sep**-tik) A substance that prevents the growth of microorganisms.

antitussive (an-tih-**tus**-iv) A substance that suppresses coughing.

anxiety disorders Psychiatric conditions characterized by persistent worry.

apical (**ap**-ih-kal) Pertaining to the pointed portion of the heart that faces downward and to the right.

apitherapy (ap-eh-**ther**-ah-pee) The use of products derived from honeybees to promote health and healing.

apothecary system (ah-**poth**-e-kayr-ee) A historical system of medication measurement that is now rarely used.

aqueous humor The fluid in the anterior cavity of the eye that is responsible for maintaining pressure within the eye.

aromatherapy (ah-rO-mah-**ther**-ah-pee) The inhalation or application of essential oils distilled from various plants to heal the body, mind, and spirit.

arteriograms (angiograms) (ahr-**tee**-ree-O-gramz) X-rays of arteries of the brain made more visible by the injection of dye.

arthritis An inflammation of one or more joints.

arthroscopy (ahr-**thrOs**-kah-pee) Examination of the interior of a joint by inserting a specially designed endoscope through a small incision.

artifacts Unwanted voltage or interference in an ECG recording.

artificially acquired active immunity Immunity to a specific infectious disease that results from exposure to a harmless "cue" that prepares the body's defenses.

artificially acquired passive immunity The introduction of preformed antibodies into an unprotected individual by injection.

art therapy A mind-body therapy that uses art media, images, the creative art process, and patient response to artwork as tools for healing.

asepsis (ay-**sep**-sis) The condition of being free from pathogenic microorganisms.

assault A threat to inflict harm.

assertiveness Displaying assurance and confidence without being aggressive.

assessment Analysis and synthesis of subjective and objective data.

asset Anything of value that is owned.

assignment of benefits Agreement by the patient to the insurance company's payment of benefits directly to the physician.

assisted living facilities Long-term-care facilities, used primarily by the elderly, which provide living assistance and a range of available healthcare services on a continuum of care. A resident who requires more services as time passes can arrange to increase the level of care given.

assistive devices Items that help the patient perform the activities of daily living.

astringent (ah-**strin**-jent) A substance that constricts or binds proteins on a cell's surface to stop hemorrhage.

asystole (ay-**sis**-tO-lee) Lack of ventricular depolarization, and therefore no contractions of the heart.

attenuation (ah-ten-yoo-**ay**-shun) The absorption of electromagnetic radiation in direct relation to the density of a material.

atrioventricular block (ay-tree-O-ven-**trik**-yoo-ler blok) A rhythm in which the electrical conduction system of the heart is blocked or delayed at any point.

atrioventricular (AV) node (ay-tree-O-ven-**trik**-yoo-ler nOd) A group of specialized conductive cells on the bottom of the right atrium, near the septum separating the two atria, that receives the electrical impulse traveling through the atria.

atrium (**ay**-tree-um) One of the upper chambers of the heart; the right chamber receives blood from the body tissues, and the left chamber receives it from the lungs.

audiologist A health professional with at least a master's degree who studies the sense of hearing, detects and diagnoses hearing loss, and works to rehabilitate individuals with hearing loss.

audiometer An electrical device used to test hearing.

audiometry Testing of the sensitivity of hearing.

aural (**aw**-ral) Tympanic, relating to the ear.

auricle The visible, external portion of the ear.

auscultation (aw-skyool-**tay**-shun) Act of listening for the sounds of the body.

autoclave (**aw**-tO-klayv) An apparatus for sterilizing materials by steam and pressure.

autoimmune disorders Disorders in which antibodies attack the patient's own tissues.

automated external defibrillators Devices for sensing a patient's heart rhythm and delivering electrical shocks to start the heart pumping again, if needed.

automaticity (aw-tO-mah-**tis**-ih-tee) The property of cardiac cells that enables them to initiate activity and maintain the rhythmic activity of the heart.

autonomic nervous system (ANS) The portion of the peripheral nervous system that consists of autonomic nerve fibers which are stimulated by involuntary actions.

axilla (ak-**sil**-ah) Armpit.

ayurveda (ah-yoor-**vay**-dah) An Indian holistic system of healing that stresses the interdependence of the individual's body, mind, and spirit and the importance of balancing these aspects.

B

bacilli (bah-**sih**-lI) Rod-shaped bacteria.

bacteria Single-celled microorganisms that do not join together, do not have a cell wall, divide asexually, and can cause infection.

bactericidal (bak-teer-ih-**sI**-dal) Destructive to bacteria.

bacteriology The study of bacteria.

balance sheet A statement of the financial condition of a business on a given date based on the accounting equation.

ballottement (bah-**lot**-ment) Passive movement of the fetus elicited by the examiner's inserting a finger in the vagina and tapping gently forward, causing the fetus to rise, followed by the sinking of the fetus producing a gentle tap on the examiner's finger.

bandage Gauze or elastic used to wrap a body part.

bandage scissors Scissors with one sharp point and one flat, blunt one. The blunt probe is inserted under a dressing or bandage to avoid injuring the skin while the scissors are used to remove it.

bankruptcy A legal proceeding that allows a debtor to free himself of financial obligations or resolve debts through a supervised plan.

barium sulfate A liquid contrast agent that is opaque to x-rays. It is commonly used for upper and lower gastrointestinal series.

barrel The part of a syringe that holds the medication and has calibrated markings.

basal metabolism (**bay**-sal meh-**tab**-O-liz-em) The amount of energy required to sustain the body's normal processes.

basal nuclei (**bay**-sal **new**-clE-eye) Islands of gray matter found throughout the white matter of the cerebrum that assist in the control of motor function.

basophils (**bay**-sO-filz) A type of white blood cell that contributes to allergic and inflammatory reactions. It also stimulates other white blood cell activity.

battery Bodily contact with another person without permission.

beneficiary A person designated by an insurance policy to receive benefits or funds.

benefits Payments made by an insurance company.

benign neoplasm A growth that does not invade surrounding tissue or spread to distant sites.

bevel (**bev**-el) The slant at the tip of a needle at the end of the shaft.

bilateral agreement An agreement between two parties.

bile A substance secreted by the liver to help in the breakdown of fats.

bilirubin (bil-ih-**roo**-bin) A normal breakdown product of hemoglobin in red blood cells. It is not usually present in the urine and may indicate biliary obstruction or liver dysfunction.

bilirubinuria (bil-ih-roo-bih-**nyoo**-ree-ah) The presence of bilirubin in the urine.

binge Increased eating of food in general or of certain categories of foods.

bioelectromagnetics (BEM) The study of the interaction of living organisms with electromagnetic fields.

bioethics The study of moral and ethical questions evolving from new research and medical advances.

biohazard (**bi**-O-haz-rd) A substance or object that may contain microorganisms that can spread disease.

biomedical ethics An area of academic research that studies the intersection between science and morality.

bipolar disorder A depressive disorder in which the patient swings from a depressive phase to a manic phase of feeling very happy, agitated, irritable, or energized. Also termed manic-depressive illness.

blepharitis (blef-ah-**rI**-tis) Inflammation of the eyelid edges.

bloodborne pathogen An organism that can be transmitted by direct contact with blood.

bloodborne pathogen disease Infection caused by microorganisms that may be present in human blood, other specific fluids, and tissue.

blood pressure Force that the flow of blood being pumped by the heart exerts against the walls of blood vessels.

blood smear A droplet of blood that has been spread out over a slide for examination under a microscope.

Blue Cross/Blue Shield A nationwide association of independent healthcare insurers; many are non-profit organizations.

bonding The close relationship and interaction between parent and child.

bone conduction Transmission of sound through the bones of the skull to the cochlea and auditory nerve.

bone marrow aspiration Removal of samples of bone marrow from the iliac crest or sternum to determine the types and numbers of cells present, their phase of cellular development, and the presence of any abnormal cells.

bookkeeping The keeping of systematic records of financial transactions.

bradycardia (bray-dee-**kar**-dee-ah) Slowness of heartbeat, usually fewer than sixty beats per minute.

brain stem The midbrain, pons, and medulla oblongata, areas of the brain that are involved with visual and auditory reflexes and serve as a relay station for sensory stimuli.

brainstorming A process in which all ideas for solving a problem are initially considered and no criticism of them is allowed.

brand name The name under which a pharmaceutical manufacturer patents a drug, also called the trade name.

Braxton Hicks contractions Uterine contractions that can be felt through the abdominal wall.

bronchodilator (brong-kO-**dIh**-lay-tor) A substance that dilates the bronchi.

bronchoscopy (bron-**kos**-kO-pee) Endoscopic examination of one or both bronchi.

buccal (**buk**-al) The route of medication administration in which the drug is placed between the cheek and gums to be absorbed into the bloodstream.

budget A financial document showing estimated revenues and expenditures for a given period of time, usually a year.

buffy coat The gray, opaque layer found between the red blood cells and serum after blood has been centrifuged. It contains white blood cells and platelets.

bulimia nervosa (buh-**lee**-mee-ah ner-**vO**-sah) A psychological disorder involving repeated secretive episodes of eating large quantities of food followed by self-induced vomiting, use of laxatives or diuretics, and/or vigorous exercise to prevent weight gain.

bulla A vesicle that is larger than 1 cm.

Bundle of His (**AV bundle**) A group of conductive cells adjacent to the AV node through which the wave of cardiac electrical current flows (named for physician Wilhelm His).

bursae (**bur**-see) Pad-like sacs between certain tendons and the bones beneath them.

C

calcitonin (kal-sih-**tO**-nin) The thyroid hormone that regulates the level of calcium phosphate in the blood.

call-director A touch-tone phone with up to thirty buttons that is used to direct incoming calls.

caloric test (ka-**lor**-ik test) A procedure to evaluate the function of the vestibular system.

calorie (**kal**-O-ree) A unit of heat measuring the amount of energy required to heat one gram of water one degree Celsius.

cancer An uncontrolled growth of abnormal cells that originate from normal tissues and eventually can cause death by spreading from the original site to other sites.

candidiasis (can-di-**dI**-a-sis) An inflammatory reaction caused by *Candida albicans* infection of the epidermis.

capillary blood specimen A droplet of blood obtained from the cutting of the skin with a lancet.

capitation The type of plan in which healthcare providers contract to provide care for a group at a fixed amount per person per month.

carbohydrates (kahr-bO-**hI**-drayts) Food substances consisting of relatively small molecules. Fruits, whole-grain breads, and cereals are complex carbohydrates; sugars, syrup, fructose, and dextrose are simple carbohydrates.

carbuncle A collection of furuncles that drains pus-containing fluid.

carcinoma A type of cancer affecting the epithelial cells that form the outer surface of the body and line the body cavities and passages leading to the exterior of the body.

cardiac murmurs Heart sounds heard by auscultation with a stethoscope that indicate ineffective closing and opening of heart valves.

cardiologist A physician who treats conditions caused or characterized by dysfunction of the heart.

cardiology The study of the anatomy, normal functions, and disorders of the heart.

cardiopulmonary arrest The stoppage of both heartbeat and respiration.

cardiopulmonary resuscitation A lifesaving technique of chest compression and artificial respiration that mimics the body's own actions of heartbeat and breathing.

cardiotonic (kahr-dee-O-**ton**-ik) A substance that works directly on the heart muscle to increase the force of contraction.

carotid duplex A procedure that uses high-frequency ultrasound waves to show the carotid artery walls and their lumen.

carpal tunnel syndrome A common painful disorder of the wrist and hand, induced by compression of the median nerve.

carrier A human reservoir who may show no signs or symptoms of disease but harbors a specific pathogenic organism and can spread it to others. Also, an insurance company that underwrites healthcare policies.

cartilaginous joints (kahr-tih-**laj**-ih-nus joynts) Joints that permit slight movement but have no joint cavity.

cashier's check A check purchased from a bank.

cash method of accounting The accounting method in which income and expenses are recorded only when they have been received or paid out.

casts Impressions of a portion of a nephron made by red or white blood cells, epithelial cells, or other proteins.

catabolism (kah-**tab**-O-liz-em) The release of energy resulting from chemical reactions within the body.

cataract (**kat**-ah-rakt) Opacity of the crystalline lens of the eye.

catecholamines (kat-eh-**kol**-am-eenz) Epinephrine and norepinephrine, the adrenal medulla hormones that prepare the body in times of anger, fear, and defense.

cathartic (kah-**thar**-tik) A substance that promotes or hastens evacuation of the bowels.

cauterization Destruction of tissue with a heated instrument.

cell differential (sel dif-er-**en**-shal) The description of the percentages of white blood cells in blood. These include neutrophils, band cells, lymphocytes, basophils, eosinophils, and monocytes.

cell-mediated immune response A form of response to infection in which the cells responsible are destroyed by T-cells.

cell-mediated immunity system An immunity system based in the blood and lymph system tissue that defends against bacteria and viruses.

cellulitis Deep infection of the skin involving the subcutaneous tissue.

central nervous system (CNS) The brain and spinal cord.

central processing unit (CPU) The main chip that runs a computer and directs its processing of data.

centrifugation (sen-trif-yoo-**gay**-shun) The process of spinning a sample at very high speeds to separate the blood into layers based on the density of the particles.

cephalocaudal (sef-ah-lO-**kaw**-dl) Pertaining to the body in a head-to-toe direction.

cerebellum (ser-ih-**bel**-um) The portion of the brain that assists in the maintenance of balance, muscle coordination, and equilibrium.

cerebrospinal fluid (CSF) A clear fluid normally containing protein, glucose, chloride, and white blood cells which bathes the brain and spinal cord and acts to nourish and cushion them.

cerebrospinal fluid analysis A diagnostic test in which spinal fluid is withdrawn for analysis; also known as a spinal tap or lumbar puncture.

cerebrovascular accident (CVA) A stroke; any of a group of disorders involving loss of brain function that occurs when the blood supply to part of the brain is interrupted.

cerebrum (ser-**E**-bruhm) The largest part of the brain; it receives sensory impulses from the peripheral nerves and initiates motor impulses.

certification Usually a voluntary credential, most commonly national in scope and sponsored by a non-governmental agency, that indicates that the healthcare practitioner has acquired exemplary knowledge and skills in the field.

certified check A personal check that has been guaranteed by a bank.

Certified Medical Assistant (CMA) Title used by medical assistants with a national credential awarded by the Certifying Board of the American Association of Medical Assistants. These graduates have completed a program accredited by the Commission on Accreditation of Allied Health Education Programs.

cerumen (seh-**roo**-men) Earwax.

ceruminous Secreting cerumen; done by glands to protect the ear from bacterial invasion.

Chadwick's sign A bluish color of the uterus and cervix due to increased uterine blood flow, lymph congestion, and edema. It occurs during the early weeks of pregnancy.

chain of infection A relationship of factors that must be intact for infection to take place. It consists of infectious agents, reservoirs, portals of exit, modes of transmission, portals of entry, and hosts.

CHAMPUS/TRICARE/CHAMPVA CHAMPUS is a government health insurance program covering mainly dependents of military personnel; TRICARE is a managed care program to control costs and standardize benefits for CHAMPUS members; CHAMPVA is a program similar to CHAMPUS covering dependents of veterans with total, permanent, service-related disabilities.

chart of accounts A detailed listing of all the accounts a business uses.

check A written order on a printed form directing a bank to pay money from a specific account to a designated recipient.

chemical name The name of a drug that describes its chemical make-up.

Chemiclave® (**kem**-ih-klayv) A sterilization process using pressure, temperature, and a proprietary chemical.

chief complaint Concise description of the main reason the patient is seeking healthcare.

chiropractic therapy (kI-rO-**prak**-tik **ther**-ah-pee) A therapeutic system based on the belief that most medical problems are caused by misalignments of the vertebrae and can be corrected by manipulating the spine.

chloasma (klO-**az**-mah) The "mask of pregnancy;" blotchy, brownish pigmentation over the forehead.

cholesterol (kO-**les**-ter-ol) A substance consumed in foods, primarily those of animal origin, and also produced by the body, which is associated with the risk of heart disease and atherosclerosis.

chorionic villi sampling (**core**-e-on-ick **vil**-I **samp**-ling) A procedure to obtain a specimen for prenatal diagnosis of disease or other conditions.

choroid (**kor**-oyd) The portion of the eye that absorbs light rays to prevent reflection within the eyeball and provides the blood supply to the retina.

Chvostek's sign (**khvos**-teks sIn) A sign of hypocalcemia in which a tapping on the patient's facial nerve just in front of the earlobe and below the zygomatic arch results in responses ranging from a twitching of the corner of the mouth to a twitching of all facial muscles on the side tested.

chyme (kIm) Food moving through the gastrointestinal tract that has been broken down into a semi-solid state.

cilia (**sil**-E-ah) Hairlike structures that protect the inside of the body by filtering outside elements. Includes the small hairs that line the mucous membranes of the nose to filter dirt and other impurities from inhaled air.

ciliary body The portion of the eye surrounding the iris which changes the shape of the lens to focus light on the retina.

circular turn A bandaging technique in which each turn exactly covers the previous turn.

circulator A person who moves around the operating room and supplies the sterile field as needed.

circumduction Moving a body part in a cone-shaped motion.

civil law The body of law dealing with the rights of individuals in their relationships with each other rather than with government.

claim A request for payment from an insurance carrier.

claim status The status of a claim that has been filed to which there has been no response.

clean technique Disinfection.

clearinghouse A third-party administrator who reformats medical claims according to the requirements of various insurance carriers and distributes them to the carriers electronically.

clinical competencies Skills that the medical assistant usually uses in the "back office," which may include assisting the physician with physical examinations, obtaining and processing diagnostic tests, and interviewing patients for medical histories.

clinical impression An objective evaluation of a patient's health status.

closed questions Questions that ask for a specific fact or particular piece of information.

cluster scheduling A method of scheduling in which similar appointments are grouped together at an established time of day or day of the week to allow for efficient use of personnel and equipment.

coarse focus The adjustment control on a microscope that makes large changes in the focal distance to sharpen an image.

cocci (**kok**-sl) Spherical bacteria.

cochlea (**kok**-lee-ah) A bony, tubelike structure of the middle ear which resembles a snail shell and transfers sound waves to the brain for interpretation.

coding Translating words that describe a diagnosis or procedure into numeric designations.

coinsurance An arrangement in which the insured must pay a percentage of the cost of medical services covered by the insurer.

colonies Dense collections of bacteria that can be seen as spots on a culture medium without magnification.

colonization The growth of invading microorganisms in a host. It can occur without the person either becoming a carrier or contracting the infection.

colonoscopy (kO-lon-**os**-kah-pee) Examination of the colon with an endoscope.

colostomy (kO-**los**-tah-mee) A surgically created opening between the colon and the abdominal wall through which fecal matter is expelled.

comedo (**kOm**-ee-dO) A blackhead.

Commission on Accreditation of Allied Health Education Programs (CAAHEP) An agency that grants accreditation to programs in medical assisting upon recommendation of its Curriculum Review Board.

common bile duct The outlet through which bile is passed into the duodenum.

communicable disease A disease that can be transmitted directly or indirectly from one individual to another.

communication The exchange of thoughts, opinions, or information between two or more people.

complete blood count (CBC) The most common laboratory test. It is a hematologic test that describes the number of white blood cells, red blood cells, and platelets, among other values.

compound fracture A fracture that results in the bone penetrating the skin; also called an open fracture.

computed tomography (CT) (kom-**pyoo**-ted tO-**mog**-rah-fee) A radiographic technique in which the x-ray source revolves around the patient to create cross-section images of the body.

computer peripherals Equipment connected to the main unit of the computer, such as scanners or printers.

concept mapping A process in which circles and lines are used to represent problems and solutions.

cones The structures of the retina responsible for visual acuity and color vision.

conference calling A telephone conversation linking three to fourteen phones in which all parties can fully participate simultaneously.

conjunctiva (kon-junk-**tI**-vah) Mucous membranes lining the inner surfaces of the eyelids and the anterior portion of the sclera.

conjunctivitis (kon-junk-tih-**vI**-tis) An infection or irritation of the conjunctiva.

consent Permission from a patient, expressed either in oral or written form or implied, for medical examination, testing, or treatment.

constructive criticism Criticism aimed at helping a person perform better.

consultation report Report prepared by a physician for a referring physician.

contingency fee basis A fee based on successful completion of a job.

continuous suture A suture consisting of one thread running in a series of stitches that is tied at only the beginning and the end of the run.

contraception Prevention of pregnancy by use of a medication, device, or method that blocks or alters a process of reproduction; birth control.

contraceptive (kon-trah-**sep**-tiv) Something that prevents conception.

contract A voluntary agreement between two or more parties in which specific promises are made in exchange for something of value.

contractility The property of cardiac cells that allows them to pump in response to electrical stimuli.

contracture (kon-**trak**-cher) The state of a joint that is fixed in a flexed position.

contraindications (kon-trah-in-dih-**kay**-shunz) Conditions under which a drug should not be administered.

contrast agents Liquid or gaseous substances administered to the patient to enhance the visibility of bodily structures during radiography.

Controlled Substances Act The 1970 law that established "schedules," or categories, for controlled substances according to the probability of their abuse.

convalescent phase The period of infection when the symptoms subside.

coordination of benefits A process to prevent duplication of payment when a patient is covered under more than one insurance plan.

copayment An arrangement in which the patient pays a fixed fee when medical service is rendered and the insurer pays the rest of the cost.

cope To manage or adapt to a situation.

coping mechanism A defense strategy that an individual adopts to reduce anxiety or stress.

cornea A transparent portion of the external layer of the eyeball.

cortisol A glucocorticoid hormone involved in the metabolism of carbohydrates, fats, and proteins; also known as hydrocortisone.

courtesy Conduct that provides respect for and consideration of the dignity and needs of others.

cover-uncover test A method of screening the muscle function of the eye.

cranial nerves Twelve pairs of nerves that emerge from the brain bilaterally to innervate the muscles of the head, neck, and trunk.

credit A transaction that decreases assets and increases liabilities.

criminal law The legal area dealing with offenses committed against the safety and welfare of society.

crossover claim Automatic forwarding of a bill by Medicare after it has paid its portion of the costs to a Medigap insurer that will pay the remainder.

crust A thickened, dry area resulting from fluid leakage of vesicles, pustules, or bullae.

cryosurgery (krI-O-**ser**-jer-ee) Destruction of tissue by application of extreme cold.

crystals Chemicals transformed into a crystalline form which may make the urine cloudy.

culture A collection or population of microorganisms grown in the clinical laboratory with a growth medium. A sample of fluid or tissue from a patient is used to start the population of microorganisms. Also, ways of living developed by a group of people and passed down from one generation to another.

culture medium A liquid or gelatin substance that provides the nutrients to help bacteria grow in a culture.

curative drugs (**kyoo**-rah-tiv drugs) Drugs used to kill organisms causing disease.

Cushing's syndrome A condition in which there is an overproduction of adrenal hormones, specifically the glucocorticoid hormones.

customer service Efficient, helpful, and high-quality service provided to the consumer.

cutting edge needle A suturing needle whose sharp point is needed to get through tissue.

cyanosis (sI-ah-**nO**-sis) Blue discoloration of the skin indicating low oxygen saturation or diminished circulation.

cycle billing Distribution of billing throughout the month based on the patients' last names.

cycloplegic A medication used to temporarily paralyze accommodation (ciliary) muscles of the eye to facilitate examination.

cyst A raised, solid mass filled with liquid or semisolid expressible material.

D

day sheet (daily journal, daily log, daily record) A cumulative listing of all patient-related financial transactions recorded on a daily basis in chronological order.

debit A transaction that increases assets and decreases liabilities.

debris (de-**bree**) Foreign or waste matter.

decongestant (dee-kon-**jes**-tant) A substance that reduces nasal congestion and swelling.

deductible The amount of a bill that the patient must pay before insurance begins payment for medical services.

defamation of character Damaging a person's reputation by making false and malicious statements.

deferred payment price Total cost including finance charges.

deltoid A site for intramuscular injection on the upper outer arm just below the shoulder.

delusions False beliefs that are inconsistent with an individual's culture, knowledge, and experience, and do not change in the face of facts.

dementia (dih-**men**-shuh) A condition characterized by chronic personality disintegration, confusion, disorientation, deterioration of intellectual ability, and impaired control of memory, judgment, and impulses.

dependence Physical and/or psychological need for a substance.

deposit slip (deposit ticket) A form that is completed and submitted with funds to ensure that they are credited to the right bank account.

depressant A substance that reduces functional activity.

depression A mood disturbance characterized by sadness, despair, and discouragement resulting from and normally proportionate to a personal loss or tragedy; also, an abnormal emotional state characterized by exaggerated feelings of sadness, melancholy, dejection, worthlessness, emptiness, and hopelessness that are inappropriate and out of proportion to reality.

dermatitis Inflammation of the skin characterized by erythema and pain or pruritis.

dermatologist A physician specializing in the evaluation, diagnosis, and treatment of skin disorders.

dermis The inner layer of the skin.

diabetes insipidus (DI) A posterior pituitary disorder caused by a deficiency of ADH secretion and resulting in polyuria and polydipsia.

diabetes mellitus (dI-ah-**bee**-teez **mel**-ih-tus) A disorder related to carbohydrate metabolism that requires patients to be on a lifelong special diet; also called diabetes. The disease is characterized by decreased production of insulin or decreased ability to use insulin.

diabetic retinopathy A long-term complication of diabetes in which the tiny blood vessels of the retina receive decreased blood and oxygen, sometimes resulting in vision changes and blindness.

diagnosis-related group (DRG) A system of patient classification used in hospitals for reimbursement based on a fixed fee instead of fee-for-service.

diagnostic drugs Drugs used to identify the cause or location of a disease.

diagnostic imaging The use of diagnostic radiology and other imaging technologies such as ultrasound and magnetic resonance imaging to aid in diagnosis.

diagnostic radiology The use of x-rays to aid in diagnosis.

diaphoresis (dI-ah-fO-**ree**-sis) Excessive sweating.

diaphragm (**dI**-ah-fram) The main muscle involved with breathing. It is located at the floor of the thoracic cavity. Also, the part of the operative microscope that controls the amount of light passing through from the light source. It is used to adjust the intensity of the light striking the object being studied.

diastole (dI-**as**-tO-lee) (**diastolic phase**) The portion of the cardiac cycle in which the heart muscle relaxes, exerting the least amount of pressure against the walls of the arteries, and allowing blood to fill the chambers of the heart.

diathermy (**dI**-ah-ther-mee) Deep heat treatment originating in electrical energy.

diencephalon (dI-en-**sef**-ah-lon) The phase of the brain consisting of the thalamus and hypothalamus.

differential diagnosis (dif-er-**en**-shul dI-ag-**nO**-sis) A list of possible explanations for a patient's clinical condition. And the process of ruling out alternative diagnoses.

digestion The process that turns food into substances the body can use for energy, growth, and well-being.

diplomacy Tact; communicating in such a way that there is little or no ill will.

disability Physical or mental impairment that considerably limits one or more of the major life activities of the individual.

discharge summary A summary of the course of the patient's stay in the hospital, including condition and diagnoses at admission, tests, procedures, treatments, observations, progress, and condition upon discharge.

discoid lupus erythematosus (DLE) (**dis**-koyd **loo**-pus er-ith-uh-mah-**tO**-sis) A benign skin disorder in which the patient experiences chronic skin eruptions consisting of round red or purple scaling plaques with follicular plugging.

discrimination Acting toward others in a prejudiced manner; treating one group or person differently than another.

disinfecting Reducing or eliminating infectious organisms.

disinfection Use of chemical or physical methods to destroy disease-producing microorganisms.

diskette A small circle of magnetized material, housed in a plastic casing, that provides for permanent data storage; often called a "disk."

diskette drives Drives that write or store information on a diskette.

dislocation Displacement of a part of the body from its normal position.

distribution The process by which drugs move from the bloodstream into other body fluids and tissues.

diuretic (dI-yoo-**ret**-ik) A substance that increases the production of urine.

diversity Variety; the state of being different.

DME Durable medical equipment used by patients at home such as hospital beds, commodes, oxygen, and wheelchairs.

dorsal recumbent position A position in which the patient lies on her back with knees bent and feet flat on the examining table. This enables a physician to examine the rectum, vagina, or both.

dorsogluteal (dor-sO-**gloo**-tee-al) An intramuscular injection site on the buttocks.

double-booking A method of scheduling in which more than one patient is given an appointment for the same time.

double-contrast study The use of both gas and liquid as contrast media to provide more detail in diagnostic imaging than liquid contrast would alone.

double-entry bookkeeping A system in which each financial transaction must be recorded in at least two accounts.

drape Sterile fabric used to surround the surgical field.

dressing Materials used to cover and protect a wound or incision.

drug abuse The use of a drug for purposes other than those prescribed and/or in amounts that were not directed.

Drug Enforcement Administration (DEA) The branch of the U. S. Justice Department that regulates the use and sale of specified (controlled) drugs.

drugs Medicinal substances that alter or modify the functioning of living organisms.

durable power of attorney for healthcare A legal document that allows another person to make healthcare decisions on behalf of a person who is physically or mentally impaired.

dysmenorrhea (dis-men-O-**ree**-ah) Pain during menstruation.

dyspepsia (dis-**pep**-see-ah) Indigestion, heartburn.

dysphagia (dis-**fay**-jee-ah) Difficulty swallowing.

dyspnea (disp-**nee**-ah) Difficulty breathing.

dysthymia (dis-**thih**-mee-ah) A milder but more lasting form of depression in which the individual has a generally depressed mood for most of the day, on most days, for at least two years.

E

ectopic beats (ek-**top**-ik beets) Cardiac electrical beats that originate at a spot other than the SA node.

ectopic pregnancy (ek-**top**-ik) Development of an ovum outside the uterus, such as in the fallopian tubes.

eczema (**ek**-zeh-mah) A superficial inflammation of the skin of unknown cause characterized initially by itching, erythema, and edema and later becoming crusted, scaly, thickened, and lichenified.

EDTA Ethylenediaminetetraacetic acid, an additive to blood samples that acts as an anticoagulant and preservative.

efferent nerves Motor nerves, those that receive messages from the brain.

elastic bandage A stretchable roll of bandaging material.

elective procedures Optional procedures that are not medically necessary.

electrocardiogram (ee-lek-trO-**kar**-dee-O-gram) **(ECG)** A tracing that graphically represents the electrical activity of the heart.

electrocautery (ee-**lek**-trO-**kaw**-ter-ee) Use of an electrical apparatus to destroy tissue by burning.

electroencephalograph (EEG) (ee-lek-trO-en-**sef**-ah-lO-graf) A machine that records brain electrical activity.

electrolytes Minerals found in body fluids and cells whose measurement may give information on disease states. The most common are sodium, potassium, chloride, and bicarbonate.

electromagnetic fields Electrical potentials that may be created either within or outside the body.

electromagnetic radiation Invisible waves of energy that are found throughout the environment. They differ by the wavelength of the radiation. Visible light and radio waves are common forms; shorter wavelengths produce x-rays.

electromyography (EMG) (ee-lek-trO-mI-**og**-rah-fee) Recording of electrical impulses of muscle fibers and peripheral nerves after the insertion of teflon-coated needle electrodes into skeletal muscles.

electroneurodiagnostic technologist (ee-lek-trO-noo-rO-dI-ag-**nost**-ik tek-**nol**-O-gist) An allied healthcare practitioner who operates an electroencephalograph.

electronystagmogram (ee-lek-trO-nis-**tag**-mO-gram) A method of assessing and recording eye movements by measuring the electric activity of the extraocular muscles.

E-mail Electronic mail sent and received by computer.

emancipated minor A person younger than the age of majority who is married, in the armed services, self-supporting, or no longer living under parental control. Such a person does not need the consent of a parent or guardian to obtain medical treatment.

emergency appointments Appointments for patients with acute symptoms who need to be seen soon but do not require immediate care in a hospital emergency room.

emergent conditions Those requiring treatment or intervention in less than fifteen minutes.

emetic (ee-**met**-ik) A substance that induces vomiting.

empathy An attitude marked by conscious awareness of and insight into another person's actions and behavior. Understanding and being sensitive to another person's feelings.

endocrinologist (**en**-dO-krih-**nol**-O-jist) The medical specialist practicing in the field of endocrinology.

endocrinology (**en**-dO-krih-**nol**-O-jee) The medical specialty involved with the pathology of the endocrine system and the treatment of endocrine problems.

endogenous defenses (en-**doj**-en-us dee-**fens**-ez) Chemical defenses made by the body that are normally found in the body.

endometriosis (en-dO-mee-tree-**O**-sis) A condition in which tissue that is similar to the endometrium is present outside the uterus.

endometrium (en-dO-**mee**-tree-um) The innermost lining of the uterus which is shed each month during menstruation.

endorphins (en-**dor**-finz) Neurochemicals released in the brain that can relieve pain.

endoscope (**en**-dO-skOp) An instrument used to visualize internal organs or structures.

endoscopy (en-**dos**-kO-pee) Visualization of the inside of a body cavity by means of a lighted tube.

endospore (**en**-dO-spor) Highly resistant capsules that some bacteria form to protect themselves.

enteric-coated (en-**ter**-ik **kOt**-ed) Describing a medication that is coated to delay absorption or prevent the drug from irritating the stomach.

environmental medicine A form of alternative medical intervention concerned with the responses of individuals to substances in the environment that include chemicals, dust, molds, and certain foods.

eosinophils (ee-O-**sin**-O-filz) White blood cells that travel from the bloodstream to areas of lining in the body. They can ingest microorganisms and increase in a number of conditions such as cancer, parasitic infection, and allergy.

epidermis The outer layer of skin.

epiglottis A cartilaginous structure overhanging the larynx that prevents food from entering the larynx and trachea while being swallowed.

epilepsy A brain disorder involving recurrent seizures.

epinephrine (ep-ih-**nef**-rin) Adrenalin, a hormone secreted by the adrenal medulla in response to stress.

epistaxis Nosebleed.

Equal Credit Opportunity Act A federal law prohibiting discrimination against persons seeking credit.

equilibrium Balance.

erosion A scraped-out, shallow, open lesion that does not reach the dermal layer.

erysipelas (ayr-ih-**sip**-ih-las) An acute inflammatory form of cellulitis involving the lymphatics.

erythema (er-ih-**thee**-mah) Redness or inflammation of the skin.

erythrocyte (ee-**rith**-rO-sIt) A red blood cell.

erythrocyte sedimentation rate (ESR) A blood test that measures the height of red blood cells that settle in a tube after a specified amount of time. The result gives information about inflammatory conditions.

esophagogram (ee-**sof**-ah-gO-gram) A radiographic study in which a contrast agent is swallowed and fluoroscopic images of the esophagus are obtained.

established patient A patient who has seen the physician within the last three years.

ethics Principles governing the right thing to do.

ethnicity The cultural or racial background of a people or country.

ethylene oxide (**eth**-eh-leen **ox**-Id) A toxic, penetrating gas used for sterilization.

eupnea (**Up**-nee-a) Normal breathing.

eustachian tube (yoo-**stay**-shun toob) The hollow tube connecting the middle ear with the throat.

evaluation A determination of how well the patient learned the information presented in a teaching session and how well the information was presented.

eversion A turning out, as of the foot at the ankle.

evoked potential test A measurement of brain waves to determine cerebral response to peripheral sensory stimulation.

exacerbation (eg-zas-er-**bay**-shun) Increased intensity of signs and symptoms.

examination suite The "back office" area of a medical facility where the patient is interviewed to determine the reason for the visit, is then examined, and appropriate care is planned.

exclusions Conditions and circumstances for which the insurance company will not pay benefits.

Exclusive Provider Organization (EPO) A healthcare plan that provides coverage only when services are provided by contracted or preferred providers.

excretion (ek-**skree**-shun) The elimination of waste from the body.

exogenous defenses (ex-**ah**-jen-us dee-**fens**-ez) Chemical defenses administered from outside the body that help its defense system prevent or destroy pathogens.

expectorant (ek-**spek**-tO-rant) A substance that facilitates the removal of secretions from the bronchopulmonary tree.

explanation of benefits (EOB) An explanation of the payments made for services which the insurer sends to the patient and the provider.

extension Movement of a joint that increases the angle between two adjoining bones, such as straightening the elbow.

external customers Those individuals and organizations outside the medical office that supply necessary information and products or specialized services to the office.

external fixation device A frame of metal rods that connects skeletal pins.

external urinary meatus (eks-**ter**-nal **yoo**-rin-ayr-ee mee-**ay**-tus) The opening to the outside of the body through which urine flows.

F

face sheet The first page of a patient's hospital chart, containing demographic data.

fallopian tubes Hollow tubes that transport the ova from the ovaries to the uterus; also referred to as uterine tubes.

false imprisonment The unlawful restraint of another person's freedom of movement.

family medicine A practice in which the doctor is concerned with maintaining the health of individuals across their entire life span: children, adults, and the elderly.

fats Food substances that serve as a concentrated source of heat production and energy, furnish essential fatty acids, and promote the absorption of certain vitamins.

Federal Insurance Contributions Act (FICA) The law establishing the Social Security tax and setting its rates.

Federal Unemployment Tax Act (FUTA) The law establishing federal unemployment taxes and setting the rate.

feedback The oral or nonverbal response of one person to another person's actions or words.

fee-for-service A payment method in which the patient is charged a specific fee each time a specific service is provided.

fee schedule A list of services and procedures that a physician usually performs, with the amount charged for each.

fibrinogen (fI-**brin**-O-jen) A protein found in plasma which aids in the clotting process.

fibrous joints (**fI**-brus joyntz) Joints that permit no movement, since there is no joint cavity and only a small amount of connective tissue.

figure-of-eight turn A bandaging technique that allows limited motion in a joint.

final diagnosis The conclusion a physician reaches after receiving the results of all diagnostic tests and procedures.

finance charge The total cost of credit.

fine focus The adjustment control on a microscope that makes minor changes in the focal length to sharpen an image.

fingernail drill A surgical instrument used to relieve pressure under a fingernail.

fiscal agent (fiscal intermediary) An organization that has a contract to process claims for Medicaid, Medicare, or CHAMPUS.

fissures (**fish**-ers) Thin, linear cracks in the skin. Also, grooves that divide the cerebrum into lobes.

flange The rim at the end of the barrel of a syringe.

flexion Movement that decreases the angle between two adjoining bones, such as bending the elbow.

focused questions Questions that narrow or define the topic by isolating or concentrating on one specific aspect of the communication.

Foerster forceps Forceps with ring-shaped tips for grasping sponges and other objects.

fluoroscopy (floo-**ros**-kO-pee) An x-ray technology that provides a "live" view of a body structure to allow for evaluation of its functioning as well as its anatomy.

folliculitis Infection of a hair follicle.

follow-up appointments Appointments made for the physician to recheck the condition of an established patient.

Food and Drug Administration (FDA) The U.S. government agency that regulates food, drug, and cosmetic safety.

forceps A two-bladed instrument with a handle used to compress tissues in surgical procedures or for handling sterile dressings or other objects.

formaldehyde (for-**mal**-de-hId) A powerful disinfectant and antiseptic which is also used as a preservative for pathologic specimens.

four Ds of negligence The elements necessary to meet the legal definition of negligence: duty, dereliction, direct cause, and damages.

Fowler's position The position of a patient sitting on the examination table with the backrest elevated to a ninety-degree angle. The legs are extended flat on the table. This position lets the physician examine the patient's lower extremities.

fracture An injury in which the tissue of a bone is disrupted.

fungi (**fun**-jI) A simple plant that depends on other life forms for growth. Examples include yeasts, molds, and *Candida.*

furuncle (**foo**-rung-kl) A boil; deep folliculitis.

G

galvanometer A recording device that converts the electrical activity of the heart into the mechanical action of a stylus.

ganglia Groups of nerve cell bodies outside the brain and spinal cord.

gastroenterologist (gas-trO-en-ter-**ol**-O-jist) A physician specializing in disorders and conditions of the gastrointestinal tract.

gastrointestinal (GI) tract (gas-trO-in-**tes**-tih-nal trakt) Part of the digestive system in which food is converted into usable products for the body. The tube that goes from the mouth to the anus.

gatekeeper A primary care provider who controls patients' access to specialists.

gauze A common bandaging material that is light, porous, and easily molds to the body. It allows air circulation to the dressing and wound.

gene (jeen) A single segment of the body's hereditary material.

general chemistry A field of laboratory medicine that evaluates the components dissolved in the liquid portion of the blood or serum. These include fats, sugars, proteins, and chemicals.

general (transdisciplinary) competencies Skills that are used in both the administrative and clinical areas of the medical office, including professionalism, communication ability, knowledge of legal concepts, instructing, and operational functions.

general (systemic) infection An infection that involves the whole body and produces symptoms such as fever, fatigue, and headache.

general ledger A record of all the accounts of a business.

generic name The name given a drug by its manufacturer, often a shortened version of the chemical name.

genetic engineering The modification of organisms to produce compounds they would not otherwise produce.

genome (**jee**-nOm) All of the DNA in an organism, including its genes.

genuineness The ability to express oneself honestly, without hiding behind a facade.

germicidal (jer-mih-**sId**-al) Lethal to pathogens.

gestation Pregnancy.

gestational diabetes Diabetes that first occurs during pregnancy.

Glascow Coma Scale A tool to measure levels of consciousness.

glaucoma A condition in which there is increased intraocular pressure.

glucagon (**gloo**-kah-gon) A hormone secreted by the alpha cells of the islets of Langerhans in the pancreas to regulate the amount of sugar in the blood.

glucocorticoid hormones Hormones secreted by the two inner layers of the cortex of the adrenal gland.

gluconeogenesis (**gloo**-kO-nee-O-**jen**-ih-sis) The process of synthesizing glucose and glycogen from fats and proteins.

glucose tolerance test A test of the body's ability to metabolize carbohydrates in the form of glucose.

glucosuria (gloo-kO-**syoo**-re-ah) The presence of glucose in the urine.

glutaraldehyde (gloo-tah-**ral**-de-hId) A room-temperature chemical sterilizer.

glycogen (**glI**-kO-jen) A form of glucose stored in the liver.

glycogenolysis (**glI**-kO-je-**nol**-ih-sis) The process of converting glycogen to glucose.

glycosuria (glI-kO-**soo**-ree-ah) Excretion of sugar into the urine.

goiter Enlargement of the thyroid gland.

goniometer (gO-nee-**om**-e-ter) An instrument used to measure joint motion.

Goodell's sign (goo-**delz** sIn) A cervical softening that occurs during pregnancy.

Good Samaritan law A statute protecting a volunteer who administers emergency medical treatment from liability in most circumstances.

gout A form of arthritis in which uric acid is commonly deposited in the joints, usually of the feet and legs.

grain The basic unit of weight in the apothecary system.

Gram-negative Describing bacteria that do not retain crystal violet from Gram's stain because of their cell wall. They are counter-stained and appear red.

Gram-positive Describing bacteria whose cell wall retains crystal violet when exposed to Gram's stain, giving them a purple color.

grams A metric measurement of weight.

Gram stain A method of differentiating bacteria based on the color that results from the staining procedure.

Graves' disease Hyperthyroidism caused by overproduction of thyroid hormone.

gravida A pregnant woman.

gross pay The amount earned before deductions.

group climate The atmosphere or comfort level in a group of people or a team.

guided imagery A mind-body therapy that uses consciously chosen positive and healing images along with deep relaxation to reduce or manage stresses, prevent illness, and help patients deal with the effects of disease.

gynecology (gI-neh-**kol**-ah-jee) The branch of medicine concerned with the healthcare of women, including their sexual and reproductive functioning and diseases of the reproductive organs.

gyri (**jI**-rI) Bulges within the gray matter of the cerebrum.

H

hallucinations Sensory perceptions that occur without external stimulation.

halo traction Traction that stabilizes and supports fractured cervical vertebrae.

hard disk or **hard drive** The computer's main drive, offering a large amount of permanent storage.

hardware The physical parts, or machinery, that make up a computer system.

HCPCS The Health Care Financing Administration Common Procedure Coding System, an alphanumeric coding system developed for Medicare.

healthcare proxy A document transferring the authority to make medical decisions for a patient who cannot reason or communicate.

Health Maintenance Organizations (HMOs) Managed care in which the patient must use the plan's physicians and generally needs a primary care physician's referral or plan approval before visits to specialists, tests, surgery, or hospitalization.

Hegar's sign (**hay-**garz sIn) Softening of the lower portion of the uterus and the isthmus that occurs during pregnancy.

hematocrit (hee-**mat**-O-krit) The percentage of red blood cell volume relative to total blood volume.

hematology (hee-mah-**tol**-O-jee) The field of laboratory medicine that studies blood and its components, such as erythrocytes, leukocytes, and thrombocytes.

hematoma (hee-mah-**tO**-mah) A collection of blood under the skin caused by leakage of blood from a blood vessel into surrounding tissues. It is a common complication of blood drawing.

hematuria (hee-mah-**tyoo**-ree-ah) The presence of red blood cells in the urine.

hemiplegia (heem-ih-**plee**-jee-ah) Paralysis of one side of the body.

hemocytometer (hee-mO-sI-**tom**-ih-ter) A glass slide containing a microscopic grid on which a sample of blood is placed so that cells can be counted under a microscope.

hemoglobin (**hee**-mO-glO-bin) The iron-protein portion of a red blood cell that binds oxygen in the cell.

hemoglobinuria (hee-mO-glO-bih-**nyoo**-ree-ah) The presence of hemoglobin, a breakdown product of red blood cells, in the urine.

hemolysis (hee-**mol**-ih-sis) Rupture of red blood cells.

hemostasis (hee-mo-**stay**-sis) The stoppage of bleeding.

hemostatic (hee-mO-**stat**-ik) A substance that controls or stops bleeding.

hemostats (**hee**-mO-stats) Forceps with serrated tips that are used to clamp off blood vessels.

hepatitis (hep-ah-**tI**-tis) An inflammation of the liver that may be caused by a variety of agents including viral infections, bacterial invasion, and physical or chemical agents.

herbal remedies The use of various herbs to treat minor health problems.

herpes simplex 1 Cold sores or fever blisters.

herpes zoster Shingles.

hirsutism (**her**-soot-iz-em) Excessive body hair in a masculine distribution pattern.

holistic healthcare Healthcare that emphasizes the fundamental wholeness and integrity of the individual and views the body, mind, and spirit as inseparable and interdependent.

homebound Describing a patient who cannot walk without assistance or requires a device to aid with walking, moving, or breathing.

home healthcare agencies Long-term-care agencies that provide a combination of medical and social services in the patient's home, including changing dressings, monitoring medications, and assisting with bathing and cooking.

homeopathy (hO-mee-**op**-ah-thee) An alternative medical approach based on the notion that "like cures like;" treatment includes the administering of minute doses of a remedy that would, in healthy persons, produce symptoms similar to those of the disease.

homeostasis (hO-mee-o-**stay**-sis) The balancing in the body of various functions and of the chemical composition of fluids and tissues.

hordeolum (hor-**dee**-O-lum) A stye.

hormones Chemical substances that initiate or regulate the activity of an organ or group of cells in another part of the body.

hospice Long-term care that emphasizes the management of pain and other symptoms when conventional treatment is no longer of value and the patient is dying.

hub The part of a needle that fits onto the tip of the syringe.

human chorionic gonadotropin (**hyoo**-men kor-ee-**on**-ik gO-nad-O-**trop**-in) A hormone that becomes elevated after conception.

Human Immunodeficiency Virus (HIV) (**hyoo**-men im-myoon-O-deh-**fish**-in-see **vI**-rus) The virus that causes Acquired Immune Deficiency Syndrome (AIDS).

humoral immune response An immune response in which antibodies are formed in reaction to antigens.

humoral immunity system (**hyoo**-mor-ahl im-**myoon**-ih-tee) The body system that produces B cells to defend against bacteria, toxins, and viruses.

hydrocortisone Cortisol.

hydrotherapy The use of water in physical therapy treatment.

hypercalcemia (**hI**-per-kal-**see**-mee-ah) A condition in which the serum calcium level is above 10.5 mg/dl.

hyperglycemia (hI-per-glI-**see**-mee-ah) An abnormally increased level of blood glucose.

hyperopia (hI-per-**O**-pee-ah) Farsightedness resulting from an error of refraction in which rays of light entering the eye are brought into focus behind the retina.

hypersensitivity reaction An excessive response of the immune system to an allergen.

hypertension (hI-per-**ten**-shun) High blood pressure.

hypertext Icons or highlighted text in a computer document that open related documents.

hypnosis Mind-body therapy that produces a relaxed yet heightened state of awareness during which individuals are more open to suggestion.

hypnotic A substance that produces sleep.

hypocalcemia (hI-pO-kal-**see**-mee-ah) A condition in which the serum calcium level is below 8.5 mg/dl.

hypodermic (hI-pO-**der**-mik) A type of syringe used for subcutaneous and intramuscular injections.

hypoglycemic (hI-pO-glI-**see**-mik) A substance that lowers blood glucose levels.

hypotension (hI-pO-**ten**-shun) Low blood pressure.

hypothalamus (hI-pO-**thal**-ah-mus) The portion of the brain that helps maintain homeostasis of appetite, thirst, temperature, and water. The central endocrine gland located within the brain which produces releasing factors, antidiuretic hormone, and oxytocin.

hypothermia Overall lowering of body temperature to the point where the victim is at risk of death.

hypoxemia (hI-pok-**see**-mee-ah) Low levels of oxygen in the blood.

hysterosalpingogram (his-ter-O-sal-**ping**-gO-gram) A radiographic study in which the uterus and fallopian tubes are visualized with the aid of a contrast agent instilled through the cervix.

I

ICD-9-CM The International Classification of Diseases, Ninth Revision, Clinical Modification, which is used for coding diagnoses on insurance claims.

immunity The body's ability to prevent tissue and organ damage by resisting invading organisms and toxins.

immunization The process of creating immunity to a specific disease in an individual.

immunocompromised (im-myoon-O-**com**-prO-mIzd) A state in which an individual is at increased risk for infection because his or her immune system cannot provide adequate protection.

immunologist The medical specialist who treats conditions of the immune system.

immunosuppression (im-myoon-O-sup-**presh**-un) Decreased functioning of the immune system caused by introduction of chemicals.

immunosuppressive (im-yoo-nO-suh-**pres**-iv) A substance that suppresses the body's natural immune response.

impetigo (im-pih-**tI**-gO) A superficial bacterial skin infection.

implied consent Willingness to undergo a medical procedure that the patient indicates by appearing for the procedure at the scheduled time and place.

inactive files Files of patients who have not been a patient of a medical practice for a specified period (usually six months or more).

incineration Destruction by burning.

incubation phase The stage of an infection in which the offending microorganism enters the patient and proliferates until symptoms develop.

indemnity Compensation paid by an insurance carrier for damage, loss, or services rendered.

indemnity health insurance Traditional health insurance plans for major medical expenses that include coinsurance paid by the individual.

induration A raised, firm region of skin whose size indicates the patient's reaction to a tuberculin test.

infarction An area of tissue that undergoes necrosis, caused by interruption of the blood supply.

infection The condition resulting when the body or a part of it is invaded by a pathogenic agent which, under favorable conditions, multiplies and produces harmful effects.

infertility Inability to conceive and bear a child.

informed consent The patient's permission for a procedure given with a full understanding of its nature, risks, and alternatives.

innervate Stimulate.

inoculation The application of a microbiologic specimen to culture medium.

inscription The part of a prescription that includes the name of the drug and the quantity prescribed.

instillation Administering a drug by drop.

insulin A pancreatic hormone secreted by the beta cells of the islets of Langerhans which, along with glucagon, regulates the amount of sugar in the blood.

insulin-dependent diabetes mellitus (IDDM) A form of diabetes in which no insulin or an insufficient amount is secreted to enable the body to use glucose; also termed Type I.

insurance A contract whereby one party agrees to compensate or reimburse another for any loss due to a specified cause.

insured A person or organization covered by insurance.

insurer A company or underwriter that provides insurance coverage.

integument (in-**teg**-yoo-ment) The skin.

integumentary system (in-teg-yoo-**men**-tar-ee **sis**-tem) The skin, hair, nails, and sweat and sebaceous glands.

interaction The action of a substance to diminish or increase that of another.

intercostal spaces The spaces between the ribs.

interdisciplinary healthcare team A group of workers from different disciplines who bring together diverse skills and expertise to provide coordinated, high-quality services for the patient.

intermediate care facility A nursing home that provides care for patients who need minimal professional nursing care.

internal customers Patients and colleagues of the medical assistant in the medical office.

internal medicine The medical specialty that focuses on diseases and disorders of the body's internal organs.

internist A doctor who specializes in internal medicine.

interrupted suture A suture in which each stitch is tied and knotted separately.

interventional radiology A field of radiology in which x-ray techniques are used to treat, rather than diagnose, disorders.

intradermal test A form of allergy testing in which the allergen is injected intradermally to determine the patient's response.

intramuscular Administration of drugs into a muscle.

intravenous (in-trah-**vee**-nus) Administration of drugs into a vein.

intravenous pyelogram (in-trah-**vee**-nus **pI**-eh-lO-gram) A radiographic exam in which a contrast agent that is injected intravenously is concentrated in the kidneys and used to visualize the kidneys, ureters, and bladder.

invasion of privacy Interference in a person's private affairs, encroachment on a person's right to be left alone.

inventory A count of all items on hand.

inverse square law The principle governing rapid decrease in energy with increasing distance from the source. X-ray energy decreases exponentially as this distance grows.

inversion Turning inward, as the turning of the foot at the ankle.

iris The colored area of the eye consisting of muscles that change the size of the pupil.

ischemia (is-**kee**-mee-ah) Reduced blood flow.

ischemic (is-**kee**-mik) Relating to pain caused by insufficient oxygen supply, usually affecting a large area of the chest.

islets of Langerhans Endocrine cells located in clusters within the pancreas.

J

jaundice A yellowish or greenish skin color.

Joint Commission on Accreditation of Healthcare Organizations (JCAHO) A voluntary accrediting agency that establishes quality standards and surveys hospitals and other healthcare organizations to ensure that the standards are met.

joints The points where bones meet (articulate).

journal A sheet or book in which each business transaction is recorded from source documents.

Journal of Continuing Education A professional journal published by American Medical Technologists.

K

keratin (**ker**-ah-tin) A fluid that gives the outer portion of the skin its hard, tough, water-resistant character.

ketonuria (kee-tO-**nyoo**-ree-ah) The presence of a breakdown product of fat metabolism in the urine that indicates poorly controlled diabetes or starvation.

kilocalorie (**kil**-O-kal-O-ree) The amount of energy required to heat one kilogram of water one degree Celsius.

kinesics The study of the role of body movements in interpersonal communication.

Kling A type of gauze bandage that will stretch and mold to the body.

knee-chest position A position in which the patient kneels on the examining table and raises the buttocks while the head and chest remain flat on the table. The patient's arms should be extended above the head with the elbows bent. This position allows for examination of the rectum.

Korotkoff sounds (kO-**rot**-kof sowndz) Sounds auscultated through a stethoscope when assessing blood pressure.

L

laceration A wound in which tissue is torn.

lactation The secretion of milk from the breasts to nourish an infant or child.

lancet A bladed instrument used for performing capillary puncture.

laparoscopic examination (lap-a-rO-**scop**-ic eg-zam-ih-**nay**-shun) Examination of the abdominal cavity with a scope through a small incision in the abdominal wall.

laryngectomy (lar-in-**jek**-tO-mee) Surgical removal of the larynx.

laryngitis A condition in which the vocal cords become inflamed or irritated and swollen, causing hoarseness.

larynx The voice box.

laser An acronym for **l**ight **a**mplification by **s**timulated **e**mission of **r**adiation. Surgical lasers emit an intense beam of light to cut away tissues.

law A rule established by authority, society, or custom.

laxative (**lak**-sah-tiv) A substance that stimulates bowel emptying.

ledger cards Individual patient account records.

legal incompetent A person under the legal age or one who is cognitively delayed or under the influence of mind-altering drugs.

legend drug A drug sold by prescription only.

leiomyoma (lee-O-mI-**O**-mah) A benign, smooth muscle tumor in the wall of the uterus; also called myoma, fibroma, and fibroid.

letter of withdrawal A letter informing a patient of the physician's intent to withdraw from care of the patient and setting a deadline by which the patient must find alternative medical care.

leukemia A form of cancer that affects the blood-forming tissues.

leukocyte (**loo**-kO-sIt) A white blood cell.

leukorrhea (loo-kO-**ree**-ah) A white mucoid discharge from the vagina.

liability Debt owed.

libel The damaging of a person's reputation through written words or pictures.

libido (lih-**bee**-dO) Sex drive.

licensure A mandatory credential for some healthcare workers, established by government processes, usually at the state level, which grants individuals who successfully meet the statutory requirements authority to practice in a particular field of endeavor. Also, a limited legal permission to use a product such as a computer software program.

lichenification (lI-ken-ih-fih-**kay**-shun) A palpable thickened area formed on the skin as a result of chronic rubbing or scratching.

lightening The dropping of the uterus near the end of pregnancy as the fetal head begins descent into the pelvic canal.

light therapy Use of exposure to various forms of artificial light to treat illness.

linea nigra (**lin**-ee-ah **nee**-gra) A pigmented line that occurs during pregnancy extending from the symphysis pubis to the top of the fundus in the midline.

lipoproteins (lip-O-**prO**-teen) Carriers of fat and cholesterol through the bloodstream. Some are "good," others are "bad," depending on where they leave the cholesterol they carry.

liters (**lee**-terz) A metric measurement of volume.

lithotomy position (lith-**Ot**-O-mee pO-**zih**-shun) A position in which the patient lies on her back with her buttocks at the end of the examining table and her feet placed in stirrups. It is used for pelvic examinations and Pap smears.

living will An advanced directive in which the individual specifies the types of treatment he or she would want to have and, more importantly, not have if the individual can no longer provide that information.

local effect The effect of a drug in the immediate area of administration.

localized infection Infection restricted to a limited area of the body.

log A book used to record the arrival of each patient.

long-term care A range of health and social services that compensate for the functional disabilities of people or care for the chronically ill.

lower gastrointestinal series A radiographic exam in which a contrast agent is instilled into the colon through the rectum.

lumen (**loo**-men) The hollow space inside the shaft of a needle.

Lyme disease A disorder with multisystem immune effects that is transmitted to humans by the bite of a deer tick.

lymphocyte (**lim**-fO-sIt) A white blood cell produced by the lymph nodes, spleen, bone marrow, and thymus. It is responsible for the immune response to infection and some types of allergic response.

lymphocytosis (lim-fO-sI-**tO**-sis) An elevated number of lymphocytes.

M

macrophage (**mak**-rO-fayj) A type of white blood cell that ingests and destroys microorganisms, removes dead or damaged cells, and stimulates other white blood cells.

macula lutea (**mak**-yoo-lah **loo**-tee-ah) The yellow spot at the center of the retina.

macular degeneration A progressive degeneration of the macula of the retina and the choroid of the eye resulting in blurred central vision and inability to see fine detail.

macule (**mak**-yool) A round, flat, pigmented area.

magnetic resonance imaging (MRI) An imaging technique that uses a strong magnetic field instead of x-rays. The field aligns the atoms in a patient's body, then a radio frequency signal disturbs the alignment so that the atoms give off their own radio frequency, yielding data that can be viewed as three-dimensional, cross-sectional "slices" of the body.

malignant Cancerous.

mammogram X-ray of the breast to reveal tumors too small to be detected by breast self-exam.

mammography (mah-**mog**-rah-fee) The use of x-rays to image structures in the breasts. It is often used in screening for breast malignancies.

managed care Healthcare plans that provide services and stress early intervention in the disease process, avoidance of complications of illness, and managing catastrophic episodes in a cost-effective manner.

manic-depressive illness See bipolar disorder.

manipulation Movement of a joint to determine the range of extension or flexion of a part of the body.

Mantoux tuberculin test (man-**too** too-**ber**-kyoo-lin test) A method for checking for exposure to tuberculosis by introducing tuberculin under the skin.

manual healing therapies Alternative therapies in which the practitioner uses his or her hands to treat the patient and, in some cases, diagnose the patient's condition.

marketing Activities designed to promote the medical practice and inform the public about its services.

Maslow's Hierarchy of Needs A theory developed by psychologist Abraham Maslow listing human needs and their sequential importance to the individual.

massage Organized, intentional touch to increase circulation, relieve pain, and stretch tight muscles.

mast cell A cell found in connective tissue that contains chemicals to produce an allergic reaction.

matrix The basic format of an appointment book.

Mayo stand A moveable, adjustable stainless steel table.

McDonald's sign Softening and slight fullness of the fundus near the area in the uterus where the fetus has been implanted.

mechanical defenses Primary defenses against infection, including skin, mucous membranes, and cilia.

Medicaid Governmental medical insurance for individuals with reduced incomes.

medical asepsis (**med**-ih-kal ay-**sep**-sis) Techniques, culminating in sterilization, that eliminate varying levels of microorganisms. The destruction of microorganisms after they leave the body.

medical ethics Principles of right or wrong conduct that apply in the medical setting.

medical record The record of individual medical diagnoses and treatments; also called the patient chart.

Medicare Federal medical insurance for the elderly and some disabled recipients.

Medicare intermediary A private insurance company that has a contract with the federal government to handle Medicare claims.

Medicare Part A A national health insurance program that covers hospitalization of the elderly and other qualified persons.

Medicare Part B A national health insurance program that covers physicians' services and other medical services for the elderly and other qualified persons.

Medigap A health insurance plan offered by private entities to supplement Medicare benefits by filling in gaps not covered by Medicare.

meditation A profound form of deep relaxation during which attention is focused on one thing at a time.

medulla oblongata (med-**ul**-ah ob-long-**gah**-tah) The part of the brain containing the cardiac, circulatory, and respiratory centers. The primary respiratory center, located at the base of the brain.

melanin (**mel**-ah-nin) A dark brown or black pigment that occurs naturally in the hair, skin, and iris and choroid of the eye.

melanocytes (mah-**lan**-O-sIts) Body cells capable of producing melanin.

melatonin (mel-ah-**tO**-nin) A hormone secreted by the pineal gland.

Ménière's disease (men-**yayrz** dih-**zeez**) A recurrent and usually progressive disorder of the inner ear that affects hearing and balance.

meninges (men-**in**-jeez) Membranes that protect the brain and spinal cord.

menopause (**men**-O-pawz) The period in a woman's life cycle when ovulation ceases, eliminating reproductive ability, and menstruation becomes less frequent and eventually stops; also termed "change of life."

menstruation (men-stroo-**ay**-shun) Sloughing off of the uterine lining and its passage through the vagina approximately fourteen days after ovulation.

mensuration (men-syoo-**ray**-shun) The process of taking measurements such as height, weight, and circumference of the head.

mentor A knowledgeable person who counsels and guides less experienced employees.

meridians (meh-**rid**-ee-anz) Channels that run up and down the surface of the body, as well as deeper inside, along which acupuncture and acupressure is performed.

metabolism (meh-**tab**-O-liz-em) The cellular process that produces energy from the foods we eat. Also, the chemical alteration or breaking down of a drug in the body.

metastasize (meh-**tas**-tah-sIz) Spread, as cancer, to sites other than the site of origin.

metered dose inhaler (MDI) A device that delivers a specific amount of medication with each actuation; also called a "puffer."

metric system The primary system of measurement in the medical field.

microbial antagonism Inhibiting of pathogens by competing with them for living areas.

microbiology A field of clinical medicine that studies microorganisms such as viruses, bacteria, and parasites, and their relationship to infectious disease.

microorganism (mI-krO-**org**-ah-niz-um) A germ, a minute living body invisible to the naked eye.

midbrain The part of the brainstem involved with visual and auditory reflexes.

midstream clean-catch specimen A sterile urine sample taken for analysis after the urinary meatus has been cleaned and a portion of urine has been voided.

migraine headaches Severe headaches usually preceded by fatigue, depression, and visual disturbances.

mind-body therapies A form of non-traditional medicine based on the theory that stress leads to illness and stress reduction helps restore health.

mineralocorticoid hormones The hormones secreted by the outer layer of the adrenal cortex that regulate the resorption of sodium and the excretion of potassium by the kidneys.

minerals Inorganic material necessary for the proper functioning of the body.

Mini Mental State Exam (MMSE) A tool used to evaluate a person's cognitive state.

miotic (mI-**ot**-ik) A substance that constricts the pupils of the eye.

modem A device that transmits data electronically through a telephone line.

modified cash method of accounting The accounting method in which revenue is recorded only when money is received and expenses are recorded only when paid out, but adjustments are made for expenditures for items having an economic life of more than one year.

money order A form of check that may be purchased from post offices and certain businesses.

monocyte A type of leukocyte that is responsible for removing dead tissue and bacteria.

morals Personal codes of conduct based on individual beliefs, religion, and cultural values.

mosquito forceps Small hemostats for small blood vessels.

motherboard The primary circuit board of the computer that holds or has connections for all other computer components.

mucus plug The collection of mucus that closes off the uterus at the cervical opening during pregnancy to prevent bacterial invasion.

multiple sclerosis (MS) A progressive, degenerative disease characterized by demyelination of nerve fibers of the brain and spinal cord.

musculoskeletal system The system that includes the bones, joints, ligaments, tendons, muscles, and nerves that allow the body to move, work, and be active.

music therapy An alternative therapy that uses creating, singing, moving to, and/or listening to music to address a patient's physical and emotional needs.

mycobacterium A slow-growing bacterium that does not stain as a result of Gram's stain. Infection by a mycobacterium causes tuberculosis.

mydriatic (mId-ree-**at**-ik) A medication that dilates the pupils of the eye.

myelinated (**mI**-eh-lin-ay-ted) Having a sheath of myelin, a fatty substance covering nerve fibers in the brain and spinal cord.

myelogram (**mI**-eh-lO-gram) An x-ray of the spinal canal taken after the injection of dye.

myocardium The muscular tissue of the heart.

myopia (mI-**O**-pee-ah) Nearsightedness caused by elongation of the eyeball or by an error in refraction so that rays of light entering the eye are focused in front of the retina.

myringotomy (mer-ing-**got**-ah-mee) See tympanostomy.

myxedema (mik-se-**dee**-mah) Hypothyroidism.

N

Nägele's rule (**nay**-guh-leez rool) A formula for determining the estimated date of delivery.

narcotics Substances that produce sleep, relieve pain, and allay anxiety.

nares (**nay**-reez) Nostrils.

National Center for Complementary and Alternative Medicine (NCCAM) Office established by the National Institutes of Healthin 1991 to investigate alternative and holistic methods of healthcare. It was originally called the Office of Alternative Medicine.

naturally acquired active immunity Immunity acquired by coming in contact with an infectious disease and developing antibodies to it.

naturally acquired passive immunity Immunity acquired by receiving antibodies through the placenta or breast milk.

naturalness The ability to speak and act in an authentic, rather than contrived, manner.

naturopathy (nay-chur-**op**-ah-thee) An alternative therapy that emphasizes health maintenance, disease prevention, patient education, and the patient's responsibility for his or her own health; the overriding principle is vitalism, the belief that the body naturally strives for a maximum level of health.

nebulizer A device that changes a liquid medication into tiny droplets that can be breathed deep into the lungs.

needle holder An instrument to hold and manipulate a needle and suture material.

negligence Failure to meet the standards of reasonable care.

neoplasms (**nee**-O-plaz-emz) Abnormal growth of new tissue.

nerve conduction times A study of the speed of conduction of motor and sensory peripheral nerves.

nervous system The network transmitting messages to and from the brain that activates, coordinates, and controls the body's functions.

net pay The amount earned after deductions.

neurologist A physician specializing in neurology.

neurology The field of medicine dealing with the nervous system and its disorders.

neurosurgeon A physician specializing in surgery involving the brain, spinal cord, and peripheral nerves.

neutrophil (**noo**-trO-fil) A type of leukocyte that is responsible for ingesting bacteria and cellular debris. It is usually elevated early in a bacterial infection.

neutrophilia (noo-trO-**fil**-ee-ah) An elevation of neutrophils.

new patient A patient who has never seen the physician or has not seen the physician in the last three years.

nitrites (**nI**-trItz) A urinary component whose presence suggests a urinary tract infection because the bacteria that often cause such infections convert nitrates to nitrites.

nodule (**nod**-yool) A raised, solid mass.

non-insulin-dependent diabetes mellitus (NIDDM) A form of diabetes in which the pancreas is producing insufficient insulin or the body has a resistance to the insulin which is produced.

nonverbal communication Messages that are sent and received without using spoken words.

noradrenalin Norepinephrine.

norepinephrine (nor-ep-ih-**nef**-rin) A hormone secreted by the adrenal medulla in response to stress.

normal flora Microorganisms that inhabit the body and do not cause disease under normal circumstances.

no-shows Patients who do not show up for their appointments at the scheduled time.

nosocomial infection (nos-O-**kO**-mee-al) Infection acquired from a healthcare environment.

nuclear medicine A field of medicine in which radioactive agents are administered to specific parts of the body to provide data or therapy.

nurse-midwives Registered nurses with additional education in obstetrics and gynecology, usually on the master's level.

nurse practitioner A registered nurse with a master's degree who has received advanced education in a specific field such as family practice or pediatrics and works under the supervision of a medical doctor.

nutrients (**noo**-tree-ents) Essential food elements.

nystagmus (nis-**tag**-mus) Jerking movements of the eye.

O

objective data Information the healthcare practitioner can perceive through the external senses.

objectives The lenses on a microscope that increase the visualized size of an object.

obstetrics (ob-**stet**-riks) The branch of medicine concerned with pregnancy and childbirth, including the study of the physiologic and pathologic functioning of the reproductive tract.

occult Not visibly detectable.

occupational therapy A medical specialty area that analyzes a patient's everyday activities and helps the person develop the skills or use the devices that will lead to an independent, productive, and satisfying lifestyle.

ocular (**ah**-kyoo-lar) The eyepiece of a microscope. It has its own magnification which is usually a factor of ten.

oncologist A physician specializing in the treatment of patients with cancer.

oncology The medical specialty dealing with the diagnosis and treatment of cancer.

open-ended questions Questions asked in a way that invites the receiver to respond at length.

open office hours A system in which appointments are not scheduled but the physician sees patients in the order in which they arrive.

operative report An accounting of a patient's surgery and response to the operation.

ophthalmic (of-**thal**-mik) The route by which medications are administered into the conjunctival sac.

ophthalmologist (of-thal-**mol**-ah-jist) A medical practitioner specializing in ophthalmology.

ophthalmology (of-thal-**mol**-ah-jee) The branch of medicine concerned with the physiology, anatomy, and pathology of the eye and the diagnosis and treatment of disorders of the eye.

ophthalmoscope (of-**thal**-mah-skOp) An instrument used to examine the lens, vitreous body, and retinal structures of the eye.

opportunistic infections Those that usually do not cause infection but do so in a host with a depressed immune system.

optician A person who grinds and fits eyeglasses and contact lenses by prescription.

optometrist A practitioner of optometry.

optometry The practice of testing the eyes for visual acuity, prescribing corrective lenses, and recommending eye exercises.

oral communication Communication using spoken words.

orientation The process by which new employees are introduced to the work environment.

orphan drugs Drugs used to treat rare conditions.

orthopedics The medical specialty concerned with diagnosis, treatment, rehabilitation, and prevention of injuries and diseases of the musculoskeletal system.

orthopedic surgeon A surgeon who operates on disorders of the musculoskeletal system.

orthopedist A specialist in musculoskeletal diseases, injuries, and conditions.

orthopod An orthopedist.

orthosis (or-**thO**-sis) A device used to protect, restore, or improve function by supporting, assisting, resisting, or aligning a moveable part of the body.

ossicular chain The three smallest bones in the body—the malleus, incus, and stapes—located in the middle ear.

osteoarthritis (os-tee-O-ar-**thrI**-tis) The most common form of arthritis, involving degenerative changes in the joints.

osteomalacia (os-tee-O-mah-**lay**-shuh) A condition involving impaired calcification of newly formed, abnormal osteoid matrix which results in softening of the bone.

osteomyelitis (os-tee-O-mI-ee-**lI**-tis) A local or generalized infection of the bone or bone marrow, usually caused by bacteria introduced by trauma or surgery.

osteopathic physicians Physicians who emphasize structural manipulation in additional to using the usual tools of medical therapy; also known as osteopaths.

osteopathy (os-tee-**op**-ah-thee) A therapeutic approach to medicine that uses all the usual forms of medical therapy and diagnosis but also places greater emphasis on the influence of the relationship between the organs and the musculoskeletal system.

osteoporosis (os-tee-O-pah-**rO**-sis) A condition characterized by a progressive loss of bone density and thinning of the bone tissue.

otalgia (O-**tal**-jah) Earache.

otic route (**O**-tik) The route by which medications are administered into the ear canal.

otitis (O-**tI**-tis) Inflammation of the ear.

otitis media Internal or middle ear infection.

otolaryngology (O-tO-lar-in-**gol**-O-jee) The branch of medicine dealing with the diagnosis and treatment of diseases and disorders of the ears, nose, throat, and adjacent structures of the head and neck.

otologist (O-**tol**-O-jist) A physician specializing in the diagnosis and treatment of diseases and disorders of the ear.

otosclerosis (O-tO-skluh-**rO**-sis) An overgrowth of bone around the oval window and stapes that prevents movement of the stapes in the oval window and results in chronic, progressive, conductive hearing loss.

otoscope (**O**-tO-skOp) An instrument used to examine the external auditory canal and the tympanic membrane.

out guides Brightly colored cards used to mark where files have been removed.

ova (**O**-vah) Eggs, the female cells of reproduction.

ovary (**O**-vah-ree) One of the two glands in the female reproductive system that produce ova.

overbooking Scheduling too many patients for the amount of time available, resulting in a day that is too crowded and a schedule that cannot be kept.

over-the-counter (OTC) drugs Medications that can be purchased without a prescription.

ovulation (ov-yoo-**lay**-shun) Release of the ovum by the ovary.

owner's equity The owner's share of the assets of a business.

oxytocin (ok-see-**tO**-sin) A hormone produced by the hypothalamus that stimulates the secretion of breast milk in response to the infant's sucking on the mother's nipple.

P

pager A messaging device that displays a phone number for the recipient to call.

palliative (**pal**-ee-ah-tiv) Affording relief.

pallor Decreased skin color.

palpation An examination that uses touch to detect abnormalities such as movement, size, shape, temperature, texture, and tenderness.

pancreas An organ located behind the stomach that produces endocrine (insulin) and exocrine (digestive enzymes) secretions.

pancreatic juice (pan-kree-**at**-ic joos) A combination of enzymes that can digest proteins, fats, and carbohydrates.

panel A group of complementary laboratory tests that are presented together to give information about a patient's condition.

panic value A laboratory result that deviates far beyond the normal range and may represent an emergency medical situation.

papule (**pap**-yool) A raised, palpable lesion less than 1 cm in diameter.

paraffin A form of wax that is used to provide heat to joints to relieve pain and inflammation.

paraplegia (par-ah-**plee**-jee-ah) Paralysis of the lower body.

parasites Organisms that live on nourishment from other organisms.

parasympathetic nervous system A portion of the autonomic nervous system whose impulses have an inhibitory effect on the body, preparing it for rest and relaxation.

parathormone (par-ah-**thor**-mOn) Parathyroid hormone that works in conjunction with calcitonin to regulate calcium and phosphate levels in the blood.

parathyroid glands Peripheral endocrine glands embedded behind the thyroid gland that secrete parathormone.

parenteral (pah-**ren**-ter-al) Administration of medication by some means other than through the gastrointestinal tract, generally, through the skin via needle.

Parkinson's disease A degenerative neurologic disorder characterized by bradykinesia, muscle rigidity, postural instability, and tremors.

paronychia (par-O-**nik**-ee-ah) Infection of the nail fold.

passive ROM Range of motion exercises performed totally by the practitioner because the patient lacks sufficient muscle strength and/or control to participate.

pasteurization Process of killing microorganisms to increase food safety or preservation.

past history (PH) Information about previous major health problems, experiences with the healthcare delivery system, and attitude toward healthcare.

pathogenicity (path-O-jen-**is**-ih-tee) The ability of a microorganism to enter, survive in, and produce disease in a host.

pathogens (**path**-O-jenz) Microorganisms or other agents capable of producing disease.

patient-centered listening Using good listening skills to understand what the patient is saying and feeling, and then communicating back in your own words what you think is being said and felt.

patient data sheet A form containing demographic data about the patient; sometimes called the patient information sheet.

patient ledger cards Individual patient account records.

Patient Self-Determination Act A federal law requiring that patients receive written information about their right to make medical decisions and execute advance directives.

patient teaching An active process between teacher and patient that aims to produce an observable change in the patient's attitude or behavior.

payee The person or entity receiving money from a check.

payer The person or entity writing out a check.

payroll The total paid out to all employees for a pay period.

pediatrician (pee-dee-ah-**trish**-un) A physician who specializes in the care of children.

pediatrics (pee-dee-**at**-riks) The medical practice focused on the care of children.

pegboard See write-it-once.

percussion Striking a body part with short, sharp blows to diagnose internal conditions.

percutaneous (per-kyoo-**tay**-nee-us) Through the skin; describing procedures performed in this way.

performance assessment/evaluation/review A formal process in which a supervisor examines the quality of an employee's work and informs the employee of the conclusion.

peripheral nervous system (PNS) The nervous system component consisting of the cranial and spinal nerves.

peristalsis (per-ih-**stal**-sis) The action of the muscular walls of the digestive tract that propels food forward through the tract.

PERRLA Pupils, equal, round, react to light and accommodation.

petri dish (**pee**-tree dish) A flat, clear, glass or plastic, circular plate in which a culture medium is present for the growing of microorganisms.

pH The acidity or alkalinity of a substance.

phagocytes (**fay**-go-sIts) "Eating cells" that engulf and break apart invading microorganisms, part of the body's second line of defense against infection.

phagocytosis (fag-O-sI-**tO**-sis) The process by which certain cells engulf and destroy microorganisms and cellular debris.

pharmacist A person licensed to mix and dispense drugs upon written order from a licensed practitioner.

pharmacogenetics (far-mah-kO-jih-**net**-iks) Study of the actions of drugs based on genetic factors.

pharmacognosy (far-mah-**kog**-nO-see) The area of pharmacology concerned with the natural and botanical sources of drugs.

pharmacokinetics (far-mah-kO-kih-**net**-iks) The area of pharmacology dealing with the movement of drugs through the body.

pharmacology (far-mah-**kol**-O-jee) The science that deals with the preparation, use, and effects of drugs.

pharyngeal tonsils (fah-**rin**-jee-al **ton**-silz) The adenoids.

pharyngitis (far-in-**jI**-tis) An infection of the throat which may be caused by viral or bacterial organisms. Infection of the pharynx.

pharynx (**far**-inks) The muscular tubular structure where the esophagus and trachea jointly open into the throat.

pheochromycytoma (fee-O-krO-mee-sI-**tO**-mah) A rare, usually benign, tumor of the adrenal medulla which results in hypersecretion of epinephrine and/or norepinephrine.

phlebitis (fleh-**bI**-tis) Inflammation of a vein.

phlebotomy (fleh-**bot**-O-mee) Commonly used to describe obtaining blood specimens by performing a capillary puncture or by venipuncture.

physical therapy A medical specialty involved with the prevention, correction, and alleviation of the effects of disease and injury by relieving pain and restoring function.

physician's assistant A practitioner who is formally trained to provide diagnostic, therapeutic, and preventive healthcare services and must graduate from an accredited program and work under the supervision of a medical doctor.

pineal gland An endocrine gland located in the brain that secretes melatonin.

pituitary The central endocrine gland within the brain that is considered the master gland of the body and is responsible for releasing most of the hormones in the body.

plain film The use of x-rays without a contrast agent to produce a radiographic image.

plaque A raised lesion, larger than a papule.

plasma The liquid portion of blood. It has a characteristic straw color.

platelet A cellular particle that assists in clotting; also called a thrombocyte.

pledget (**plej**-et) A long-handled swab with twisted cotton at the top used in cryosurgery.

plunger The movable cylinder that is inserted into the barrel of a syringe and moved back and forth to draw up and administer medication.

PMA (Professional Medical Assistant) A professional journal published by the American Association of Medical Assistants.

point-of-care testing (POCT) Laboratory tests that are performed where the patient is. The testing includes retrieval of a specimen, performing the test, and recording the result.

poison Any substance whose swallowing, inhalation, or injection causes harm.

poison ivy dermatitis A common Type IV hypersensitivity in which sensitized T-cells cause cell damage.

policy manual A document listing the organization's guiding principles.

polydipsia Increased thirst.

polyphagia (pol-ee-**fay**-jah) Excessive eating.

polysomnographic technologists Experts who monitor and study brain waves and respiratory and heart activity during sleep.

polyuria (pol-ee-**yoo**-ree-ah) Increased urinary output.

pons A relay station for sensory stimuli on their way to the brain.

positron emission tomography (PET) The use of a radionuclide to show the functioning of a specific organ in which it concentrates. Positrons that produce an image on radiographic film are emitted from the organ.

posting Transferring amounts from the journal to the ledger.

postpartum (post-**par**-tum) The period of about six weeks after giving birth during which a woman's body returns to its non-pregnant state.

postprandial (post-**pran**-dee-al) After having eaten.

practice information sheet Information for patients about office hours, payment policies, emergency procedures, and other aspects of the medical practice.

preauthorization (precertification) Submission of a treatment plan to an insurance carrier for approval before proceeding with the plan.

precision Reproducibility.

pre-existing condition A condition or disease that was present before an insurance policy was issued.

Preferred Provider Organizations (PPO) A loose form of managed care that arranges with providers to serve a defined group of patients who pay reduced fees (plus a copayment) and also can see other providers if they pay more.

prejudice Unreasonable feelings, opinions, or attitudes directed against others.

premiums The fees paid periodically to keep insurance in force.

presbyopia (prez-bee-**O**-pee-ah) Loss of close-up visual accommodation due to the lens becoming more rigid and unable to bend and focus light properly. Farsightedness that commonly develops with advancing age.

prescription A written order for a drug or treatment.

press release Information for an article about the medical practice that is submitted to a newspaper for publication.

prick test A form of allergy testing in which the patient's skin is pricked with a needle to introduce the allergen.

primary care Medical care that is oriented toward the daily, routine needs of the patient.

primary care physician A physician who manages the healthcare of patients in an HMO or PPO plan and serves as a gatekeeper.

primary lesions Lesions that appear initially in response to an alteration in the environment of the skin.

primary payer The insurance company or health plan that assumes initial responsibility for paying benefits when the patient is covered under more than one plan.

primary practitioner A medical practitioner who provides routine care for non-emergency conditions and acts as a "gatekeeper" for specialists.

primary survey The first evaluation of an injury or sudden illness.

problem-oriented medical record (POMR) A systematized process of documentation, centered on the patient's specific health problems, that provides a logical and organized approach to patient care management.

procedure manual A document listing the steps for performing specific tasks.

prodromal phase The period of an infection in which the patient feels the onset of symptoms indicating that an illness is developing.

professional courtesy The practice of treating colleagues or employees at no charge or a reduced rate.

professionalism Being skilled at a job that requires advanced educational training; an on-the-job attitude that includes adhering to ethical principles, working as a team member, and adapting to change.

professional liability insurance Insurance that physicians buy to protect themselves against damages resulting from a malpractice suit.

professional organization An organization that exists to support and provide continuing education for a certain profession.

proficiency testing The examination of standardized samples provided by an external lab or manufacturer that a clinical lab uses to establish the reliability of its test results.

progress notes Information provided by the patient and observations and examination results from healthcare personnel.

pronation (prO-**nay**-shun) Rotation of the forearm so that the palm turns up.

prone position A position in which the patient lies face down with hands at the sides and head facing to one side. This allows for examination of the spine and legs.

prophylactic drugs (prO-fih-**lak**-tik drugz) Drugs used to prevent or decrease the severity of disease; also called preventative drugs.

proportion Two or more equivalent ratios.

proprioception (prO-pree-O-**sep**-shun) The sensation of the movement and position of the body, especially the limbs.

prostate gland The gland that secretes seminal fluid. It surrounds the urethra at the neck of the urinary bladder.

prosthesis (pros-**thee**-sis) An artificial substitute for a missing body part, such as an eye, leg, or tooth, that is used for functional or cosmetic reasons or both.

proteins (**prO**-teenz) Large molecules consisting of amino acids that form the building blocks of the human body.

proteinuria (prO-tee-**nyoo**-ree-ah) Protein in the urine.

provider A person, organization, or institution that delivers healthcare services.

provocative Causing (a symptom).

proximodistal (prok-sih-mO-**dis**-tal) Moving from the center of the body toward the extremities.

pruritus (proo-**rI**-tus) Itching.

psoriasis (sO-**rI**-eh-sis) A common, chronic skin disorder characterized by circumscribed red patches covered with thick, dry, silvery, adherent scales.

psychiatric nurse practitioner A registered nurse with a master's degree in theoretical and clinical study and expert knowledge in the treatment and prevention of mental disorders.

psychiatric nursing The branch of nursing concerned with the prevention and cure of mental disorders and their complications.

psychiatric social worker A social worker who usually has a master's degree that includes experience in counseling patients and their families in dealing with social, emotional, or environmental problems pertaining to mental illness.

psychiatrist A physician who specializes in psychiatry.

psychiatry The branch of medical science dealing with the causes, treatment, and prevention of mental, emotional, and behavioral disorders.

psychologist A licensed professional with an academic degree (e.g., Psy.D. or Ph.D) in psychology.

psychology The profession that focuses on the interaction between the individual and the physical and social environment in an effort to treat and prevent individual or social problems.

psychotherapy The use of specific psychological techniques to modify feelings, attitudes, and behaviors.

psychotropic Describing drugs that can affect the mind, emotions, and behavior.

public relations Activities designed to create a favorable public view of the medical practice.

pulmologist A physician who specializes in diseases and treatment of the pulmonary system.

pulmonary artery The blood vessel that carries unoxygenated blood from the right atrium to the lungs for oxygenation.

pulmonary function testing Evaluation of airway and lung functioning.

pulmonary vein The blood vessel that carries oxygenated blood from the lungs to the left atrium.

pulse oximetry An inexpensive and portable, non-invasive monitoring device that estimates the saturation of erythrocytes' hemoglobin with oxygen.

pupil The dark central portion of the eye.

purified protein derivative (PPD) A concentration of the tuberculin antigen found on *Mycobacterium tuberculosis*. It is used in tuberculin skin testing.

purulent (**pyoo**-roo-lent) Emitting pus. Wound drainage consisting of spent white blood cells that indicates infection.

pustule (**pust**-yool) A cavity filled with pus.

P wave The first ECG waveform, representing atrial depolarization.

pyramidal tract The pathway composed of groups of nerve fibers in the white matter of the spinal cord through which motor impulses are conducted.

Q

QRS complex The tracing on an electrocardiogram that represents ventricular depolarization.

QT interval The time from the beginning to the end of ventricular depolarization.

quadraplegia (quah-drah-**plee**-jee-ah) Paralysis from the neck down.

quickening Maternal recognition of fetal movements, usually in the fourteenth to sixteenth week for multiparous women and the eighteenth or later for nulliparous women.

R

R.A.C.E. Acronym for a method of dealing with fire emergencies: Rescue, Alarm, Contain, and Evacuate (or Extinguish).

radiation therapy The application of x-ray energy to regions of the body to treat disease, frequently used in cancer therapy.

radioallergosorbent test (RAST) (ray-dee-O-al-er-gO-**sor**-bent test) A form of allergy testing using a sample of blood to determine the presence of allergen-specific IgE antibodies.

radiopharmaceutical (ray-dee-O-fahr-mah-**soo**-tih-kl) A radioactive substance used in nuclear medicine to create radiographic images of bodily organs.

random access memory (RAM) A part of the computer that stores information temporarily.

range of motion (ROM) Exercises involving the movement of each joint through as full a range of motion as possible without pain.

ratio The relationship between two numbers.

read only memory (ROM) A part of the computer that stores information permanently.

Recommended Dietary Allowances (RDAs) The levels of intake of essential nutrients that are known to meet the needs of most healthy people as defined by the Food and Nutrition Board.

reconciled Made to agree, referring to the balances on a bank statement and in a checkbook.

reconstituted Made into a liquid drug by adding sterile water or saline to a powder.

recreational therapists Healthcare specialists who employ medically approved activities that provide enjoyment, as well as opportunities for exercise and social participation, to help restore the patient's physical and psychological well-being.

rectus femoris (**rek**-tus **fem**-oris) A site for intramuscular injection on the anterior aspect of the thigh.

recurrent turn A bandaging technique used for the top of the head.

red bone marrow The specialized, soft tissue filling the spaces in various bones where blood cells are produced.

reference range A set of test values that represent 95% of the values occurring in the normal population.

reflective listening A type of active listening in which the listener asks the speaker questions that mirror the speaker's own statements.

reflexes Involuntary responses to stimuli.

reflexology (ree-fleks-**ol**-O-gee) A form of manual healing based on the principle that reflexes in the feet and hands correspond to various organs and glands within the body.

refractometer A device to measure the specific gravity of a urine specimen.

Registered Medical Assistant (RMA) Title used by medical assistants with a national credential awarded by the Certifying Board of American Medical Technologists. These graduates have completed a program accredited by the Accrediting Bureau of Health Education Schools.

rehabilitation The process of restoring a patient with an acute or chronic disability to the highest possible level of physical, psychological, social, and economic functioning; also called restorative care.

rehabilitation counselor A healthcare specialist who helps patients deal with social, personal, and vocational aspects of their disabilities or injuries.

reimbursement Repayment for expenses or losses incurred.

releasing factors Substances that are produced in the hypothalamus and sent to the pituitary gland to stimulate or inhibit the production and release of hormones.

reliability Trustworthiness; capability of being dependable or responsible in action or performance. Also, the quality of being accurate and precise.

remission Partial or complete disappearance of signs and symptoms.

replacement drug A drug used as a substitute for a body substance that is no longer available.

repolarization The electrical recovery of cardiac cells.

reportable injuries Injuries that concern the public welfare because they were caused by lethal weapons or resulted from abuse.

reservoir A source of supply of an infectious agent or disease.

res ipsa loquitur "The thing speaks for itself." Indicates obvious negligence.

Resource-Based Relative Value Scale (RBRVS) A system of determining medical fees developed by the federal government in which each service is assigned a unit value based on time, skill, expenses involved, and geographic location.

respondeat superior "Let the master answer," a legal doctrine that holds the employer physician responsible for acts performed by employees acting within the scope of their duties.

retention Inability to urinate.

retina The inner layer of the eye, covering the choroid, which forms the visual image.

review of systems (ROS) The portion of a patient's health history that includes a review of the physical and psychological health status.

review status The status of a claim on which the insurer's action is being appealed or for which a review is requested.

rheumatoid arthritis A chronic, systemic, commonly progressive, inflammatory disease that chiefly affects the synovial membranes of multiple joints in the body.

rhinitis (rI-**nI**-tis) Inflammation of the mucous membranes of the nose.

R.I.C.E. Acronym for a first aid technique for sprains: Rest, Ice, Compression, and Elevation.

Rinne test (**rihn**-ee test) A hearing test used to determine air and bone conduction.

rods The cells of the retina that allow for vision in dim light.

role delineation study A 1996 study by the American Association of Medical Assistants that defined the competencies medical assistants must have to practice.

rotation A range of motion in which the joint moves around an axis outwardly (external rotation) or inwardly (internal rotation).

route of administration The means by which a drug enters the body.

Rule of Nines A method of estimating how much body surface area is involved in an injury, especially a burn.

∫

salaries The pay for employees who earn the same amount per period regardless of the number of hours worked.

sanguineous (sang-**gwin**-E-us) Describing wound drainage that is red and consists mainly of blood.

sanitization Washing and scrubbing of the body or instruments to remove microorganisms.

sarcoidosis (sar-koy-**dO**-sis) A chronic multisystem Type IV hypersensitivity that affects the lungs, spleen, skin, mucous membranes, and lacrimal and salivary glands, usually with involvement of the lymph glands.

sarcoma (sar-**kO**-mah) A classification of cancer that affects the connective tissue, blood and blood vessels, and the lymphatic system.

scale A dry, silvery, often white area on the skin that flakes.

scalpels Specially designed knives to make surgical incisions.

scanner A device that inputs text or graphics into the computer.

scheduled drugs Drugs that have been designated by the DEA as having potential for addiction or abuse; also called controlled substances.

schizophrenia (skit-sO-**freh**-nee-ah) A mental condition characterized by disordered thinking which usually includes delusions and hallucinations.

sclera (**sklee**-rah) The white portion of the external layer of the eyeball.

scoliosis (skO-lee-**O**-sis) A skeletal deformity involving a lateral deviation of the spine.

scratch test A form of allergy testing in which the skin is scratched to determine the patient's reaction to the allergen being tested.

screening The use of a test or exam to identify a disease state before it is clinically noticed.

sebaceous Secreting sebum.

sebum (**see**-bum) An oily secretion that keeps the hair pliable and the skin soft and waterproof.

secondary lesions Lesions resulting from changes in the primary lesion.

secondary payer The insurance carrier that pays benefits after the primary payer has paid the portion of the bill for which it is responsible.

sedatives Substances that produce a calming effect.

sediment Solid particles in the urine that settle out over time, such as crystals, casts, cells, and microorganisms.

self-actualization A feeling of wellness and wholeness that allows a person to turn from the needs of the self and commit to a vocation or to serving others. This is the ultimate goal of people, according to Maslow's Hierarchy of Needs.

semicircular canals The portion of the inner ear that aids in adjustment of the body to changes in direction.

sensitivity testing A bacterial culture technique in which the response of bacteria to particular antibiotics is evaluated.

sensorineural hearing loss A hearing loss whose cause lies with the inner ear or cranial nerve VIII.

serology (suh-**rol**-ah-jee) The use of antigen-antibody interaction for laboratory testing. Typical tests describe blood types or past or present infections.

serosanguineous (**seer**-O-sang-**gwin**-E-us) Describing wound drainage that is pink and contains both serum and blood.

serous drainage (**see**-rus **drayn**-aj) Describing clear wound drainage that consists of serum and is considered normal.

serum Plasma from which solids and fibrinogen have been separated out.

sexually transmitted diseases (STDs) Infections passed from person to person through sexual contact; also termed venereal disease.

shaft The part of a needle that is inserted into the patient's body tissue; also called the cannula.

sharps container Clearly marked receptacle for needles, blades, or any other sharp instruments.

shock The inability of the body to maintain a blood pressure that is compatible with life.

side effect An undesirable—but not detrimental—result of taking a drug; also called an untoward reaction.

sighted guide A person who assists a visually-impaired person by offering an elbow. The guided person can feel the guide's body moving up or down elevations and left or right to avoid obstacles.

sigmoidoscopy Endoscopic examination of the sigmoid colon of the large intestine.

signature (sig) The part of a prescription that provides directions for the patient.

signs Objective data or evidence of disease.

Sims' position An examination position in which the patient lies on one side with the top leg sharply bent and the other leg slightly bent. This allows for examination of the rectum.

single-entry bookkeeping The bookkeeping method in which a transaction is recorded in only one account.

sinoatrial (SA) node (sI-nO-**ay**-tree-al nOd) The main cardiac pacemaker, consisting of a group of specialized cells in the right atrium.

sinusitis Inflammation of one or more of the paranasal sinuses.

sinus rhythms Cardiac rhythms that originate at the SA node, normally from sixty to a hundred beats per minute.

sitting position An examination position in which the patient sits upright on the examining table with legs over the end of the table and feet resting on the footrest. This allows auscultation of the heart and lungs and examination of the head, eyes, ears, nose, and throat.

six "rights" Guidelines for administering medication: right medication, right dosage, right route, right time, right patient, and right documentation.

skeletal muscles Voluntary muscles generally located between the skin and bones.

skeletal system The 206 bones and the joints connecting them that support and protect the body and allow it to move.

skeletal traction Application of traction through the use of wires, pins, or rods that are surgically attached to or placed through bones.

skilled nursing care Home healthcare that requires the services of a registered nurse.

skilled nursing facility A nursing home that provides twenty-four-hour professional nursing services.

skin traction Traction applied to muscles or bones by pulling on the skin using adhesive, tapes and harnesses.

skip A person who moves without leaving a forwarding address to avoid paying a debt.

slander The damaging of a person's reputation through spoken words.

Snellen eye chart A commonly used means of testing vision. Letters on the chart are arranged in rows from largest to smallest.

SOAP format Documenting information by listing subjective data, objective data, assessment, and plan for each medical problem.

software Instructions that tell a computer how to process information; also called "applications" or "programs."

somatic nervous system (SNS) The portion of the peripheral nervous system whose fibers stimulate the skeletal muscles.

source documents Documents containing the information needed to record transactions.

source-oriented medical record (SOMR) A record-keeping format in which data in the file are organized according to their source; also called narrative or diary format.

specific gravity A measurement of the density of urine relative to water, which is used to indicate the kidney's ability to concentrate urine and the volume status of the body.

speculum (**spek**-yoo-lum) An instrument used to open and visualize an orifice.

speech and language pathologists Healthcare practitioners who diagnose and treat patients experiencing speech or language problems.

sphygmomanometer (sfig-mO-mah-**nom**-ee-ter) An instrument that measures the pressure of blood in an artery.

spina bifida (**spI**-nah **bif**-ih-dah) A congenital defect in which the vertebrae of the fetus fail to close.

spinal cord The nerves of the central nervous system within the spinal canal.

spiral reverse turn A bandage wrapping technique in which each turn includes a backward redirection of the material to accommodate an increasing diameter.

spiral turn A bandage wrapping technique in which each turn overlaps the preceding one by two-thirds of the width of the bandage.

spirochetes (spI-rO-**keet**-eez) Spiral bacteria.

spirometry Measurement of breath volume.

splinter forceps Forceps with fine tips to grasp objects embedded in tissue.

spreadsheet A software program for inputting and manipulating numerical data to facilitate a wide variety of financial activities.

stage The platform on which a microscope slide rests. It often has control knobs that can move the slide forward or backward and side to side.

Standard Precautions Precautions designed to reduce the risk of transmitting recognized or unrecognized sources of infection.

standard reagent A sample substance from an outside lab or manufacturer that has a known value. It is used for proficiency testing.

stapedectomy (stay-peh-**dek**-tah-mee) Surgical removal of the stapes and insertion of a graft and prosthesis.

stat Notation on a lab request indicating that a test result should be processed immediately.

statute of limitations A time limit fixed by state laws within which a lawsuit must be filed.

statutory laws Laws enacted by a legislative body.

stereotypes The mistaken concept that all members of a cultural, ethnic, or other group are the same and lack substantial individual differences.

sterile field The sterile area for a surgical procedure and surgical supplies.

sterile scrub assistant A medical assistant who assists the surgeon in the sterile field by handing instruments, applying traction, and cutting off excess suture material.

sterile technique Maintaining a process or area free of all microorganisms.

sterilization The use of heat or chemicals to destroy all microorganisms.

Steri-Strips® Sterile adhesive strips for wound closure.

stethoscope (**steth**-O-skOp) An instrument used to amplify sounds.

stream scheduling A system for scheduling patients based on their status and need.

stress Physical and/or psychological tension caused by events or situations.

striae gravidarum (**strI**-E grav-i-**dar**-um) Stretch marks in pregnancy that result from greater fragility of the skin's elastic tissues.

stricture The narrowing of a tube-like structure.

ST segment The time from the beginning of ventricular depolarization to the beginning of ventricular repolarization.

subacute care Healthcare that falls between the level of care provided in an acute care hospital setting and the various forms of long term healthcare.

subarachnoid space (sub-ah-**rak**-noyd spAs) The area between the middle and innermost meningeal membranes.

subcutaneous (sub-kyoo-**tay**-nee-us) Administration of drugs into the tissue beneath the skin.

subjective data Data perceived only by the affected individual.

sublingual (sub-**ling**-gwal) Administration of a drug by placing it under the tongue for absorption into the bloodstream.

submucous resection Surgery to straighten and reduce the nasal septum.

subpoena duces tecum A court order to produce documents.

subscriber (policyholder) A person who takes out an insurance policy or is covered through an employer or other group plan.

subscription The part of a prescription that gives directions to the pharmacist, including the size of the dosage and the form of the drug.

substance abuse Regular misuse of alcohol or a drug that affects the central nervous system and causes behavioral changes.

sudoriferous (soo-dO-**rif**-er-us) Producing sweat.

sulci (**sul**-sI) Deep grooves or fissures within the cerebrum.

superscription The part of a prescription with the symbol "Rx," meaning "take" in Latin.

supination (soo-pih-**nay**-shun) Rotation of the forearm so that the palm turns down.

supine position (soo-**pIn** pO-**zih**-shun) An examination position in which the patient lies on his back with face upward, arms at sides, and legs extended.

surgical asepsis Creation and maintenance of a sterile environment.

surgical field The sterile area within which surgical procedures are performed.

sustained-release Medication that is released into the bloodstream over time.

suture (**soo**-cher) Surgical stitches or the material used for such stitching.

swabs Sterile cotton-tipped sticks used to collect tissue fluid samples.

sympathetic nervous system A portion of the autonomic nervous system whose impulses have an excitatory effect on the body, increasing the rate of organ activity.

symptoms Subjective data perceived by the patient indicating deviation from the normal state.

syncope Fainting.

synovial joints Joints that contain a cavity and are freely movable.

synthesized (**sin**-theh-sIzd) Produced by the body.

syringe (ser-**inj**) A device used to inject medications or extract fluids.

systemic effect A generalized, all-inclusive drug effect on the entire body.

systemic lupus erythematosus (SLE) (sis-**tem**-ik **loo**-pus er-ith-uh-ma-**tO**-sis) A multisystem autoimmune disorder characterized by the presence of various autoantibodies.

systole (**sis**-tO-lee) (**systolic phase**) The phase of the heart cycle in which the ventricles contract and push blood into the pulmonary system and throughout the body.

T

T-account A skeleton version of the standard accounting form.

tachycardia (tak-i-**kar**-dee-ah) Rapid beating of the heart, usually more than 100 beats per minute.

tai chi (tI-**chee**) A form of exercise built upon the mind-body connection that combines physical movement, meditation, and breathing.

taper-tipped needle A needle whose tip tapers to a point or blunt tip.

teamwork The ability to work interdependently with others toward a goal.

telangiectatic angiomas (te-**lan**-jee-ek-**tA**-tic an-jee-**O**-maz) Tiny, branched, slightly raised and pulsating end-arterioles, commonly called vascular spiders. They sometimes develop during pregnancy.

telemedicine Using video and computer technology to let physicians in one location see patients in another, providing an expanded means for patients to access healthcare.

templates Basic files that are used repeatedly to speed up work.

temporomandibular joint (TMJ) dysfunction (tem-pO-rO-man-**dib**-yoo-lar) Painful dysfunction of the lower jaw, sometimes with clicking of the joint and limitation of movement.

tension headaches Common headaches, which may or may not be associated with psychological stress, that are usually felt in the back of the head and neck.

tentative diagnosis An assumption about the cause of an illness or condition that is held until further

information is received from diagnostic studies and laboratory tests.

texture The fineness or coarseness of the skin.

thalamus (**thal**-ah-mus) A portion of the brain that acts as a relay station for sensory nerve impulses.

thallium stress test Imaging of the myocardium's blood flow during an exercise stress test.

therapeutic communication An exchange between the patient and healthcare worker that provides support, information, and hope to the patient with the goal of overcoming distress.

therapeutic drugs (ther-ah-**pyoo**-tik) Drugs used to relieve symptoms of disease.

therapeutic environment A setting in which a patient can express himself or herself comfortably, be heard, and be understood.

therapeutic exercise The prescription of body movement to correct impairment, improve musculoskeletal functioning, or maintain a state of well-being.

therapeutic massage The use of various motions and pressures on the body to improve circulation and remove toxins.

therapeutic touch A complementary therapy used to relieve pain and anxiety in which the practitioner moves her hands over the patient's body without touching the skin to detect any alterations in the patient's energy field.

thermosensor A thermometer that registers temperature by the heat of the skin.

thrombocyte (**throm**-bO-sIt) A cellular particle that assists in clotting; also called a platelet.

thrombus An aggregation of platelets, fibrin, clotting factors, and the cellular elements of the blood that attach to the interior wall of a blood vessel and sometimes occlude the lumen.

thumb forceps Forceps that are used by grasping the blades between the thumb and fingers.

thyroid gland The peripheral endocrine gland located in the neck below the larynx that secretes the two thyroid hormones.

thyrotoxicosis (**thI**-rO-tox-sih-**kO**-sis) Hyperthyroidism causing signs and symptoms.

tickler file A system the medical assistant can use as a reminder of time-sensitive activities such as sending or paying bills.

tidal volume The air inhaled and exhaled in a normal respiratory cycle.

time-specific appointments (**time-specific scheduling**) A system for scheduling appointments at an established time or within a relatively narrow range of time to meet specific medical requirements.

tinea barbae Ringworm of the beard area.

tinea capitis Ringworm of the scalp.

tinea corporis (**tin**-ee-ah kor-**por**-is) Ringworm of the body.

tinea cruris Ringworm of the groin.

tinea pedis Ringworm of the feet.

tinea unguium Ringworm of the nails.

tinea versicolor A common, chronic disorder resulting in loss of skin color.

tinnitus (tih-**nI**-tus) A noise heard in one or both ears that is not caused by external stimulus.

tip The end of the barrel of a syringe; the place where the needle is attached.

tissue forceps Thumb forceps with teeth.

TNM staging A method of classifying a malignancy based on the size of the tumor (T), characteristics of regional lymph nodes and presence or absence of malignant cells in the lymph nodes (N), and absence or presence of metastasis (M).

tolerance Decrease in a drug's effects because of continued use.

tonometer (tO-**nom**-ee-ter) An instrument used to measure intraocular pressure.

topical The route of administration in which medication is absorbed through the skin or mucous membrane.

tort A wrongful act committed by one person against another person or against property that results in damage or injury but does not involve a breach of contract.

towel clamp An instrument used to grasp a sterile towel or drape and hold it in place.

traction Treatment of musculoskeletal injuries and conditions through use of a device that provides a pulling force on bones, immobilization, and alignment of fractures.

Traditional Chinese Medicine (TCM) An alternative therapy in which the patient is responsible for his own health and the doctor serves as a guide and role model, offering aid in the form of herbs, acupuncture, and massage.

tranquilizer A substance that reduces mental anxiety and tensions.

transaction A financial action or event that changes the amount of a business's assets, liabilities, or owner's equity.

transient ischemic attacks (TIAs) Episodes of cerebrovascular insufficiency that are similar to a cerebrovascular accident but last only a few minutes.

traveler's checks Checks purchased from a bank or other institution to use when personal checks are not accepted.

triage The ranking of patients for treatment by the priority of their needs.

trial balance A listing of the balances of all accounts in the ledger, as of a specific date, to check the equality of debits and credits.

Trousseau's sign (troo-**sOz** sIn) A sign of hypocalcemia which is elicited by inflating a blood pressure cuff to a level above the patient's systolic pressure and maintaining the inflation for at least two minutes, resulting in a carpal spasm lasting five to ten seconds after deflation.

Truth in Lending Act Regulation Z of the federal Consumer Protection Act, protecting consumers who use credit.

Truth in Lending Disclosure Statement A written agreement between the physician and patient stating the terms under which a fee will be paid in more than four installments.

Tubegauz® A seamless tubular gauze bandage.

tuberculin The antigen on *Mycobacterium tuberculosis* that is responsible for the hypersensitivity reaction from a tuberculosis infection.

tuberculin syringe A syringe used to administer very small doses of medication for allergy testing and tuberculin skin testing.

tuberculosis (TB) (too-ber-kyoo-**lO**-sis) An infectious disease caused by the bacillus *Mycobacterium tuberculosis*, most commonly affecting the respiratory system.

tuning fork An instrument used to determine if the patient has a conductive or a sensorineural hearing loss.

turgor Elasticity of the skin.

T wave The portion of the ECG tracing showing repolarization of the ventricles.

twenty-four-hour urine specimen The collection of all of a patient's urine throughout a twenty-four-hour period, usually to measure protein and glucose content.

tympanic membrane (tim-**pan**-ik **mem**-brayn) The eardrum.

tympanostomy A surgical procedure performed to drain fluid through an incision in the eardrum and insertion of tubes; also called a myringotomy.

U

ulcer A deep, open lesion that extends into the dermis.

ultrasound The use of extremely high frequency sound waves to determine the anatomy of internal structures. The waves are reflected in varying amounts according to the make-up of the structures, creating an image of the part of the anatomy being studied.

Also, the use of high-frequency sound waves as an application of heat to aid in the healing of tissues.

underbooking Scheduling that allows too much time for patients, resulting in large gaps in the schedule.

Uniform Anatomical Gift Act State laws facilitating the donation of bodies or body parts for use in transplant surgery, tissue banks, or medical research or education.

Universal Precautions Precautions that involve treating all blood and all body fluids except sweat as if they are infected by bloodborne pathogens. They are practiced for all patients regardless of diagnosis and infectious status.

upgraded Enhanced or improved computer software programs.

upper gastrointestinal series A radiographic examination in which a contrast agent is swallowed and pictures of the esophagus, stomach, and upper intestines are taken using a fluoroscope.

ureters (**yoo**-ree-terz) The long, slender tubes connecting the kidneys with the urinary bladder.

urethra (yoo-**ree**-thrah) The tube that leads from the bladder to the outside of the body.

urgent conditions Those requiring treatment or intervention in fifteen to sixty minutes, though for some, intervention in much less than fifteen minutes is desirable.

urinalysis (yoo-rih-**nal**-ih-sis) An evaluation of the physical, chemical, and microscopic properties of urine.

urinary meatus (mee-**ay**-tus) The opening of the urethra.

urinary studies Laboratory tests that use urine as the test specimen.

urinometer A device to measure the specific gravity of urine.

urobilinuria (yoo-rO-bil-ih-**nyoo**-ree-ah) The presence of a breakdown product of red blood cells in urine that indicates increased destruction of red blood cells or liver dysfunction.

urologist (yoo-**rol**-ah-jist) A medical specialist who deals with conditions of the male and female urinary tract and the male genital tract.

urology (yoo-**rol**-ah-jee) The branch of medicine dealing with the anatomy, physiology, disorders, and care of the urinary tract in men and women and of the male genital tract.

urticaria (**er**-ti-**kar**-ee-ah) A pruritic skin eruption characterized by transient wheals of varying shapes and sizes with well-defined erythematous margins and pale centers.

usual, customary, and reasonable rates (UCR) Maximum amounts that insurance companies will pay based on prevailing fees in a geographic area.

uterine soufflé (**yoo**-ter-in soo-**flay**) or **bruit** (broo-**ee**) The rushing sound of the maternal blood going to the placenta. It is synchronous with the woman's pulse.

uterus (**yoo**-ter-us) The pear-shaped organ, about the size of a fist, in which the product of conception is implanted.

V

vaccine A substance that promotes resistance to infectious disease.

varicella (var-ih-**sel**-ah) Chickenpox.

vasoconstrictor (vas-O-kon-**strik**-tor) A substance that constricts blood vessels, resulting in decreased blood flow.

vasodilator (vas-O-**dlh**-lay-tor) A substance that relaxes blood vessels, resulting in increased blood flow.

vasopressor (vas-O-**pres**-or) A substance that increases blood pressure by contracting capillaries and arteries.

vastus lateralis (**vas**-tus lat-er-**ah**-lis) The intramuscular injection site on the anterolateral aspect of the thigh.

vendor A company that sells supplies.

venereal disease (VD) Infections passed from person to person through sexual contact; also termed sexually transmitted diseases.

venipuncture (**veen**-ih-pungk-shur) Accessing a vein with a needle to collect blood.

ventricle (**ven**-trih-kl) One of the lower chambers of the heart; the right chamber pumps blood to the lungs, and the left chamber pumps it to the other body tissues.

ventrogluteal (ven-trO-**gloo**-tee-al) The intramuscular injection site in the hip region.

verrucae (vuh-**roo**-see) Warts.

vertigo Dizziness.

vesicle A small skin cavity, less than 1 cm in size, that contains free fluid.

vestibule The portion of the inner ear that responds to slow movements of the head, straight-ahead movements, and gravity.

vials (**vI**-alz) Small bottles of medication with a rubber stopper.

villi (**vil**-I) Fingerlike projections in the small intestine through which nutrients are absorbed.

virology The study of viruses.

virulence (**veer**-yoo-lens) The relative ability of an infectious agent to produce disease.

viruses Microorganisms smaller than bacteria that require a host cell to survive or replicate.

visceral muscles (**vis**-er-al **mus**-ahls) The smooth muscles in the body's organs.

visual acuity Sharpness or clearness of vision.

visual fields Peripheral vision.

visual inspection An examination that involves looking at body areas for the presence of any abnormalities of size, color, continuity, shape, position, or symmetry.

vital signs Objective data indicating the patient's condition, including temperature, pulse, respiratory rate, and blood pressure.

vitamins (**vI**-tah-minz) Organic substances found in foods that are essential for normal metabolism and health.

voice mail A messaging system that provides a recorded greeting for callers and records their messages to be retrieved later.

voucher check A check with a detachable portion that explains the purpose of the check.

vulva A woman's external genital organs, consisting of the mons pubis, labia majora, labia minora, clitoris, vaginal vestibule, hymen, and Bartholin's glands.

W

wages Pay earned on an hourly basis.

waiting period The time that must pass before a subscriber's pre-existing condition will be covered by an insurance policy.

waived-complexity testing Testing that does not require inspections from outside the laboratory or medical office to perform proficiency testing, specially trained personnel to perform tests, or a formal method of quality control.

wave scheduling A system in which a given number of patients is scheduled for each hour and they are seen in the order of arrival.

Weber test (**vay**-ber test) A test used to determine conductive-type deafness.

wheal (weel) A transient, irregularly shaped elevation.

Wood's lamp An ultraviolet light used to diagnose certain scalp and skin conditions; also called a black light.

worker's compensation insurance A government program providing benefits for employees suffering from job-related accident or illness, and their dependents.

World Wide Web (**web**) The collection of Internet information connected by hypertext links.

write-it-once (**pegboard**) A manual method of bookkeeping in which information is recorded on several forms simultaneously.

X

x-rays Invisible electromagnetic radiation of very short wavelength that can penetrate solid objects. The rays create images because of the way in which objects of varying density impede them.

Y

yoga (**yO**-guh) A Hindu mind-body therapy that involves the integration of physical, mental, and spiritual energies to promote health and wellness.

Z

z-track technique A form of intramuscular injection that prevents irritation and staining of the subcutaneous tissue.

References

CHAPTER 1

American Association of Medical Assistants. *Bylaws 1997–1998*. Chicago: American Association of Medical Assistants.

Balasa, Donald. *Certification and Licensure Facts You Should Know*. [Fact Sheet] Chicago: American Association of Medical Assistants.

Balasa, Donald. "Growing Demand for MSHPs Expands Opportunities for the Medical Assisting Profession." *Professional Medical Assistant* 28, no. 2 (March/April 1995).

CMA vs. RMA and CAAHEP vs. ABHES—What's the Difference? American Association of Medical Assistants.

Commission on Accreditation of Allied Health Education Programs. "Standards and Guidelines for an Accredited Educational Program for the Medical Assistant." 1999. < http://www.caahep.org/standards/ma-st_99.htm > (October 16, 2000).

Melchionno, Rick, and Michael Steinman. "The 1996–2006 Job Outlook in Brief." *Occupational Outlook Quarterly*. U. S. Department of Labor Bureau of Labor Statistics. Spring (1998): 2–36.

CHAPTER 2

Administration on Aging. "Aging into the Twenty-first Century." May 31, 1996. < www.aoa.dhhs.gov/aoa/stats/aging21/ > (October 16, 2000).

Agency for Healthcare Research and Quality. "Consumers and Patients." n.d. < www.ahcpr.gov/consumer/index.html#plans > (October 16, 2000).

Center for the Health Professions at the University of California, San Francisco. "Interview with Mark D. Smith, MD, MBA." *Front and Center* 2, no. 4 (Summer 1998): 1–5.

Eldredge, Janice, and Darrell Buono. *150 Careers in the Healthcare Field*. New Providence, NJ: U. S. Directory Service, 1993.

Feldstein, Paul. *Healthcare Economics*. Albany, NY: Delmar Publishers, 1999.

Harris, Mark. "Helping Patients Through the Maze of Managed Care Plans." *Professional Medical Assistant* (November/December 1999): 16–18.

Raffel, Marshall, and Norma Raffel. *The U. S. Health System: Origin and Functions*. Albany, NY: Delmar Publishers, 1994.

Simmers, Louise. *Diversified Health Occupations*. Albany, NY: Delmar Publishers, 1998.

Spector, Rachel. *Cultural Diversity in Health and Illness*. Stamford, CT: Appleton and Lange, 2000.

Stanfield, Peggy. *Introduction to the Health Professions*. Boston: Jones and Bartlett, 1995.

CHAPTER 3

American Association of Medical Assistants. *Law for the Medical Office*. Chicago: American Association of Medical Assistants, 1984.

Centers for Disease Control. "Notice to Readers: Changes in National Notifiable Disease Data Presentation." *Morbidity and Mortality Weekly Report*, June 4, 1999. < www.cdc.gov/epo/mmwr/preview/mmwrhtml/mm4821a4.htm > (October 10, 2000).

Dorland's Illustrated Medical Dictionary. 26th ed. Philadelphia: W. B. Saunders Co., 1981.

Flight, Myrtle. *Law, Liability, and Ethics for Medical Office Professionals*. Albany, NY: Delmar Publishers, 1998.

Judson, Karen, and Sharon Blesie. *Law and Ethics for Health Occupations*. New York: Glencoe/McGraw-Hill, 1994.

Lewis, Marcia A., and Carol D. Tamparo. *Medical Law, Ethics, and Bioethics in the Medical Office*. 3rd ed. Philadelphia: F. A. Davis Co., 1993.

Lewis, Martha A., and Carol D. Warden. *Law and Ethics in the Medical Office, Including Bioethical Issues*. 2nd ed. Philadelphia: F. A. Davis Co., 1988.

CHAPTER 4

The Alan Chapman Consultancy. "Empathy and Trust: Empathy Communications—the Key to Successful Relationships." n.d. < http://ds.dial.pipex.com/alan.chapman/empathy.htm > (October 11, 2000).

Cabrera, James, and Charles Albrecht. "The Techniques of Active Listening." *The Lifetime Career Manager: New Strategies for a New Era*. Madison, WI: Adams Publishing, 1995. < http://www.dbm.com/career/leading/paths/new19.html > (October 11, 2000).

Ettinger, Alice G., and Pamala F. Burch. *Medical Terminology for Health Careers*. St. Paul, MN: Paradigm Publishing Inc., 1999.

Forman, Judy. "Many Men Resist Seeing Doctors: Staying Away Doesn't Make Them Less Healthy, But It Can Still Cost Them Dearly." *Minneapolis Star Tribune*, June 20, 1999. < http://startribune.com.html > (October 11, 2000).

Gardenswartz, L., and L. Rowe. *Managing Diversity in Health Care*. San Francisco: Jossey-Bass, 1998.

Hicks, D. J., B. S. Innes, and W. L. Shores. *Patient Care Techniques*. Indianapolis: Bobbs-Merrill, 1975.

Ismail, Norhayati. "Communicating Across Cultures" (Part 1). *Pertinent Information Ltd.* n.d.

< http://pertinent.com/pertinfo/business/ yaticom.html > (October 11, 2000).

Ismail, Norhayati. "Communicating Across Cultures" (Part 2). *Pertinent Information Ltd.* n.d. < http:// pertinent.com/pertinfo/business/yaticom1.html > (October 11, 2000).

Kolbe, David A. "Adult Learning Theory and Model." *Experiential Learning.* New York: Prentice-Hall, 1984. < http://www.arl.org/training/ilcso/ adultlearn.html > (October 11, 2000).

Morgan, Clifford T., Richard A. King, and Nancy M. Robinson. *Introduction to Psychology.* 6th ed. New York: McGraw-Hill, 1979.

"Overview of Models and Strategies for Overcoming Linguistic and Cultural Barriers to Health Care." *Diversity Rx,* August 6, 2000. < http://www. diversityrx.org/html/movera.htm > (October 11, 2000).

Paplia, D. E., and S. W. Olds. *Psychology.* 2nd ed. New York: McGraw-Hill, 1988.

Roberts, Barry S., and Richard A. Mann. "Sexual Harassment in the Workplace: A Primer." n.d. < http://www.uakron.edu/lawsrev/robert1.html > (June 4, 1999).

Rockwell, Jay. "Common Focus Unites Team Members." *Teamwork.* Dartnell Corporation, 1998. < http://www.dartnellcorp.com/traintool/ article17.html > (June 6, 1999).

Sullivan, E. J., and P. J. Decker. *Effective Management in Nursing.* 2nd ed. Menlo Park, CA: Addison-Wesley, 1988.

CHAPTER 5

American Medical Association. *Health Professions Education Directory.* 27th ed. Chicago: Medical Education Products, 1999.

Center for Health Professions at the University of California, San Francisco. "Growth of Managed Care." *Front and Center* 2, no. 4 (Summer 1998): 1, 3, 5.

Center for Health Professions at the University of California, San Francisco. "Interview with Mark D. Smith, MD, MBA." *Front and Center* 2, no. 4 (Summer 1998): 4–6.

Clark, Carolyn. "A Complementary Potpourri." *Nursing Spectrum,* May 17, 1999: 14–16.

Cowley, Geoffrey, and Anne Underwood. "Finding the Right Rx." *Newsweek,* September 20, 1999: 66–7.

Dossey, Barbara. "Holistic Modalities and Healing Moments." *American Journal of Nursing* 98, no. 6 (June 1998): 44–7.

Fetrow, Charles, and Juan Avila. *Complementary and Alternative Medicines.* Springhouse, PA: Springhouse Corp., 1999.

Greenley, Hough, and Anne Banas. *The Directory of Complementary and Alternative Medicine.* Marblehead, MA: Opus Communications, 2000.

Harvard Medical School. "Yoga—The Mind-Body Workout." *Harvard Health Letter* 24, no. 2 (1998): 4–5.

Miller, Anne. "Documentation in the Alternative Care Setting." *Advance for Health Information Professionals,* December 8, 1997: 16–18.

Mulcahy, Robert. *Diseases: Finding the Cure.* Minneapolis, MN: The Oliver Press, Inc., 1996.

Porter, Roy, ed. *The Cambridge Illustrated History of Medicine.* Cambridge: Cambridge University Press, 1996.

Raffel, Marshall, and Norma Raffel. *The U. S. Health System.* 4th ed. Albany, NY: Delmar Publishers, 1994.

Salvo, Susan. *Massage Therapy Principles and Practice.* Philadelphia: W. B. Saunders Co., 1999.

Tidwell, John. "House Calls of the Future." *Modern Maturity* (November/December 1998).

Williams, Stephen, and Paul Torrens. *Introduction to Health Services.* 4th ed. Albany, NY: Delmar Publishers, 1993.

Yaglinski, Marion. "Nurses Discover Reiki." *Nursing Spectrum,* June 1, 1999: NJ9.

CHAPTER 7

Chicago Manual of Style. 14th ed. Chicago: University of Chicago Press, 1998.

Miller-Keane Encyclopedia and Dictionary of Medicine, Nursing, and Allied Health. 6th ed. Philadelphia: W. B. Saunders Co., 1997.

Oxford American Dictionary. New York: Oxford University Press, 1990.

Physician's Desk Reference. 1999 ed. Montvale, NJ: Medical Economics Co., 1999.

Roget's 21st Century Thesaurus. Nashville: Thomas Nelson Publishers, 1992.

CHAPTER 8

Clark, Jonathan, and Susan Clark. *Prioritize, Organize: The Art of Getting It Done.* Shawnee Mission, KS: National Press Publications, 1992.

Covey, Stephen R. *The 7 Habits of Highly Effective People.* New York: Simon and Schuster, 1989.

Covey, Stephen R. *First Things First.* New York: Simon and Schuster, 1994.

Merriam Webster Secretarial Handbook. 3rd ed. Springfield, MA: Merriam Webster Inc., 1998.

CHAPTER 9

Ettinger, Alice, and Pamala Burch. *Medical Terminology for Health Careers.* St. Paul, MN: Paradigm Publishing Inc., 1998.

Ettinger, Blanche, and Alice Ettinger. *Medical Transcription*. St. Paul, MN: Paradigm Publishing Inc., 1996.

Fast File. St. Paul, MN: Paradigm Publishing Inc., 1991.

CHAPTER 10

Dansby, Robert L., Burton S. Kaliski, and Michael D. Lawrence. *Paradigm College Accounting*. 4th ed. St. Paul, MN: Paradigm Publishing Inc., 2000.

Fordney, Marilyn T., and Joan J. Follis. *Administrative Medical Assisting*. 3rd ed. Albany, NY: Delmar, 1993.

Holmes, A. W., G. P. Maynard, J. D. Edwards, and R. A. Meier. *Elementary Accounting*. 3rd ed. Homewood, IL: Richard D. Irwin, 1962.

Internal Revenue Service. "Recordkeeping." *Publication 583, Starting a Business and Keeping Records*. March 11, 1999. < http://www.irs.gov/forms_pubs/pubs/p58310.htm > (October 11, 2000).

Legal Information Institute of Cornell University. "Bankruptcy: An Overview." *Law About....* n.d. < http://www.law.cornell.edu/topics/bankruptcy.html > (October 11, 2000).

Sanderson, S. M. *Computers in the Medical Office: Using Medisoft for Windows*. New York: Glencoe/McGraw-Hill, 1999.

Siegel, J. G., and J. K. Shim. *Dictionary of Accounting Terms*. 2nd ed. New York: Barron's, 1995.

Stein, J., ed. *The Random House College Dictionary*. Revised ed. New York: Random House, 1998.

U. S. Treasury Department. Internal Revenue Service. *Circular E, Employer's Tax Guide*. Washington, DC: U. S. Government Printing Office, 1999.

CHAPTER 11

Federal Trade Commission. *Staff Commentary on the Fair Debt Collection Practices Act: Statements of General Policy or Interpretation*. Washington, DC: U. S. Government Printing Office, 1988.

Fordney, Marilyn T., and Joan J. Follis. *Administrative Medical Assisting*. 3rd ed. Albany, NY: Delmar, 1993.

Frailey, L. E. *Handbook of Business Letters*. 3rd ed. Englewood Cliffs, NJ: Prentice Hall, 1989.

Hamburg, J., ed. *Merriam-Webster's Medical Office Handbook*. 2nd ed. Springfield, MA: Merriam-Webster, 1996.

Harrison, Mary N. "Disclosures." *Consumer Credit Contracts*. Fact Sheet FCS 5002, University of Florida, Institute of Food and Agricultural Sciences: July 1999. < http://hammock.ifas.ufl.edu/txt/fairs/41017.html > (October 11, 2000).

Lane, Karen. *Saunders Manual of Medical Assisting Practice*. Philadelphia: Saunders, 1993.

Legal Information Institute of Cornell University. "Bankruptcy: An Overview." *Law About....* n.d. < http://www.law.cornell.edu/topics/bankruptcy.html > (October 11, 2000).

Low, R. J. *Bottom Line Basics: Understand and Control Business Finances*. Grants Pass, OR: Oasis Press, 1995.

Sanderson, S. M. *Computers in the Medical Office: Using Medisoft for Windows*. New York: Glencoe/McGraw-Hill, 1999.

U. S. Postal Service. *Publication 221, Make Your Mail Machinable and Readable...The Right Way*. Washington, DC: U. S. Government Printing Office, 1995.

CHAPTER 12

American Medical Association, eds. *Current Procedural Terminology CPT 2000*. Chicago: American Medical Association, 1999.

Blue Cross Blue Shield Association. "Who We Are: Understanding the Blue Cross Blue Shield System." n.d. < http://64.37.231.116/whoweare.index.html > (October 11, 2000).

Colorado Health Site. "Overview of the Principal Types of Health Care Plans: An Introduction to HMOs." n.d. < http://www.coloradohealthnet.org/insurance/hmo.html > (October 11, 2000).

Colorado Health Site. "Overview of the Principal Types of Health Care Plans: An Introduction to PPOs/EPOs." n.d. < http://www.coloradohealthnet.org/insurance/ppo.html > (October 11, 2000).

Colorado Health Site. "Overview of the Principal Types of Health Care Plans: What Is Indemnity Health Insurance?" n.d. < http://www.coloradohealthnet.org/insurance/ind.html > (October 11, 2000).

Fordney, M. T. *Insurance Handbook for the Medical Office*. 5th ed. Philadelphia: W. B. Saunders Co., 1997.

Hamburg, J., ed. *Merriam-Webster's Medical Office Handbook*. 2nd ed. Springfield, MA: Merriam-Webster, 1996.

ICD-9-CM Alphabetic Index to Diseases. Duke University Health System Corporate Information Services. July 10, 2000. < http://www.mcis.duke.edu/standards/termcode/icd9/2index.html > (October 11, 2000).

ICD-9-CM Codes. Duke University Health System Corporate Information Services. July 10, 2000. < http://www.mcis.duke.edu/standards/termcode/icd9/1tabular.html > (October 11, 2000).

ICD-9-CM Easy Coder. 1999 ed. Montgomery, Ala.: Unicor Medical, 1999.

Medicare Computer-Based Training. Health Care Financing Administration. August 30, 2000. < http://www.medicaretraining.com/ cbt_download.htm > (September 5, 2000).

Medicare Provider News. No. 038. Richmond, VA: United Healthcare, September 1997.

CHAPTER 13

Cunningham, William H., Ramon J. Aldag, and Stanley B. Block. *Business in a Changing World.* Cincinnati, OH: South-Western Publishing Co., 1993.

H and R Block 2000 Income Tax Guide. New York: Simon and Schuster, 1999.

Lyons, Art, Patricia Seraydarian, and Marie Longyear. *The Paradigm Reference Manual.* St. Paul, MN: Paradigm Publishing Inc., 1995.

Quibble, Zane K. *Administrative Office Management: An Introduction.* Upper Saddle River, NJ: Prentice Hall, Inc., 1996.

Robbins, Stephen P., and Phillip L. Hunsaker. *Training in InterPersonal Skills: TIPS for Managing People at Work.* Upper Saddle River, NJ: Prentice Hall, Inc., 1996.

Seraydarian, Patricia E. *Proofreading and Editing Business Documents.* St. Paul, MN: Paradigm Publishing Inc., 1996.

Shepherd, Robert D. *Introduction to Computers and Technology.* St. Paul, MN: Paradigm Publishing Inc., 1998.

Timm, Paul R., and Kristen Bell DeTienne. *Managerial Communication.* Upper Saddle River, NJ: Prentice Hall, Inc., 1995.

CHAPTER 14

Bayer Corporation. "A Brief History of Infectious Disease," *Health Care 101.* n.d. < http://www.bayerpharma-na.com/hottopics/ hc0102.asp > (October 12, 2000).

McMillan, Patricia, and Katharine McMillan. *Home Decorating for Dummies.* Foster City, CA: IDG Books Worldwide, 1998.

Thaler-Carter, Ruth. "Give the Office a Facelift." *Professional Medical Assistant* (January/February 2000): 10–12.

U. S. Census Bureau. "Table 1: Disability Status of Persons by Race and Hispanic Origin." *Americans with Disabilities, 1994–95 – Table 1.* June 22, 1999. < http://www.census.gov/hhes/www/disable/ sipp/disab9495/ds94t1.html > (October 12, 2000).

U. S. Equal Employment Opportunity Commission and U. S. Department of Justice. *Americans With Disabilities Act Handbook.* Washington, DC: U. S. Government Printing Office, 1991.

Zurlinden, Jeff. "New Bugs at the Picnic." *Nursing Spectrum,* August 9, 1999: 24–5.

Index

Page numbers followed by t refer to a table. *Italic* numbers refer to a figure.

Photo Credits

Cover Image SuperStock; **6** Custom Medical Stock Photo, Inc.; **10** SuperStock, Inc.; **11** Index Stock Imagery/Patricia Barry Levy; **16** Dynamic Graphics, Inc.; **17** The Stock Market, Inc./Chuck Savage; **21** Special thanks to Susan Zolvinski, Commonwealth Business College; **30** SuperStock, Inc.; **31** Robert Fried Photography; **35** Custom Medical Stock Photo, Inc.; **37** SuperStock, Inc.; **40** Courtesy of Mayo Clinic in Rochester, MN; **41** SuperStock, Inc.; **50** International Stock/Elliot Smith; **51** Corbis; **64** Dynamic Graphics, Inc.; **68** Index Stock Imagery/Larry George; **69** Custom Medical Stock Photo, Inc.; **73** PhotoPaq/R. Eisele; **74** Index Stock Imagery/Mathew Borkoski; **75** Index Stock Imagery/Frank Siteman; **76** Index Stock Imagery/IT Stock International; **77** Index Stock Imagery/Derek Cole; **80** International Stock/Patrick Ramsey; **81** Index Stock Imagery/Chip Henderson; **85** International Stock/Michael Paras; **91** Digital Stock Corporation; **93** Index Stock Imagery/Jacob Halaska; **97** SuperStock, Inc.; **99** Corbis/Wally McNamme; **100** Artville/LLC The Blant Group; **101** Artville/LLC The Blant Group; **112** Special thanks to Fairview Nicollet Mall Clinic; **115** Special thanks to Fairview Nicollet Mall Clinic; **116** (bottom) Custom Medical Stock Photo, Inc.; **116** (top) Special thanks to Fairview Nicollet Mall Clinic; **119** Special thanks to Fairview Nicollet Mall Clinic; **125** Custom Medical Stock Photo, Inc.; **127** Alvis Upitis Photography; **129** Stockbyte; **131** PictureQuest/Bill Gallery; **139** Digital Stock; **140** Corbis; **141** Index Stock Imagery/Fredde Lieberman; **145** The Stock Market/Rob Levine; **149** The Stock Market, Inc./Tom Stewart; **166** DoctorStock; **168** Custom Medical Stock Photo, Inc.; **170** Special thanks to Fairview Nicollet Mall Clinic; **175** The Stock Market, Inc./C/B Productions; **180** SuperStock, Inc; **187** Special thanks to Fairview Nicollet Mall Clinic; **190** SuperStock, Inc.; **191** Index Stock Imagery; **192** Custom Medical Stock Photo, Inc.; **202** SuperStock, Inc.; **205** The Image Bank/Romilly Lockyer; **207** Eyewire; **219** International Stock/Peter Russel L'femens; **228** Custom Medical Stock Photo, Inc.; **229** Special thanks to Fairview Nicollet Mall Clinic; **237** Corbis; **246** International Stock/Patrick Ramsey; **251** Custom Medical Stock Photo, Inc.; **255** Corbis; **270** SuperStock, Inc.; **273** SuperStock, Inc.; **276** SuperStock, Inc.; **280** SuperStock, Inc.; **293** (top) The Stock Market, Inc./Rob Lewine; **293** (bottom) Special thanks to Fairview Nicollet Mall Clinic; **294** (top right) Special thanks to Fairview Nicollet Mall Clinic; **294** (bottom left) Index Stock Imagery/BSIP Agency; **296** Special thanks to Fairview Nicollet Mall Clinic; **298** Special thanks to University of Minnesota School of Nursing; **299** Special thanks to Fairview Nicollet Mall Clinic; **300** Special thanks to Fairview Nicollet Mall Clinic; **302** Special thanks to Fairview Nicollet Mall Clinic;